THERAPY FOR

Ocular Angiogenesis

Principles and Practice

THERAPY FOR Ocular Angiogenesis

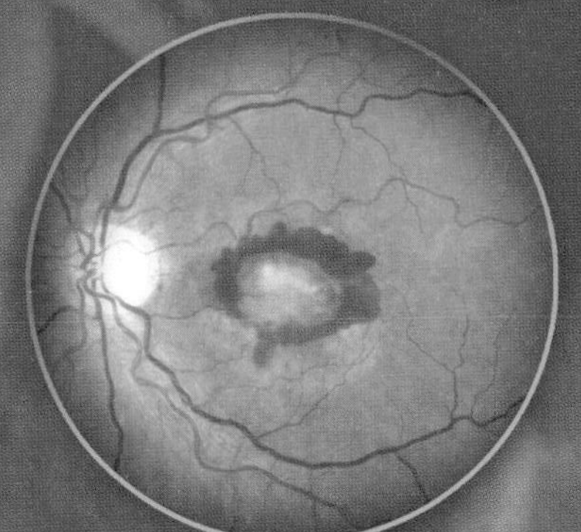

Principles and Practice

Arup Das, MD, PhD
Professor of Ophthalmology
Cell Biology and Physiology
University of New Mexico School of Medicine
NM VA Health Care System
Albuquerque, New Mexico

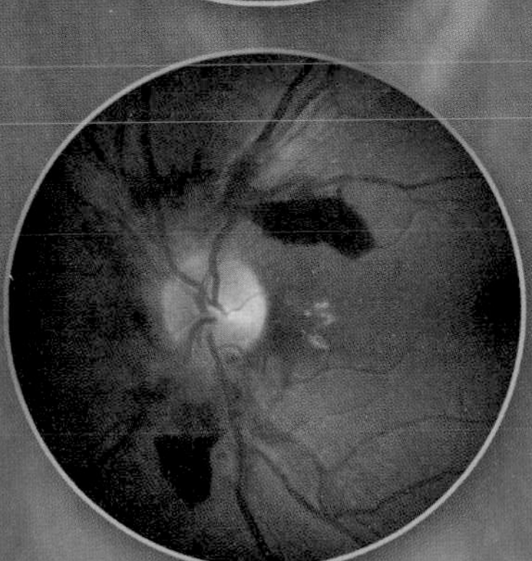

Thomas R. Friberg, MS, MD
Professor of Ophthalmology
UPMC Eye Center
University of Pittsburgh
Pittsburgh, Pennsylvania

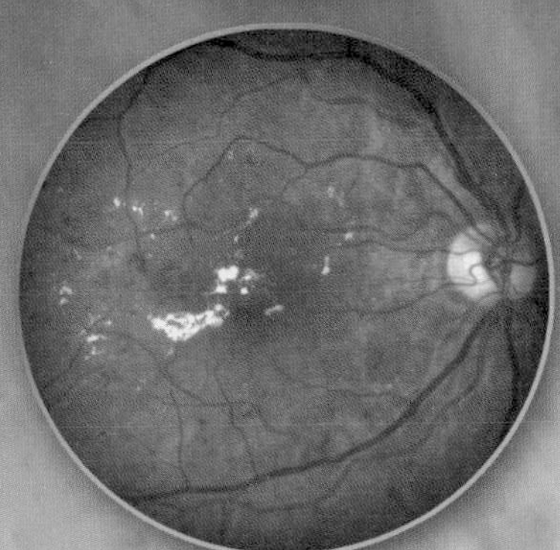

Wolters Kluwer Health | Lippincott Williams & Wilkins
Philadelphia • Baltimore • New York • London
Buenos Aires • Hong Kong • Sydney • Tokyo

Senior Executive Editor: Jonathan W. Pine, Jr
Senior Product Manager: Emilie Moyer
Vendor Manager: Bridgett Dougherty
Senior Manufacturing Manager: Benjamin Rivera
Marketing Manager: Lisa Lawrence
Design Coordinator: Teresa Mallon
Production Service: SPi Technologies

Two Commerce Square, 2001 Market Street
Philadelphia, PA 19103 USA
LWW.com

Printed in China.

Library of Congress Cataloging-in-Publication Data
Therapy for ocular angiogenesis : principles and practice / [edited by] Arup Das, Thomas Friberg.
p. ; cm.
Includes bibliographical references and index.
Summary: "Ocular angiogenesis, or the abnormal growth of blood vessels in the eye, is the cause of major neovascular eye diseases. In addition, retinal and choroidal neovascularization are the major causes of vision loss in this country. With the new era of anti-angiogenic therapies already in practice, ophthalmologists have started treating many ocular diseases including macular degeneration, diabetic retinopathy, and retinal vascular occlusion using anti-angiogenic drugs. This book covers the basic pathophysiology of ocular angiogenesis and strategies for inhibition. The authors discuss the "Principles" of anti-angiogenic therapy, pre-clinical studies, future drugs on the horizon, drug delivery, and the "Practice" of the therapy in many ocular diseases. Vision researchers in both academia and industry, as well as clinician scientists, have contributed chapters on different aspects of the angiogenic process, and clinical strategies to fight it. The book also includes chapters that deal with diabetic macular edema, and various therapeutic options for this condition. A companion website includes the fully searchable text and an image bank"—Provided by publisher.
ISBN 978-1-60547-640-7 (alk. paper)
1. Eye—Blood-vessels—Diseases—Chemotherapy. 2. Neovascularization. I. Das, Arup. II. Friberg, Thomas.
[DNLM: 1. Eye Diseases—drug therapy. 2. Angiogenesis Inhibitors—therapeutic use. 3. Eye—blood supply. 4. Neovascularization, Pathologic—drug therapy. 5. Neovascularization, Pathologic—physiopathology. WW 140]
RE720.T44 2010
616.99'484—dc22

2010030537

DISCLAIMER
Care has been taken to confirm the accuracy of the information presented and to describe generally accepted practices. However, the authors, editors, and publisher are not responsible for errors or omissions or for any consequences from application of the information in this book and make no warranty, expressed or implied, with respect to the currency, completeness, or accuracy of the contents of the publication. Application of the information in a particular situation remains the professional responsibility of the practitioner.

The authors, editors, and publisher have exerted every effort to ensure that drug selection and dosage set forth in this text are in accordance with current recommendations and practice at the time of publication. However, in view of ongoing research, changes in government regulations, and the constant flow of information relating to drug therapy and drug reactions, the reader is urged to check the package insert for each drug for any change in indications and dosage and for added warnings and precautions. This is particularly important when the recommended agent is a new or infrequently employed drug.

Some drugs and medical devices presented in the publication have Food and Drug Administration (FDA) clearance for limited use in restricted research settings. It is the responsibility of the health care provider to ascertain the FDA status of each drug or device planned for use in their clinical practice.

To purchase additional copies of this book, call our customer service department at (800) 638-3030 or fax orders to (301) 223-2320. International customers should call (301) 223-2300.

Visit Lippincott Williams & Wilkins on the Internet: http://www.lww.com. Lippincott Williams & Wilkins customer service representatives are available from 8:30 am to 6:00 pm, EST.

10 9 8 7 6 5 4 3 2 1

We dedicate this book to ***Judah Folkman, MD,*** *the father of the field of angiogenesis, whose contributions and achievements are reflected virtually in each chapter.*

To our dear friend and colleague, ***Yasuo Tano, MD,*** *whose wisdom was as boundless as his sense of humor, and whose contributions to ophthalmology were monumental and numerous.*

—*Editors*

To my wife, ***Moushumi*** *and son,* ***Arinjoy****.*

—*Arup*

Foreword

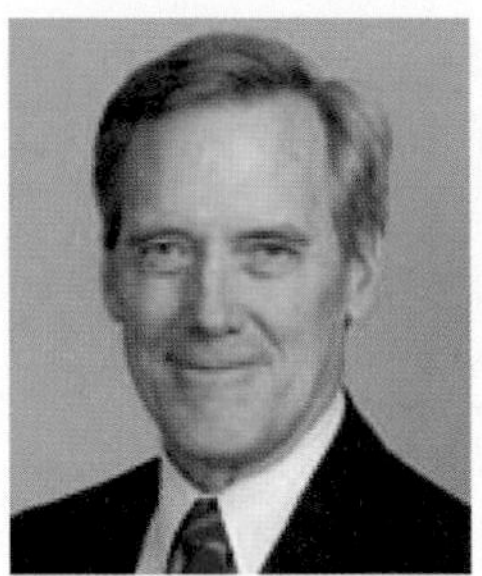

Over the last decade, there has been tremendous progress in the field of ocular angiogenesis. Advances in cell biology, biochemistry, immunology, and pharmacology have revolutionized our management of retinal vascular and macular diseases. Many clinical trials on the use of anti-angiogenic drugs have been completed, many more are in progress now. With this rapid development in the field, clinicians now have one book that compiles the information and covers a broad area of topics.

Drs. Arup Das and Thomas R. Friberg have made an important contribution to the therapy for ocular angiogenesis, based on sound principles and current clinical trials. Both editors have extensive experience in the field of ocular angiogenesis, and are recognized as leading experts in this field. They and their contributing authors have provided treatment guidelines based on up-to-date results.

The principles of angiogenic therapy and pre-clinical studies are provided in the first nine chapters. From these principles, the basis of therapy, including the most up-to-date clinical trials as they relate to age-related macular degeneration, diabetic retinopathy, retinopathy of prematurity, and retinal vein occlusions, are provided in the next 21 chapters. In addition to the focus on angiogenesis, the authors consider macular edema resulting from diabetes as well as from retinal vein occlusions.

This book is convenient, easily accessible to the reader interested in clinical trials and has the most up-to-date information. The principles underlying angiogenesis are presented in a way which makes it easy to understand the pathways of potential new drugs and their benefits.

The editors and authors have provided a book that will be very useful to clinicians in their day-to-day practice.

Stephen J. Ryan, MD
President, Doheny Eye Institute
Keck School of Medicine,
University of Southern California
Los Angeles

Preface

In the last five years, ophthalmology has undergone a revolution with the introduction of anti-angiogenic drugs. These compounds have radically altered our therapeutic approaches to age-related macular degeneration, diabetic retinopathy, and many other retinal diseases. A multitude of clinical trials were launched to evaluate these agents, and many have been completed or are ongoing, and more are in planning stages. Currently, no concise written work covering this expanding and broad topic is available. Our book addresses this void. In *Therapy for Ocular Angiogenesis: Principles and Practices*, the pathophysiology of ocular angiogenesis and related morbidities such as macular edema are discussed, as are the scientific principles of therapy. The clinical trials that led to the common usage of this new class of drugs are summarized, and ongoing clinical investigations searching for more optimal agents are highlighted. We also include ocular drug delivery, as this topic has great relevance to our patients and their families, and to future treatment strategies.

We have assembled numerous experts in this nascent field, and all are passionate about sharing their knowledge with the reader. Our book begins with a cogent discussion of the basic pathophysiology of ocular angiogenesis, and strategies for its inhibition. The **Principles** of anti-angiogenic therapy, including the different steps of the angiogenic cascade, are covered first by nine chapters which address many pre-clinical studies. We then transition to the **Practice** of ophthalmology, which integrates the concepts into therapeutic approaches. Many ocular diseases are addressed in the 21 subsequent chapters, including age-related macular degeneration, diabetic retinopathy, retinopathy of prematurity, and retinal venous occlusive diseases.

We trust that this book will assist ophthalmologists, retina specialists, researchers, residents, fellows, and anyone with an interest in the field. We also wish to express our sincere appreciation to the late Judah Folkman, the father of the field of angiogenesis. He inspired us to publish this concise book, and he intended to contribute a chapter. While his untimely passing precluded this specific wish, we pay tribute to this maestro for his remarkable and unwavering efforts that served as the foundation of our understanding. His achievements are reflected in virtually every chapter.

We are indebted to our colleagues for their scholarly contributions, made inspite of many other commitments, and we are especially appreciative of their friendship. We are particularly indebted to Ms. Jackie Cremar for her help in preparing and editing the manuscripts.

Arup Das, MD, PhD
Thomas R. Friberg, MS, MD

Contributors

Salwa Abdel-Aziz, MD, MPH
John Moran Eye Center
University of Utah
Salt Lake City, Utah
Chapter 24

Anthony P. Adamis, MD
Vice-President, Global Head, Genentech, Inc.
Adjunct Professor of Ophthalmology and Visual Sciences
University of Illinois College of Medicine
Chicago, Illinois
Chapters 1, 30

L.P. Aiello, MD, PhD
Associate Professor
Ophthalmology
Harvard Medical School
Director
Beetham Eye Institute
Joslin Clinic
Boston, Massachusetts
Chapter 15

Balamurali K. Ambati, MD, PhD
Associate Professor
Department of Ophthalmology
John Moran Eye Center
University of Utah
Salt Lake City, Utah
Chapter 24

Jayakrishna Ambati, MD
Professor and Vice Chair
Departments of Ophthalmology and Visual Science
Professor of Physiology
Dr. E Vernon Smith and Eloise C. Smith Endowed Chair
University of Kentucky
Lexington, Kentucky
Chapter 3

Albert Augustin, MD
Professor
Department of Ophthalmology
University of Mainz
Mainz, Germany
Director
Department of Ophthalmology
Klinikum Karlsruhe
Karlsruhe, Germany
Chapter 22

Ashay Bhatwadekar, PhD
Department of Pharmacology and Therapeutics
University of Florida
Gainesville, Florida
Chapter 27

David Boyer, MD
Clinical Professor of Ophthalmology
Department of Ophthalmology
University of Southern California, Keck School of Medicine
Los Angeles, California
Chapter 12

Peter M. Brennen, MD
UPMC Eye Center
University of Pittsburgh
Pittsburgh, Pennsylvania
Chapter 21

Antonio Capone, Jr., MD
Clinical Associate Professor
Oakland University
Associated Retinal Consultants
Royal Oak, Michigan
Chapter 17

Siobhan M. Cashman, PhD
Research Assistant Professor
Department of Ophthalmology
Tufts University School of Medicine
Boston, Massachusetts
Chapter 26

J.D. Cavallerano, OD, PhD
Assistant Professor
Department of Ophthalmology
Harvard Medical School
Staff Optometrist
Beetham Eye Institute
Joslin Diabetes Center
Boston, Massachusetts
Chapter 15

Roomasa Channa, MD
Postdoctoral Fellow
Wilmer Eye Institute
Johns Hopkins University School of Medicine
Baltimore, Maryland
Chapter 11

Felix Y. Chau, MD
Vitreoretinal Fellow
Department of Ophthalmology
University of Illinois Eye and Ear Infirmary
Chicago, Illinois
Chapter 16

Kip M. Connor, PhD
Instructor
Department of Ophthalmology
Harvard Medical School
Children's Hospital Boston
Boston, Massachusetts
Chapter 5

Karl G. Csaky, MD, PhD
Retina Foundation of the Southwest
Dallas, Texas
Chapter 13

Patricia A. D'Amore, PhD
Schepens Eye Research Institute
Professor of Ophthalmology and Pathology
Harvard Medical School
Boston, Massachusetts
Chapter 4

Arup Das, MD, PhD
Professor of Ophthalmology
Department of Cell Biology and Physiology
University of New Mexico School of Medicine
NM VA Health Care System
Albuquerque, New Mexico
Chapters 7, 9

Diana V. Do, MD
Assistant Professor,
Wilmer Eye Institute
Johns Hopkins University School of Medicine
Baltimore, Maryland
Chapter 11

Michael Engelbert, MD
Vitreous, Retina, and Macula Consultants of New York
LuEsther T. Mertz Retinal Research Center
Manhattan Eye, Ear, and Throat Hospital
Edward S. Harkness Eye Institute
Columbia University, New York
Chapter 23

Robert N. Frank, MD
Professor
Departments of Ophthalmology and Anatomy/Cell Biology
Kresge Eye Institute
Wayne State University School of Medicine
Senior Staff
Department of Ophthalmology
Harper-Hutzel Hospital
Detroit, Michigan
Chapter 2

Thomas R. Friberg, MS, MD
Professor of Ophthalmology
UPMC Eye Center
University of Pittsburgh
Pittsburgh, Pennsylvania
Chapters 12, 21

Maria Grant, MD
Professor
Department of Pharmacology and Therapeutics
University of Florida
Gainesville, Florida
Chapter 27

Jonathan B. Gunther, MD
Departments of Ophthalmology and Visual Sciences
University of Wisconsin
Madison, Wisconsin
Chapter 18

Z.A. Haddad
Department of Ophthalmology
Joslin Diabetes Center
Boston, Massachusetts
Chapter 15

Jeffrey S. Heier, MD
Assistant Professor
Department of Ophthalmology
Tufts University School of Medicine
Clinical Instructor
Department of Ophthalmology
Harvard Medical School
Boston, Massachusetts
Chapter 10

Ann Hellstrom, MD, PhD
Professor
Section of Pediatric Ophthalmology
Queen Silvia Children's Hospital
Sahlegrenska Academy at University of Gothenburg
Gothenburg, Sweden
Chapter 5

David R. Hinton, MD, FARVO
Professor
Departments of Ophthalmology and Pathology
Keck School of Medicine of the University of Southern California
Arnold and Mabel Beckman Macular Research Center
Doheny Eye Institute
Los Angeles, California
Chapter 8

Allen C. Ho, MD
Professor
Department of Ophthalmology
Thomas Jefferson University School of Medicine
Associate Surgeon
Wills Eye Institute
Wyndmoor, Pennsylvania
Chapter 14

Derick Holt, MD, PhD
John Moran Eye Center
University of Utah
Salt Lake City, Utah
Chapter 24

Jason Hsu, MD
Clinical Instructor
Retina Service
Wills Eye Institute
Department of Ophthalmology
Thomas Jefferson University Hospital
Wyndmoor, Pennsylvania
Chapter 14

Mohamed Ibrahim, MD
Postdoctoral Fellow
Wilmer Eye Institute
Johns Hopkins University School of Medicine
Baltimore, Maryland
Chapter 11

Michael S. Ip, MD
Associate Professor
Department of Ophthalmology and Visual Sciences
University of Wisconsin School of Medicine
Madison, Wisconsin
Chapter 18

Grant P. Janzen, MD
Retina Fellow
Department of Ophthalmology
Tufts University School of Medicine
Ophthalmic Consultants of Boston
Boston, Massachusetts
Chapter 10

Ram Kannan, PhD
Professor of Research
Department of Ophthalmology
Doheny Eye Institute
Keck School of Medicine of the University of Southern California
Los Angeles, California
Chapter 8

Pearse A. Keane, MRCOphth MSc
Clinical Research Fellow
Doheny Eye Institute
Keck School of Medicine of the University of Southern California
Los Angeles, California
Chapter 20

Muge Kesen, MD
Wilmer Eye institute
Johns Hopkins University School of Medicine
Baltimore, Maryland
Chapter 13

Daniel F. Kiernan, MD
Vitreoretinal Fellow
Department of Ophthalmology
University of Illinois at Chicago
Chicago, Illinois
Chapter 16

Mark E. Kleinman, PhD
Departments of Ophthalmology and Visual Sciences
University of Kentucky
Lexington, Kentucky
Chapter 3

Amol D. Kulkarni, MD
Departments of Ophthalmology and Visual Sciences
University of Wisconsin School of Medicine
Madison, Wisconsin
Chapter 18

Rajendra Kumar-Singh, PhD, BSc
Associate Professor
Department of Ophthalmology
Tufts University School of Medicine
Boston, Massachusetts
Chapter 26

Leanne T. Labriola, DO
Department of Ophthalmology
University of Pittsburgh Medical Center
Eye and Ear Institute
Pittsburgh, Pennsylvania
Chapter 13

Jennifer I. Lim, MD
Professor of Ophthalmology
Director of Retina Service
Department of Ophthalmology and Visual Sciences
University of Illinois Eye and Ear Infirmary
Chicago, Illinois
Chapter 16

Alexander Ljubimov, PhD
Professor
Department of Medicine
David Geffen School of Medicine at University of California, Los Angeles
Director, Ophthalmology Research Laboratories
Department of Surgery
Cedars-Sinai Medical Center
Los Angeles, California
Chapter 7

Hylton R. Mayer, MD
Assistant Clinical Professor
Department of Ophthalmology
Yale University School of Medicine
Associate Physician
Department of Ophthalmology
Yale-New Haven Hospital
New Haven, Connecticut
Chapter 25

Gary W. McCollum, PhD
Senior Research Scientist
Departments of Ophthalmology and Visual Sciences
Vanderbilt University School of Medicine
Nashville, Tennessee
Chapter 6

Paul McGuire, PhD
Professor
Department of Cell Biology & Physiology
University of New Mexico School of Medicine
Albuquerque, New Mexico
Chapters 7, 9

Reinhold Medina, PhD
Centre for Vision Science
Queen's University Belfast
Belfast, Ireland
Chapter 27

Bryan K. Monson, MD
John Moran Eye Center
University of Utah
Salt Lake City, Utah
Chapter 24

Prithvi Mruthyunjaya, MD
Assistant Professor of Ophthalmology
Vitreoretinal Surgery and Ocular Oncology
Duke University Eye Center
Durham, North Carolina
Chapter 28

Matthew Neu
Undergraduate Student
Department of Pharmacology and Therapeutics
University of Florida
Research Lab Volunteer
Gainesville, Florida
Chapter 27

Quan Dong Nguyen, MD, MSc
Associate Professor
Wilmer Eye institute
Johns Hopkins University School of Medicine
Baltimore, Maryland
Chapter 11

John S. Penn, PhD
Professor
Departments of Cell and Developmental Biology
Ophthalmology and Visual Sciences
Vanderbilt Eye Institute
Vanderbilt University School of Medicine
Nashville, Tennessee
Chapter 6

Tushar Ranchod, MD
Vitreoretinal Fellow
Associated Retinal Consultants
Royal Oak, Michigan
Chapter 17

Sampathkumar Rangasamy, PhD
Research Associate
Departments of Cell Biology and Physiology
University of New Mexico School of Medicine
Albuquerque, New Mexico
Chapters 7, 9

Sarah Parker Read, PhD
Department of Ophthalmology
Tufts University School of Medicine
Boston, Massachusetts
Chapter 26

Elias Reichel, MD
Associate Professor
Department of Ophthalmology
Tufts Medical Center
Boston, Massachusetts
Chapter 19

Sayon Roy, PhD
Professor
Departments of Medicine and Ophthalmology
Boston University School of Medicine
Boston, Massachusetts
Chapter 7

Srinivas R. Sadda, MD
Associate Professor
Department of Ophthalmology
University of Southern California
Los Angeles, California
Chapter 20

P.S. Silva, MD
Fellow
Department of Ophthalmology
Harvard Medical School
Beetham Eye Institute
Joslin Diabetes Center
Boston, Massachusetts
Chapter 15

Lois E.H. Smith, MD, PhD
Professor
Department of Ophthalmology
Harvard Medical School
Children's Hospital Boston
Boston, Massachusetts
Chapter 5

Shozo Sonoda, MD
Department of Ophthalmology
Keck School of Medicine of the University of Southern California
Arnold and Mabel Beckman Macular Research Center
Doheny Eye Institute
Los Angeles, California
Department of Ophthalmology
Kagoshima University
Graduate School of Medical and Dental Sciences
Kagoshima, Japan
Chapter 8

Richard F. Spaide, MD
Vitreous, Retina, and Macula Consultants of New York
LuEsther T. Mertz Retinal Research Center
Manhattan Eye, Ear, and Throat Hospital
Edward S. Harkness Eye Institute
Columbia University
New York, New York
Chapter 23

Parameswaran G. Sreekumar, PhD
Department of Ophthalmology
Keck School of Medicine of the University of Southern California
Arnold and Mabel Beckman Macular Research Center
Doheny Eye Institute
Los Angeles, California
Chapter 8

Ramprasad Srinivasan, PhD
Research Associate
Departments of Cell Biology and Physiology
University of New Mexico School of Medicine
Albuquerque, New Mexico
Chapter 9

Alan Stitt, PhD
Professor
Centre for Vision Science
Queen's University Belfast
Belfast, Ireland
Chapter 27

J.K. Sun, MD, MPH
Instructor
Department of Ophthalmology
Harvard Medical School
Research Associate and Ophthalmologist
Beetham Eye Institute
Joslin Diabetes Center
Boston, Massachusetts
Chapter 15

James C. Tsai, MD, MBA
Robert R. Young Professor and Chair
Department of Ophthalmology and Visual Sciences
Yale University School of Medicine
Chief of Opthalmology
Yale-New Haven Hospital
New Haven, Connecticut
Chapter 25

George A. Williams, MD
Clinical Professor
Departments of Ophthalmology and Biomedical Sciences
Oakland University, William Beaumount School of Medicine
Chairman, Department of Ophthalmology
Director, Beaumont Eye Institute
Vice Chief of Surgical Services for Academic Affairs
William Beaumont Hospital
Royal Oak, Michigan
Chapter 29

Susan E. Yanni, PhD
Postdoctoral Fellow
Departments of Cell and Developmental Biology
Vanderbilt University School of Medicine
Nashville, Tennessee
Chapter 6

Brian Zaugg, BS
John Moran Eye Center
University of Utah
Salt Lake City, Utah
Chapter 24

Contents

SECTION I
Principles

PART A
Angiogenesis

CHAPTER

1

Judah Folkman and Angiogenesis

Anthony P. Adamis

Judah Folkman, MD, was the person who conceived the idea of angiogenesis and revolutionized the field 40 years ago. Today, angiogenesis inhibitors are being used in clinical practice in many fields of medicine including ophthalmology, and many are in clinical trials. ***Anthony Adamis, MD****, a student of Folkman, recollects his memories and pays tribute to the maestro.*

—Editors

When Judah Folkman was a young boy, he would accompany his father, a noted rabbi, on visits to the hospital to provide comfort to ailing members of his congregation. Years later, when he declared his interest in medicine, his father encouraged him to become a "rabbi-like doctor." Judah Folkman took that request to heart.

It is said that one can tell the measure of a man's character by the things he does when no one is looking. On most nights before leaving the laboratory, Judah Folkman MD, Harvard Professor, pediatric surgeon, and renowned scientist, would return the calls of—five to ten cancer patients seeking his advice. They would call from all over the world. He would patiently spend time with them, dispensing advice and helping in any way he could. When he was traveling, he would carry their names and phone numbers with him and would call from his hotel room. He did this for many years, without any fanfare or publicity. I learned about it from his secretary. He never talked about it.

Judah Folkman is best known for his work on angiogenesis. In 1971, he put forth a hypothesis that proved very controversial at the time—namely that tumors deprived of new blood vessels cannot grow beyond a very small size. Such tumors, he reasoned, would not kill their hosts. Via angiogenesis inhibition, cancer could become a chronic, but manageable, disease. His novel ideas were published in an essay in the *New England Journal of Medicine*. To his surprise, his ideas were scorned by many, or worse yet, ignored. He was advised to change the focus of his research. Students were discouraged from working with him. But Judah Folkman persisted. In the 1970s, he was almost alone in studying the tumor vasculature. His earliest experiments were descriptive, yet elegant and powerful in their design. Using the eye as a model system, he showed that tumors placed in the avascular compartments, that is, cornea, anterior chamber or vitreous, would remain viable but fixed in size as long as they were not invaded by a vasculature.

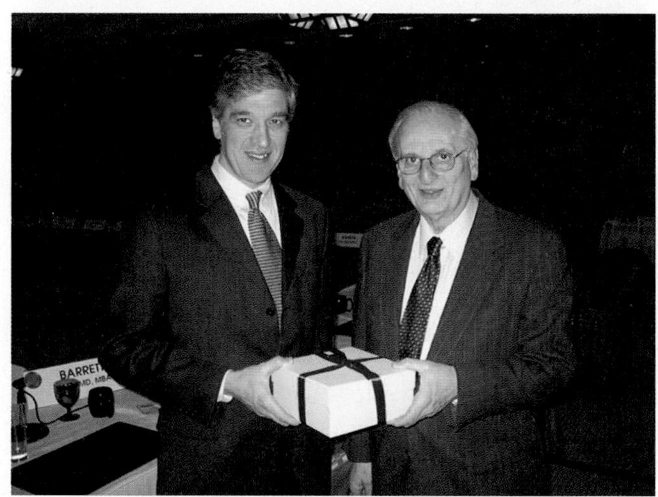

However, when new blood vessels grew into the small tumors from the adjacent vascularized tissues of the eye, for example, retina or iris, the tumors grew quickly and overtook the eye. Because the new vessels were elicited at a distance, Folkman hypothesized that the tumors secreted a diffusible, angiogenic growth factor. He termed the soluble hypothetical substance "tumor angiogenesis factor (TAF)." Using the eye as a model and observing the angiogenic response of the vascularized ocular tissues, Folkman further speculated that TAF was also operative in ocular neovascularization. If TAF could be blocked with an antibody, he reasoned, a new way of treating cancer and neovascular eye disease would emerge.

For more than a decade, Folkman had difficulty obtaining grant support. The reasons varied—the lack of direct proof for TAF, his competing surgical and administrative responsibilities, and his lack of a PhD. In later years, he often joked about this difficult period, and frequently quoted one particularly stinging NIH study section review. It concluded with the following sentence, "If TAF exists, it is solely in the mind of the applicant."

Folkman knew that if he were to silence his critics, he would have to provide direct proof for the existence of TAF. Before the search for TAF could begin though, Folkman had to develop the tools to discover it. Thus, his laboratory established the first capillary endothelial cell cultures; the first endothelial DNA synthesis assay; and proliferation, migration, and tube formation assays. These quantitative methods replicated the key steps in angiogenesis in vitro. His laboratory also developed the first in vivo angiogenesis models—the chicken choroiallantoic membrane and the corneal angiogenesis assays.

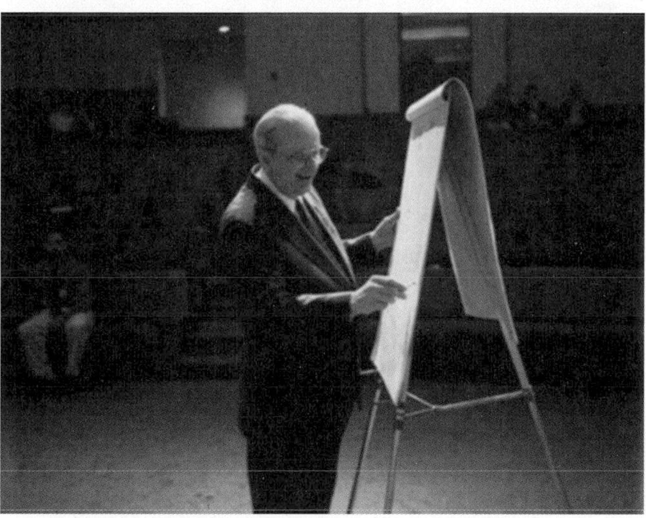

With these methods in hand, Folkman's group went on to isolate and characterize the first angiogenic growth factor (basic fibroblast growth factor) and the first angiogenesis inhibitor (TNP-1470; ultimately one of many). By the early 1990s, the stage had finally been set for the definitive proof of his hypothesis. Napoleone Ferrara, MD, a young Folkman collaborator at Genentech, created an antibody against vascular endothelial growth factor (VEGF)—his newly discovered angiogenesis factor—and used it to block tumor growth. After decades of research, incontrovertible proof was finally provided in 1993 that tumors are angiogenesis dependent. VEGF was TAF, and blockade via an antibody prevented tumor growth—just as Judah Folkman had predicted in 1971.

Today, Judah Folkman's theory is a scientific fact. Like many great ideas, in retrospect, it seems almost self-evident. And just as he predicted, the same factor is operative in angiogenic eye disease, for example, wet age-related macular degeneration, retinal vein occlusion, and diabetic retinopathy. Angiogenesis inhibitors are now first-line therapy for many cancers and are used to restore the vision of thousands of patients.

Judah Folkman was well served by his curiosity, intellect, and persistence. He possessed the traits that made for a world-class scientist—all the while possessing a child-like enthusiasm for science and the process of discovery. What is less well known is his generosity and humanity. This was by design as he never wished to draw attention to these things.

I have two personal anecdotes. The first occurred when I was a fellow in his laboratory, around 1994. Our group was delineating the role of VEGF in ocular disease and I brought to him a draft of a manuscript to review. He had been on the first four papers we published on the role of VEGF, and me being his student, it was protocol to review manuscripts together. He read the draft carefully, made some important suggestions, and then asked that his name be removed from the paper. I was taken aback and didn't know how to respond. "Is there something wrong with the paper?" I asked. He paused, looked at me and said, "No, no, no. The paper is excellent! This is important work! But you want your name associated with it, not mine." Despite my protestations, he insisted on removing his name. In academia, where authorship and publication are the most important currencies, his gesture was uniquely generous.

The second event occurred around the same time. My new wife and I secretly took a few days off one weekend, without leaving any forwarding information with anyone—we wanted to be completely alone. Ensconced in our secret hideaway, the phone rang in the hotel room. It was Dr. Folkman! How he found us remains a mystery to this day. Stammering, I tried to talk science and act normally, but Dr. Folkman got right to point. "I am creating a small lab to give you more space." he said. He went on to describe how he would give me some of his own lab space and expand it further by knocking down a wall and putting in two wet benches. I subsequently learned that he used his own funds to finish the renovations. I never asked him for lab space (really!). But he thought it was important and just did it.

These gestures happened without any public knowledge or fanfare. Many of his students have similar stories to tell. These things all happened when no one else was looking. They were the measure of the man's character.

CHAPTER

2

Pathophysiology of Retinal Neovascularization

Robert N. Frank

INTRODUCTION

The human retinal vasculature is essentially complete at birth in the full-term infant. These vessels elongate with growth of the eye through childhood and adolescence, but new vessel sprouts do not appear. Mitogenesis of cells of the capillaries in the adult retina is very infrequent,[1] and all postnatal retinal blood vessel sprouting in the human eye, called *neovascularization*, is abnormal.

NORMAL AND PATHOLOGICAL RETINAL VASCULAR GROWTH

Despite this major temporal difference between normal and pathological retinal blood vessel development, many of the molecular mechanisms of these two processes are, to the best of our present understanding, similar. The initial formation of primitive vessels in the developing retina from vascular precursors is called *vasculogenesis*, while sprouting of new vascular endothelial cells from these early vessels is termed *angiogenesis*.[2] Although retinal vascular development was initially thought to proceed by vasculogenesis, more recent investigations[2–4] indicate that, at least in some species (mouse, primates including humans), angiogenesis plays a highly important role. By these definitions, all pathologic retinal neovascularization involves angiogenesis. There has been a considerable amount of recent work dealing with the recruitment of bone marrow–derived stem cells into both retinal and choroidal neovascular lesions in experimental animals, which, by the definition above, indicates that vasculogenesis may also be involved in pathologic neovascularization.[5–7] How frequently this actually occurs in retinal and choroidal neovascularization that is observed clinically in humans is, however, unknown (Box 2.1).

BOX 2.1 Retinal Neovascularization Cascade

The flow chart below describes the mechanisms of retinal angiogenesis. The capillary nonperfusion results in hypoxia, which then upregulates the expression of growth factors either directly or through HIF-1. Growth factors then increase the expression of integrins and proteinases, which results in endothelial cell migration. These factors also promote endothelial cell proliferation directly. Both cell migration and proliferation are essential steps in angiogenesis. There is a critical balance between angiogenesis promoters and endogenous inhibitors. Any destabilization in this balance may lead to angiogenesis.

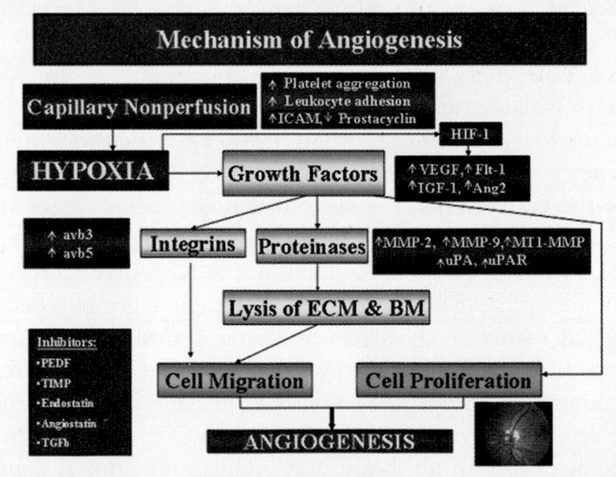

Reproduced from Das A, McGuire P. Retinal and choroidal angiogenesis: pathophysiology and strategies for inhibition. *Progr Ret Eye Res.* 2003; 22:721–748. Copyright (2003) with permission from Elsevier.

ROLE OF GROWTH FACTORS IN PROMOTING NEOVASCULARIZATION: VEGF

Both normal retinal vessels and pathologic neovascularization develop through the elaboration of specific peptides, called growth factors, that are elaborated primarily by nonvascular cells and stimulate the proliferation of vascular endothelium. While there are a number of growth factors that are elaborated in the retina and that appear to contribute to the process, the most prominent of these is vascular endothelial growth factor-A (VEGF-A), a family of polypeptides derived from a single gene but with alternative splicing, resulting in several isoforms having different molecular weights and with somewhat different properties.[8,9] Other closely related peptides are VEGF-B, -C, and -D and placental growth factor, all of which are mitogens for vascular endothelial cells, though with much reduced potency by comparison with VEGF-A. There are three cell membrane receptors for VEGF-A, designated VEGFR-1, VEGFR-2, and VEGFR-3. Of these, VEGFR-2, also designated Kdr (kinase domain receptor), is the one responsible for both normal and abnormal vascular proliferation.

It has long been recognized, in part on the basis of clinical findings in diseases in which retinal neovascularization occurs (Figs. 2.1A, B and 2.2A–C), that such neovascularization occurs largely adjacent to regions of retinal ischemia.[10,11] One of the early findings regarding the production of VEGF is that it is strongly upregulated by hypoxia.[12,13] A similarity of pathologic neovascularization in the adult retina and fetal development of the retinal vessels is, therefore, that both seem to be mediated by hypoxia, with the hypoxic stimulus arising from neurons in the immature retina stimulating glial cells to produce VEGF and the VEGF-producing glia leading the advancement of the vascular precursors through the fetal retina. Similarly, in the retinas and optic nerves of humans with diabetes and of animals with experimental galactosemia (a condition that produces a diabetic-like retinopathy), VEGF is substantially upregulated in glial cells,[14–16] which in turn stimulates production of VEGFR-2 (Figs. 2.3 and 2.4) in retinal vascular endothelial cells.[17] With maturation of the fetal retinal vasculature, the hypoxic stimulus is reduced and VEGF production decreases.[16–18] Because pathologic neovascularization in the adult retina does not revascularize the hypoxic tissue, but rather migrates inward through the inner limiting membrane of the retina and onto this inner retinal surface, or into the vitreous cavity, the hypoxic stimulus in such cases continues unless it is aborted either by some therapeutic intervention or by another process.

The hypoxic stimulus to VEGF production appears to be mediated by hypoxia inducible factor (HIF-1), a transcription factor that is itself highly regulated by tissue oxygenation and binds to the hypoxia response element of the VEGF gene, thereby stimulating upregulation of VEGF protein.[19] The importance of VEGF, and HIF-1, to fetal development is evident from the fact that fetal mice with knockouts either of the VEGF gene or of the HIF-1 gene

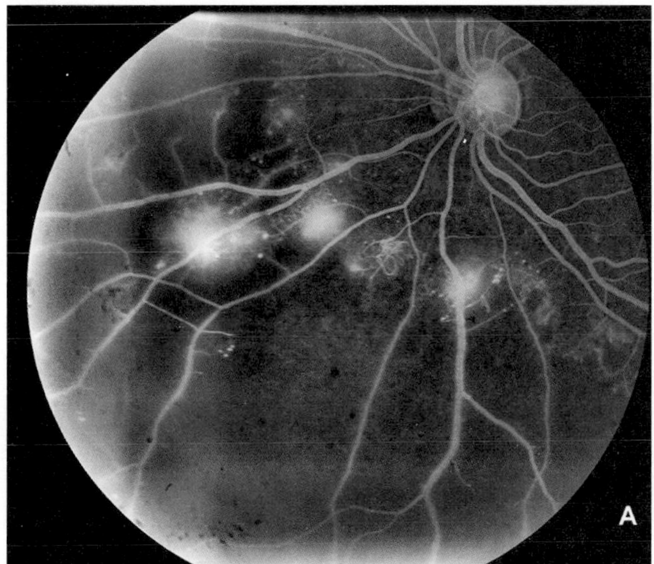

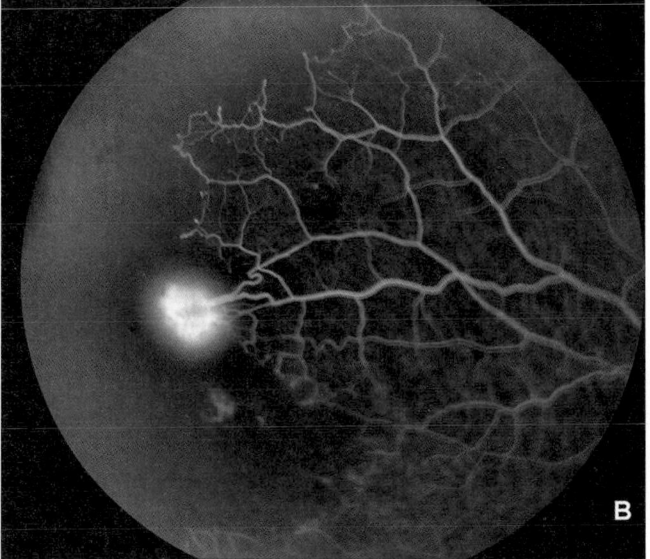

FIGURE 2.1. A: Frame from a fluorescein angiogram in a case of proliferative diabetic retinopathy showing new vessels (areas of intense dye leakage) next to nonperfused area, which appears *black* at the lower right of the image. **B:** Frame from a fluorescein angiogram in a case of proliferative sickle retinopathy. Note the intense leakage from the single neovascular tuft and the entirely nonperfused (*black*) peripheral retina in the portion of the photograph to the left. Note also the arteriovenous shunts, typical of sickle cell retinopathy, at the border of the nonperfused area.

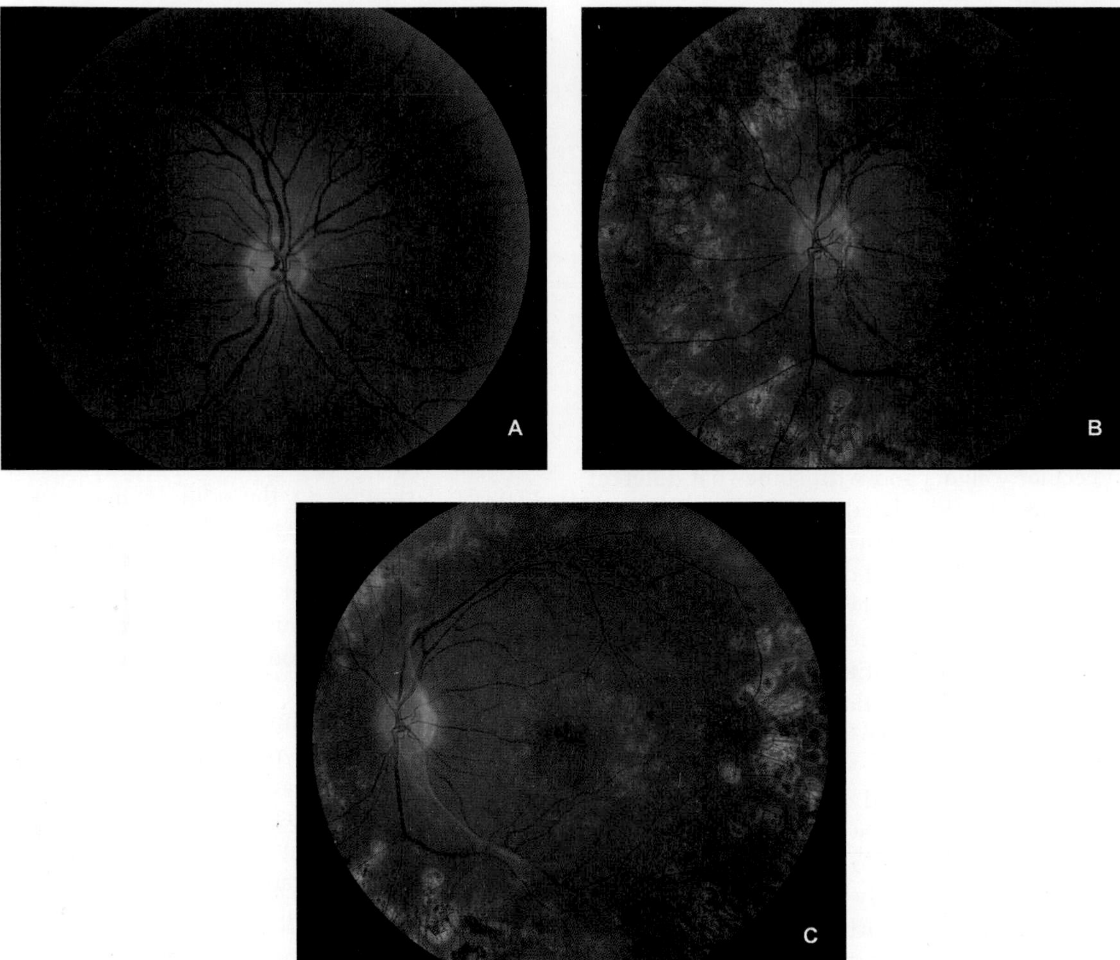

FIGURE 2.2. **A:** Normal right eye of a 50-year-old woman with a 12-year history of type 2 diabetes. Her left eye **(B)** had proliferative retinopathy with neovascularization of the optic nerve head that increased despite extensive panretinal argon laser photocoagulation. Subsequently, she was found to have an atherosclerotic lesion that greatly reduced blood flow through the left common carotid artery. She underwent successful carotid endarterectomy, following which the neovascularization dramatically regressed **(C)**. Presumably, retinal hypoxia due to the carotid atherosclerosis was an important contributor to her persistent proliferative diabetic retinopathy.

die *in utero* because they are unable to develop a vascular system.[20,21] Although hypoxia itself is a major stimulus to HIF-1 production, this transcription factor, and VEGF, can also be upregulated by a variety of molecular stimuli, such as cytokines and other growth factors,[19] and perhaps other molecules as well.[22–24] In addition to hypoxia, growth factors and cytokines that are increased in the inflammatory process may, therefore, also contribute to retinal neovascularization in diabetic retinopathy and in inflammatory diseases that involve the retina and choroid.[25–27]

Even after long duration (>25 years) of type 1 diabetes, proliferative retinopathy appears in not more than 50% to 60% of diabetic individuals.[28] This, together with evidence from epidemiologic studies that there is familial clustering both of diabetic retinopathy and of nephropathy,[29–31] indicates the likelihood of a genetic predisposition to these complications of the disease. Attempts to determine what gene(s) may be involved, through genome-wide scans of multiplex families of several different ethnicities with proliferative or severe nonproliferative retinopathy and nephropathy, using genome-wide scanning and other methods, are still underway.[31] Several reports have appeared describing the association of specific single nucleotide polymorphisms (SNPs) and haplotypes within the VEGF gene with proliferative and severe nonproliferative diabetic retinopathy.[32–34] A problem with these and several other papers on the same topic is that they are not all in agreement about the particular SNPs and/or haplotypes that each study is reporting as associated with proliferative and severe nonproliferative disease, even with quite high probability values. Of particular interest is the report from the very large and well-characterized DCCT/EDIC study cohort, in which several VEGF gene variants in this population with type 1 diabetes were highly

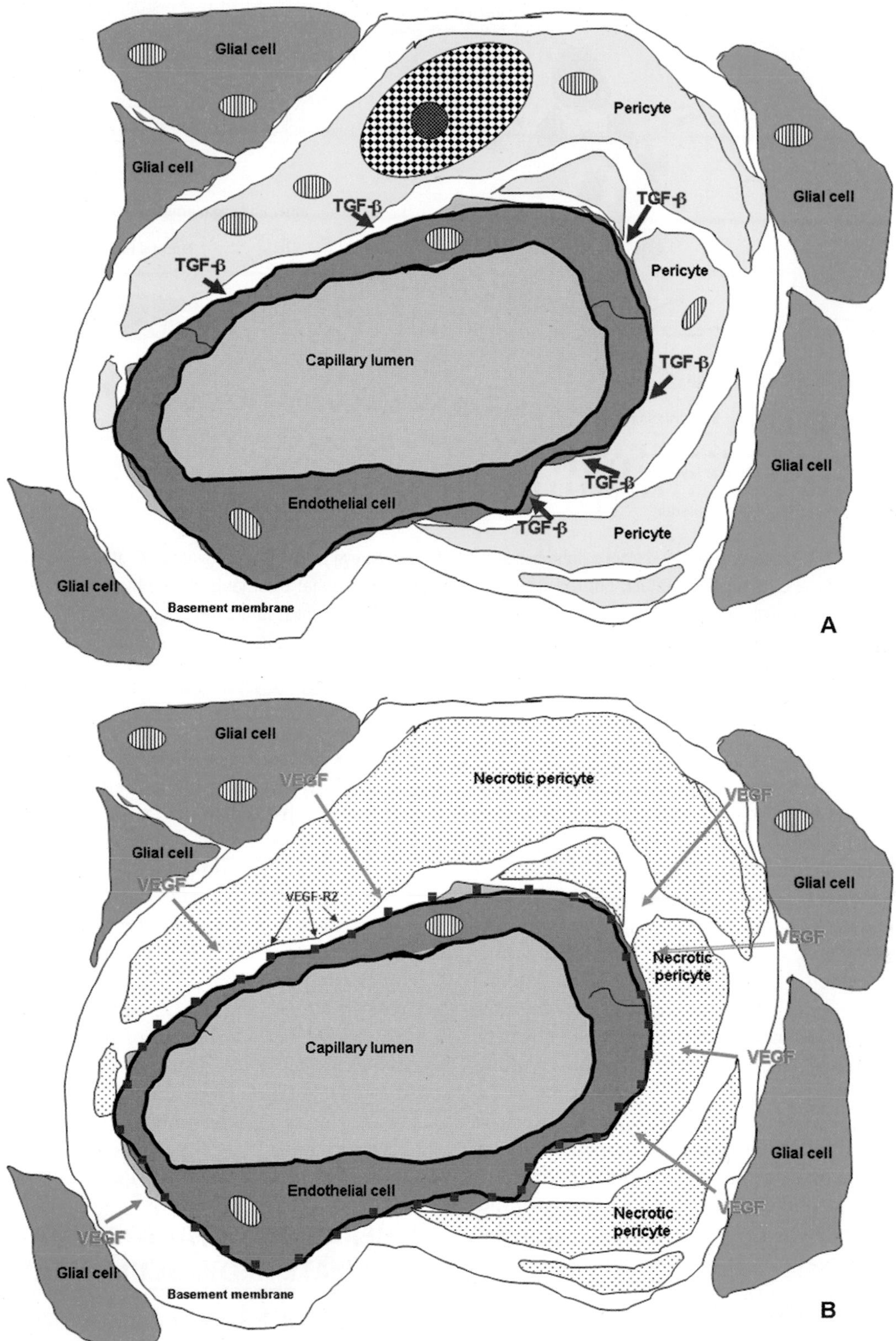

FIGURE 2.3. A: Diagram adapted from an electron micrograph of a human retinal capillary. Pericyte processes, shown in *yellow*, envelop the endothelial cell tube, shown in *beige*. The pericytes, together with the endothelial cells, produce transforming growth factor-β, which acts to prevent endothelial cell proliferation. Pericytes and endothelial cells of the capillaries are surrounded by a thick basement membrane, which is not shown in color, and the entire capillary is enveloped in glial processes (*green*). **B:** In the diabetic retina, pericytes are lost, removing the inhibitory stimulus and, perhaps, contributing to reduced blood flow with consequent hypoxia to regions of the retina. The hypoxic glial cells produce VEGF, which upregulates the receptor, VEGFR-2, on endothelial plasma membranes stimulating endothelial proliferation and neovascularization.

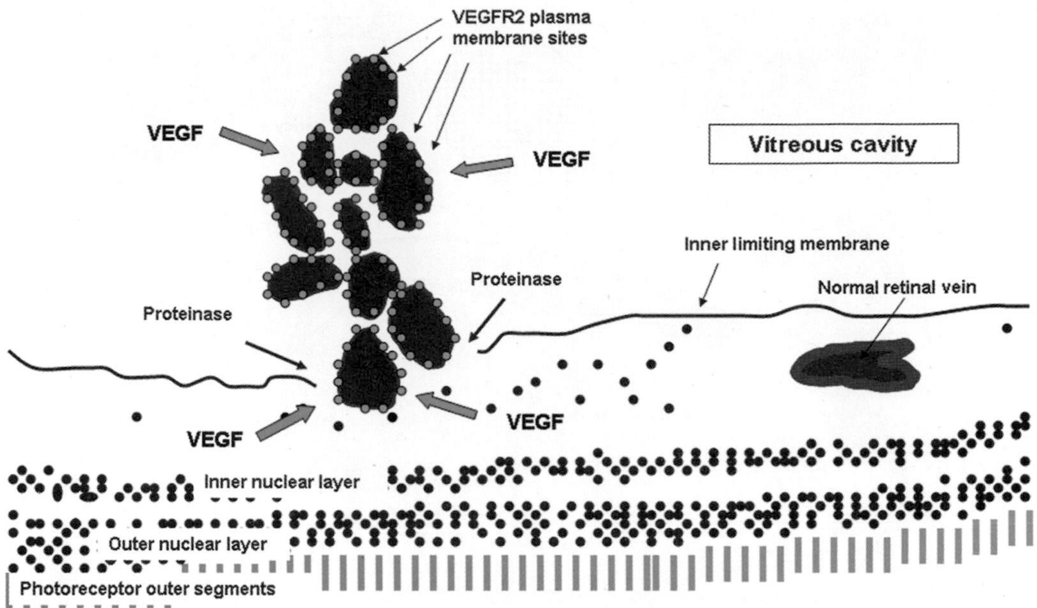

FIGURE 2.4. Drawing adapted from a light micrograph of a human eye with retinal neovascularization. The outer retinal layers are relatively intact, but the ganglion cell layer is somewhat disorganized. The hypoxic retina, in particular its glial cells, is producing greatly increased amounts of VEGF, which stimulates neovascularization. The new vessels grow inward, and the proteinases they produce allow them to digest the inner limiting membrane and break through into the vitreous.

associated with proliferative and severe nonproliferative diabetic retinopathy, but not with diabetic macular edema. Although VEGF has been strongly linked to proliferative diabetic retinopathy for a number of years,[35,36] there has also been considerable recent interest in a pathogenic role for VEGF in diabetic macular edema.[37–39] This derives from the initial discovery of VEGF (then called "vascular permeability factor") as a molecule that enhanced permeability of blood vessels.[40–42] The role of VEGF in macular edema in diabetes and other retinal diseases may be more complex than it is in retinal neovascularization, however. Questions that must be resolved are, first, the observations of Al-Kateb et al.[32] that SNPs and haplotypes of the VEGF gene that are significantly associated with proliferative and severe preproliferative diabetic retinopathy are not associated with macular edema and, second, that macular edema may occur in diabetes and other diseases without retinal neovascularization and, conversely, that neovascularization may occur without macular edema.[43]

VEGF, THE BLOOD-RETINAL BARRIER, AND PROTEINASE ACTIVITY

The breakdown of the blood-retinal barrier, and the proliferation of retinal new blood vessels, require the production of enzymes or other substances that can, first, break down the junctional complexes that form the gates between retinal vascular endothelial cells or retinal pigment epithelial cells, thereby separating retinal vascular lumina or the choriocapillaris and the neural retina, and, second, digest the basement membranes that encase the endothelial cells and pericytes or smooth muscle cells of the retinal blood vessels, or that comprise the inner limiting membrane that comprises the boundary between the neural retina and the vitreous (Fig. 2.4). VEGF stimulates an initial step in blood-retinal barrier breakdown by promoting the phosphorylation of specific sites on the cellular tight junction proteins zonula occludens-1 and occluding.[44,45] Second, VEGF upregulation in the hypoxic retina stimulates production of matrix metalloproteinase enzymes (MMPs)[46,47] that enhance blood-retinal barrier breakdown.[48] These enzymes (MMPs) have been reported in excess in neovascular membranes from the retinas of diabetic humans,[49] and experimental retinal neovascularization can be suppressed by MMP inhibitors.[50]

OTHER GROWTH FACTORS THAT MAY STIMULATE NEOVASCULARIZATION

Although VEGF has been the most widely studied growth factor involved in retinal neovascularization, there has been considerable interest in other growth factors in this process. The upregulation of insulin-like growth factor-1 (IGF-1) following the imposition of "tight" blood glucose control in previously poorly controlled individuals with type 1 diabetes and early retinopathy has been claimed to be responsible for the "early worsening" of retinopathy that has been observed in that situation.[51]

However, Wang et al.[52] have reported that serum IGF-1 levels did not correlate with proliferative diabetic retinopathy either in type 1 or in type 2 diabetics in their large, population-based series. The elegant work of Lois Smith and her co-workers strongly suggests that IGF-1 serves primarily as a "permissive" factor for neovascularization occurring in the presence of VEGF, rather than as the principal angiogenic factor itself.[53]

Angiopoietin-1 (Angl) and angiopoietin-2 (Ang2), acting through the receptor Tie2, also serve as permissive factors for vascular growth. In a series of transgenic mice that can express Angl or Ang2 and VEGF, stimulated by different promoters that are engineered to respond to dosing with the antibiotic doxycycline, Campochiaro and colleagues[54] have been able to show differential regulation of vascular sprouting from the superficial or deep retinal capillary beds, governed by the expression of Angl or Ang2 at different postnatal times during the development of the retinal vasculature in these mice. Although a role for Angl or Ang2 in the adult eye, or in pathological processes such as the proliferative retinopathies, has not been delineated, Campochiaro speculates that increased expression of one of these molecules may be necessary to permit neovascularization in the retinas of diabetic humans or experimental animals, in which VEGF has been upregulated but new vessels have not appeared.[8,15,54] Additional evidence for permissive, or accessory, roles for Ang2 and the Tie2 receptor in retinal neovascularization has been presented by other authors.[55,56]

Members of the fibroblast growth factor family were initially thought to be important contributors to retinal neovascularization. However, subsequent work and a variety of arguments (summarized in Ref. 57) suggest that this is not likely to be the case.

Impressive recent work[53,58,59] indicates that erythropoietin contributes importantly to the pathogenesis of proliferative diabetic retinopathy and, perhaps, to other proliferative retinopathies. A single SNP in the promoter of the erythropoietin gene was found, in three separate patient series, to be significantly associated with proliferative diabetic retinopathy and with end-stage diabetic nephropathy.[59]

INHIBITORY GROWTH FACTORS

Using the technique that they had developed for preparing flat mounts of the isolated human retinal vascular tree following digestion of the neural retina with concentrated trypsin solutions, Cogan, Kuwabara and their colleagues in the 1960s showed that an early vascular lesion in eyes from diabetic human subjects was loss of the pericytes, or "mural cells," from the retinal capillaries.[60] Selective early loss of pericytes in diabetic eyes has been considered a cardinal lesion of early diabetic retinopathy, although Kern[61] has recently argued that capillary pericyte loss is not selective and that both pericytes and endothelial cells are lost equally in diabetic retinas. While this argument may be valid with consideration to vascular cell loss over the entire retina, it is certainly the case that there are some regions in which pericyte loss precedes that of endothelial cells, as Kuwabara and Cogan initially reported. While the metabolic processes that lead to this cellular loss are still unclear, it has been demonstrated that cells of the retinal capillaries in diabetic humans and laboratory animals do undergo apoptosis or programmed cell death.[62] Subsequent work has shown that retinal neurons and glia in diabetic eyes also undergo apoptosis,[63] a process that must be extremely slow, or else the cellular content of the retinas of diabetic individuals would soon become depopulated.

What are the consequences of capillary cell loss? Studies of trypsin digest preparations of human eyes in which, fortuitously, fluorescein angiograms had been performed shortly before the individual's death have demonstrated that capillaries that have become totally acellular and are recognizable only as empty basement membrane tubes do not carry blood and therefore contribute to the retinal ischemia that is a stimulus to VEGF upregulation and neovascularization.[64] However, the selective removal of pericytes appears to remove an inhibitory "brake," permitting endothelial cells to proliferate, as Orlidge and D'Amore[65] showed some years ago. They subsequently showed that the inhibitory molecule was another growth factor, transforming growth factor-β (TGF-β; Fig. 2.3A).[66] Microaneurysms would, therefore, appear to be localized endothelial cell proliferations, likely in areas where pericytes have been lost (Fig. 2.3B).

While details of the mechanism(s) by which pericytes and endothelial cells eventually undergo apoptosis in the retinas of diabetics are not completely clear, a finding that appears to be relevant is that in fetal mice in which the gene for platelet-derived growth factor (PDGF) has been knocked out, capillary pericytes do not develop and the fetus dies.[67] In the developing fetal eye, PDGF, therefore, appears to be important for recruiting pericytes to the developing retinal vessels and for subsequent maintenance of the vasculature.[68] Whether hyperglycemia or other metabolic abnormalities in the diabetic eye interfere with PDGF production or its interaction with the cells of the retinal capillaries, leading to pericyte loss, has not been described.

Another inhibitory growth factor is pigment epithelium–derived factor (PEDF). Although many cells throughout the retina produce PEDF, its major site of biosynthesis is, as its name implies, the retinal pigment epithelium (RPE).[69] In addition to its ability to inhibit blood vessel proliferation, PEDF also appears to facilitate retinal neuronal differentiation.[70] The RPE is a major site of synthesis of both PEDF and VEGF, and both of these molecules are released constitutively by normal RPE cells but, remarkably, in opposite directions (Fig. 2.5). VEGF is released from the basal surface of the RPE layer,[71] thereby

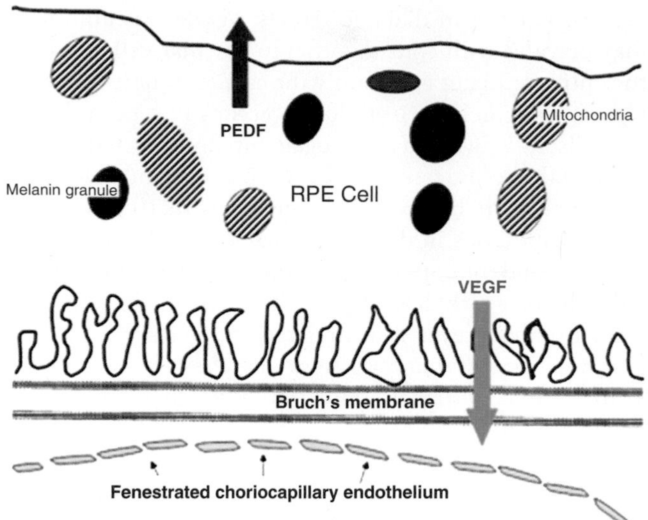

FIGURE 2.5. Drawing made from an electron micrograph, showing polarized secretion of VEGF from the basal plasma membrane of the RPE cells toward the choriocapillaris, maintaining the anatomy and function of that vascular layer and inducing the asymmetrical choriocapillary plasma membrane, which is fenestrated on the retinal side. PEDF is secreted from the apical side of the PRE, presumably acting to maintain the normal avascularity of the outer retina.

facilitating the maintenance of the choriocapillaris and also the asymmetrical anatomy of the choriocapillary endothelium, with a thin, fenestrated surface facing the RPE and a thicker endothelial lining facing the deeper layers of the choroid. VEGF interacts with cellular junction proteins,[44,45] leading to their disruption with breakdown of the blood-retinal barrier, and facilitates the development of endothelial fenestrations.[72] By contrast, PEDF is released from the apical surface of RPE cells,[73] which may be the reason that the outer layers of the vertebrate retina normally are avascular and also, perhaps, explains why retinal neovascularization nearly always grows inward, toward the inner limiting membrane and the vitreous. Could exceptions,[74–76] in which the new vessels grow *outward*, toward the RPE, be the result of aberrant secretion of PEDF and/or VEGF in localized regions of the RPE?

As demonstrated in the Key Points, which summarizes the major points of this chapter, we have learned a great deal about the pathophysiology of retinal neovascularization. Much of this knowledge has already been put to good use in developing therapeutic methods, as described in other chapters in this volume. But there is clearly much more to be learned. The therapies that we have inhibit the process far downstream, at the level of the growth factors that actually stimulate the process. But future developments toward therapy, and prevention, will be even more effective if they act at targets further upstream, before the neovascular process has a chance to get underway.

KEY POINTS

- Many features of pathologic retinal neovascularization are similar to those of fetal vascular development.
- Both processes are stimulated by hypoxia. In fetal life, the developing vasculature alleviates the hypoxia, while in the diseased adult retina, the hypoxic stimulus is maintained.
- The major growth factor that is upregulated by hypoxia is VEGF (or, more strictly, VEGF-A). In hypoxia and some other conditions, HIF-1, a transcription factor, binds to the VEGF gene and increases its activity.
- VEGF is produced in nonvascular cells of the retina, primarily glial cells. It in turn upregulates VEGFR-2 on the plasma membranes of vascular endothelial cells, facilitating VEGF binding to those cells and stimulating both endothelial cell proliferation and breakdown of the blood-retinal barrier.
- Proliferating endothelial cells elaborate proteinases that help them to digest vascular basement membranes and also the inner limiting membrane of the retina as they break through into the vitreous.
- Other molecules may also facilitate retinal neovascularization. Among these are erythropoietin and possibly the Ang1 and Ang2.
- Still other growth factors may act to prevent neovascularization. Among these are PEDF and TGF-β. The latter molecule is elaborated by pericytes and activated by endothelial cells. Loss of pericytes in diabetic retinopathy, thus, removes an inhibitory stimulus to neovascular proliferation.
- PDGF is required in fetal life for the development and maturation of pericytes and in adult life for their maintenance. Its malfunction may facilitate pericyte loss.

REFERENCES

1. Engerman RL, Pfaffenbach D, Davis MD. Cell turnover of capillaries. *Lab Invest*. 1967;17:738–743.
2. Chan-Ling T. Vasculogenesis and angiogenesis in formation of the human retinal vasculature. In: Penn JS, ed. *Retinal and Choroidal Angiogenesis*. Dordrecht, the Netherlands: Springer; 2008:chap 6, 119–138.
3. Fruttiger M. Development of the mouse retinal vasculature: angiogenesis versus vasculogenesis. *Invest Ophthalmol Vis Sci*. 2002;43:522–527.
4. Gariano RF. Cellular mechanisms in retinal vascular development. *Prog Retin Eye Res*. 2003;22:295–306.
5. Kramerov AA, Saghizadeh M, Caballero S, et al. Inhibition of protein kinase CK2 suppresses angiogenesis and hematopoietic stem cell recruitment to retinal neovascularization sites. *Mol Cell Biochem*. 2008;316:177–186.

6. Sengupta N, Caballero S, Mames RN, et al. The role of adult bone marrow-derived stem cells in choroidal neovascularization. *Invest Ophthalmol Vis Sci*. 2003;44:4908–4913.
7. Ljubimov AV, Caballero S, Aoki AM, et al. Involvement of protein kinase CK2 in angiogenesis and retinal neovascularization. *Invest Ophthalmol Vis Sci*. 2004;45:4583–4591.
8. Campochiaro PA and the First ARVO/Pfizer Working Group. Ocular versus extraocular neovascularization: mirror images or vague resemblances. *Invest Ophthalmol Vis Sci*. 2006;47:462–474.
9. Ferrara N. VEGF and EG-VEGF. *Invest Ophthalmol Vis Sci* 2006;47(suppl 1):462–474. Available online at: http://www.iovs.org/cgi/data/47/2/462/DC1/10
10. Henkind P. Ocular neovascularization. *Am J Ophthalmol*. 1978;85:287–301.
11. Ashton N. Oxygen and the retinal blood vessels. *Trans Ophthalmol Soc U K*. 1980;100:359–362.
12. Shweiki D, Itin A, Soffer D, et al. Vascular endothelial growth factor induced by hypoxia may mediate hypoxia-initiated angiogenesis. *Nature*. 1992;359:843–845.
13. Aiello LP, Northrup JM, Keyt BA, et al. Hypoxic regulation of vascular endothelial growth factor in retinal cells. *Arch Ophthalmol*. 1995;113:1538–1544.
14. Amin RH, Frank RN, Kennedy A, et al. Vascular endothelial growth factor is present in glial cells of the retina and optic nerve of human subjects with nonproliferative diabetic retinopathy. *Invest Ophthalmol Vis Sci*. 1997;38:36–47.
15. Frank RN, Amin R, Kennedy A, et al. An aldose reductase inhibitor and aminoguanidine prevent vascular endothelial growth factor expression in rats with long-term galactosemia. *Arch Ophthalmol*. 1997;115:136–147.
16. Zahs K, Esguerra M. Glial cells in the developing retina. In: *Retinal Development*. Sernagor E, Eglen S, Harris B, Wong R, eds. Cambridge, UK: Cambridge University Press; 2006: 172–192.
17. Witmer AN, Blaauwgeers HG, Weich HA, et al. Altered expression patterns of VEGF receptors in human diabetic retina and in experimental VEGF-induced retinopathy in monkey. *Invest Ophthalmol Vis Sci*. 2002;43:849–857.
18. Provis JM. Development of the primate retinal vasculature. *Prog Retin Eye Res*. 2001;20:799–821.
19. Semenza GL. Hypoxia and HIF-1. *Invest Ophthalmol Vis Sci*. 2006;47(suppl 12):462–474. Available online at http://www.iovs.org/cgi/data/47/2/462/DC1/20
20. Carmeliet P, Ferreira V, Breier G, et al. Abnormal blood vessel development and lethality in embryos lacking a single VEGF allele. *Nature*. 1996;380:435–439.
21. Iyer NV, Kotch LE, Agani F, et al. Cellular and developmental control of O_2 homeostasis by hypoxia-inducible factor 1α. *Genes Dev*. 1998;12:149–162.
22. Lu M, Kuroki M, Amano S, et al. Advanced glycation end products increase retinal vascular endothelial growth factor expression. *J Clin Invest*. 1998;101:1219–1224.
23. Lu M, Amano S, Miyamoto K, et al. Insulin-induced vascular endothelial growth factor expression in retina. *Invest Ophthalmol Vis Sci*. 1999;40:3281–3286.
24. Kuroki M, Voest EE, Amano S, et al. Reactive oxygen intermediates increase vascular endothelial growth factor expression in vitro and in vivo. *J Clin Invest*. 1996;98:1667–1675.
25. Adamis AP. Is diabetic retinopathy an inflammatory disease? *Br J Ophthalmol*. 2002;86:363–365.
26. Ushio-Fukai M, Alexander RW. Reactive oxygen species as mediators of angiogenesis signaling: role of NAD(P)H oxidase. *Mol Cell Biochem*. 2004;264:85–97.
27. Al-Shabrawey M, Rojas M, Sanders T, et al. Role of NADPH oxidase in retinal vascular inflammation. *Invest Ophthalmol Vis Sci*. 2008;49:3239–3244.
28. Klein R, Klein BEK, Moss SE, et al. The Wisconsin Epidemiologic Study of Diabetic Retinopathy. II. Prevalence and risk of diabetic retinopathy when age at diagnosis is less than 30 years. *Arch Ophthalmol*. 1984;102:520–526.
29. DCCT Research Group. Clustering of long-term complications in families with diabetes in the diabetes control and complications trial. *Diabetes*. 1997;46:1829–1839.
30. Seaquist ER, Goetz FC, Rich S, et al. Familial clustering of diabetic kidney disease: evidence for genetic susceptibility to diabetic nephropathy. *N Engl J Med*. 1989;320:1161–1165.
31. Arar NH, Freedman BI, Adler SG, et al. Family Investigation of Nephropathy and Diabetes Research Group. Heritability of the severity of diabetic retinopathy: the FIND-Eye study. *Invest Ophthalmol Vis Sci*. 2008;49:3839–3845.
32. Al-Kateb H, Mirea L, Xie X, et al. and the DCCT/EDIC Research Group. Multiple variants in vascular endothelial growth factor (VEGFA) are risk factors for time to severe retinopathy in type 1 diabetes: the DCCT/EDIC genetics study. *Diabetes*. 2007;56:2161–2168.
33. Churchill AJ, Carter JG, Ramsden C, et al. VEGF polymorphisms are associated with severity of diabetic retinopathy. *Invest Ophthalmol Vis Sci*. 2008;49:3611–3616.
34. Errera FI, Canani LH, Silva ME, et al. Functional vascular endothelial growth factor -634G>C SNP is associated with proliferative diabetic retinopathy: a case-control study in a Brazilian population of European ancestry. *Diabetes Care*. 2007;30:275–279.
35. Aiello LP, Avery RL, Arrigg PG, et al. Vascular endothelial growth factor in ocular fluid of patients with diabetic retinopathy and other retinal disorders. *N Engl J Med*. 1994; 331:1480–1487.
36. Adamis AP, Miller JW, Bernal M-T, et al. Increased vascular endothelial growth factor levels in the vitreous of eyes with proliferative diabetic retinopathy. *Am J Ophthalmol*. 1994; 118:445–450.
37. Shimada H, Akaza E, Yuzawa M, et al. Concentration gradient of vascular endothelial growth factor in the vitreous of eyes with diabetic macular edema. *Invest Ophthalmol Vis Sci*. 2009;50:2953–2955.
38. Khurana RN, Do DV, Nguyen QD. Anti-VEGF therapeutic approaches for diabetic macular edema. *Int Ophthalmol Clin*. 2009;49:109–119.
39. Aiello LP. Targeting intraocular neovascularization and edema—one drop at a time. *N Engl J Med*. 2008;359:967–969.
40. Senger DR, Galli SJ, Dvorak AM, et al. Tumor cells secrete a vascular permeability factor that promotes accumulation of ascites fluid. *Science*. 1983;219:983–985.
41. Brown LF, Detmar M, Claffey K, et al. Vascular permeability factor/vascular endothelial growth factor: a multifunctional angiogenic cytokine. *EXS*. 1997;79:233–269.
42. Dvorak HF. Discovery of vascular permeability factor (VPF). *Exp Cell Res*. 2006;312:522–526.
43. Frank RN. Treating diabetic retinopathy by inhibiting growth factor pathways. *Curr Opin Investig Drugs*. 2009;10: 327–335.

44. Murakami T, Felinski EA, Antonetti DA. Occludin phosphorylation and ubiquitination regulate tight junction trafficking and vascular endothelial growth factor (VEGF)-induced permeability. *J Biol Chem*. 2009 May 28; [Epub ahead of print].
45. Antonetti DA, Barber AJ, Hollinger LA, et al. Vascular endothelial growth factor induces rapid phosphorylation of tight junction proteins occludin and zonula occluden 1. A potential mechanism for vascular permeability in diabetic retinopathy and tumors. *J Biol Chem*. 1999;274:23463–23467.
46. Hoffmann S, He S, Ehren M, et al. MMP-2 and MMP-9 secretion by RPE is stimulated by angiogenic molecules found in choroidal neovascular membranes. *Retina*. 2006;26:454–461.
47. Ottino P, Finley J, Rojo E, et al. Hypoxia activates matrix metalloproteinase expression and the VEGF system in monkey choroid-retinal endothelial cells: involvement of cytosolic phospholipase A2 activity. *Mol Vis*. 2004;10:341–350.
48. Giebel SJ, Menicucci G, McGuire PG, et al. Matrix metalloproteinases in early diabetic retinopathy and their role in alteration of the blood-retinal barrier. *Lab Invest*. 2005;85:597–607.
49. Das A, McGuire PG, Eriqat C, et al. Human diabetic neovascular membranes contain high levels of urokinase and metalloproteinase enzymes. *Invest Ophthalmol Vis Sci*. 1999;40:809–813.
50. Das A, McLamore A, Song W, et al. Retinal neovascularization is suppressed with a matrix metalloproteinase inhibitor. *Arch Ophthalmol*. 1999;117:498–503.
51. Chantelau E, Kohner EM. Why some cases of retinopathy worsen when diabetic control improves. *Br Med J*. 1997;315:1105–1106.
52. Wang Q, Dills DG, Klein R, et al. Does insulin-like growth factor I predict incidence and progression of diabetic retinopathy? *Diabetes*. 1995;44:161–164.
53. Smith LE. Through the eyes of a child: understanding retinopathy through ROP the Friedenwald lecture. *Invest Ophthalmol Vis Sci*. 2008;49:5177–5182.
54. Campochiaro P. Ocular neovascularization. *Invest Ophthalmol Vis Sci*. 2006;47(suppl 21):462–474. Available online at: http://www.iovs.org/cgi/data/47/2/462/DC1/7
55. Takagi H, Koyama S, Seike H, et al. Potential role of the angiopoietin/tie2 system in ischemia-induced retinal neovascularization. *Invest Ophthalmol Vis Sci*. 2003;44:393–402.
56. Das A, Fanslow W, Cerretti D, et al. Angiopoietin/Tek interactions regulate MMP-9 expression and retinal neovascularization. *Lab Invest*. 2003;83:1637–1645.
57. Frank RN. Etiologic mechanisms in diabetic retinopathy. In: RyanSJ, Schachat AP, Wilkinson CP, Hinton D, eds. *Retina*, 4th ed. London: Elsevier; 2006:chap 66, 1240–1270.
58. Watanabe D, Suzuma K, Matsui S, et al. Erythropoietin as a retinal angiogenic factor in proliferative diabetic retinopathy. *N Engl J Med*. 2005;353:782–792.
59. Tong Z, Yang Z, Patel S, et al. and the Genetics of Diabetes and Diabetic Complication Study Group. Promoter polymorphism of the erythropoietin gene in severe diabetic eye and kidney complications. *Proc Natl Acad Sci U S A*. 2008;105:6998–7003.
60. Kuwabara T, Cogan DG. Retinal vascular patterns. VI. Mural cells of the retinal capillaries. *Arch Ophthalmol*. 1963;69: 492–502.
61. Kern TS. Animal models of diabetic retinopathy. In: Penn JS, ed. *Retinal and Choroidal Angiogenesis*. Dordrecht, the Netherlands: Springer; 2008:chap 4, 81–102.
62. Mizutani M, Kern TS, Lorenzi M. Accelerated death of retinal microvascular cells in human and experimental diabetic retinopathy. *J Clin Invest*. 1996;97:2883–2890.
63. Barber AJ, Lieth E, Khin SA, et al. Neural apoptosis in the retina during experimental and human diabetes. Early onset and effect of insulin. *J Clin Invest*. 1998;102:783–791.
64. Kohner EM, Henkind P. Correlation of fluorescein angiogram and retinal digest in diabetic retinopathy. *Am J Ophthalmol*. 1970;69:403–414.
65. Orlidge A, D'Amore PA. Inhibition of capillary endothelial cell growth by pericytes and smooth muscle cells. *J Cell Biol*. 1987;105:1455–1462.
66. Antonelli-Orlidge A, Saunders KB, Smith SR, et al. An activated form of transforming growth factor β is produced by cocultures of endothelial cells and pericytes. *Proc Natl Acad Sci U S A*. 1989;86:4544–4548.
67. Lindahl P, Johansson BR, Levéen P, et al. Pericyte loss and microaneurysm formation in PDGF-B-deficient mice. *Science*. 1997; 77:242–245.
68. Betsholtz C, Lindblom P, Gerhardt H. Role of pericytes in vascular morphogenesis. *EXS*. 2005;94:115–125.
69. Dawson DW, Volpert OV, et al. Pigment epithelium-derived factor: a potent inhibitor of angiogenesis. *Science*. 1999;285:245–248.
70. Steele FR, Chader GJ, Johnson LV, et al. Pigment epithelium-derived factor: neurotrophic activity and identification as a member of the serine protease inhibitor gene family. *Proc Natl Acad Sci U S A*. 1993;90:1526–1530.
71. Blaauwgeers HG, Holtkamp GM, Rutten H, et al. Polarized vascular endothelial growth factor secretion by human retinal pigment epithelium and localization of vascular endothelial growth factor receptors on the inner choriocapillaris. Evidence for a trophic paracrine relation. *Am J Pathol*. 1999;155:421–428.
72. Esser S, Wolburg K, Wolburg H, et al. Vascular endothelial growth factor induces endothelial fenestrations in vitro. *J Cell Biol*. 1998;140:947–959.
73. Becerra SP, Fariss RN, Wu YQ, et al. Pigment epithelium-derived factor in the monkey retinal pigment epithelium and interphotoreceptor matrix: apical secretion and distribution. *Exp Eye Res*. 2004;78:223–234.
74. Eliassi-Rad B, Green WR. Histopathologic study of presumed parafoveal telangiectasis. *Retina*. 1999;19:332–335.
75. Lafaut BA, Aisenbrey S, Vanden Broecke C, et al. Clinicopathological correlation of deep retinal vascular anomalous complex in age related macular degeneration. *Br J Ophthalmol*. 2000;84:1269–1274.
76. Yannuzzi LA, Negrão S, Iida T, et al. Retinal angiomatous proliferation in age-related macular degeneration. *Retina*. 2001;21:416–434.

CHAPTER 3

Choroidal Neovascularization: Pathophysiology

Mark E. Kleinman • Jayakrishna Ambati

INTRODUCTION

The chorioretinal architecture is a heterogeneous assembly of specialized tissues derived from neuroectoderm and mesenchyme. The dual-layered blood-retina barrier, which incorporates the retinal pigment epithelium (RPE), serves as a sentry for the vital cellular circuitry that integrates visual data while the underlying choroid provides the hypermetabolic photoreceptor segments with one of the richest nutrient exchange networks in the human body. In multiple inflammatory, infectious, and immune-mediated diseases, these tissues undergo specific cellular transformations, for which nature intended to protect and repair the choroid and retina, but which paradoxically lead to blindness. This chapter addresses the clinical and molecular pathogenesis of choroidal neovascularization (CNV) with a particular emphasis on critical growth factors and newly discovered cell signaling pathways that will yield an armamentarium of targeted therapeutics in the 21st century.

The choroid is a highly vascularized pigmented tissue layer engineered to provide efficient nutrient and metabolic exchange for the RPE and outer two thirds of the retina. In the setting of choroidal inflammation or injury, cellular components of the RPE and choroid activate in order to contain the wound, destroy any invading pathogens, and initiate the repair process. As a result of the subsequent proinflammatory surge, newly formed blood vessels invade the wound bed to revascularize hypoxic areas and provide growth factors to the damaged cells. Typically, as in several other peripheral tissues in the human body such as skin, this neovascular response allows for tissue healing and scar remodeling; however, in the delicate architecture of the chorioretinal interface, these abnormal vessels grow in an unregulated fashion beneath the retina and are susceptible to leakage and rupture. CNV and the resultant extravascular leakage of fluid into the subretinal space are hardly suitable for the highly specialized function of photoreceptors and lead to significant loss of visual quality. Through centuries of clinical observations and scientific investigation, critical insights into the biology of CNV in injury and repair have modernized our current understanding of the cellular and molecular pathways that drive this pathological process.

PATHOGENIC MECHANISMS OF CNV IN AGE-RELATED MACULAR DEGENERATION

The most common forms of CNV are due to a combination of inflammation, oxidative stress, and photochemical damage secondary to age-related macular degeneration (AMD), which is the leading cause of blindness among the elderly on three continents and affects 30 to 50 million people worldwide.[1–3] CNV is a public health epidemic as its prevalence (~2 million) and annual incidence (~200,000) are as great as those of breast or prostate cancer in the United States.[4,5] Between 10% and 20% of people with AMD will progress to the neovascular form, which is responsible for about 90% of vision loss in patients with AMD. Recent evidence suggests that the gradual accumulation of inflammatory debris in drusen beneath the RPE and within the choroid ultimately leads to the production of proangiogenic cytokines and retinal invasion by abnormal and leaky vasculature.[6] Some of these inflammatory components are comprised of photochemically altered proteins that are linked to intermediate or terminal products of the vitamin A cycle or lipid breakdown products released by dying photoreceptors and RPE.[7] There is now sufficient scientific evidence that drusen do not simply precede neovascular AMD but in fact promote pathologic angiogenesis in the setting of AMD. CNV can wreak havoc on visual acuity via leakage into the subretinal, intraretinal, or vitreous spaces near the macula. Overtime, these CNV membranes remodel into fibrotic scars that may still harbor abnormal vasculature and be sites of recurrently active neovascularization (NV).

The original diagnostic classification of neovascular AMD presented by Gass described two patterns of CNV as determined by fluorescein angiography and histopathologic examination (Fig. 3.1).[8] Type I or occult CNV was characterized by late leakage of fluorescein, suggesting that the neovascular lesion was contained beneath the RPE layer. In Type II or classic CNV, fluorescein angiography demonstrates early, lacey hyperfluorescence and subsequent pooling in the subretinal space (Fig. 3.2). In these lesions, the CNV has grown through Bruch membrane and the RPE layer into the subretinal space. More recently, a third type of CNV termed retinal angiomatous proliferation (RAP) was described in which a pathologic anastomosis develops between the choroidal and retinal circulation via CNV growth through the RPE/Bruch membrane complex.[9] These lesions usually occur later in the remodeling stages of CNV but are frequently noted on detailed angiographic studies. Another pattern of CNV, polypoidal choroidal vasculopathy (PCV), has also been associated with AMD and is currently an area of active investigation.[10]

Type I or sub-RPE CNV

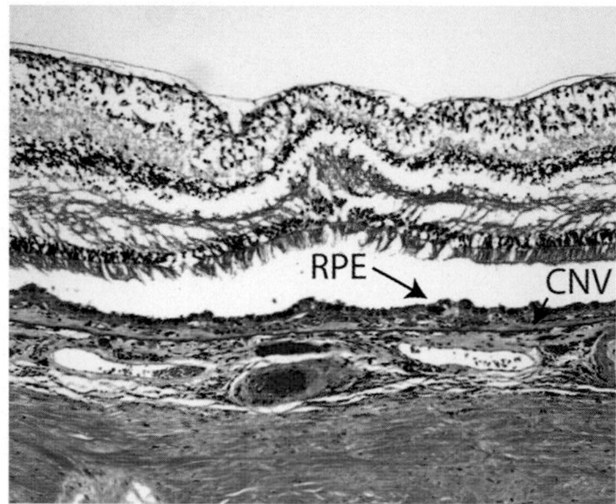

Type II or sub-retinal CNV

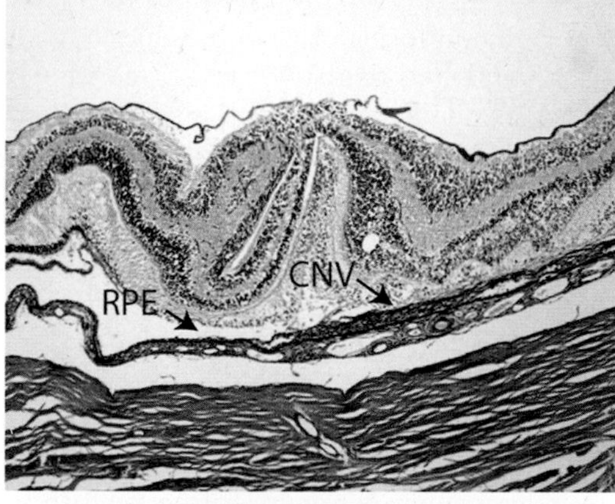

Mixed Type CNV

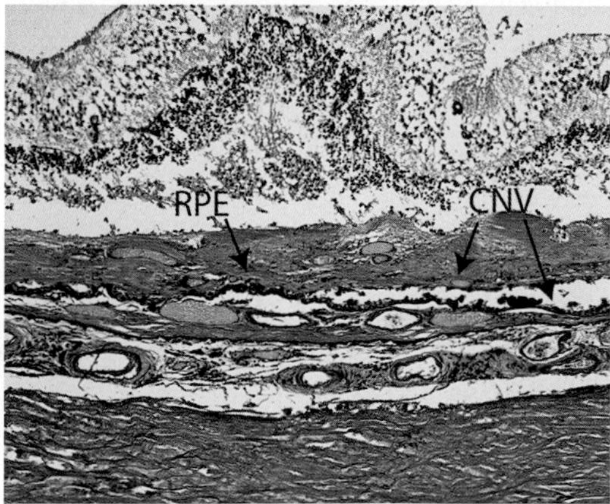

FIGURE 3.1. Histopathology of AMD-related CNV. Light micrographs of tissue sections from eyes with neovascular AMD demonstrated sub-RPE, subretinal, and mixed forms of CNV formation (hematoxylin and eosin). (Images courtesy of Dr. Hans Grossniklaus.)

OTHER PATHOGENIC MECHANISMS OF CNV

CNV may be caused by a wide-range of mechanical, cellular, physiologic, photochemical, and iatrogenic processes that disrupt the chorioretinal interface and lead to inflammation of the posterior segment. Each of these instigating factors, either individually or in concert with one another, is capable of setting off the intricate cascade of factors leading to CNV. While AMD is the most common etiology of CNV, below is a partial list of some of the other disorders that may also result in CNV formation:

Structural and Inflammatory Choroidal Diseases

There are several ophthalmologic disorders in which fractures develop within Bruch membrane such as angioid streaks and pathologic myopia, which allow for the ingrowth of choroidal vasculature, subsequent NV, and leakage into the subretinal space. Presumed ocular histoplasmosis syndrome (POHS) is hypothesized to result from choroidal seeding of *Histoplasma capsulatum*, a fungal organism endemic to the Ohio and Mississippi River Valleys. Infected choroidal tissue undergoes cycles of inflammation and quiescence leading to localized areas of CNV, which eventually scar over with RPE and glial cells.

Choroidopathies are a group of rare disorders that affect the tissues around the RPE due to either immune system dysregulation or infectious disease. Multifocal choroiditis (MFC), multiple evanescent white-dot syndrome (MEWDS), bird-shot choroidopathy, serpiginous choroidopathy, and diffuse unilateral subacute neuroretinitis (DUSN) have all been associated with CNV, which is hypothesized to be secondary to chronic inflammation or immune dysregulation.

Laser-Induced Injury of RPE and Bruch Membrane

The use of laser photocoagulation for targeted thermal injury in the treatment of extrafoveal CNV and proliferative diabetic retinopathy (DR) has been widely used with success for several decades. In the treatment of CNV, focal

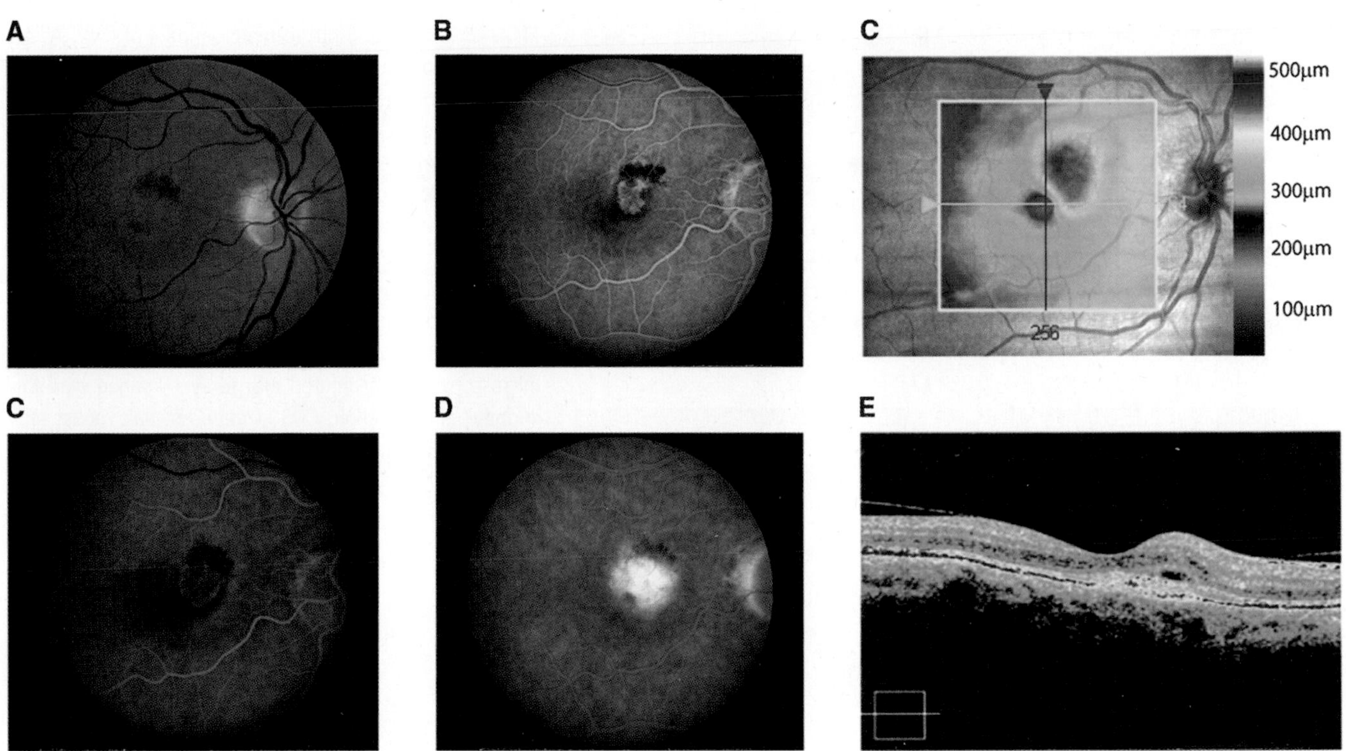

FIGURE 3.2. CNV formation in human eye with AMD. **A:** Color fundus photograph of patient with AMD and acute decrease in vision showed large CNV membrane with subretinal heme and fluid. **B:** Fluorescein angiogram of same eye at 18 seconds exhibited early lacey hyperfluorescence with large semicircular frond of predominantly classic CNV. **C:** Summed voxel projection image of retina on SD-OCT with significant retinal elevation in juxtafoveal area. **D:** An early fluorescein angiogram (21 seconds) from the same eye acquired 10 days later demonstrated the rapid growth of the CNV membrane. A late image revealed significant fluorescein leakage with pooling consistent with features of a predominantly classic CNV membrane. **E:** SD-OCT of the same eye confirmed the presence of subretinal fluid and disruption of the RPE. (Images courtesy of Drs John Kitchens and Scott Westhouse.)

laser injury is able to inhibit growth and decrease leakage from abnormal microvasculature. With panretinal photocoagulation, laser is used to ablate large swaths of the peripheral retina in DR that would otherwise be ischemic, producing proangiogenic factors. It is through the destruction of this pathologic tissue that NV is spared in the precious visual real estate in the macula. Laser-injured tissues will commonly remodel into small areas of RPE hyperpigmentation with fibrosis and only go on to develop CNV when high-energy laser photocoagulation ruptures Bruch membrane. It is critical to note that laser-induced injury, which fractures Bruch membrane, serves as a very well-described animal model of CNV, which is addressed in the following section.

Mechanical Trauma

Blunt trauma to the eye disorganizes the retinal architecture to varying degree. Choroidal rupture may induce neovascular invasion of the subretinal space via fractures in Bruch membrane. Over time, these lesions eventually involute but do leave behind a residual fibrotic scar that significantly decreases visual acuity in the area.

ANIMAL MODEL OF LASER-INJURY–INDUCED CNV

In order to study the natural history of CNV in vivo, several experimental models[11–13] have been developed to mimic the disease process that occurs in humans. However, it is the laser injury model of CNV that is the longest standing and most widely used experimental model of CNV and is accepted as a surrogate, accelerated model of neovascular AMD. Over 25 years ago, Stephen Ryan described the laser-induced injury model of CNV in rhesus monkeys.[14,15] The same technology has since been used to develop similar models in a variety of research animals, including the mouse and rat. In this model, high-energy laser photocoagulation is used to fracture Bruch membrane, which results in the formation of CNV (Fig. 3.3). The laser-induced model captures many of the important features of the human condition including migration of choroidal endothelial cells into the subretinal space via defects in Bruch membrane, accumulation of subretinal fluid, congregation of leukocytes adjacent to neovascular tufts, gliosis, leakage of fluorescein from immature

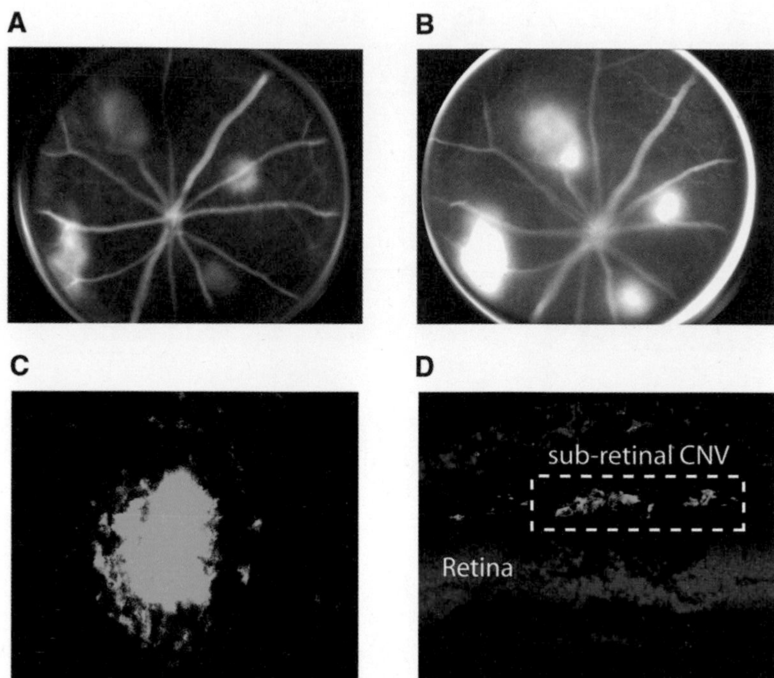

FIGURE 3.3. Laser-induced mouse model of CNV. **A:** An early time-point fundus fluorescein angiogram 7 days after laser-injury of the retina, RPE, and Bruch membrane showing hyperfluorescent areas. **B:** Later time-point fluorescein angiogram of the same mouse eye exhibiting significant fluorescein leakage similar to the human form of CNV. **C:** Choroidal flatmount of laser-induced CNV stained with fluorescent lectin to identify blood vessels showing a dense vascular lesion in choroid. Z-stacks of these entire lesions are acquired in order to measure the total CNV volume in preclinical therapeutic studies. **D:** Immunofluorescent microscopy of laser-injured mouse eyes stained with the endothelial cell marker, CD31 (*green*), reveals robust subretinal CNV. Nuclei are shown in blue.

new vessels into the subretinal space, and increased expression of angiogenic growth factors and their receptors in cells and ocular tissues. This model has provided a powerful system in which we can dissect the molecular mechanisms of CNV formation and test potential targeted therapeutics.

VEGF-A IS A CRITICAL MEDIATOR IN THE PATHOGENESIS IN NEOVASCULAR AMD

The growth factor hypothesized as the "Factor X" in angiogenesis some 60 years ago was isolated and characterized as vascular endothelial growth factor (VEGF) in 1989.[14–18] VEGF belongs to the highly conserved platelet-derived growth factor (PDGF) family along with several other related proteins that constitute the VEGF subfamily including placental growth factor (PlGF), VEGF-B, VEGF-C, and VEGF-D. For nomenclature purposes, the original VEGF protein was designated VEGF-A. Multiple isoforms of VEGF-A exist due to alternative splicing of the *Vegfa* gene; however, the 165 amino acid variant in humans (VEGF-A_{165}) is the most potent and prevalent among the major isoforms expressed during pathologic NV.[19] The potential roles for VEGF-A signaling in the pathophysiology of CNV have become the focus of numerous translational investigations. CNV membranes surgically excised from patients with AMD were strongly reactive with anti–VEGF-A antibody,[20,21] and pharmacological inhibition of VEGF-A decreased experimental laser-induced CNV in animal studies.[22,23] These data ushered in an era of rapid development of VEGF-A-targeted therapies for use in patients with neovascular AMD. Further details on VEGF biology and VEGF-targeted therapies will be addressed in subsequent chapters.

REGULATION OF ANGIOGENESIS DURING CNV BY THE EXTRACELLULAR MATRIX

The pathogenesis of CNV requires the invasion of pre-existing extracellular matrix (ECM) and the formation of new avenues of vasculature. During this process, specific enzymes are expressed, which degrade the basement membranes allowing for subsequent vascular in-growth. Surgically excised CNV tissue contained fibrin and fibronectin,[24] both of which are important in ECM-guided angiogenesis. Integrin receptors, which regulate cell signaling through interaction with various components of the ECM, are also important in CNV formation[25] and have been successfully targeted in animal models of CNV.[26,27] Several years ago, a link was discovered between proangiogenic factors found in CNV membranes and the upregulation of specific matrix-metalloproteinases (MMP-2 and MMP-9), which are capable of ECM breakdown.[28–30] Tissue inhibitors of MMPs (TIMPs), which prevent dissolution of ECM by MMPs, are also expressed in CNV membranes and have provided a novel therapeutic target.[31,32] Another proteinase mechanism known to be involved in CNV progression is the urokinase plasminogen activator pathway, which is also being evaluated as an alternative treatment modality.[33–35]

More novel ECM proteins are being discovered that may be involved in VEGF-A signaling and CNV pathogenesis (Fig. 3.4). The matricellular protein SPARC (secreted protein, acidic and rich in cysteine) is induced

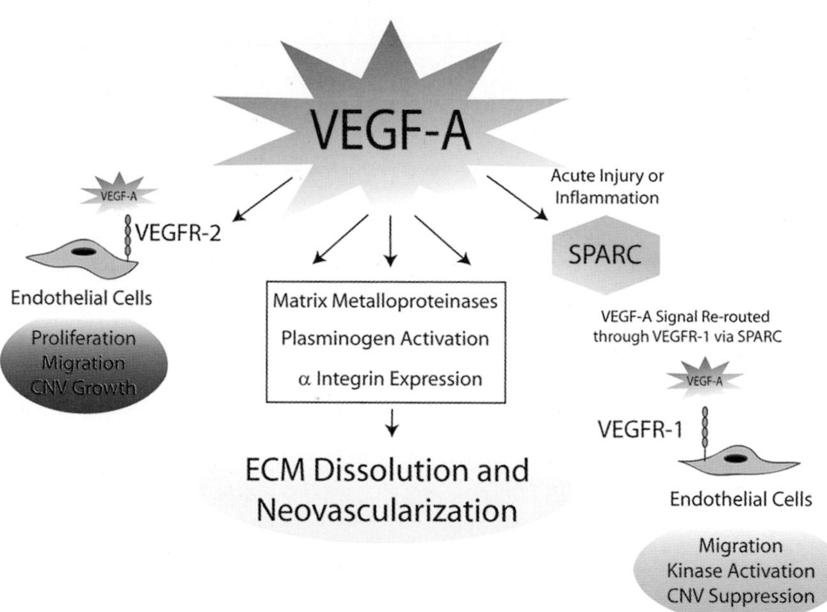

FIGURE 3.4. Modulation of the ECM with injury and VEGF-A upregulation. VEGF-A is a major factor in the pathogenesis of CNV through its direct effects on endothelial cell proliferation and modulation of the ECM. Integrins, plasminogen factors, and MMPs are all upregulated in response to VEGF-A, contributing to ECM degradation that promotes neovascular invasion. VEGF-A is also able to curb the endothelial cell responses through its interaction with SPARC, which reroutes signal transduction away the proangiogenic pathways of VEGFR-2 to the nonproliferative cellular pathways of VEGFR-1.

by VEGF-A and affects remodeling, cellular migration, and angiogenesis.[36,37] SPARC decreased the stimulatory activity of VEGF-A on endothelial cell proliferation,[38] but at this time, the exact mechanism of interaction between SPARC and VEGF-A is unknown. Further investigations showed that intravitreous VEGF-A paradoxically suppressed CNV when injected after laser injury, whereas mouse eyes treated with VEGF-A prior to laser injury exhibited the typical proangiogenic response and enhanced CNV.[39] This unexpected biphasic VEGF-A activity may be due to decreased SPARC levels during the acute phase of laser-induced injury. These data may dually help improve the scheduling and dosing of VEGF-A targeted therapeutics in order to restrict pharmacologic effects to the intended action of suppressing and reversing CNV. In addition, SPARC expression is restricted to the macula in primates, which may help explain the macular predilection of CNV in humans.[40]

MULTICELLULAR RESPONSES IN CHOROIDAL NEOVASCULARIZATION

Similar to epithelial wound healing, CNV is preceded by an orchestrated arrival of various inflammatory cell types. Pathogenic invasion or physical disruption of the blood-retina barrier initiates this multicellular response through the activation of resident cells and infiltration of circulating leukocytes. Detailed histologic analyses of postmortem eyes detected several inflammatory cells, especially macrophages, localized to areas of subretinal lesions associated with neovascular AMD.[41,42] The precise function of these cells has not been completely defined, but significant progress has been made in delineating the individual contributions of immune/inflammatory cell types and their signal transduction pathways to AMD using transgenic mouse models and the laser injury model of CNV.

Neutrophils

There are data suggesting that neutrophils may play a role in CNV progression.[43] With laser injury and breakdown of the blood-retina barrier, there is an acute increase in VEGF-A–driven expression of ICAM-1 on the retinal and choroidal endothelia, and an immediate and rampant neutrophil extravasation into the choroidal and retinal tissues, which is maximal at 24 hours.[44] Acute elevations in C5a, IL-1β, and TNF-α may upregulate IL-8, which acts as a potent neutrophil chemoattractant.[45,46] These cells serve as a potent proinflammatory stimulus by secreting more VEGF-A along with numerous proangiogenic cytokines into the wound. Without neutrophil participation in wound healing, there is only a partial abrogation of the CNV response in the laser injury model.

Macrophages

Subsequent to neutrophil invasion, the next major influx of circulating proinflammatory leukocytes is the macrophage, which is driven by the enhanced expression of monocyte chemoattractant protein-1 (MCP-1) that peaks at 2 days after injury.[47] These professional inflammatory cells home to sites of increased MCP-1 gradients via the expression of its cognate receptor, CCR2. This signaling axis is responsible for maximal macrophage infiltration into the choroid at 3 days postinjury.[48] Macrophages are able to respond to the proinflammatory milieu of vascular growth factors and secrete even more VEGF-A in order to aid revascularization and tissue repair. After the arrival of macrophages, endothelial cells continue to increase their mitotic activity with peak proliferation at 5 days postinjury

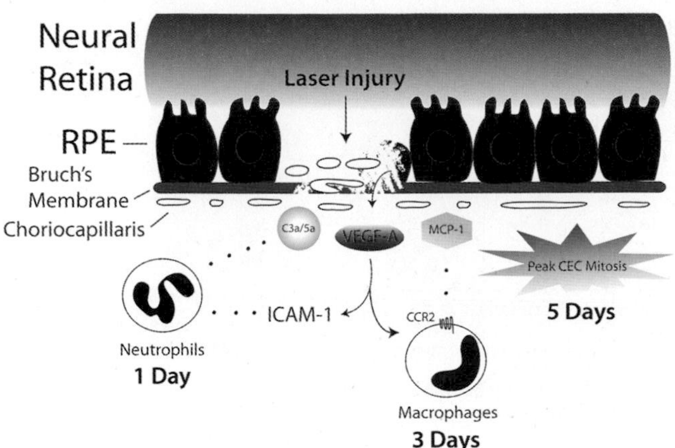

FIGURE 3.5. Critical mediators in CNV formation after acute and chronic injury. The initiating step of CNV is often an injury or disease process that induces local inflammation in the retina, RPE, and choroid. Locally produced leukocyte chemoattractants and provascular growth factors are secreted in the wound bed, resulting in peak neutrophil infiltration at 1 day, maximal macrophage influx at 3 days, and a spike in choroidal endothelial cell proliferation at 5 days.

(Fig. 3.5). Approximately 1 week after injury, organized CNV membranes are formed, which can be visualized in vivo with fluorescein angiography. Without macrophage influx, the ability of laser-injured areas to fully develop CNV is completely eliminated.

Several laboratories have independently demonstrated the critical involvement of macrophages in the proangiogenic response after laser injury.[48–50] While most of these studies suggest that the macrophage is the dominant proangiogenic cell type in CNV pathogenesis, there are other models, which suggest that macrophages may serve a beneficial role in the early stages of AMD[51] and in some CNV models.[52] Recently, an animal model for AMD was characterized in mice deficient in either MCP-1 or CCR2 wherein over the course of a year, these transgenic mice developed the major clinical findings found in AMD in humans including drusen formation beneath the RPE, photoreceptor atrophy, and CNV.[51] Similar findings in mice deficient in either MCP-1 or CCR2 have now been reported by other investigators.[53–55] Furthermore, the ocular phenotypes of mouse strains deficient in an alternate macrophage chemotaxis receptor, CX3CR, or both CX3CR1 and CCR2 were consistent with AMD-like features.[56,57] In combination, these studies conclude that severe derangements in the recruitment and in situ function of macrophage progenitors may be contributory to AMD progression and CNV pathogenesis.

Microglia

Microglia are tissue macrophages dispersed throughout the normal retina, choroid, and central nervous system. Their primary functions are to respond to the local invasion of pathogens through activation of the innate immune system, promotion of inflammation, and phagocytosis of bacteria and virus-laden cells. Microglia express a unique set of surface markers, as well as the chemokine receptor CX3CR1, which binds to fractalkine (or CX3CL1), a cytokine that is secreted preferentially by inflamed retinal and endothelial cells. CX3CR1 is present on a number of differentiated cell types derived from myeloid progenitor cells such as dendritic cells, infiltrating macrophages, neutrophils, and some endothelial cells, thus providing another signaling axis for the infiltration of professional inflammatory cells after laser injury. As previously mentioned, CX3CR1-deficient mice develop many of the cardinal features of AMD, further supporting the paramount contribution of macrophages and microglia to choroidal and retinal health.

Microglia also serve as an important component of the immune system and express a series of innate immune receptors, called toll-like receptors (TLRs), that recognize pathogen-associated molecular patterns. TLR activation initiates rapid immune responses by alarming other immune system components, mediating cellular infiltration, and selectively inducing apoptosis to prevent infectious spread. Several TLRs, including TLR 2–9, all of which are expressed on microglia,[58] are likely to be involved in modulating angiogenesis in the setting of injury, thus creating a significant link between the innate immune response and NV. This immunovascular phenomenon is an area of great interest at this time, given the strong evidence that several neovascular-related diseases, including AMD, may be driven by immune system activation.

VEGF-A, once thought to be a pure vascular mediator, has been discovered to impart significant cellular effects on neural cells including microglia. Similar to blood-derived macrophages, microglia express VEGF receptor-1 (VEGFR-1), enabling their migration toward areas of VEGF-A production.[59] With injury, microglia switch from their quiescent state to become activated, demonstrated by increased cytokine secretion, immune receptor expression, and proliferation, thereby promoting CNV growth.

Progenitor/Stem Cells

Stem/progenitor cells are also recruited to sites of CNV and incorporate into pathologic vasculature. Animal studies have now demonstrated that interfering with stem/progenitor cell homing to the sites of CNV through the modulation of the cytokine stromal-derived factor-1 and its receptor, CXCR4, inhibits neovascular growth,[60,61] a finding that offers another potential treatment for the human condition.

Other Infiltrating Cell Types

Although mast cells and eosinophils are able to generate significant proinflammatory stimuli, their contribution to CNV is negligible. Moreover, B lymphocytes and T lymphocytes as well as natural killer cells are also able to infiltrate retina injuries, yet their particular effects and contribution to NV are still unclear but also thought to be minimal at most.[44]

OTHER PROANGIOGENIC FACTORS INVOLVED IN CNV

Several other molecular factors have been implicated in the development of CNV through descriptive expression analyses in human specimens including transforming growth factor-beta 1 (TGF-β1), PDGF, fibroblast growth factor-2 (FGF-2), insulin-like growth factor-1 (IGF-1), and estrogen.[3] Hepatocyte growth factor (HGF) is produced by RPE, upregulated as early as 6 hours after laser injury, and hypothesized to mediate RPE proliferation during tissue repair.[62,63] Endogenous antiangiogenic molecules have also been identified such as pigment epithelium-derived factor (PEDF) and thrombospondin-1 that are decreased in CNV lesions[64,65] and are capable of regulating retinal and CNV in animal studies.[66,67] More recently, the chemokine receptor 3 (CCR3), which was previously believed to be solely involved in eosinophil and mast cell trafficking in allergic disease, was discovered to be specifically expressed on pathological choroidal endothelial cells in CNV membranes in human eyes with neovascular AMD.[68] CCR3 inhibition in the mouse model of laser-injury resulted in significantly greater CNV suppression than with anti–VEGF-A blockade, suggesting that this receptor may be a potential target for future pharmacologic development. Fortunately, this is one of many candidate pathways currently under active investigation, as a multitude of molecular mechanisms have been identified in the increasingly complex system of vascular regulation.

NEOVASCULAR PROGRESSION VIA COMPLEMENT ACTIVATION

Many of the currently identified drusen components are inflammatory mediators and may directly upregulate cytokines that are required for CNV. Over a decade of scientific research has supported the importance of complement activation in the pathogenesis of neovascular AMD.[69] The complement pathways are comprised of multiple complex domino-like cascades engineered to generate massive proinflammatory induction via cytokine expression and leukocyte invasion in addition to promoting the self-assembly of molecular components that are capable of cellular destruction. The two main active by-products of complement activation, C3a and C5a, are predominantly responsible for the anaphylactic response. Recent data have directly linked C3a and C5a, known components of AMD drusen, to the upregulation of VEGF-A.[70] RPE cell cultures treated with C3a or C5a secreted significantly more VEGF-A, whereas choroidal endothelial cells did not. In animal studies, VEGF-A concentrations in the RPE and choroid peaked just 4 hours after intravitreous C3a/C5a administration. This well-localized and rapid response suggests that the RPE, and perhaps other resident cells, plays a major role in VEGF-A production after complement activation. Functional blockade of complement activation may be a valuable preventative therapy to arrest CNV progression and is currently being evaluated in clinical trials. Rapid complement activation may also help explain the abrupt switch like progression to neovascular AMD in patients with previously dry fundus exams.

KEY POINTS

- The choroid is a highly vascularized pigmented tissue layer engineered to provide efficient nutrient and metabolic exchange for the RPE and outer two thirds of the retina.
- In the setting of choroidal inflammation or injury, cellular components of the RPE and choroid activate in order to contain the wound, destroy any invading pathogens, and initiate the repair process.
- The most common forms of CNV are due to a combination of inflammation, oxidative stress, and photochemical damage secondary to AMD.
- *VEGF-A is a critical mediator in the pathogenesis of neovascular ARMD.*
- The pathogenesis of CNV requires the invasion of preexisting ECM and cell migration, which is facilitated through expression of MMPs and urokinase (uPA).
- The matricellular protein SPARC (secreted protein, acidic and rich in cysteine) is induced by VEGF-A and affects remodeling, cellular migration, and angiogenesis.
- CNV is preceded by an orchestrated arrival of various inflammatory cell types: neutrophils, macrophages, microglia, and progenitor/stem cells.
- Several other molecules have been implicated in the development of CNV: transforming growth factor-beta 1 (TGF-β1), PDGF, fibroblast growth factor-2 (FGF-2), insulin-like growth factor-1 (IGF-1), and estrogen.
- More recently, the chemokine receptor 3 (CCR3), which was previously believed to be solely involved in eosinophil and mast cells, has been discovered to be specifically expressed on pathological choroidal endothelial cells in CNV membranes in human eyes with neovascular AMD.
- CCR3 inhibition in the mouse model of laser-injury resulted in significantly greater CNV suppression than with anti–VEGF-A blockade, suggesting that this receptor may be a potential target for future pharmacologic development.
- Complement activation (C3a and C5a) plays an important role in the pathogenesis of neovascular AMD.

CONCLUSION

As further molecular research is conducted on the pathogenesis of CNV, more mechanisms will be revealed, thus providing additional therapeutic targets for this debilitating disease. Already, we are within reach of a detailed map of critical proteins and cells that mediate the formation and growth of CNV, a feat that has taken over 20 years of dedicated science. The wide use of VEGF-A–specific therapies and their proven efficacy demonstrate the incredible power of this modernized approach to pharmacologic design and solidify the utility of the current animal models designed to mimic the human form of neovascular AMD. With these novel molecular tools and predictive models, future scientific investigations into this disease process will continue to yield invaluable insight with the hope of offering clinicians the information necessary to improve the outcomes of their patients.

REFERENCES

1. Friedman DS, O'colmain BJ, Munoz B, et al. Prevalence of age-related macular degeneration in the United States. *Arch Ophthalmol*. 2004;122(4):564–572.
2. Smith W, Assink J, Klein R, et al. Risk factors for age-related macular degeneration: Pooled findings from three continents. *Ophthalmology*. 2001;108(4):697–704.
3. Ambati J, Ambati BK, Yoo SH, et al. Age-related macular degeneration: etiology, pathogenesis, and therapeutic strategies. *Surv Ophthalmol*. 2003;48(3):257–293.
4. RPB. *Research to Prevent Blindness, Incidence of Exudative AMD in the United States*. 2004 [cited August 20, 2006]; Available from: www.rpb.org
5. ACS. *2006 American Cancer Society Statistics*. 2006 [cited August 20, 2006]; Available from: http://www.cancer.org/
6. Hageman GS, Luthert PJ, Victor Chong NH, et al. An integrated hypothesis that considers drusen as biomarkers of immune-mediated processes at the RPE-Bruch's membrane interface in aging and age-related macular degeneration. *Prog Retin Eye Res*. 2001;20(6):705–732.
7. Zhou J, Jang YP, Kim SR, et al. Complement activation by photooxidation products of A2E, a lipofuscin constituent of the retinal pigment epithelium. *Proc Natl Acad Sci U S A*. 2006;103(44):16182–16187.
8. Gass JD. *Stereoscopic Atlas of Macular Diseases*, 4th ed. St. Louis: C.V. Mosby, 1997.
9. Yannuzzi LA, Negrao S, Iida T, et al. Retinal angiomatous proliferation in age-related macular degeneration. *Retina*. 2001;21(5):416–434.
10. Yannuzzi LA, Wong DW, Sforzolini BS, et al. Polypoidal choroidal vasculopathy and neovascularized age-related macular degeneration. *Arch Ophthalmol*. 1999;117(11):1503–1510.
11. Elizabeth Rakoczy P, Yu MJ, Nusinowitz S, et al. Mouse models of age-related macular degeneration. *Exp Eye Res*. 2006;82(5):741–752.
12. Edwards AO, Malek G. Molecular genetics of AMD and current animal models. *Angiogenesis*. 2007;10(2):119–132.
13. Marmorstein AD, Marmorstein LY. The challenge of modeling macular degeneration in mice. *Trends Genet*. 2007;23(5):225–231.
14. Ryan SJ. Subretinal neovascularization after argon laser photocoagulation. *Albrecht Von Graefes Arch Klin Exp Ophthalmol*. 1980;215(1):29–42.
15. Ryan SJ. Subretinal neovascularization. Natural history of an experimental model. *Arch Ophthalmol*. 1982;100(11):1804–1809.
16. Folkman J, Merler E, Abernathy C, et al. Isolation of a tumor factor responsible for angiogenesis. *J Exp Med*. 1971;133(2):275–288.
17. Ferrara N, Henzel WJ. Pituitary follicular cells secrete a novel heparin-binding growth factor specific for vascular endothelial cells. *Biochem Biophys Res Commun*. 1989;161(2): 851–858.
18. Gospodarowicz D, Abraham JA, Schilling J. Isolation and characterization of a vascular endothelial cell mitogen produced by pituitary-derived folliculo stellate cells. *Proc Natl Acad Sci U S A*. 1989;86(19):7311–7315.
19. Usui T, Ishida S, Yamashiro K, et al. VEGF164(165) as the pathological isoform: differential leukocyte and endothelial responses through VEGFR1 and VEGFR2. *Invest Ophthalmol Vis Sci*. 2004;45(2):368–374.
20. Lopez PF, Sippy BD, Lambert HM, et al. Transdifferentiated retinal pigment epithelial cells are immunoreactive for vascular endothelial growth factor in surgically excised age-related macular degeneration-related choroidal neovascular membranes. *Invest Ophthalmol Vis Sci*. 1996;37(5):855–868.
21. Kvanta A, Algvere PV, Berglin L, et al. Subfoveal fibrovascular membranes in age-related macular degeneration express vascular endothelial growth factor. *Invest Ophthalmol Vis Sci*. 1996;37(9):1929–1934.
22. Saishin Y, Takahashi K, Silva RL, et al. VEGF-TRAPR1R2 suppresses choroidal neovascularization and VEGF-induced breakdown of the blood-retinal barrier. *J Cell Physiol*. 2003;195(2):241–248.
23. Krzystolik MG, Afshari MA, Adamis AP, et al. Prevention of experimental choroidal neovascularization with intravitreal anti-vascular endothelial growth factor antibody fragment. *Arch Ophthalmol*. 2002;120(3):338–346.
24. Grossniklaus HE, Martinez JA, Brown VB, et al. Immunohistochemical and histochemical properties of surgically excised subretinal neovascular membranes in age-related macular degeneration. *Am J Ophthalmol*. 1992;114(4):464–472.
25. Friedlander M, Theesfeld CL, Sugita M, et al. Involvement of integrins alpha v beta 3 and alpha v beta 5 in ocular neovascular diseases. *Proc Natl Acad Sci U S A*. 1996;93(18):9764–9769.
26. Kamizuru H, Kimura H, Yasukawa T, et al. Monoclonal antibody-mediated drug targeting to choroidal neovascularization in the rat. *Invest Ophthalmol Vis Sci*. 2001;42(11): 2664–2672.
27. Fu Y, Ponce ML, Thill M, et al. Angiogenesis inhibition and choroidal neovascularization suppression by sustained delivery of an integrin antagonist, EMD478761. *Invest Ophthalmol Vis Sci*. 2007;48(11):5184–5190.
28. Steen B, Sejersen S, Berglin L, et al. Matrix metalloproteinases and metalloproteinase inhibitors in choroidal neovascular membranes. *Invest Ophthalmol Vis Sci*. 1998;39(11): 2194–2200.

29. Hoffmann S, He S, Ehren M, et al. MMP-2 and MMP-9 secretion by rpe is stimulated by angiogenic molecules found in choroidal neovascular membranes. *Retina*. 2006;26(4):454–461.
30. Das A, Fanslow W, Cerretti D, et al. Angiopoietin/Tek interactions regulate mmp-9 expression and retinal neovascularization. *Lab Invest*. 2003;83(11):1637–1645.
31. Das A, Mclamore A, Song W, et al. Retinal neovascularization is suppressed with a matrix metalloproteinase inhibitor. *Arch Ophthalmol*. 1999;117(4):498–503.
32. Della NG, Campochiaro PA, Zack DJ. Localization of TIMP-3 mRNA expression to the retinal pigment epithelium. *Invest Ophthalmol Vis Sci*. 1996;37(9):1921–1924.
33. Rakic JM, Lambert V, Munaut C, et al. Mice without uPA, tPA, or plasminogen genes are resistant to experimental choroidal neovascularization. *Invest Ophthalmol Vis Sci*. 2003;44(4):1732–1739.
34. Das A, McGuire P. Role of urokinase inhibitors in choroidal neovascularization. *Semin Ophthalmol*. 2006;21(1):23–27.
35. Lambert V, Munaut C, Carmeliet P, et al. Dose-dependent modulation of choroidal neovascularization by plasminogen activator inhibitor type I: Implications for clinical trials. *Invest Ophthalmol Vis Sci*. 2003;44(6):2791–2797.
36. Kato Y, Lewalle JM, Baba Y, et al. Induction of SPARC by VEGF in human vascular endothelial cells. *Biochem Biophys Res Commun*. 2001;287(2):422–426.
37. Hasselaar P, Sage EH. SPARC antagonizes the effect of basic fibroblast growth factor on the migration of bovine aortic endothelial cells. *J Cell Biochem*. 1992;49(3):272–283.
38. Kupprion C, Motamed K, Sage EH. SPARC (BM-40, osteonectin) inhibits the mitogenic effect of vascular endothelial growth factor on microvascular endothelial cells. *J Biol Chem*. 1998;273(45):29635–29640.
39. Nozaki M, Sakurai E, Raisler BJ, et al. Loss of SPARC-mediated VEGFR-1 suppression after injury reveals a novel antiangiogenic activity of VEGF-A. *J Clin Invest*. 2006;116(2):422–429.
40. Rodriguez IR, Moreira EF, Bok D, et al. Osteonectin/SPARC secreted by RPE and localized to the outer plexiform layer of the monkey retina. *Invest Ophthalmol Vis Sci*. 2000;41(9):2438–2444.
41. Grossniklaus HE, Miskala PH, Green WR, et al. Histopathologic and ultrastructural features of surgically excised subfoveal choroidal neovascular lesions: submacular surgery trials report no. 7. *Arch Ophthalmol*. 2005;123(7):914–921.
42. Grossniklaus HE, Cingle KA, Yoon YD, et al. Correlation of histologic 2-dimensional reconstruction and confocal scanning laser microscopic imaging of choroidal neovascularization in eyes with age-related maculopathy. *Arch Ophthalmol*. 2000;118(5):625–629.
43. Zhou J, Pham L, Zhang N, et al. Neutrophils promote experimental choroidal neovascularization. *Mol Vis*. 2005;11: 414–424.
44. Tsutsumi-Miyahara C, Sonoda KH, Egashira K, et al. The relative contributions of each subset of ocular infiltrated cells in experimental choroidal neovascularisation. *Br J Ophthalmol*. 2004;88(9):1217–1222.
45. Engelhardt E, Toksoy A, Goebeler M, et al. Chemokines IL-8, GROalpha, MCP-1, IP-10, and Mig are sequentially and differentially expressed during phase-specific infiltration of leukocyte subsets in human wound healing. *Am J Pathol*. 1998;153(6):1849–1860.
46. Crane IJ, Wallace CA, Mckillop-Smith S, et al. Control of chemokine production at the blood-retina barrier. *Immunology*. 2000;101(3):426–433.
47. Yamada K, Sakurai E, Itaya M, et al. Inhibition of laser-induced choroidal neovascularization by atorvastatin by downregulation of monocyte chemotactic protein-1 synthesis in mice. *Invest Ophthalmol Vis Sci*. 2007;48(4):1839–1843.
48. Sakurai E, Anand A, Ambati BK, et al. Macrophage depletion inhibits experimental choroidal neovascularization. *Invest Ophthalmol Vis Sci*. 2003;44(8):3578–3585.
49. Caicedo A, Espinosa-Heidmann DG, Pina Y, et al. Blood-derived macrophages infiltrate the retina and activate Muller glial cells under experimental choroidal neovascularization. *Exp Eye Res*. 2005;81(1):38–47.
50. Tsutsumi C, Sonoda KH, Egashira K, et al. The critical role of ocular-infiltrating macrophages in the development of choroidal neovascularization. *J Leukoc Biol*. 2003;74(1): 25–32.
51. Ambati J, Anand A, Fernandez S, et al. An animal model of age-related macular degeneration in senescent Ccl-2- or Ccr-2-deficient mice. *Nat Med*. 2003;9(11):1390–1397.
52. Apte RS, Richter J, Herndon J, et al. Macrophages inhibit neovascularization in a murine model of age-related macular degeneration. *PLoS Med*. 2006;3(8):e310.
53. Chowers I, Deleon E, Obolensky A, et al. *Iron-Associated Oxidative Injury as a Novel Therapeutic Target in Age Related Macular Degeneration. Toward the Prevention of Age Related Macular Degeneration*. In: *ARVO 2006 Summer Eye Research Conference (SERC)*. Fort Myers, Florida, 2006.
54. Shen D, Wen R, Tuo J, et al. Exacerbation of retinal degeneration and choroidal neovascularization induced by subretinal injection of matrigel in CCL2/MCP-1-deficient mice. *Ophthal Res*. 2006;38(2):71–73.
55. Chan CC. *Findings Similar to AMD in CCl2 Knockout Mice*. Personal Communication to Ambati J, 2006.
56. Combadiere C, Feumi C, Raoul W, et al. CX3CR1-dependent subretinal microglia cell accumulation is associated with cardinal features of age-related macular degeneration. *J Clin Invest*. 2007;117(10):2920–2928.
57. Tuo J, Bojanowski CM, Zhou M, et al. Murine ccl2/cx3cr1 deficiency results in retinal lesions mimicking human age-related macular degeneration. *Invest Ophthalmol Vis Sci*. 2007;48(8):3827–3836.
58. Jack CS, Arbour N, Manusow J, et al. TLR signaling tailors innate immune responses in human microglia and astrocytes. *J Immunol*. 2005;175(7):4320–4330.
59. Forstreuter F, Lucius R, Mentlein R. Vascular endothelial growth factor induces chemotaxis and proliferation of microglial cells. *J Neuroimmunol*. 2002;132(1–2):93–98.
60. Sengupta N, Caballero S, Mames RN, et al. Preventing stem cell incorporation into choroidal neovascularization by targeting homing and attachment factors. *Invest Ophthalmol Vis Sci*. 2005;46(1):343–348.
61. Lima e Silva R, Shen J, Hackett SF, et al. The SDF-1/CXCR4 ligand/receptor pair is an important contributor to several types of ocular neovascularization. *FASEB J*. 2007;21(12):3219–3230.
62. He PM, He S, Garner JA, et al. Retinal pigment epithelial cells secrete and respond to hepatocyte growth factor. *Biochem Biophys Res Commun*. 1998;249(1):253–257.

63. Hu W, Criswell MH, Fong SL, et al. Differences in the temporal expression of regulatory growth factors during choroidal neovascular development. *Exp Eye Res*. 2009;88(1):79–91.
64. Uno K, Bhutto IA, Mcleod DS, et al. Impaired expression of thrombospondin-1 in eyes with age related macular degeneration. *Br J Ophthalmol*. 2006;90(1):48–54.
65. Bhutto IA, Mcleod DS, Hasegawa T, et al. Pigment epithelium-derived factor (PEDF) and vascular endothelial growth factor (VEGF) in aged human choroid and eyes with age-related macular degeneration. *Exp Eye Res*. 2006;82(1):99–110.
66. Mori K, Duh E, Gehlbach P, et al. Pigment epithelium-derived factor inhibits retinal and choroidal neovascularization. *J Cell Physiol*. 2001;188(2):253–263.
67. Zamiri P, Masli S, Kitaichi N, et al. Thrombospondin plays a vital role in the immune privilege of the eye. *Invest Ophthalmol Vis Sci*. 2005;46(3):908–919.
68. Takeda A, Baffi JZ, Kleinman ME, et al. CCR3 is a target for age-related macular degeneration diagnosis and therapy. *Nature*. 2009;460(7252):225–230.
69. Gehrs KM, Anderson DH, Johnson LV, et al. Age-related macular degeneration—emerging pathogenetic and therapeutic concepts. *Ann Med*. 2006;38(7):450–471.
70. Nozaki M, Raisler BJ, Sakurai E, et al. Drusen complement components C3a and C5a promote choroidal neovascularization. *Proc Natl Acad Sci U S A*. 2006;103(7):2328–2333.

SECTION I

Principles

PART B

Molecular Mechanisms

CHAPTER

4

VEGF: The Major Player

Patricia A. D'Amore

INTRODUCTION

As early as 1948, Michaelson posited the existence of a diffusible factor, which he termed "factor x," released by nonperfused (and therefore hypoxic) retina that could cause angiogenesis.[3] Early efforts to identify this agent led to the isolation and purification of acidic and basic fibroblast growth factors,[5,6] but the fibroblast growth factors' lack of a conventional signal sequence and their high level of constitutive expression in the adult retina made these growth factors less likely to be the elusive retinal angiogenic factor. However, in 1992, there were two reports of an angiogenic factor, called vascular endothelial growth factor (VEGF), that not only mediated tumor neovascularization but could be regulated by hypoxia.[7,8] The unusual feature (at this point in time) of hypoxic regulation of this growth factor was a characteristic that was perfectly suited for the long sought-after "factor x" as it was hypothesized to be produced by retinal tissue made ischemic during the progression of diabetic retinopathy. A body of work published over the next 15 years, and reviewed below, proved this to be the case and has earned VEGF the place it holds today—as the major player.

VEGF BIOLOGY

VEGF is a member of a family of cysteine knot growth factors that includes VEGF-A, VEGF-B, placental growth factor (PlGF), VEGF-C, VEGF-D, viral VEGF (also known as VEGF-E), and snake venom VEGF (also known as VEGF-F) and binds the receptor tyrosine kinases, VEGFR-1, VEGFR-2, and VEGFR-3. VEGF-A, also known as vascular permeability factor[9] (hereafter referred to simply as VEGF), is well known as an endothelial cell (EC) hemoattractant, mitogen, and as a potent angiogenic fac- (for review see Ref. 10). VEGF is encoded by a single hat gives rise to multiple isoforms depending on the three in the mouse[11] and up to nine in humans,[12] a splice variant that reportedly functions as an VEGF inhibitor.[13] VEGF binds VEGFR1 with igher affinity than VEGFR2.[14,15] VEGF165, VEGF206, but not VEGF121, which lacks exons 6 and 8, also bind to heparan sulfate as well as neuropilin-1[16] and neuropilin-2,[17] receptors that lack tyrosine kinase activity. Significant progress has been made in understanding the downstream pathways that mediate many of VEGF biological effects. The reader is referred to a recent review for further reading in this area.[18]

VEGF Isoforms

Murine VEGF-A encodes three biochemically distinct protein isoforms generated through alternative splicing of a single gene.[19,20] These different gene products exhibit tissue-specific expression during embryogenesis[21] and in the adult organism.[22–24] For instance, early murine lung development is characterized primarily by the expression of VEGF120 and VEGF164; at E18 around the time of lung alveolarization and vascularization, there is a dramatic increase in VEGF188 that persists through out adulthood.[21] In contrast, brain development is associated with relatively constant levels of VEGF120 and VEGF164, which are also the predominant isoforms seen in the adult.[21]

The biochemical investigations of VEGF isoforms have focused on the distinct heparan sulfate–binding properties of the different proteins, which are encoded by exons 6 and 7. The affinity of each VEGF isoform for heparan sulfate correlates with that isoform's level of interaction with cell surface and extracellular matrix molecules upon secretion from the cell.[24] VEGF120 does not bind heparan sulfate and is therefore freely soluble. VEGF164 binds heparan sulfate with moderate affinity, and protein released from cells is found bound to the matrix and soluble in the media. VEGF188 has a strong affinity for heparan sulfate and is nearly completely sequestered to the cell surface and extracellular matrix after its secretion.[25] These binding characteristics influence their availability in vivo and thus their relative contributions to various processes in different tissues.

Studies of the mitogenic effects of the VEGF isoforms indicate that they differ in their biological potency with VEGF165 100-fold more mitogenic than VEGF121.[26] Identification of a receptor, termed neuropilin, that binds VEGF164 (and VEGF188) but not VEGF121,[27] further supports the hypothesis that the various VEGF isoforms are not functionally equivalent. Functional evidence to support distinct roles for the isoforms comes from mice that have been genetically engineered to express single VEGF isoform where the relative contributions of the isoforms during development are revealed. Mice that express only VEGF120 live to term but die either at birth or within 2 weeks of birth (at the latest) as a result of a variety of vascular defects, including defective pulmonary development and the absence of postnatal cardiac angiogenesis.[28] Mice that express only VEGF188 are viable but are born at a reduced ratio and display a number of defects including abnormal vascular remodeling in the retina.[29]

Distinct roles for VEGF isoforms postnatally have also been suggested. Studies using the murine oxygen-induced retinopathy (OIR) model suggest that the expression of VEGF164 is increased to a greater extent during the ischemia-induced neovascularization than during normal vascularization.[30] Furthermore, this study also reported leukocyte involvement in vessels associated with pathologic, but not normal, angiogenesis. Interestingly, inhibition of the heparan sulfate–binding isoforms (VEGF164 and VEGF188) using an aptamer blocked the abnormal vessels without influencing the developmental vascularization of the retina. The targeted inactivation of monocyte lineage cells with clodronate-liposomes led to the suppression of pathological neovascularization, whereas blockade of T-lymphocyte–mediated immune responses with an anti-CD2 antibody exacerbated pathological neovascularization. These data highlight important molecular and cellular differences between physiological and pathological retinal neovascularization and suggest that during pathological neovascularization, VEGF164 selectively induces inflammation and cellular immunity. They further imply that new therapeutic approaches for selectively targeting pathological, but not physiological, retinal neovascularization are possible.

ROLES OF VEGF

VEGF in Development

A role for VEGF in the development of the vascular system is clearly indicated by the fact that mice with targeted disruption of the VEGF gene die at midgestation due to abnormalities in vascular development, including impaired formation of blood island in the yolk sac (i.e., early vasculogenesis) and the virtual absence of the aorta.[31,32] In fact, mice with just a single targeted allele (VEGF–/+) die around the same time and display similar defects, pointing to a critical dose-dependence for the actions of VEGF. Not surprisingly, VEGF has been shown to be involved in the vascularization of virtually every organ examined to date. Disruption of VEGF expression and/or signaling has been shown to interfere with vascularization of lung,[33,34] kidney,[35] skeletal muscle,[36] and bone.[37,38]

The fact that the rodent retina is entirely vascularized postnatally has allowed the examination of the role and regulation of VEGF in that process. In situ hybridization revealed the expression of VEGF by astrocytes as they migrate in from the optic disc across the developing ganglion cell layer[39]; this was followed closely by the formation of the superficial retinal vessels (Fig. 4.1). Vessel ingrowth into the inner nuclear layer was shown to be associated with VEGF expression by Müller cells. In vitro studies demonstrating hypoxic induction of VEGF in glial cells led to the hypothesis that retinal vascularization was controlled by a "physiologic" hypoxia that developed as the retina differentiated and thickened so that the inner retina could no longer be nourished by the choroidal circulation.[40] Support for a role for hypoxia in retinal normal retinal vascularization came from studies using the feline and rodent models of the retinopathy of prematurity (ROP). In this model, newborn mouse or rat pups (postnatal day 7) are placed into hyperoxia for 5 days and then returned to room air at which time new vessels grow out of the superficial retina into the vitreous.[41] Analysis of VEGF revealed reduced expression in mice exposed to hyperoxia but increased on return to room air.[42] Thus, the vaso-obliterative phase of ROP due to the suppression of VEGF expression by neuroglial cells followed by vessel regression was shown to occur via apoptosis, pointing to a role for VEGF as a survival factor in vivo.[43] During the proliferative phase of ROP, VEGF levels were increased beyond what were seen in the normal controls. Examination of hypoxia inducible factor-1 (HIF-1) by immunohistochemistry or in situ hybridization during normal retinal vascularization as well as in the ROP

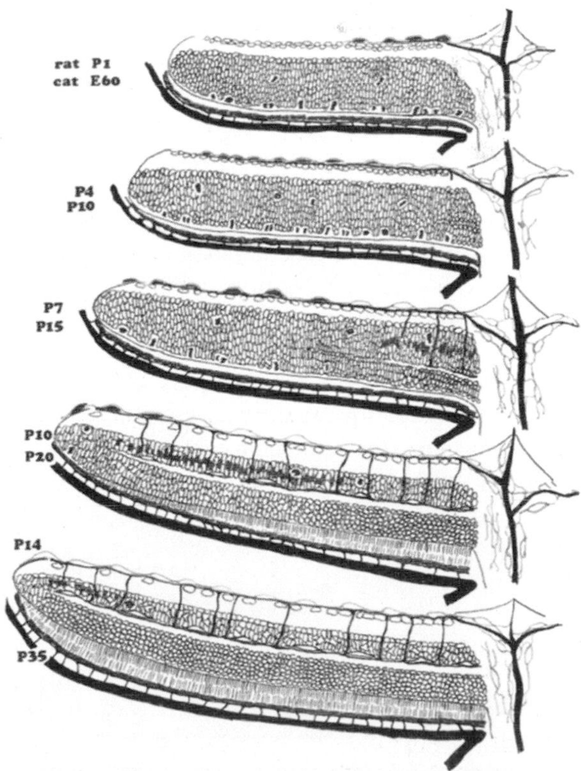

FIGURE 4.1. Summary diagram of VEGF expression in the developing retina. (Reprinted from Stone et al. *J Neurosci.* 1995;15:4738–4747, with permission.)

BOX 4.1 Role of VEGF in the Adult Retina

The use of immunohistochemistry and mice with a LacZ reporter introduced into the VEGFR2 locus has revealed the expression of VEGFR2 in specific cells throughout the retina.[2] VEGFR2 is expressed by the retinal microvascular EC and by astrocytes in the ganglion cell layer, on Müller cells and on photoreceptors. On the other hand, use of mice with a LacZ reporter in the VEGF locus shows VEGF to be produced by scattered cells in the ganglion cell layer and by Müller and amacrine cells. The proximity between the VEGF-producing Müller cells and VEGFR2-expressing photoreceptors is indicative of a paracrine interaction. A possible role for VEGF in the adult retina was addressed by systemically expressing a VEGF-neutralizing soluble Flt-1 via adenoviral delivery. Interestingly, the inner retinal vessels appeared unaltered at the light and ultrastructural level as well as in terms of barrier functions.[2] In contrast, there was significant thinning of the inner and outer nuclear layers that was associated with significant apoptosis and with reduced visual acuity. Defects in the RPE layer were also evident in the form of vacuolization, separation form the photoreceptor layers, and breakdown of intercellular junctions. These findings provide strong support for a role for VEGF as a neuroprotectant for photoreceptors and suggest that long-term intravitreal should be conducted with caution.

model revealed an increase in HIF-1 alpha at P4, which was sustained during retinal vascularization and then decreased in the adult.[44] In the ROP model, HIF-1 alpha peaked at 2 hours and returned to normal by 24 hours. In light of the convincing evidence for a role for hypoxia in normal retinal vascularization, mice null for HIF1-alpha exhibited normal retinal vascularization,[45] suggesting an alternative means for hypoxic upregulation of VEGF during retinal vascularization.

In addition to the well-studied transcriptional induction of VEGF and other hypoxia-regulated genes such as erythropoietin,[46] mRNA stability is another mechanism for increasing message, and hence protein, levels. As is the case for many other growth factors and cytokines, the half-life of the VEGF mRNA in cultured retinal pigment epithelium (RPE) is quite short—at 45 minutes—and incubation of cells under hypoxic conditions leads to a dramatic increase of the half-life to 8 hours.[47] This effect has been shown to be mediated by a region of the 3' untranslated region of the VEGF transcript. Using a tumor cell system, RNA-binding/electrophoretic mobility shift assays identified a single 125-bp AU-rich element in the 3' untranslated region that formed hypoxia-inducible RNA-protein complexes.[48] Moreover, two proteins of 90-88-kDa and 60-kDa were found to specifically bind this hypoxia stability region element.

Although it is clear from both experimental OIR models and from human pathology (i.e., ROP) that VEGF is required for the formation of retinal vessels, the retinal vasculature in the adult appears to be less dependent on sustained VEGF signaling than other vascular beds. As described below in the "Role of VEGF in the Adult Retina," robust systemic VEGF neutralization did not result in changes in the inner retinal vasculature though significant vascular regression was noted in many other vessel beds. A clue into the mechanism(s) that may mediate this relative VEGF-independence may come from the unique association of the pericyte with the retinal microvasculature (Box 4-1) and (Fig. 4.2).

Of all microvascular beds examined, the retinal microvasculature has the highest ratio of pericytes to ECs with one pericyte for each EC.[49] The concept that the presence of the pericyte might stabilize the EC is suggested by the fact that pericyte loss is known to precede the development of proliferative diabetic retinopathy (PDR). To gain insight into how the pericyte might serve a stabilizing role, coculture models were used to examine the nature of the interactions between EC and undifferentiated mesenchymal cells (i.e., pericyte precursors). These studies revealed that proliferating EC synthesize and secrete PDGF-B, which stimulates mesenchymal proliferation[50] and acts as chemoattractant, directing the migration of undifferentiated mesenchymal cells toward the nascent vessel.[51] It was also demonstrated that upon contact with the endothelium, the mesenchymal cells were induced to differentiate toward a pericyte/smooth muscle cell phenotype and to produce VEGF[52] via contact-activated TGF-ß1, events that contribute to microvessel stabilization. Thus, it

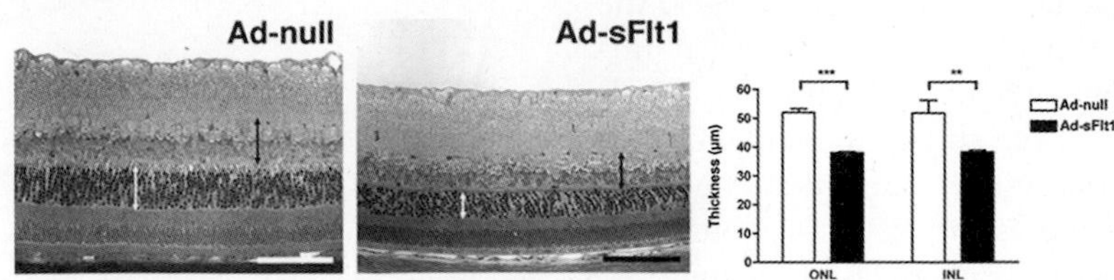

FIGURE 4.2. Decreased retina thickness and loss of visual function in sFlt1-expressing mice. **A:** Semithin epon sections from retinas of experimental mice expressing sFlt1 for 28 days showed substantial thinning of the INL (*black double arrowheads line*) and the ONL (*white double arrowheads line*) ($n = 3$ for Ad-null and $n = 4$ for Ad-sFlt1). (Reproduced from Saint-Geniez M, Maharaj AS, Walshe TE, et al. Endogenous VEGF is required for visual function: evidence for a survival role on muller cells and photoreceptors. *PLoS One*. 2008;3:e3554. with permission.)

is possible that the VEGF that is locally produced by some pericytes (not all retinal pericytes make VEGF) is not accessible to the sFlt1 used in the experimental models.[2] Moreover, the TGF-β that is generated upon local EC-pericyte interactions and the angiopoietin-1 that is produced by pericytes may also contribute to making the retinal vascular the stable vascular bed that it appears to be.

VEGF has similarly been demonstrated to mediate the formation of the choriocapillaris. RPE-specific deletion of VEGF led to the absence of the choriocapillaris, micropthalmia, and loss of visual function.[53] Mice heterozygous for RPE-specific VEGF deletion displayed significant defects in the RPE, in spite of normal choroidal vessel formation. The use of mice in which the RPE was null for HIF-1alpha indicated that VEGF expression in RPE was not mediated by hypoxia-induced transcriptional activation. The latter is not a surprising finding, however, since VEGF expression by RPE begins very early during ocular development when, in contrast to retinal vascularization, retinal differentiation has yet to commence.[54]

Role of VEGF in Ocular Angiogenesis

Under normal circumstances, the blood vessels of the retina, though metabolically active, are quiescent with respect to growth.[55] Studies of the labeling index of retinal capillary EC indicate that the turnover time for these cells

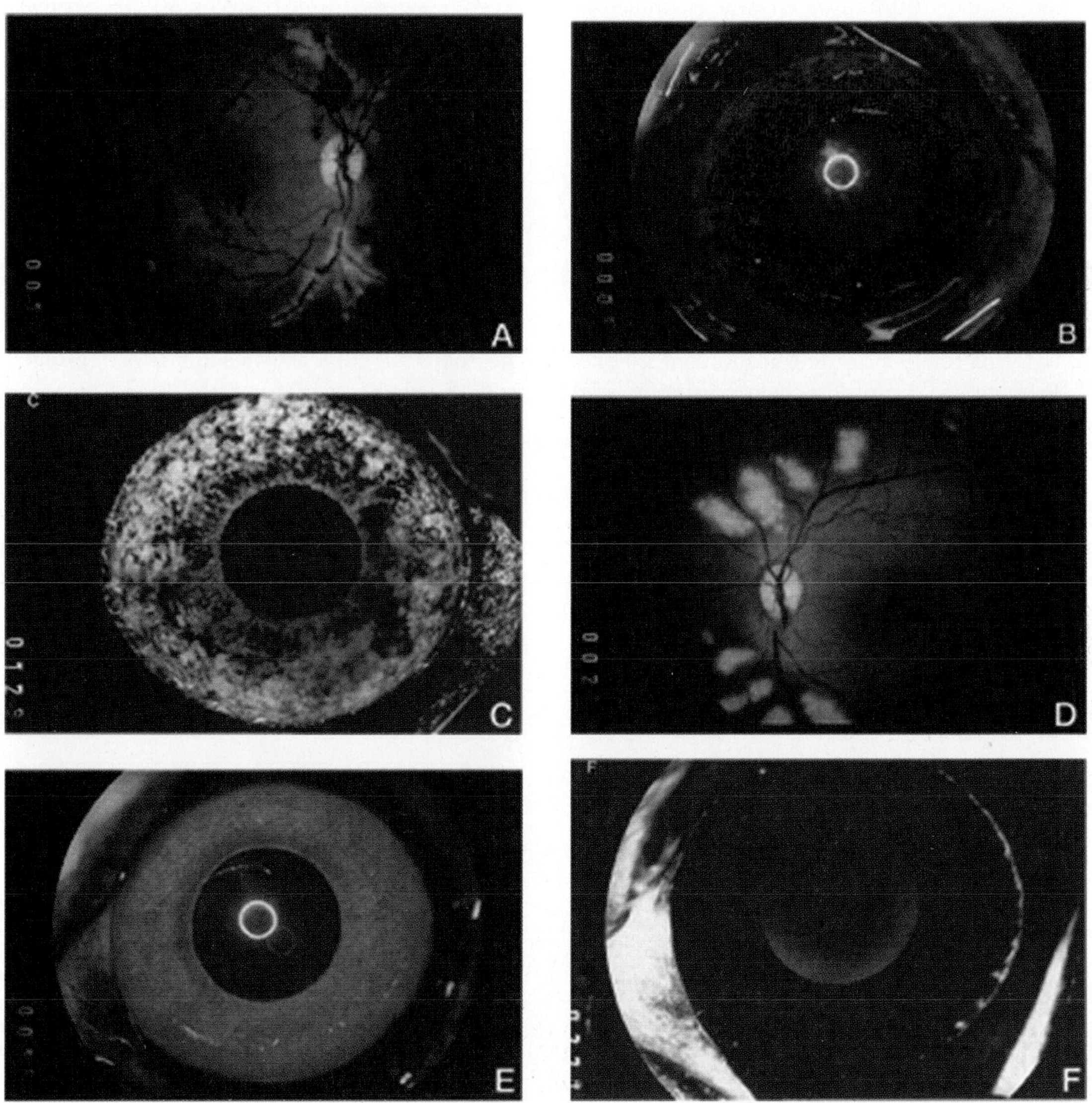

FIGURE 4.3. Experimental iris neovascularization. **A:** Fundus photograph immediately after laser vein occlusion. **B:** New vessels are seen on the surface of the iris. Iris neovascularization appears 4 to 7 days after laser vein occlusion, increases, and persists for an average of 24 days, or leads to the development of neovascular glaucoma. **C:** Fluorescein angiography demonstrates new vessels on the surface of the iris, with a characteristic tortuous pattern, and abundant leakage of fluorescein into the anterior chamber (grade 3). **D:** Fundus photograph immediately after sham laser, in which laser spots were placed adjacent to the retinal vessels, to produce retinal injury while preserving normal retinal vasculature. **E:** The iris appears normal 12 days after sham laser. **F:** Fluorescein angiography of the iris in **(E)** demonstrates no leakage of fluorescein from the normal iris vessels (grade 0). (Reprinted from Miller et al. *Am J Pathol.* 1994;145:574–584, with permission.)

(i.e., the time it takes to replace the entire population) is in the range of years.[55] To put this in perspective, the turnover time of EC in tumor blood vessels is days to weeks.[56] However, there are a variety of retinal pathologies that have rapid vessel proliferation as a component including PDR, retinal venous occlusion, and ROP. These pathologies are all characterized by the presence of nonperfused, and therefore hypoxic, retinal tissue as a precedent to the neovascularization. Realizing the central role that ischemia plays in the pathogenesis of the disease process and knowing that local oxygen levels can regulate VEGF expression, a number of laboratories, using various animal models, have examined the role of VEGF in neovascular retinopathies.[57]

Using a modification of a model of retinal ischemia-induced iris neovascularization,[57] VEGF was examined in the cynomologous monkey retina, which had been rendered ischemic by laser occlusion of the branch retinal veins[20,58] (Fig. 4.3). Seven to fourteen days following the occlusion, new blood vessels grow on the surface of the iris. (This is similar to rubeosis iridis, which occurs in diabetics and is associated with retinal capillary nonperfusion). VEGF protein and mRNA levels were shown to correlate with the timing and severity of iris angiogenesis (Fig. 4.4). PCR analysis revealed that the retina was producing the 121 and 165 amino acid isoforms of VEGF, the more diffusible forms relative to the third known isoform VEGF189.[20] (Primate VEGF isoforms have one amino acid more than the rodent counterparts.) In situ hybridization demonstrated VEGF mRNA expression by the ganglion cells of the retinal ganglion cell layer and by another cell type, possibly amacrine cells, in the inner nuclear layer. This expression pattern is consistent with the concept that expression is regulated by hypoxia because these cells are located in the inner retina, which is the tissue normally served by the occluded vessels.

A necessary role for VEGF in this process was demonstrated by studies in which neutralizing monoclonal antibodies against VEGF were administered intravitreally at the time of vein occlusion and every other day thereafter for 14 days.[59] The vitreous of eyes with PDR has been shown to have levels of VEGF significantly higher than vitreous of eyes without proliferative retinopathy[60–62] and neovascular membranes were shown to have VEGF mRNA.[62]

VEGF has been similarly implicated in the neovascularization that characterizes the ROP. The retinas of neonatal mice incubated in high oxygen and then returned to room air had elevated levels of VEGF mRNA that were localized to Muller cells in the inner nuclear layer.[63] A causal link between VEGF expression and the observed neovascularization was demonstrated when the vessel growth was shown to be suppressed by the injection of soluble VEGF receptor chimeric proteins that block VEGF activity.[21] Since the neovascularization had been shown to be due to hypoxia-induced VEGF, it was suspected that oxygen levels might be titrated to be high enough to prevent hypoxic damage to the retina but not so high as to suppress the VEGF expression required for normal retinal vascularization. This balance was shown to be effective in the kitten model of ROP[64] and is now the focus of clinical trials for the treatment of human ROP. Further insight into the involvement of VEGF in the pathogenesis of ROP came from studies using a cat model of the disease.

VEGF in the Adult

There is no doubt that VEGF plays a critical and central role in vascular development and in pathologic angiogenesis such occurs in proliferative retinopathies and choroidal neovascularization. In contrast, the role of VEGF in

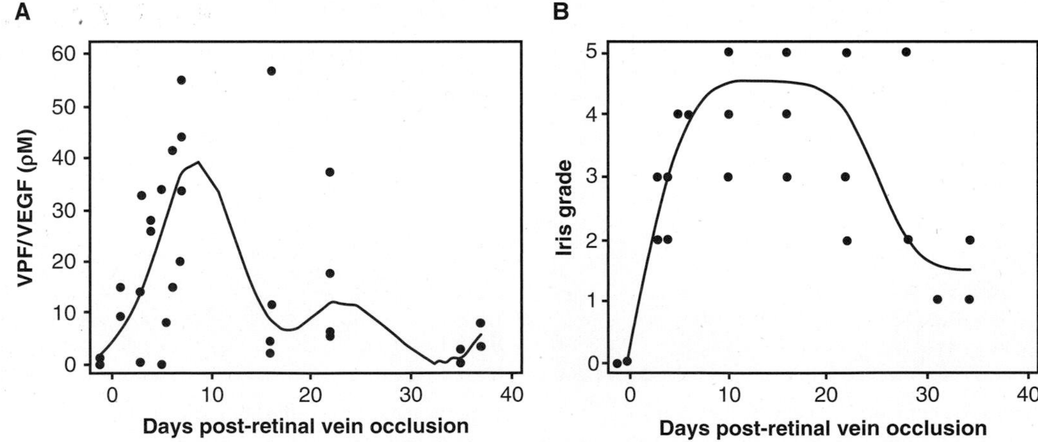

FIGURE 4.4. Aqueous VEGF levels in eyes with iris neovascularization. **A,B:** VEGF levels in the aqueous **(A)** and grade of iris neovascularization **(B)** of four monkey eyes are compared over time after laser vein occlusion as a scatterplot with best-fit curves. Although there is substantial variability between eyes, there seems to be an association between VEGF level and iris neovascularization. VEGF was undetectable in the aqueous before laser, the levels rise as neovascularization develops, and fall as the neovascularization regresses. (Reprinted from Miller et al. *Am J Pathol.* 1994;145:574–584, with permission.)

the adult is relatively uninvestigated. Virtually all adult tissues express VEGF[21] and examination of the expression pattern of VEGF in the adult using a VEGF-LacZ mouse has revealed that VEGF expression is localized to specific cell types in each tissue/organ.[65] In the retina, VEGF is expressed by a subset of pericytes and astrocytes[52] as well as by the RPE.[1,66] In the lung, VEGF is expressed by type 2 pneumocytes,[21] and in the kidney, it is expressed by podocytes and some ductal cells.[67] It is increasingly clear that VEGF in the adult contributes to the stabilization of the tissue microvasculature. Evidence that the VEGF is signaling the EC of adult vessels is provided by the fact that VEGFR2 is constitutively phosphorylated in a number of tissues including the lung,[68] retina,[1] and choroid.[1]

Systematic VEGF inhibition in mice achieved using a small molecule VEGF tyrosine kinase inhibitor or soluble VEGF receptors led to the regression of capillaries in normal tissues as well as in tumors. Among the normal tissues examined, significant vessel loss was measured in pancreatic islets, thyroid, adrenal cortex, pituitary, choroid plexus, small-intestinal villi, and epididymal and adipose tissue after one week of VEGF neutralization.[69,70] The extent of vessel loss varied depending on the tissue, with the most significant vessel regression seen in the thyroid (66%). Of interest, all the capillary beds were fenestrated and expressed high levels of VEGF and VEGFR2 and the capillaries that remained in these beds had fewer fenestrations and lower VEGF. Vessels in the thyroid grew back within two weeks after withdrawal of the inhibitors.

A role for VEGF in renal microvascular integrity is similarly indicated by recent observations of human preeclampsia. Overexpression of soluble Flt (VEGFR1) by the placenta has been shown to be correlated with development of the symptoms of preeclampsia, including proteinuria due to loss of glomerular integrity.[71] Moreover, many of the features of preeclampsia including hypertension and proteinuria were replicated by systemic expression of sFlt-1 in pregnant rats. These studies not only generated insight into the pathogenesis of preeclampsia but also provided evidence that the most common side effects of systemic anti-VEGF therapy in human, hypertension and proteinuria, were the direct result of VEGF neutralization and supply strong evidence for a role for VEGF in the integrity and function of the adult large and small vessels.[72]

Similar studies in which VEGF was systemically neutralized in nonpregnant mice revealed a role for VEGF not only in the maintenance of the choroid plexus of the brain, a result that was expected because of its status as a fenestrated vascular bed, but also in the maintenance of the ependymal lining of the ventricles.[73] Results of these studies expanded the list of nonvascular VEGF targets and provided a possible explanation for the observation of reversible posterior leukencephalopathy as a rare side effect in patients on anti-VEGF therapy for cancer treatment.[74]

Nonvascular Targets of VEGF

In addition to its multiple roles on vascular cells, it has become apparent that VEGF targets many nonvascular cells (for review see Ref. 75). VEGFR1 and VEGF2 expressions have been demonstrated on a number of cells types including pneumocytes,[76] megakaryocytes,[77] dendritic cells,[78] monocytes, lens epithelial cells,[79] retinal pigment epithelial cells,[1] and a variety of neural cells. The preponderance of data supporting a role for VEGF outside of the vascular system is the neural system where there is significant evidence to indicate both neurotrophic and neuroprotective effects on neural cells both in vitro and in vivo.[80,81] Neural targets of VEGF include astrocytes and microglia, as well as a variety of neurons (sensory, cortical, hippocampal, etc.), with neurogenic, neuroprotective, and/or neurotrophic effects. Moreover, VEGF has been demonstrated to stimulate the proliferation of neural progenitors in parts of the brain capable of neurogenesis such as the hippocampus, the olfactory, and

BOX 4.2 Role for RPE-derived VEGF in the Maintenance of the Adult Choriocapillaris

RPE produces VEGF early during retinal development, and its production continues into adulthood.[1] On the other hand, the endothelium of the choriocapillaris expresses relatively high levels of VEGFR2 and biochemical analysis reveals that VEGFR2 is constitutively phosphorylated.[1] Since this VEGF signaling is occurring in the absence of active angiogenesis, VEGF must be serving a role other than stimulating vessel growth. RPE in vivo produced VEGF120 and VEGF164, but no detectable VEGF188.[1] Since VEGF188 is not freely diffusible, and since VEGF produced by RPE would need to diffuse through Bruch membrane to reach the target choriocapillary EC, the absence of VEGF188 production is logical. Taking advantage of the restricted VEGF isoform production by RPE, mice that had been engineered to express only VEGF188 were used to examine the effect of reduced VEGF signaling between the RPE and the choriocapillaris. Although the RPE-choriocapillaris of mice that produce only VEGF188 were normal though 4 months of age, there was significant pathology in the choriocapillaris of 6-month-old VEGF188 mice, including the replacement of the choriocapillaris with large, nonfenestrated vessels and abnormalities in the RPE such as vacuoles, separation from the photoreceptor layers, and breakdown on intercellular junctions (Fig. 4.5).[4] The defects worsen with age and lead to areas of RPE loss and reduced visual function. These findings indicate that RPE-derived VEGF is essential for the maintenance of the choriocapillaris and the RPE themselves and suggest that chronic use of anti-VEGF therapies should be applied with caution and with attention to possible unwanted side effects.

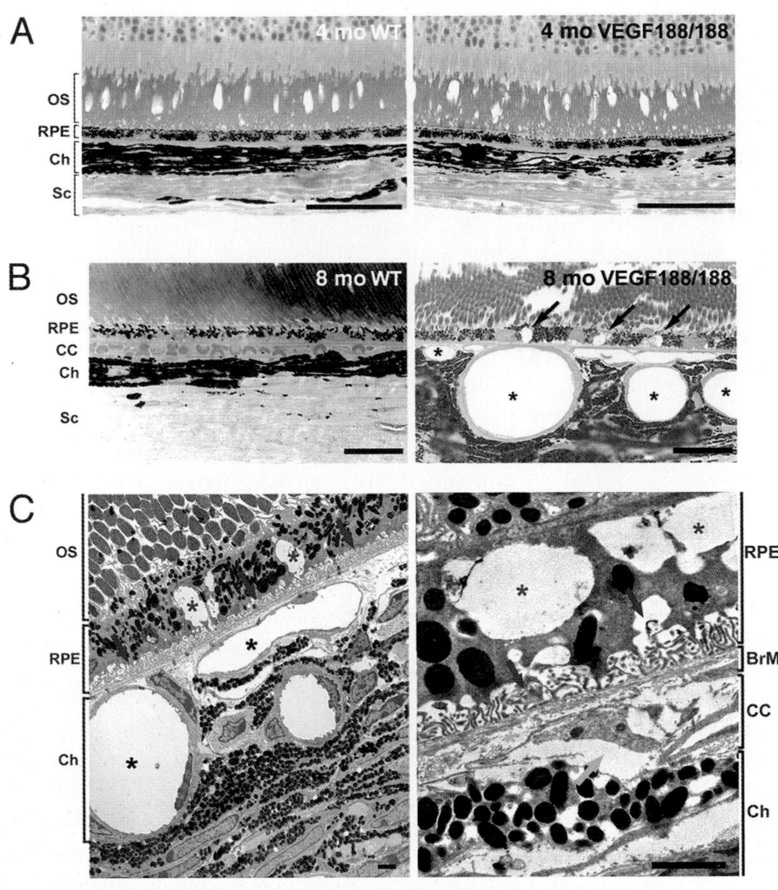

FIGURE 4.5. Abnormal choroidal vasculature and RPE defects in aged VEGF188/188 mice. **A,B:** One-micrometer-thin epon sections of 4- and 8-month-old wt (**right**) and VEGF188/188 (**left**) mice were stained with paraphenylenediamine for light microscopy (**A** and **B**) or were visualized by TEM (**C**). **A:** No changes in the organization of the retina layers were observed in 4-month-old VEGF188/188 mice. **B:** An 8-month-old, VEGF188/188 mouse eye displays major abnormalities in the RPE and choroidal vessels. Larges vacuoles were observed within the RPE (*arrows*). The choroidal vessels appear enlarged, and the CC is replaced by discontinuous vessels wrapped by pericytes (*asterisk*). **C:** Electron micrograph of the midperiphery of an 8-month-old VEGF188/188 mouse retina. Note the significant enlargement of the choroidal vessels (*black asterisk*). RPE cells displayed large vacuoles containing membranous debris (*blue asterisk*). Regression of the RPE basal infoldings is associated with accumulation of materials (*red arrow*). Higher magnification (**right**) showing discontinuous collagen and elastin layers in Bruch membrane (*green asterisk*) and a regressing CC vessel with an entrapped erythrocyte (*green arrow*). [Scale bar, 50"m (**A**); scale bar, 20"m (**B**); scale bar, 2"m (**C**).] OS, outer segment; BrM, Bruch membrane; CC, choriocapillaris; Ch, choroid; Sc, sclera. (Reproduced from Saint-Geniez M, Kurihara T, Sekiyama E, et al. An essential role for RPE-derived soluble VEGF in the maintenance of the choriocapillaris. *Proc Natl Acad Sci U S A.* 2009;106:18751–18756 with permission.)

the subventricular zones. Most recently, a conditional transgenic system was used to suppress VEGF signaling at specific site in the brain where interneurons traverse on their way to be incorporated into the existing olfactory circuits. Blockage of VEGF that is expressed by a specific type of resident olfactory neurons significantly reduced dendrite development in incoming subventricular zone–born neurons. These results point to a role for VEGF in the maturation of adult-born neurons in the brain.[82]

Of significance for this publication is the presence of VEGFR2 on retinal astrocytes, Müller cells, photoreceptors, and RPE.[1,2] These observations coupled with the production of VEGF by the Muller cells and the RPE themselves point to the presence of both paracrine (Müller-photoreceptor; RPE-choriocapillaris) and autocrine (Müller cells, RPE) in the adult retina (see Boxes 4-1 and 4-2).

CLINICAL STRATEGIES TO INHIBIT VEGF

The first demonstration that VEGF blockade would lead to reduced angiogenesis was reported in 1993 by researchers at Genentech who had developed a neutralizing monoclonal antibody against VEGF and demonstrated efficacy against experimental tumor growth.[83] Just 10 years later in 2003, press releases reported that clinical trials of the humanized form of an anti-VEGF monoclonal antibody (bevacizumab, Avastin) had extended the media survival time of patients with colorectal cancer from 15.6 to 20.3 months (http://www.highbeam.com/doc/1P2-7777109.html). The following year, the U.S. Food and Drug Administration approved Avastin for the treatment of metastatic colorectal cancer.

Ocular angiogenesis, as a target for anti-VEGF therapy, was obvious to all. The two major ocular pathologies with associated angiogenesis are PDR and the wet form of age-related macular degeneration (AMD). Panretinal photocoagulation is considered by most an effective, if not ideal, treatment for PDR, whereas the current care of wet AMD, primarily photodynamic, was minimally effective. Thus, the introduction Macugen in December 2004, the first anti-VEGF therapy FDA approved for the treatment of wet macular degeneration, was met with great excitement. Macugen is an aptamer, an oligonucleotide that binds specifically to VEGF and neutralizes its actions. Although clinical trial results were promising (reviewed in Ref. 84), the efficacy in the clinic did not prove to be as dramatic or durable.

Although there was interest in using Avastin (bevacizumab) for the treatment of wet AMD, animals studies conducted by Genentech comparing bevacizumab to ranibizumab localization following intravitreal injection in the primate eye indicated that radiolabeled full length antibody did not cross the inner limiting membrane whereas the Fab fragment diffused through to the RPE.[85] Thus, simple reformulation of the bevacizumab for ocular purposes would not be sufficient and the Fab fragment would have to go through the requisite clinical trials.

Unwilling to wait for the time that this would require, some ophthalmologists began to test Avastin for its efficacy against wet AMD. Initial tests involved systemic administration of Avastin to nine individuals in an uncontrolled trial, as was being done for oncology purposes, and showed significant improvement in visual acuity.[86] Though these observations were exciting in terms of proof-of-principle, the complications associated with systemic Avastin, such as hypertension and thrombosis, would be unacceptable in the aged, AMD population. Following this, ophthalmologists began to use Avastin intravitreally with stunning results. Several papers published around the same time reported preliminary results. In one, 3-month study of bevacizumab administration to 53 eyes, "the mean visual acuity improved from 20/160 to 20/125 ($p < 0.001$) and the mean central retinal thickness decreased by 99.6 µm ($p < 0.001$)."[87] In another publication of 81 eyes over 3 months, the mean retinal thickness was reported to be decreased by 67 µm, respectively ($p < 0.01$) and mean visual acuity was improved from 20/200 to 20/125 ($p < 0.0001$) at 8 weeks.[88] Clearly, the Avastin injected intravitreally was accessing its target at the back of the eye. In retrospect, the study suggesting that Avastin would not be sufficiently diffusible was flawed because it examined Avastin localization following injection into an intact, undiseased eye and used a humanized monoclonal antibody against HER2, and not Avastin itself.

With the July 2006 FDA approval of Lucentis (ranucizumab), ophthalmologists were faced with a dilemma. At approximately one fortieth of the cost of Lucentis, Avastin had apparently the same efficacy. Whether the two drugs do, in fact, function similarly is the subject of a clinical trial "Comparison of Age-related Macular Degeneration Treatments Trials: Lucentis-Avastin Trial (CATT)" sponsored by the National Eye Institute (http://www.nei.nih.gov/neitrials/viewStudyWeb.aspx?id=137#Results) in which the two are being compared on both a fixed and variable schedule of administration.

KEY POINTS

- VEGF is a potent stimulator of angiogenesis and vascular permeability.
- Hypoxia increases VEGF levels by gene transcription and by mRNA stabilization.
- VEGF is essential for early vascular development and for organ vascularization.
- VEGF plays an important role in the maintenance of adult fenestrated microvessels.
- A variety of nonvascular cells, including many neural cells, express VEGF receptors.
- VEGF acts a neurotrophic factor and neuroprotectant for many neural cells.
- VEGF acts as a survival factor and neuroprotectant in the adult retina including
  - Paracrine interactions between Müller cells and photoreceptors
  - Paracrine interactions between RPE and the choriocapillaris
  - Autocrine actions in Müller cells and in RPE.

REFERENCES

1. Saint-Geniez M, Maldonado AE, D'Amore PA. VEGF expression and receptor activation in the choroid during development and in the adult. *Invest Ophthalmol Vis Sci.* 2006;47:3135–3142.
2. Saint-Geniez M, Maharaj AS, Walshe TE, et al. Endogenous VEGF is required for visual function: evidence for a survival role on muller cells and photoreceptors. *PLoS One.* 2008;3:e3554.
3. Michaelson IC. The mode of development of the vascular system of the retina with some observations on its significance for certain retinal diseases. *Trans Ophthalmol Soc UK.* 1948;68:137–180.
4. Saint-Geniez M, Kurihara T, Sekiyama E, et al. An essential role for RPE-derived soluble VEGF in the maintenance of the choriocapillaris. *Proc Natl Acad Sci U S A.* 2009;106:18751–18756.
5. Glaser BM, D'Amore PA, Michels RG, et al. Identification of a vasocproliferative activity from mammalian retina. *J Cell Biol.* 1980;84:298–304.
6. D'Amore PA, Klagsbrun M. Endothelial mitogens derived from retina and hypothalamus: Biological and biochemical similarities. *J Cell Biol.* 1984;99:1545–1549.
7. Shweiki D, Itin A, Soffer D, et al. Vascular endothelial growth factor induced by hypoxia may mediate hypoxia-initiated angiogenesis. *Nature.* 1992;359:843–845.
8. Plate KH, Breier G, Weich HA, et al. Vascular endothelial growth factor is a potential tumour angiogenesis factor in human gliomas *in vivo*. *Nature.* 1992;359:845–848.
9. Leung DW, Cachianes G, Kuang W-J, et al. Vascular endothelial growth factor is a secreted angiogenic mitogen. *Science.* 1989;246:1306–1309.
10. Ferrara N, Gerber HP, LeCouter J. The biology of VEGF and its receptors. *Nat Med.* 2003;9:669–676.
11. Shima DT, Kuroki M, Deutsch U, et al. The mouse gene for vascular endothelial growth factor. Genomic structure, definition of the transcriptional unit and characterization of transcriptional and post-transcriptional regulatory sequences. *J Biol Chem.* 1996;271:3877–3883.
12. Yamazaki Y, Morita T. Molecular and functional diversity of vascular endothelial growth factors. *Mol Divers.* 2006;10:515–527.
13. Woolard J, Wang WY, Bevan HS, et al. VEGF165b, an inhibitory vascular endothelial growth factor splice variant:

mechanism of action, in vivo effect on angiogenesis and endogenous protein expression. *Cancer Res.* 2004;64:7822–7835.
14. Waltenberger J, Claesson-Welsh L, Siegbahn A, et al. Different signal transduction properties of KDR and Flt1, two receptors for vascular endothelial growth factor. *J Biol Chem.* 1994;269:26988–26995.
15. Quinn TP, Peters KG, De Vries C, et al. Fetal liver kinase 1 is a receptor for vascular endothelial growth factor and is selectively expressed in vascular endothelium. *Proc Natl Acad Sci U S A.* 1993;90:7533–7537.
16. Soker S, Takashima S, Miao H, et al. Neuropilin-1 is expressed by endothelial and tumor cells as an isoform-specific receptor for vasular endothelial growth factor. *Cell.* 1998;92: 735–745.
17. Gluzman-Poltorak Z, Cohen T, Herzog Y, et al. Neuropilin-2 is a receptor for the vascular endothelial growth factor (VEGF) forms VEGF-145 and VEGF-165 [corrected]. *J Biol Chem.* 2000;275:18040–18045.
18. Li X, Claesson-Welsh L, Shibuya M. VEGF receptor signal transduction. *Methods Enzymol.* 2008;443:261–284.
19. Tischer E, Mitchell R, Hartman T, et al. The human gene for vascular endothelial growth factor. Multiple proteins are encoded through alternative exon splicing. *J Biol Chem.* 1991;266:11947–11954.
20. Shima DT, Gougos A, Miller JW, et al. Cloning and mRNA expression of vascular endothelial growth factor in ischemic retinas of Macaca fasicularis. *Invest Ophthalmol Vis Sci.* 1996;37:1334–1347.
21. Ng Y-S, Rohan R, Sunday M, et al. Differential expression of VEGF isoforms in mouse during development and in the adult. *Dev Dyn.* 2001;220:112–121.
22. Ng YS, Ramsauer M, Loureiro RM, et al. Identification of genes involved in VEGF-mediated vascular morphogenesis using embryonic stem cell-derived cystic embryoid bodies. *Lab Invest.* 2004;84:1209–1218.
23. Bacic M, Edwards NA, Merrill MJ. Differential expression of vascular endothelial growth factor (vascular permeability factor) forms in rat tissues. *Growth Factors.* 1995;12:11–15.
24. Ferrara N, Houck K, Jakeman L, et al. Molecular and biological properties of the vascular endothelial growth factor family of proteins. *Endocr Rev.* 1992;13:18–32.
25. Houck KA, Ferrara N, Winer J, et al. The vascular endothelial growth factor family: identification of a fourth molecular species and characterization of alternative splicing of RNA. *Mol Endocrinol.* 1991;5:1806–1814.
26. Keyt BA, Berleau LT, Nguyen HV, et al. The carboxyl-terminal domain (111–165) of vascular endothelial growth factor is critical for its mitogenic potency. *J Biol Chem.* 1996;271:7788–7795.
27. Soker S, Fidder H, Neufeld G, et al. Characterization of novel vascular endothelial growth factor (VEGF) receptors on tumor cells that bind VEGF165 via its exon 7-encoded domain. *J Biol Chem.* 1996;271:5761–5767.
28. Carmeliet P, Ng Y-S, Nuyen D, et al. Impaired myocardial angiogenesis and ischemic cardiomyopathy in mice lacking the vascular endothelial growth factor isoforms VEGF164 and VEGF188. *Nat Med.* 1999;5:495–502.
29. Stalmans I, Ng YS, Rohan R, et al. Arteriolar and venular patterning in retinas of mice selectively expressing VEGF isoforms. *J Clin Invest.* 2002;109:327–336.
30. Ishida S, Usui T, Yamashiro K, et al. VEGF164-mediated inflammation is required for pathological, but not physiological, ischemia-induced retinal neovascularization. *J Exp Med.* 2003;198:483–489.
31. Ferrara N, Carver-Moore K, Chen H, et al. Heterozygous embryonic lethality induced by targeted inactivation of the VEGF gene. *Nature.* 1996;380:439–442.
32. Carmeliet P, Ferriera V, Breier G, et al. Abnormal blood vessel development and lethality in embryos lacking a single VEGF allele. *Nature.* 1996;380:435–439.
33. Compernolle V, Brusselmans K, Acker T, et al. Loss of HIF-2alpha and inhibition of VEGF impair fetal lung maturation, whereas treatment with VEGF prevents fatal respiratory distress in premature mice. *Nat Med.* 2002;8:702–710.
34. Del Moral PM, Sala FG, Tefft D, et al. VEGF-A signaling through Flk-1 is a critical facilitator of early embryonic lung epithelial to endothelial crosstalk and branching morphogenesis. *Dev Biol.* 2006;290:177–188.
35. Eremina V, Quaggin SE. The role of VEGF-A in glomerular development and function. *Curr Opin Nephrol Hypertens.* 2004;13:9–15.
36. Tang K, Breen EC, Gerber HP, et al. Capillary regression in vascular endothelial growth factor-deficient skeletal muscle. *Physiol Genomics.* 2004;18:63–69.
37. Zelzer E, McLean W, Ng YS, et al. Skeletal defects in VEGF(120/120) mice reveal multiple roles for VEGF in skeletogenesis. *Development.* 2002;129:1893–1904.
38. Maes C, Carmeliet P, Moermans K, et al. Impaired angiogenesis and endochondral bone formation in mice lacking the vascular endothelial growth factor isoforms VEGF164 and VEGF188. *Mech Dev.* 2002;111:61–73.
39. Stone J, Itin A, Alon T, et al. Development of retinal vasculature is mediated by hypoxia-induced vascular endothelial growth factor (VEGF) expression by neuroglia. *J Neurosci.* 1995;15:4738–4747.
40. Chan-Ling T, Gock B, Stone J. The effect of oxygen on vasoformative cell division. Evidence that 'physiological hypoxia' is the stimulus for normal retinal vasculogenesis. *Invest Ophthalmol Vis Sci.* 1995;36:1201–1214.
41. Smith LEH, Weslowski E, McLellan A, et al. Oxygen-induced retinopathy in the mouse. *Invest Ophthalmol Vis Sci.* 1994;35:101–111.
42. Stone J, Chan-Ling T, Pe'er J, et al. Roles of vascular endothelial growth factor and astrocyte degeneration in the genesis of retinopathy of prematurity. *Invest Ophthalmol Vis Sci.* 1996;37:290–299.
43. Alon T, Hemo I, Itin A, et al. Vascular endothelial growth factor acts as a survival factor for newly formed retinal vessels and has implications for retinopathy of prematurity. *Nat Med.* 1995;1:1024–1028.
44. Ozaki H, Yu AY, Della N, et al. Hypoxia inducible factor-1-alpha is increased in ischemic retina: temporal and spatial correlation with VEGF expression. *Invest Ophthalmol Vis Sci.* 1999;40:182–189.
45. Vinores SA, Xiao WH, Aslam S, et al. Implication of the hypoxia response element of the Vegf promoter in mouse models of retinal and choroidal neovascularization, but not retinal vascular development. *J Cell Physiol.* 2006;206:749–758.
46. Varma S, Cohen HJ. Co-transactivation of the 3 erythropoietin hypoxia inducible enhancer by the HIF-1 protein. *Blood Cells Mol Dis.* 1997;23:169–176.

47. Shima DT, Deutsch U, D'Amore PA. Hypoxic induction of vascular endothelial growth factor (VEGF) in human epithelial cells is mediated by increases in mRNA stability. *FEBS Lett*. 1995;370:203–208.
48. Claffey KP, Shih SC, Mullen A, et al. Identification of a human VPF/VEGF 3 untranslated region mediating hypoxia-induced mRNA stability. *Mol Biol Cell*. 1998;9: 469–481.
49. Tilton RG, Miller EJ, Kilo C, et al. Pericyte form and distribution in rat retinal and uveal capillaries. *Invest Ophthalmol Vis Sci*. 1985;26:68–73.
50. Hirschi KK, Rohovsky SA, Beck LH, et al. Endothelial cells modulate the proliferation of mural cell precursors via platelet-derived growth factor-BB and heterotypic cell contact. *Circ Res*. 1999;84:298–305.
51. Hirschi K, Rohovsky SA, D'Amore PA. PDGF, TGF-ß and heterotypic cell-cell interactions mediate the recruitment and differentiation of 10T1/2 cells to a smooth muscle cell fate. *J Cell Biol*. 1998;141:805–814.
52. Darland DC, Massingham LJ, Smith SR, et al. Pericyte production of cell-associated VEGF is differentiation-dependent and is associated with endothelial survival. *Dev Biol*. 2003;264:275–288.
53. Marneros AG, Fan J, Yokoyama Y, et al. Vascular endothelial growth factor expression in the retinal pigment epithelium is essential for choriocapillaris development and visual function. *Am J Pathol*. 2005;167:1451–1459.
54. Saint-Geniez M, D'Amore PA. Development and pathology of the hyaloid, choroidal and retinal vasculature. *Int J Dev Biol*. 2004;48:1045–1058.
55. Engerman RL, Pfaffenbach D, Davis MD. Cell turnover of capillaries. *Lab Invest*. 1967;17:738–743.
56. Hobson B, Denekamp J. Endothelial proliferation in tumours and normal tissues: Continuous labelling studies. *Br J Cancer*. 1984;49:405–413.
57. Virdi PS, Hayreh SS. Ocular neovascularization with retinal vascular occlusion I. Association with experimental retinal vein occlusion. *Arch Ophthalmol*. 1982;100:331–341.
58. Miller JW, Adamis AP, Shima DT, et al. Vascular permeability factor/vascular endothelial cell growth factor is temporally and spatially correlated with ocular angiogenesis in a primate model. *Am J Pathol*. 1994;145:574–584.
59. Adamis AP, Shima DT, Tolentino MJ, et al. Inhibition of VEGF prevents ocular neovascularization in a primate. *Arch Ophthalmol*. 1996;114:66–71.
60. Adamis AP, Miller JW, Bernal M-T, et al. Increased vascular endothelial growth factor levels in the vitreous of eyes with proliferative diabetic retinopathy. *Am J Ophthal*. 1994;118:445–450.
61. Aiello LP, Avery RL, Arrigg PG, et al. Vascular endothelial growth factor in ocular fluid of patients with diabetic retinopathy and other ocular disorders. *N Engl J Med*. 1994;331:1480–1487.
62. Malecaze F, Clamens S, Simorre-Pinatel V, et al. Detection of vascular endothelial growth factor messenger RNA and vascular endothelial growth factor-like activity in proliferative diabetic retinopathy. *Lab Sci*. 1994;112:1476–1482.
63. Azizkhan J, Jensen D, Pierce A, et al. Transcription from TATA-less promoters: DHFR as a model. *Crit Rev Euk Gene Exp*. 1993;3:229–254.
64. Chan-Ling T, Gock BStone J. The effect of oxygen on vasoformative cell division. *Invest Ophthal Vis Sci*. 1995;36: 1201–1214.
65. Maharaj AS, Saint-Geniez M, Maldonado AE, et al. Vascular endothelial growth factor localization in the adult. *Am J Pathol*. 2006;168:639–648.
66. Kim I, Ryan AM, Rohan R, et al. Constitutive expression of VEGF, VEGFR-1, and VEGFR-2 in normal eyes. [erratum appears in *Invest Ophthalmol Vis Sci*. 2000;41(2):368]. *Invest Ophthalmol Vis Sci*. 1999;40:2115–2121.
67. Robert B, Zhao X, Abrahamson DR. Coexpression of neuropilin-1, Flk1, and VEGF(164) in developing and mature mouse kidney glomeruli. *Am J Physiol Renal Physiol*. 2000;279:F275–F282.
68. Kasahara Y, Tuder RM, Cool CD, et al. Endothelial cell death and decreased expression of vascular endothelial growth factor and vascular endothelial growth factor receptor 2 in emphysema. *Am J Respir Crit Care Med*. 2001;163:737–744.
69. Kamba T, Tam BY, Hashizume H, et al. VEGF-dependent plasticity of fenestrated capillaries in the normal adult microvasculature. *Am J Physiol Heart Circ Physiol*. 2006;290: H560–H576.
70. Inai T, Mancuso M, Hashizume H, et al. Inhibition of vascular endothelial growth factor (VEGF) signaling in cancer causes loss of endothelial fenestrations, regression of tumor vessels, and appearance of basement membrane ghosts. *Am J Pathol*. 2004;165:35–52.
71. Maynard SE, Min JY, Merchan J, et al. Excess placental soluble fms-like tyrosine kinase 1 (sFlt1) may contribute to endothelial dysfunction, hypertension, and proteinuria in preeclampsia. *J Clin Invest*. 2003;111:649–658.
72. Hurwitz H, Saini S. Bevacizumab in the treatment of metastatic colorectal cancer: safety profile and management of adverse events. *Semin Oncol*. 2006;33:S26–S34.
73. Maharaj AS, Walshe TE, Saint-Geniez M, et al. VEGF and TGF-beta are required for the maintenance of the choroid plexus and ependyma. *J Exp Med*. 2008;205:491–501.
74. Ozcan C, Wong SJ, Hari P. Reversible posterior leukoencephalopathy syndrome and bevacizumab. *N Engl J Med*. 2006;354:980–982; discussion 980–982.
75. D'Amore PA. Vascular endothelial cell growth factor-a: not just for endothelial cells anymore. *Am J Pathol*. 2007;171: 14–18.
76. Fehrenbach H, Haase M, Kasper M, et al. Alterations in the immunohistochemical distribution patterns of vascular endothelial growth factor receptors Flk1 and Flt1 in bleomycin-induced rat lung fibrosis. *Virchows Arch*. 1999;435:20–31.
77. Casella I, Feccia T, Chelucci C, et al. Autocrine-paracrine VEGF loops potentiate the maturation of megakaryocytic precursors through Flt1 receptor. *Blood*. 2003;101:1316–1323.
78. Dikov MM, Ohm JE, Ray N, et al. Differential roles of vascular endothelial growth factor receptors 1 and 2 in dendritic cell differentiation. *J Immunol*. 2005;174:215–222.
79. Saint-Geniez M, Kurihara T, D'Amore PA. Role of cell and matrix-bound VEGF isoforms in lens development. *Invest Ophthalmol Vis Sci*. 2009;50:311–321.
80. Zachary I. Neuroprotective role of vascular endothelial growth factor: signalling mechanisms, biological function, and therapeutic potential. *Neurosignals*. 2005;14:207–221.

81. Greenberg DA, Jin K. From angiogenesis to neuropathology. *Nature*. 2005;438:954–959.
82. Licht T, Eavri R, Goshen I, et al. VEGF is required for dendritogenesis of newly born olfactory bulb interneurons. *Development*. 2010;137:261–271.
83. Kim KJ, Li B, Winer J, et al. Inhibition of vascular endothelial growth factor-induced angiogenesis suppresses tumor growth in vivo. *Nature*. 1993;362:841–844.
84. Kourlas H, Schiller DS. Pegaptanib sodium for the treatment of neovascular age-related macular degeneration: a review. *Clin Ther*. 2006;28:36–44.
85. Mordenti J, Cuthbertson RA, Ferrara N, et al. Comparisons of the intraocular tissue distribution, pharmacokinetics, and safety of 125I-labeled full-length and Fab antibodies in rhesus monkeys following intravitreal administration. *Toxicol Pathol*. 1999;27:536–544.
86. Michels S, Rosenfeld PJ, Puliafito CA, et al. Systemic bevacizumab (Avastin) therapy for neovascular age-related macular degeneration twelve-week results of an uncontrolled open-label clinical study. *Ophthalmology*. 2005;112:1035–1047.
87. Rich RM, Rosenfeld PJ, Puliafito CA, et al. Short-term safety and efficacy of intravitreal bevacizumab (Avastin) for neovascular age-related macular degeneration. *Retina*. 2006;26:495–511.
88. Avery RL, Pieramici DJ, Rabena MD, et al. Intravitreal bevacizumab (Avastin) for neovascular age-related macular degeneration. *Ophthalmology*. 2006;113:363–372, e365.

CHAPTER

5

IGF-I in Ocular Angiogenesis

Kip M. Connor • Ann Hellstrom • Lois E.H. Smith

TWO PHASES OF ROP AND DIABETIC RETINOPATHY

Retinopathy of prematurity (ROP) was first identified in the late 1940s and was associated with excessive oxygen use.[1] The number of infants with ROP has increased further despite better control of supplemental oxygen, probably because of the increased survival of very low birth weight infants.[2] This indicates the likely association of ROP with both oxygen-related growth factors and growth factors related to the degree of prematurity.

The disease pathology of both ROP and diabetic retinopathy occurs in two phases. In the first phase of ROP, there is cessation of the normal retinal vascular growth, which normally occurs in utero, as well as regression of some of the preformed vessels. As the premature infant matures, the resulting nonvascularized retina becomes increasingly metabolically active and increasingly hypoxic. Likewise, the first phase of diabetic retinopathy is associated with the slow loss of capillaries. This is most prominently linked with poor control of hyperglycemia. The second phase of both ROP and diabetic retinopathy is retinal neovascularization or proliferative retinopathy, which is hypoxia induced.[3] In ROP, the onset of neovascularization occurs at about 30 to 32 weeks postmenstrual age. The progression of neovascularization is slower in diabetic retinopathy, generally beginning 15 to 25 years after the onset of diabetes.

Currently, no rodent models exist for studying proliferative or neovascular diabetic retinopathy, so oxygen-induced retinopathy, similar to ROP, is often used to study end-stage disease. We developed a mouse model of ROP to take advantage of the genetic manipulations possible in the murine system.[4] The eyes of mice, though they are born full-term, are incompletely vascularized at birth and resemble the retinal vascular development of premature infants. Exposure of these animals to hyperoxia causes vaso-obliteration and cessation of normal retinal blood vessel development, which mimics Phase 1 of ROP.[4–6] When mice return to room air, the nonperfused portions of the retina become hypoxic, which in turn causes retinal neovascularization similar to that of the second phase of ROP and of other retinopathies.

VEGF AND PHASE 2 OF ROP

Because hypoxia is a driving force for retinal neovascularization or proliferative retinopathy, we first searched for a hypoxia-regulated factor during Phase 1 of ROP. Vascular endothelial growth factor (VEGF) is a hypoxia-inducible cytokine[7] and is a vascular endothelial cell mitogen.[8] In the mouse,[5] retinal hypoxia stimulates an increase in the expression of VEGF before the development of neovascularization.[9] Furthermore, inhibition of VEGF decreases the neovascular response,[10,11] indicating that VEGF is a critical factor in retinal neovascularization. Other investigators have also shown that VEGF is associated with ocular neovascularization in other animal models, confirming the central role of VEGF in neovascular eye disease.[12–15] These results have been corroborated clinically. VEGF is elevated in the vitreous of patients with retinal neovascularization.[16] In a patient with ROP, VEGF was found in the retina in a pattern consistent with mouse results.[15]

VEGF AND PHASE 1 OF ROP

In animal models, the first phase of ROP is also VEGF dependent. VEGF is required for normal blood vessel growth. VEGF is found anterior to the developing vasculature, in what has been described as a wave of physiological hypoxia that precedes vessel growth.[9,13] As the retina develops anterior to the vasculature, there is increased oxygen demand, which creates localized hypoxia. VEGF is expressed in response to the hypoxia, and blood vessels grow toward the VEGF stimulus. As the hypoxia is relieved by oxygen from the newly formed vessels, VEGF mRNA expression is suppressed, moving the wave forward.

Supplemental oxygen interferes with normal retinal vascular development through suppression of VEGF mRNA. Furthermore, hyperoxia-induced vaso-obliteration is caused by apoptosis of vascular endothelial cells, and vaso-obliteration can be at least partially prevented by administration of exogenous VEGF[9,17] and more specifically by placental growth factor-1 (PlGF-1), the specific agonist of VEGF receptor-1 (VEGFR-1).[18] This indicates that VEGFR-1 is required for maintenance of the immature retinal vasculature and explains at least in part the effect of hyperoxia on normal vessel development in ROP.

GH/IGF-1 IN PHASE 2 OF ROP

While the importance of VEGF has well-established role in the development of retinal blood vessels, it is clear that other biochemical mediators are also involved in the pathogenesis of ROP. Inhibition of VEGF does not completely inhibit hypoxia-induced retinal neovascularization in the second phase of ROP. In ROP, despite controlled use of supplemental oxygen, the disease persists. Infants of ever-lower gestational age continue to be saved, suggesting that other factors related to prematurity itself such as growth and development are also at work. Because growth hormone (GH) has been implicated in proliferative diabetic retinopathy,[19] we considered both GH and insulin-like growth factor-1 (IGF-1), which mediates many of the mitogenic aspects of GH, as potential candidates for postnatal regulation of ROP.

In transgenic mice expressing a GH receptor antagonist or in normal mice treated with a somatostatin analog that decreases GH release, there is a substantial reduction in the amount of proliferative retinopathy in mice subjected to the oxygen induced retinopathy (OIR) model.[20] The effect of GH inhibition is mediated through an inhibition of IGF-1, as administration of exogenous IGF-1 completely restores the neovascularization found in the control mice. The GH/IGF-1[20] inhibition occurs without diminishing hypoxia-induced VEGF production (Fig. 5.1). Proof of the direct role of IGF-1 in the proliferative phase of ROP in mice was established with an IGF-1 receptor antagonist, which suppressed retinal neovascularization without altering the vigorous VEGF response induced in the mouse ROP model.[21]

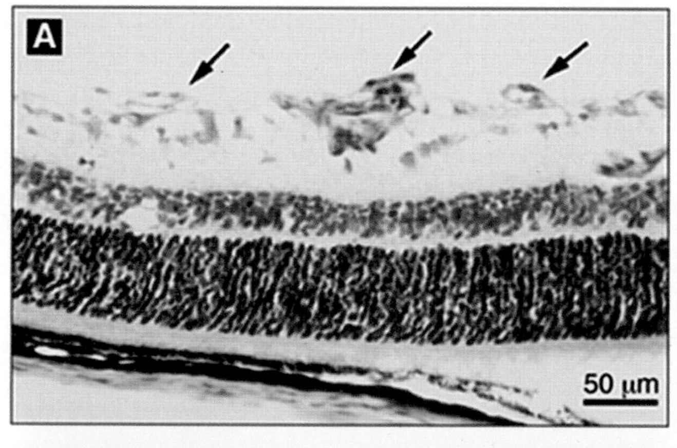

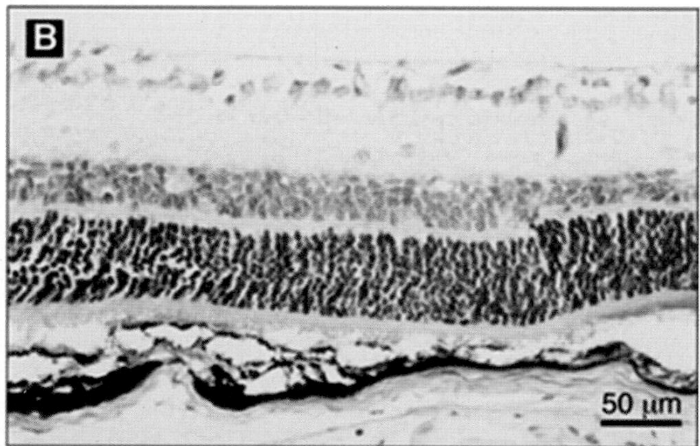

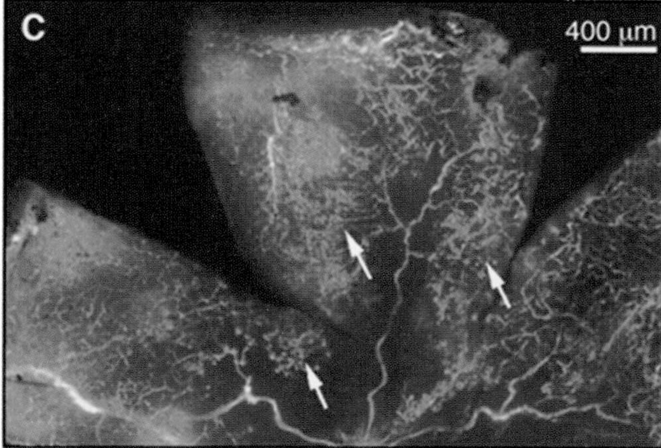

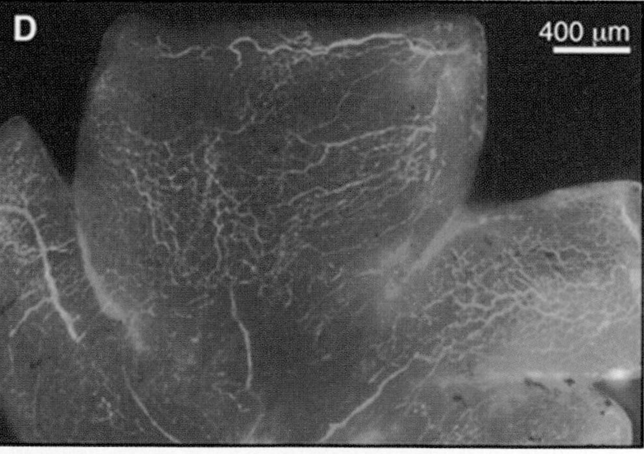

FIGURE 5.1. Effect of GH inhibition on ischemia-induced retinal neovascularization. **A:** Cross section of an eye from a nontransgenic littermate mouse, showing retinal neovascularization internal to the inner limiting membrane (*arrows*). **B:** Cross section of an eye from a GH antagonist G119K transgenic mouse. No vascular cell nuclei are apparent internal to the inner limiting membrane. **C:** Nontransgenic flat-mounted whole retina, showing extensive areas of retinal neovascularization (*bright fluorescence, indicated in part with arrows*) that is significantly reduced in the retinas from the GH antagonist G119K transgenic mice (**D**). (Reproduced from Smith et al. *Science.* 1997;276:1706–1709, with permission.)

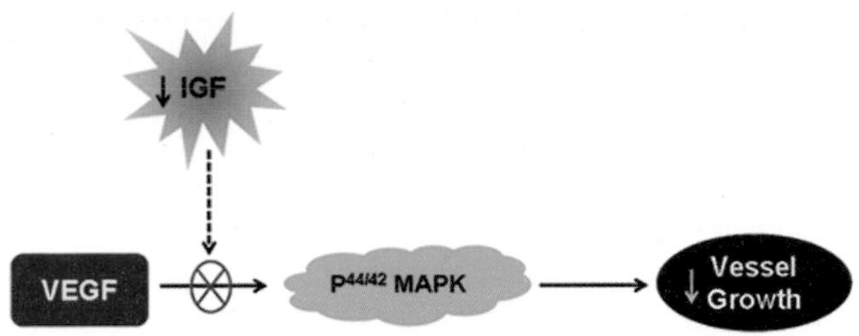

FIGURE 5.2. The relationship between IGF-I and VEGF and its effect on the growth of new blood cells.

IGF-1 regulation of retinal neovascularization is mediated at least in part through control of VEGF activation of p44/42 MAPK. IGF-1 acts permissively to allow maximum VEGF induction of new vessel growth.[21] Inadequate levels of IGF-1 inhibit vessel growth despite the presence of VEGF (Fig. 5.2).

LOW LEVELS OF IGF-1 AND PHASE 1 OF ROP

IGF-1 is also critical to the first phase of ROP[22] and to the normal development of the retinal vessels. After birth, IGF-1 is not maintained at in utero levels due to the loss of IGF-1 provided by the placenta and the amniotic fluid. We theorized that IGF-1 is critical to normal retinal vascular development and that a lack of IGF-1 in the early neonatal period is associated with a lack of vascular growth, resulting in subsequent proliferative ROP. We determined that IGF-1 is critical to normal blood vessel growth and retinal blood vessel development by examining IGF-1 null mice. We found that retinal blood vessels grew at a significantly slower rate in the IGF-1 null mice than in normal mice, a pattern very similar to that seen in premature babies with ROP. It was determined that IGF-1 controls maximum VEGF activation of the Akt endothelial cell survival pathway. This finding explains how loss of IGF-1 could cause ROP by preventing the normal survival of vascular endothelial cells.

These findings were confirmed in premature infants, where the mean IGF-1 was significantly lower in babies with ROP than babies without ROP.[22,23] These results suggest that replacement of IGF-1 to uterine levels might prevent ROP by allowing normal retinal vascular development. If vascular dropout and cessation of normal vascular growth seen in phase 1 are prevented, the destructive second phase of vaso-proliferation will not occur (Fig. 5.3).

IGF-1 IN DIABETIC RETINOPATHY

Elevated IGF-1 levels

There is a long-standing (and complex) association between IGF-1 and diabetic retinopathy,[24–26] with conflicting evidence that elevated levels of serum IGF-1 are associated with proliferative retinopathy (phase 2). The hypothesis that elevated levels of IGF-1 cause proliferative retinopathy is based in part on observations that patients with neovascular disease have very high vitreous

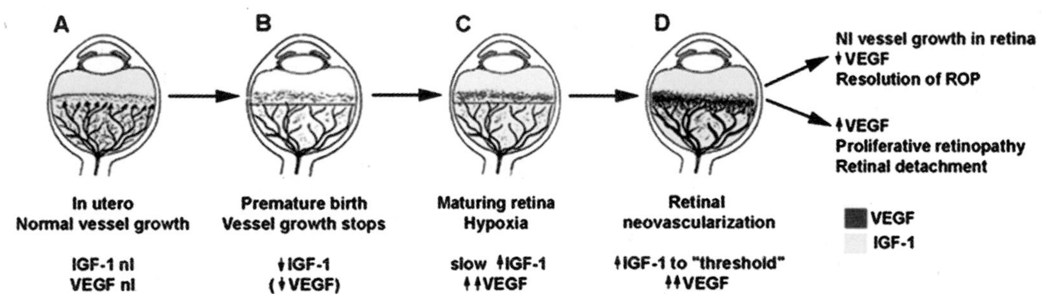

FIGURE 5.3. Schematic representation of IGF-I/VEGF control of blood vessel development in ROP. **A:** In utero, VEGF is found at the growing front of vessels. IGF-I is sufficient to allow vessel growth. **B:** With premature birth, IGF-I is not maintained at in utero levels and vascular growth ceases, despite the presence of VEGF at the growing front of vessels. Both endothelial cell survival (Akt) and proliferation (mitogen-activated protein kinase) pathways are compromised. With low IGF-I and cessation of vessel growth, a demarcation line forms at the vascular front. High oxygen exposure (as occurs in animal models and in some premature infants) may also suppress VEGF, further contributing to inhibition of vessel growth. **C:** As the premature infant matures, the developing but nonvascularized retina becomes hypoxic. VEGF increases in retina and vitreous. With maturation, the IGF-I level slowly increases. **D:** When the IGF-I level reaches a threshold at ≈34 weeks gestation, with high VEGF levels in the vitreous, endothelial cell survival and proliferation driven by VEGF may proceed. Neovascularization ensues at the demarcation line, growing into the vitreous. If VEGF vitreal levels fall, normal retinal vessel growth can proceed. With normal vascular growth and blood flow, oxygen suppresses VEGF expression, so it will no longer be overproduced. If hypoxia (and elevated levels of VEGF) persists, further neovascularization and fibrosis leading to retinal detachment can occur. (Reproduced from Hellstrom et al. *Proc Natl Acad Sci U S A.* 2001;98:5804–5808, with permission.)

levels of IGF-1.[27–31] However, it is likely that IGF system components could accumulate in the vitreous because of local production and leakage from abnormal vessels.[32,33] Specifically, it is thought that diffusion from serum plays an important role,[34] and it has been suggested that increased levels of IGF-1 in the vitreous are the result and not the cause of neovascularization. This is based on the well-established increased permeability of the blood-retina barrier in diabetic patients. Circulating IGF and IGF-binding protein-3 (IGFBP-3) levels are 10 to 100 times higher than those measured in vitreous.[34] Furthermore, patients with proliferative diabetic retinopathy show a significant positive correlation between serum and vitreous levels of IGF-1,[35] and the increase in vitreous levels of IGF-1, IGF-2, and IGFBP-3 parallels the increase in vitreous of liver-derived serum proteins. Thus, it is generally accepted that diffusion from serum plays a key role. This accumulation is caused by a nonspecific increase in leakiness of the blood-retina barrier since these same elevations are found in patients with nondiabetic causes of leaky retinal vasculature.[29,34]

Some longitudinal studies have demonstrated that intensive insulin treatment in patients with poorly controlled hyperglycemia, which rapidly increases total serum IGF-1, is associated with accelerated diabetic retinopathy.[36,37] However, the majority of investigations (cross-sectional as well as longitudinal) have found no significant correlation between circulating IGF-1 and the development of proliferative diabetic retinopathy.[38–42] An animal study of normo-glycemic/normo-insulinemic transgenic mice overexpressing IGF-1 through an insulin promoter at supraphysiological levels in the retina developed loss of pericytes (Fig. 5.4.) and thickening of basement membrane of retinal capillaries.[43] In older transgenic mice overexpressing IGF-1, neovascularization of the retina[43] (Fig. 5.5) and vitreous cavity were observed, which was consistent with increased IGF-1 induction of VEGF expression.[2] VEGF alone has been shown to cause these same effects in primates.[3] These accumulated findings suggest that once proliferative neovascular vessels occur in the retina during phase 2, leaked serum IGF-1 may further promote the proliferation of retinal vessels through stimulation of VEGF. However, it has not been established that serum IGF-1 in the absence of leaky vessels causes proliferative disease. In diabetic patients with acromegaly and elevated IGF-1 in serum and in

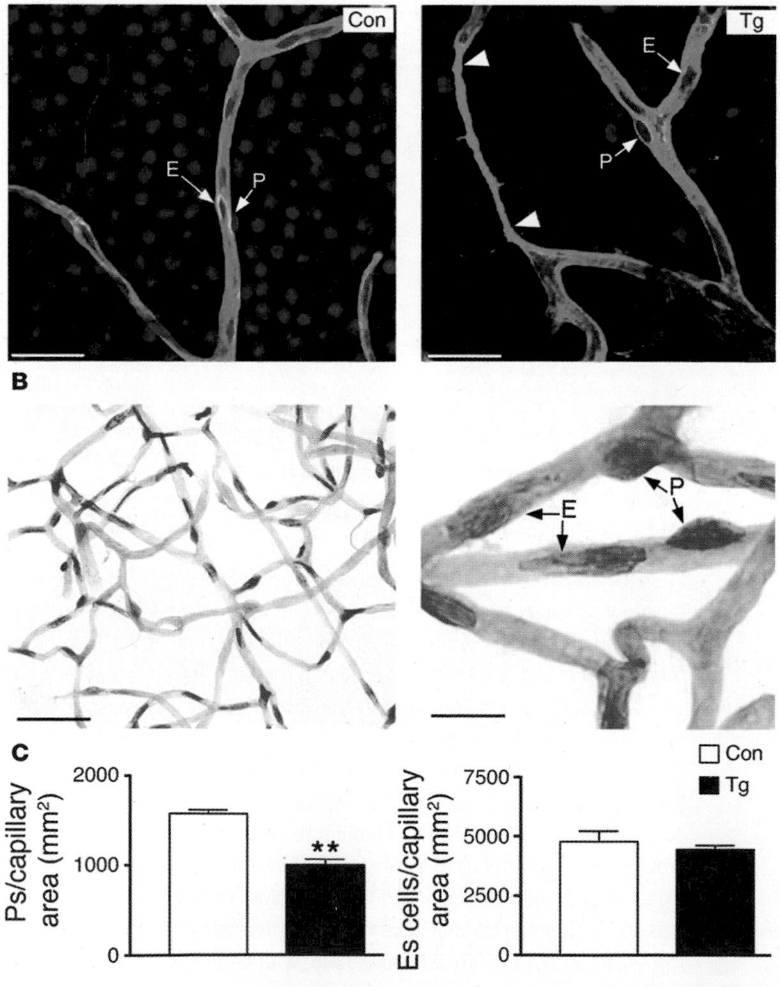

FIGURE 5.4. Pericyte loss in retinal capillaries from transgenic mice overexpressing IGF-1. **A:** Confocal analysis of retinal capillaries in flat-mounted retinas immunohistochemically marked with anticollagen IV (*green*). Nuclei were counterstained with propidium iodide (*red*). Acellular capillaries, lacking pericytes and endothelial cells, were observed (*arrowheads*) in transgenic retina. The images are single confocal sections. **B:** Retinal digest preparations were obtained. A representative area is shown (**left panel**). Endothelial cell nuclei are placed within the vessel wall, while pericyte nuclei are placed more laterally on the vessel wall (**right panel**). **C:** The number of pericytes (**left**) and endothelial cells (**right**) per square millimeter of capillary area was determined as indicated in Methods. Results are mean ± SEM of five mice in each group. $^{**}p < 0.01$. E, endothelial cell; P, pericyte. Scale bars: 35 μm (**A**), 43 μm (**B, left panel**), and 11 μm (**B, right panel**). (Reproduced from Ruberte et al. *J Clin Invest.* 2004;113:1149–1157, with permission.)

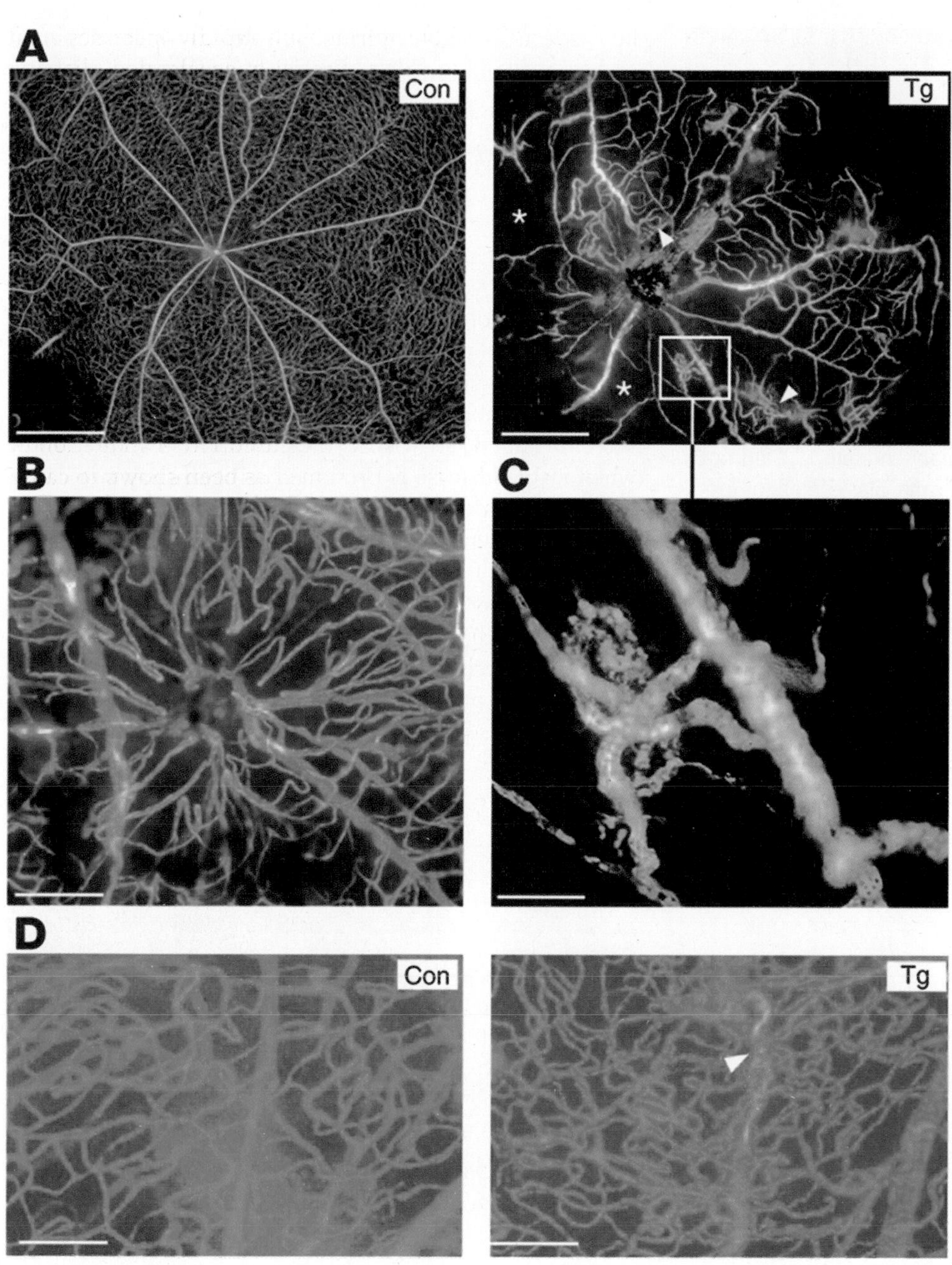

FIGURE 5.5. IRMAs (intraretinal microvascular abnormalities) and neovessels in transgenic retina. **A:** Flat-mounted, FITC-dextran–perfused retinas from transgenic eyes showed extensive areas of nonperfusion (*asterisks*) and neovessels (*arrowheads and inset*). **B:** Capillary IRMA inside the retina is shown. **C:** Neovessel originating from a venule (magnification of *inset* in **A, right panel**). This vessel had more endothelial cell nuclei after staining with propidium iodide and analysis with laser confocal microscopy (data not shown). **D:** Intraretinal dense area of neocapillaries in transgenic retina originating from a central feeding vessel (*arrowhead*). Scale bars: 630 μm (**A**), 188 μm (**B**), 87 μm (**C**), and 105 μm (**D**). (Reproduced from Ruberte et al. *J Clin Invest.* 2004;113:1149–1157, with permission.)

the vitreous, proliferative diabetic retinopathy is rare[44] (Box 5.1).

Low IGF-1 levels

While less attention has been paid to the study of the first phase of diabetic retinopathy, there is evidence that low IGF-1 is associated with vessel loss (phase 1), which could then lead to phase 2, proliferative retinopathy. There is a substantial body of work indicating that low IGF-1 is associated with the hyperglycemia of poorly controlled diabetes, which is in turn the strongest risk factor for diabetic complications. Hyperglycemia is associated with elevated GH secretion and reduced serum IGF-1 concentrations.[45,46] Low portal insulin levels are thought to lead to decreased production of IGF-1 with subsequently increased GH and IGFBP-1 levels.[47] The elevation in GH secretion, due to loss of feedback inhibition of IGF-1 resulting from low portal insulin levels, may worsen hyperglycemia by counteracting insulin action.[48] Thus, restoration of normal IGF-1 levels in insulin-treated patients with recombinant human (rh) IGF-1 or IGF-1/IGFBP-3 complex results in a concomitant reduction in GH secretion and insulin requirement to maintain euglycemia.[49–52]

A study of Laron dwarfs (with very low levels of IGF-1) found that individuals with diabetes undergo both phase 1 and phase 2 of diabetic retinopathy, suggesting that low IGF-1 may be an important contributing factor to retinopathy.[53] Low IGF-1 may also be involved in large vessel

BOX 5.1 IGF-1 Inhibitors in Clinical Trials

Octreotide

Octreotide (Sandostatin long-acting release [SLAR] Depot, Novartis Ophthalmics, East Hanover, New Jersey), a somatostatin analog, is an inhibitor of IGF-1 and GH. A randomized, controlled phase 3 trial with octreotide acetate in microspheres (30 mg intramuscular injection every 4 weeks for up to 6 years) was done in patients with severe non–proliferative diabetic retinopathy or low-risk proliferative diabetic retinopathy. Although the drug delayed the time to progression of retinopathy (primary endpoint), it did not delay time to progression to diabetic macular edema, or loss of >15 letters of vision (secondary endpoints).

Pegvisomant

A 3-month open-label trial of the GH receptor blocker, pegvisomant (Somavert, Sensus Drug Development Corporation, Austin, Texas), was done in patients with non–"high-risk" proliferative diabetic retinopathy. The trial showed no effect on regression of new vessels although there was a 50% reduction in serum levels of IGF-1.

Growth Hormone Antagonist for Proliferative Diabetic Retinopathy Study Group. The effect of a growth hormone receptor antagonist drug on proliferative diabetic retinopathy. *Ophthalmology.* 2001;108:2266–2272.

disease. Individuals with low circulating IGF-1 levels and high IGFBP-3 levels have a significantly increased risk of developing ischemic heart disease during a 15-year follow-up period.[54] Moreover, a study by Hellstrom et al. found evidence that very low IGF-1 directly causes decreased vascular density.[55]

This accumulated evidence indicates that low IGF-1 is associated with vessel loss and may be detrimental in diabetes by contributing to early vessel degeneration in phase 1. This vaso-obliteration sets the stage for hypoxia, leading later to neovascularization/proliferative retinopathy. Thus, treatment of diabetic patients with IGF-1 within the normal physiological range as an adjunct to insulin might prevent and not worsen the development of diabetic microvascular complications.[56]

CLINICAL IMPLICATIONS

These studies suggest a number of ways to intervene medically in the development of retinopathy, but they also make clear that timing is critical to any intervention. Inhibition of either VEGF or IGF-1 early after birth can prevent normal blood vessel growth and precipitate ROP, whereas inhibition at the second neovascular phase might prevent destructive neovascularization.[22,55] This also may be true in diabetic retinopathy. The choice of any intervention must be made to promote normal physiological development and survival of both blood vessels and other tissue. In particular, the proof that development of ROP is associated with low levels of IGF-1 after premature birth suggests that physiological replacement of IGF-1 to levels found in utero might prevent ROP by allowing normal vascular development.

Since it has been established that IGF-1 levels measured early after birth correlate to the degree of the later development of ROP, this information may be used to predict the development of severe disease. And since IGF-1 is related to growth, postnatal growth, which reflects IGF-1 levels might also be used to predict ROP. Currently, screening for ROP with eye examinations to determine when retinal disease is present has insufficient predictive value and is difficult in areas lacking ophthalmologists who can screen these infants. In general, only approximately 10% of screened infants require treatment. Currently, only perinatal factors such as gestational age and weight at birth are used to determine the need for ROP screening. Accumulating evidence suggests that one of the strongest predictors for ROP, in addition to low gestational age, is poor weight gain during the first weeks of

KEY POINTS

- Both ROP and diabetic retinopathy have two disease phases.
- In the first phase of ROP, there is cessation of normal retinal vascular growth, and as the baby matures, the retina becomes more hypoxic. In the first phase of diabetic retinopathy, there is also slow loss of retinal capillaries.
- In the second phase of ROP and diabetic retinopathy, there is neovascularization in the retina, which is hypoxia induced, although the progression is slower in diabetes.
- IGF-1 is critical in development of retinal blood vessels. The mean IGF-1 is significantly lower in babies with ROP than babies without ROP. Replacement of IGF-1 to uterine levels might prevent ROP by allowing normal retinal vascular development.
- Patients with proliferative diabetic retinopathy have very high vitreous levels of IGF-1. It is likely that IGF system components could accumulate in the vitreous because of local production and leakage from abnormal vessels.
- There is evidence that low IGF-1 is associated with vessel loss and may be detrimental in diabetes by contributing to early vessel degeneration in phase 1.
- Physiological replacement of IGF-1 to levels found in utero might prevent ROP by allowing normal vascular development.

life.[57,58] In these studies, the risk of sight-threatening ROP is predicted using postnatal weight gain as well as gestational age and/or weight at birth. Using an algorithm, the authors could detect early 100% of infants who developed ROP requiring treatment and correctly predicted the majority who did not require treatment. With this simple postnatal evaluation, costly and stressful eye examinations can be markedly reduced by approximately 75%. In addition, early identification of children at risk may lead to the initiation of interventions and possibly prevent sight-threatening ROP. However, before new screening guidelines can be constructed, further validation of this surveillance system has to be performed on other populations of infants.

REFERENCES

1. Patz A, Hoeck LE, De La Cruz E. Studies on the effect of high oxygen administration in retrolental fibroplasia. I. Nursery observations. *Am J Ophthalmol*. 1952;35:1248–1253.
2. Punglia RS, Lu M, Hsu J, et al. Regulation of vascular endothelial growth factor expression by insulin-like growth factor I. *Diabetes*. 1997;46:1619–1626.
3. Tolentino MJ, McLeod DS, Taomoto M, et al. Pathologic features of vascular endothelial growth factor-induced retinopathy in the nonhuman primate. *Am J Ophthalmol*. 2002;133:373–385.
4. Smith LE, Wesolowski E, McLellan A, et al. Oxygen-induced retinopathy in the mouse. *Invest Ophthalmol Vis Sci*. 1994;35:101–111.
5. Ashton N. Oxygen and the growth and development of retinal vessels. In vivo and in vitro studies. The XX Francis I. Proctor Lecture. *Am J Ophthalmol*. 1966;62:412–435.
6. Penn JS, Tolman BL, Henry MM. Oxygen-induced retinopathy in the rat: relationship of retinal nonperfusion to subsequent neovascularization. *Invest Ophthalmol Vis Sci*. 1994;35:3429–3435.
7. Plate KH, Breier G, Weich HA, et al. Vascular endothelial growth factor is a potential tumour angiogenesis factor in human gliomas in vivo. *Nature*. 1992;359:845–848.
8. Kim KJ, Li B, Winer J, et al. Inhibition of vascular endothelial growth factor-induced angiogenesis suppresses tumour growth in vivo. *Nature*. 1993;362:841–844.
9. Pierce EA, Avery RL, Foley ED, et al. Vascular endothelial growth factor/vascular permeability factor expression in a mouse model of retinal neovascularization. *Proc Natl Acad Sci U S A*. 1995;92:905–909.
10. Aiello LP, Pierce EA, Foley ED, et al. Suppression of retinal neovascularization in vivo by inhibition of vascular endothelial growth factor (VEGF) using soluble VEGF-receptor chimeric proteins. *Proc Natl Acad Sci U S A*. 1995;92:10457–10461.
11. Robinson GS, Pierce EA, Rook SL, et al. Oligodeoxynucleotides inhibit retinal neovascularization in a murine model of proliferative retinopathy. *Proc Natl Acad Sci U S A*. 1996;93:4851–4856.
12. Donahue ML, Phelps DL, Watkins RH, et al. Retinal vascular endothelial growth factor (VEGF) mRNA expression is altered in relation to neovascularization in oxygen induced retinopathy. *Curr Eye Res*. 1996;15:175–184.
13. Stone J, Chan-Ling T, Pe'er J, et al. Roles of vascular endothelial growth factor and astrocyte degeneration in the genesis of retinopathy of prematurity. *Invest Ophthalmol Vis Sci*. 1996;37:290–299.
14. Adamis AP, Shima DT, Tolentino MJ, et al. Inhibition of vascular endothelial growth factor prevents retinal ischemia-associated iris neovascularization in a nonhuman primate. *Arch Ophthalmol*. 1996;114:66–71.
15. Young TL, Anthony DC, Pierce E, et al. Histopathology and vascular endothelial growth factor in untreated and diode laser-treated retinopathy of prematurity. *J AAPOS*. 1997;1:105–110.
16. Aiello LP, Avery RL, Arrigg PG, et al. Vascular endothelial growth factor in ocular fluid of patients with diabetic retinopathy and other retinal disorders. *N Engl J Med*. 1994;331:1480–1487.
17. Alon T, Hemo I, Itin A, et al. Vascular endothelial growth factor acts as a survival factor for newly formed retinal vessels and has implications for retinopathy of prematurity. *Nat Med*. 1995;1:1024–1028.
18. Shih SC, Ju M, Liu N, et al. Selective stimulation of VEGFR-1 prevents oxygen-induced retinal vascular degeneration in retinopathy of prematurity. *J Clin Invest*. 2003;112:50–57.
19. Sharp PS, Fallon TJ, Brazier OJ, et al. Long-term follow-up of patients who underwent yttrium-90 pituitary implantation for treatment of proliferative diabetic retinopathy. *Diabetologia*. 1987;30:199–207.
20. Smith LE, Kopchick JJ, Chen W, et al. Essential role of growth hormone in ischemia-induced retinal neovascularization. *Science*. 1997;276:1706–1709.
21. Smith LE, Shen W, Perruzzi C, et al. Regulation of vascular endothelial growth factor-dependent retinal neovascularization by insulin-like growth factor-1 receptor. *Nat Med*. 1999;5:1390–1395.
22. Hellstrom A, Perruzzi C, Ju M, et al. Low IGF-I suppresses VEGF-survival signaling in retinal endothelial cells: direct correlation with clinical retinopathy of prematurity. *Proc Natl Acad Sci U S A*. 2001;98:5804–5808.
23. Hellstrom A, Engström E, Hård AL, et al. Postnatal serum insulin-like growth factor I deficiency is associated with retinopathy of prematurity and other complications of premature birth. *Pediatrics*. 2003;112:1016–1020.
24. Merimee TJ, Zapf J, Froesch ER. Insulin-like growth factors. Studies in diabetics with and without retinopathy. *N Engl J Med*. 1983;309:527–530.
25. Dills DG, Moss SE, Klein R, et al. Is insulinlike growth factor I associated with diabetic retinopathy? *Diabetes*. 1990;39:191–195.
26. Simo R, Lecube A, Segura RM, et al. Free insulin growth factor-I and vascular endothelial growth factor in the vitreous fluid of patients with proliferative diabetic retinopathy. *Am J Ophthalmol*. 2002;134:376–382.
27. Burgos R, Mateo C, Cantón A, et al. Vitreous levels of IGF-I, IGF binding protein 1, and IGF binding protein 3 in proliferative diabetic retinopathy: a case-control study. *Diabetes Care*. 2000;23:80–83.
28. Meyer-Schwickerath R, Pfeiffer A, Blum WF, et al. Vitreous levels of the insulin-like growth factors I and II, and the insulin-like growth factor binding proteins 2 and 3, increase in neovascular eye disease. Studies in nondiabetic and diabetic subjects. *J Clin Invest*. 1993;92:2620–2625.

29. Spranger J, Bühnen J, Jansen V, et al. Systemic levels contribute significantly to increased intraocular IGF-I, IGF-II and IGF-BP3 [correction of IFG-BP3] in proliferative diabetic retinopathy. *Horm Metab Res.* 2000;32:196–200.
30. Waldbillig RJ, Jones BE, Schoen TJ, et al. Vitreal insulin-like growth factor binding proteins (IGFBPs) are increased in human and animal diabetics. *Curr Eye Res.* 1994;13:539–546.
31. Boulton M, Gregor Z, McLeod D, et al. Intravitreal growth factors in proliferative diabetic retinopathy: correlation with neovascular activity and glycaemic management. *Br J Ophthalmol.* 1997;81:228–233.
32. Spoerri PE, Ellis EA, Tarnuzzer RW, et al. Insulin-like growth factor: receptor and binding proteins in human retinal endothelial cell cultures of diabetic and non-diabetic origin. *Growth Horm IGF Res.* 1998;8:125–132.
33. Lofqvist C, Willett KL, Aspegren O, et al. Quantification and localization of the IGF/insulin system expression in retinal blood vessels and neurons during oxygen-induced retinopathy in mice. *Invest Ophthalmol Vis Sci.* 2009;50:1831–1837.
34. Pfeiffer A, Spranger J, Meyer-Schwickerath R, et al. Growth factor alterations in advanced diabetic retinopathy: a possible role of blood retina barrier breakdown. *Diabetes.* 1997;46(Suppl 2):S26–S30.
35. Grant M, Russell B, Fitzgerald C, et al. Insulin-like growth factors in vitreous. Studies in control and diabetic subjects with neovascularization. *Diabetes.* 1986;35:416–420.
36. Chantelau E, Eggert H, Seppel T, et al. Elevation of serum IGF-1 precedes proliferative diabetic retinopathy in Mauriac's syndrome. *Br J Ophthalmol.* 1997;81:169–170.
37. Hyer SL, Sharp PS, Sleightholm M, et al. Progression of diabetic retinopathy and changes in serum insulin-like growth factor I (IGF I) during continuous subcutaneous insulin infusion (CSII). *Horm Metab Res.* 1989;21:18–22.
38. Wang Q, Dills DG, Klein R, et al. Does insulin-like growth factor I predict incidence and progression of diabetic retinopathy? *Diabetes.* 1995;44:161–164.
39. Sharp PS, Beshyah SA, Johnston DG. Growth hormone disorders and secondary diabetes. *Baillieres Clin Endocrinol Metab.* 1992;6:819–828.
40. Frystyk J, Bek T, Flyvbjerg A, et al. The relationship between the circulating IGF system and the presence of retinopathy in Type 1 diabetic patients. *Diabet Med.* 2003;20:269–276.
41. Feldmann B, Jehle PM, Mohan S, et al. Diabetic retinopathy is associated with decreased serum levels of free IGF-I and changes of IGF-binding proteins. *Growth Horm IGF Res.* 2000;10:53–59.
42. Feldmann B, Lang GE, Arnavaz A, et al. Decreased serum level of free bioavailable IGF-I in patients with diabetic retinopathy. *Ophthalmologe.* 1999;96:300–305.
43. Ruberte J, Ayuso E, Navarro M, et al. Increased ocular levels of IGF-1 in transgenic mice lead to diabetes-like eye disease. *J Clin Invest.* 2004;113:1149–1157.
44. van Setten G, Brismar K, Algvere P. Elevated intraocular levels of insulin-like growth factor I in a diabetic patient with acromegaly. *Orbit.* 2002;21:161–167.
45. Dunger DB, Cheetham TD, Crowne EC. Insulin-like growth factors (IGFs) and IGF-I treatment in the adolescent with insulin-dependent diabetes mellitus. *Metabolism.* 1995;44:119–123.
46. Janssen JA, Jacobs ML, Derkx FH, et al. Free and total insulin-like growth factor I (IGF-I), IGF-binding protein-1 (IGFBP-1), and IGFBP-3 and their relationships to the presence of diabetic retinopathy and glomerular hyperfiltration in insulin-dependent diabetes mellitus. *J Clin Endocrinol Metab.* 1997;82:2809–2815.
47. Moller N, Orskov H. Does IGF-I therapy in insulin-dependent diabetes mellitus limit complications? *Lancet.* 1997;350:1188–1189.
48. Holly JM, Amiel SA, Sandhu RR, et al. The role of growth hormone in diabetes mellitus. *J Endocrinol.* 1988;118:353–364.
49. Moses AC, Young SC, Morrow LA, et al. Recombinant human insulin-like growth factor I increases insulin sensitivity and improves glycemic control in type II diabetes. *Diabetes.* 1996;45:91–100.
50. Cheetham TD, Connors M, Clayton K, et al. The relationship between overnight GH levels and insulin concentrations in adolescents with insulin-dependent diabetes mellitus (IDDM) and the impact of recombinant human insulin-like growth factor I (rhIGF-I). *Clin Endocrinol (Oxf).* 1997;46:415–424.
51. Clemmons DR, Moses AC, McKay MJ, et al. The combination of insulin-like growth factor I and insulin-like growth factor-binding protein-3 reduces insulin requirements in insulin-dependent type 1 diabetes: evidence for in vivo biological activity. *J Clin Endocrinol Metab.* 2000;85:1518–1524.
52. O'Connell T, Clemmons DR. IGF-I/IGF-binding protein-3 combination improves insulin resistance by GH-dependent and independent mechanisms. *J Clin Endocrinol Metab.* 2002;87:4356–4360.
53. Laron Z, Weinberger D. Diabetic retinopathy in two patients with congenital IGF-I deficiency (Laron syndrome). *Eur J Endocrinol.* 2004;151:103–106.
54. Juul A, Scheike T, Davidsen M, et al. Low serum insulin-like growth factor I is associated with increased risk of ischemic heart disease: a population-based case-control study. *Circulation.* 2002;106:939–944.
55. Hellstrom A, Carlsson B, Niklasson A, et al. IGF-I is critical for normal vascularization of the human retina. *J Clin Endocrinol Metab.* 2002;87:3413–3416.
56. Janssen JA, Lamberts SW. Circulating IGF-I and its protective role in the pathogenesis of diabetic angiopathy. *Clin Endocrinol (Oxf).* 2000;52:1–9.
57. Lofqvist C, Andersson E, Sigurdsson J, et al. Longitudinal postnatal weight and insulin-like growth factor I measurements in the prediction of retinopathy of prematurity. *Arch Ophthalmol.* 2006;124:1711–1718.
58. Hellstrom A, Hård AL, Engström E, et al. Early weight gain predicts retinopathy in preterm infants: new, simple, efficient approach to screening. *Pediatrics.* 2009;123:e638–e645.

CHAPTER

6

Is It All VEGF? Other Angiogenic Factors

Susan E. Yanni • Gary W. McCollum • John S. Penn

Pathologic growth of new blood vessels is a common feature of ocular neovascular diseases such as age-related macular degeneration (AMD), proliferative diabetic retinopathy (PDR), and retinopathy of prematurity (ROP). These diseases often result in irreversible loss of vision. Vascular endothelial growth factor (VEGF) is the primary angiogenic factor that mediates the choroidal and retinal neovascularization (NV) occurring in these conditions. VEGF levels are elevated in the vitreous fluid of patients with active retinal NV, and VEGF induces the proliferation, migration, and tube formation of vascular endothelial (VE) cells in vitro.[1] Locally expressed VEGF is believed to play a key role in the development of choroidal NV (CNV) and its sequelae in wet AMD.[2]

This belief led to the development of a class of therapeutics for the treatment of wet AMD based on VEGF antagonism.[3,4] VEGF antagonists currently employed in clinical practice include the following: pegaptanib (Macugen, Pfizer), an RNA-like aptamer; bevacizumab (Avastin, Genentech), a humanized mouse monoclonal antibody to human VEGF that was approved for systemic administration in the treatment of cancer but is used off-label in the treatment of AMD; and ranibizumab (Lucentis, Genentech), the F(ab) fragment of an anti-VEGF similar to Avastin, which is approved for use in AMD. The therapeutic efficacy of these VEGF antagonists has been remarkable, although there are important limitations that stem, in part, from the requirement to administer the antagonists by frequently repeated intravitreal injections. In addition to the discomfort and costs associated with the procedures, this approach leads to high peak levels and prolonged trough levels of antagonist, during which time it is subtherapeutic. This unfavorable pharmacokinetic profile may contribute to reduced efficacy, as exemplified by the incomplete arrest of disease progression observed in many patients, and the frank resistance to therapy that characterizes others. Periods of very high levels of the antagonist may contribute to both local and systemic toxicity. Morbidity related to the intravitreal injections is another important limitation of the current treatment regimen.[5] The most frequent and problematic injection-related toxicity is the development of endophthalmitis, a potentially blinding condition,[6] observed at a rate as high as 1.3% per patient per year in clinical studies. This toxicity is expected to rise as the treatment becomes part of standard practice and is performed outside of the rigorous settings of clinical trials in academic centers. Finally, it remains unclear if chronic administration of anti-VEGF drugs will exert a negative influence on the retinal neurons that are known to express VEGF receptors or on the sensitivity and response of the retinal or choroidal vasculature to VEGF stimulation.

Thus, although inhibition of VEGF clearly reduces ischemia-driven NV, it does not completely eliminate it. Therefore, the involvement of other angiogenic factors in this process seems likely, and many candidate factors have been identified and are currently under consideration as therapeutic targets. Several of the most prominent of these candidates are discussed here.

BASIC FIBROBLAST GROWTH FACTOR

Basic fibroblast growth factor (bFGF; FGF-2) is one of the prototype members of the FGF family of growth factors. FGF-2 contains heparin/heparan sulfate–binding domains, which enhance receptor binding, leading to receptor dimerization, transautophosphorylation, and activation of downstream signaling cascades.[7] FGF-2 lacks a signal sequence for export out of the cell and is released only upon cell shearing or cell death.[8] Regardless of the mechanism responsible for its release, FGF-2 is a ubiquitous molecule, known to induce the proliferation and differentiation of a wide range of mesodermal and neuroectodermal cells.[9] Additionally, levels of FGF-2 are elevated in the body fluids of patients who carry large tumor burdens and hence is implicated in the angiogenic process.[10]

In the eye, FGF-2 has been localized to the astrocytes of the retinal ganglion cell layer, as well as to the inner nuclear layer.[11,12] FGF-2 has been demonstrated in the vitreous of patients with PDR, in the retinal tissue of mice that have been exposed to conditions that stimulate NV of the sort that occurs in ROP (oxygen-induced retinopathy or OIR), and in the retinal pigment epithelium (RPE) following laser-induced rupture of Bruch's membrane, resulting in CNV.[13–15] In addition, FGF-2 is routinely implanted into avascular rodent corneas in order to study the angiogenic process, because it induces potent, angiogenic ingrowth of vessels, yielding a model with which to test a compound's antiangiogenic efficacy.[16] This model of corneal angiogenesis, however, is of limited clinical relevance as the cornea is a naturally avascular tissue. In more clinically relevant models of retinal and choroidal NV, FGF-2 (unlike VEGF) does not appear to induce, or be required for, the development of NV.[17,18] However, and of importance, the cellular responses to several important growth factors can be augmented by FGF-2 addition.[19] And, recently, investigators have demonstrated that a combination of VEGF and FGF-2 inhibition led to a more significant reduction in RPE-induced angiogenic cell behaviors than did VEGF inhibition alone.[20] These findings suggest that FGF-2 plays a role in mediating ocular NV, likely acting in synergy with VEGF.

CYCLOOXYGENASE-2

The cyclooxygenase (COX) enzymes catalyze the production of prostaglandin H_2 (PGH_2) from membrane-derived arachidonic acid. The unstable intermediate PGH_2 is converted to biologically active prostanoids (PG; prostaglandins and thromboxane) by cell- and tissue-specific synthases (Fig. 6.1). COX-1 and COX-2 catalyze identical reactions and retain 60% amino acid sequence identity. COX-1, however, is typically regarded as a "housekeeping" enzyme whose constitutive expression and PG products are responsible for maintenance of the gastric mucosa, platelet aggregation, and regulation of the renal vasculature.[21] COX-2, on the other hand, is the product of an immediate early gene, inducible by mitogens, cytokines, and tumor promoters.[22] Nonsteroidal anti-inflammatory drugs (NSAIDs) inhibit the activity of the COX enzymes. The finding that regular NSAID use leads to a reduction in colorectal cancer risk and that COX-2 is elevated in this and other cancer types has led to the suggestion that COX-2 and its PG products may act as tumor promoters.[23,24] At least one tumor-promoting function of the PGs is the

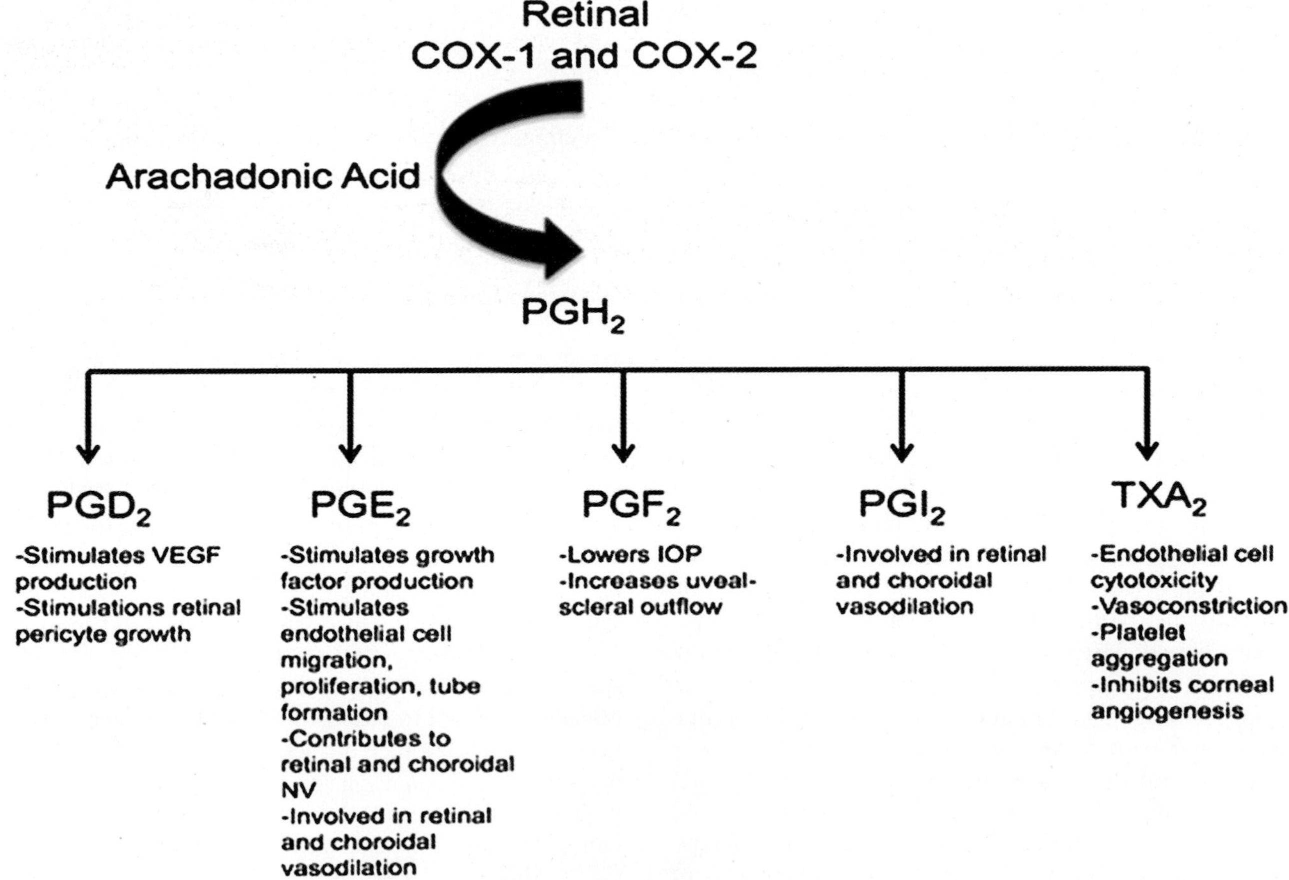

FIGURE 6.1. The cyclooxygenase cascade. COX-1 and COX-2 catalyze the biosynthesis of prostanoids (prostaglandins and thromboxane) from membrane-derived arachidonic acid. The prostanoids then bind to their cognate GPCRs (G-protein coupled receptors) on the surface of target cells, initiating and affecting a wide range of physiological and pathological processes. Some of the ocular effects are listed.

stimulation of angiogenesis.[25–27] Therefore, NSAIDs that inhibit the activity of the COX enzymes may be viable pharmacologic agents for the treatment of ocular NV.

Selective inhibition of COX-2 prevents pathological NV in the cornea, retina, and choroid. Two investigative teams have used rodent models of cautery-induced corneal NV to demonstrate that indomethacin, a nonselective COX inhibitor, and NS-398, a COX-2–selective inhibitor, significantly inhibit corneal NV and the concomitant model-induced increase in corneal PGE_2 and VEGF.[28,29] These findings suggest that COX-2 and the PGs mediate corneal NV in a VEGF-dependent manner.

COX-2 has also been implicated in the retinal NV that characterizes PDR and ROP. Several investigators have used streptozotocin (STZ)-induced diabetic rats to study the effect of COX-2 inhibition on the development of retinopathy. Treating the animals with celecoxib, an NSAID with moderate COX-2 selectivity, led to significant reductions in retinal PGE_2, VEGF mRNA expression, and vascular leakage.[30–32] Treating diabetic rats with topical nepafenac, a nonselective COX inhibitor, has been shown to inhibit the functional abnormalities and retinal vasculopathy observed in rats with STZ-induced diabetes.[33] These studies suggest a functional link between the COX pathway and PDR. Other investigators have used rodent models of ROP to define the involvement of COX-2 in retinal NV. Rodents treated with rofecoxib, etodolac, and APHS, COX-2 selective NSAIDs, and topical nepafenac demonstrate reduced retinal NV[34–36] (Fig. 6.2). In the case of etodolac, this effect was abolished by the addition of exogenous PGE_2, supporting a role for COX-derived PGs in mediating retinal NV. The same study provides data suggesting that the effect of PGE_2 is mediated through the EP_3 receptor. Signaling through EP_3 downregulates the antiangiogenic factor thrombospondin-1 (TSP-1) and its receptor, CD36. Another study demonstrates that the EP_4 receptor is involved in mediating angiogenic cell behaviors (VEGF production and endothelial cell proliferation and tube formation) and experimentally induced CNV and ROP using in vivo animal models.[37]

In rodent models of CNV, etodolac and lumiracoxib, NSAIDs with COX-2 selectivity, significantly inhibited CNV leakage, lesion size, and the development of choroidal neovascular membranes (CNVMs; angiogenic outgrowths that infiltrate the retina).[38,39] Additionally, topical ocular administration of nepafenac inhibited laser-induced CNV.[36] These studies suggest that COX-2 mediates various aspects of CNV.

In conclusion, ocular studies suggest that COX-2 and the PGs play a role in mediating NV, involving at least some degree of interaction, in some subset of cases, with VEGF.

ANGIOPOIETINS

There are four angiopoietin ligands (Ang1 to 4) and two related receptors, Tie1 and Tie2.[40] The best studied angiopoietins are angiopoietin 1 (Ang1) and angiopoietin 2 (Ang2). In vivo, Ang1 and Ang2 function in a complementary fashion to maintain vascular integrity. Ang1 promotes the integrity of vasculature by recruiting mural cells to blood vessels.[41] Transgenic mice deficient in Ang1 exhibit dissociation of endothelial cells and mural cells, severely impairing vascular function and leading to embryonic death.[42,43] Initially, Ang2 was identified as an Ang1 antagonist, inhibiting Tie2 activation by Ang1. Transgenic mice overexpressing Ang2 have phenotypes

(A)

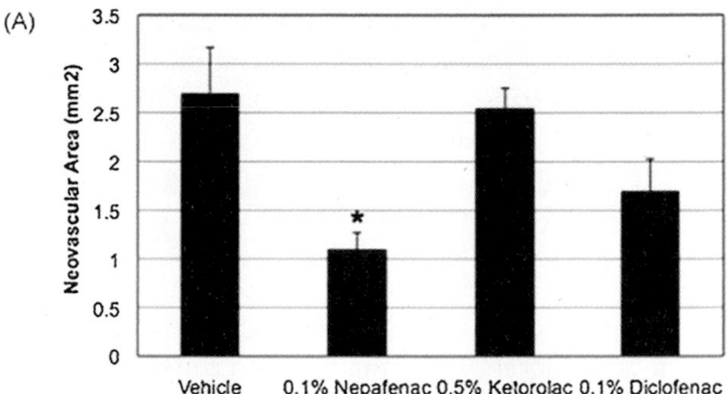

(B)

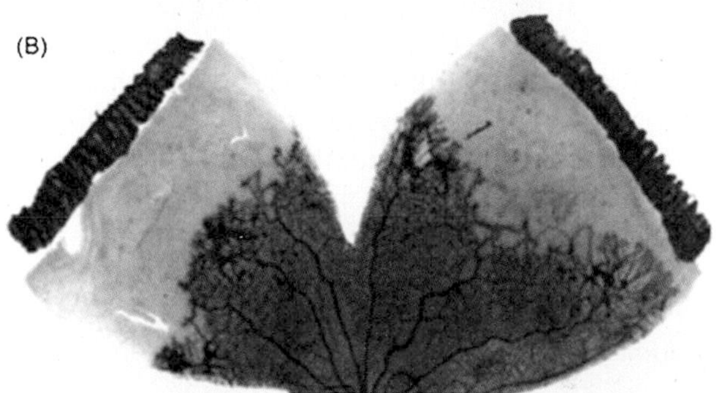

(C)

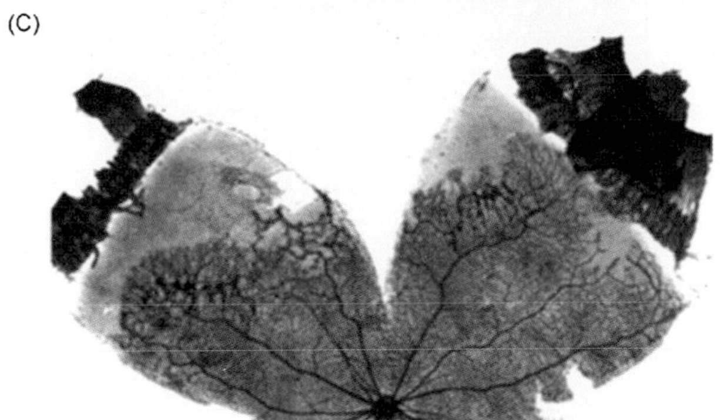

FIGURE 6.2. The effect of topical nepafenac, ketorolac, and diclofenac on the severity of OIR in the rat. **A:** Drugs were administered topically, QID, from P14-P19. Nepafenac significantly reduced (*$p \leq 0.007$) OIR-induced retinal NV. Ketorolac and diclofenac failed to demonstrate an effect. Each bar represents the mean ± SEM. **B:** A representative image of NV in vehicle-treated eyes. **C:** A representative image of NV in nepafenac-treated eyes. As demonstrated by representative ADPase-stained retinal flat mounts, nepafenac significantly reduced retinal NV. (Reproduced from Yanni et al. *Brain Res Bull.* 2010;81:310, with permission.)

similar to those of Ang1-deficient mice, where the dissociation of endothelial cells and mural cells severely disrupts blood vessel formation in the embryos. In adult mice and humans, Ang2 is expressed only at sites of vascular remodeling.[44] The primary role of Ang2 in angiogenesis appears to be in concert with VEGF. In the presence of VEGF, Ang2 destabilizes blood vessels by disrupting interactions between endothelial cells and mural cells, thus enhancing VEGF-induced endothelial cell proliferation and migration. In the absence of VEGF, however, Ang2 accelerates vessel regression.[45] This relationship was demonstrated by a study of the hyaloid vasculature. In the presence of exogenous VEGF, Ang2 promoted a rapid increase in hyaloid capillary diameter, remodeling of the basal lamina, proliferation and migration of endothelial cells, and stimulated the sprouting of new blood vessels. When VEGF was inhibited, Ang2 induced endothelial cell apoptosis, resulting in hyaloid vessel regression.[46]

In contrast to Tie2 signaling, Tie1 signaling is still poorly understood. Experiments have shown that Tie1 activation can initiate the PI3K–AKT signaling pathway to promote cell survival.[47] These findings suggest that Tie1 elicits signaling cascades similar to those initiated by Tie2. However, Tie1-specific ligands have not been identified, suggesting that Tie1 might be activated by other mechanisms. Recent work suggests that Tie1 is proteolytically cleaved following endothelial cell activation. The exposure of cultured endothelial cells to phorbol-12-myristate-13-acetate (PMA), VEGF, or shear stress induces cleavage of Tie1.[48,49] The biological consequence of this process is not understood, but the truncated form of Tie1 that is generated is thought to contribute to Tie2 signal transduction. For a review of angiopoietin-mediated signal transduction cascades and bioactivity, see Figure 6.3.

Particularly important in the context of ocular disease is the effect of hypoxia on angiopoietins. Oh and coworkers have shown that Ang1 and Tie2 are stable in microvascular endothelial cells exposed to hypoxia, whereas Ang2 expression increases.[50] Additionally, Ang2 expression in endothelial cells is tightly controlled by several angiogenic inducers including VEGF, FGF-2, and TNF-α and by environmental changes including high glucose.[50–54] In vivo,

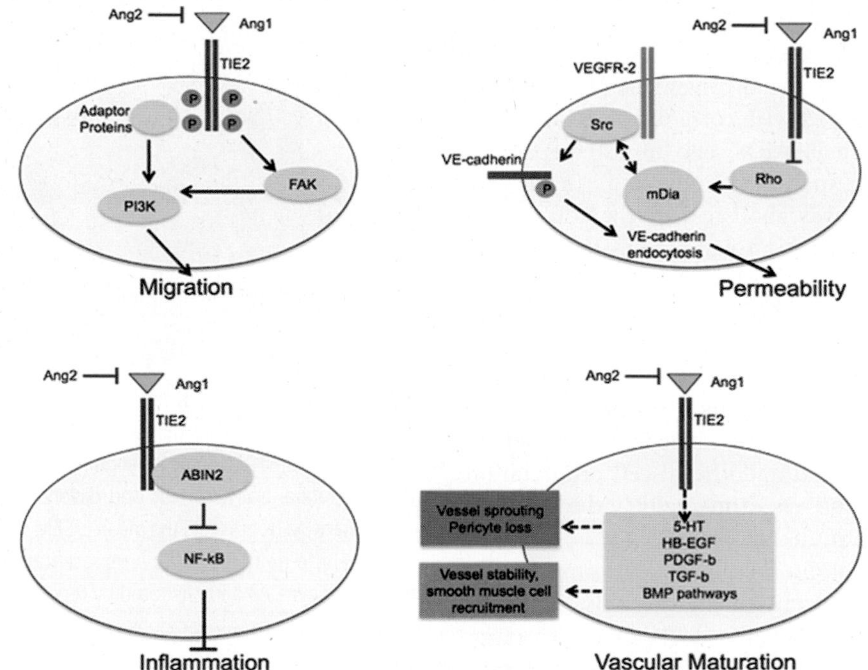

FIGURE 6.3. The effect of angiopoietins on endothelial cell (EC) signal transduction and angiogenic cell behaviors. Ang1-mediated phosphorylation of focal adhesion kinase (FAK) and other adaptor proteins leads to phosphoinositide 3-kinase (PI3K)–mediated **cell migration**. In the absence of Ang1, Src is not sequestered by mammalian diaphanous (mDia). VEGF stimulation activates Src, which leads to the internalization of VE-cadherin. This destabilizes interendothelial junctions and increases **permeability**. Tie2 activation leads to the recruitment of the intracellular protein ABIN2 (A20 binding inhibitor of NF kappa B2). This blocks the nuclear factor-kappa B (NF-κB) pathway, therefore exerting **anti-inflammatory** effects. Ang2 counteracts this response, leading to inflammation. Ang1–Tie2 signaling is required for **vascular maturation** (*purple box*). Ang2 is an antagonistic regulator of ECs and thereby leads to vessel destabilization and pericyte dropout (*red box*). The exact molecular mechanisms of this process are poorly understood. The possible regulatory molecules that are involved in this process are listed. (Adapted from Augustin HG, Koh GY, Thurston G, et al. Control of vascular morphogenesis and homeostasis through the angiopoietin-Tie system. *Nature Rev Mol Cell Biol.* 2009;10:165–177 with permission.)

Ang2 expression is greatly increased in the neovascular growth accompanying OIR in mice.[50] These findings suggest that Ang2, acting in concert with VEGF and other angiogenic inducers, contributes to the ocular NV characterizing several sight-threatening diseases. Consequently, several methods of Ang2 inhibition are currently under assessment for inhibition of tumor growth and retinal NV in preclinical tests.[55,56]

ERYTHROPOIETIN

Apart from its essential role in the regulation of red blood cell production, Erythropoietin (Epo) is involved in diverse nonhematopoietic biological functions. Various types of VE cells express the Epo receptor (EpoR), and Epo promotes the migration and proliferation of endothelial cells in different in vitro experimental models.[57–60] During development, Epo–EpoR signaling is required not only for fetal liver erythropoiesis but also for physiologic angiogenesis in the developing mouse embryo.[61,62] A series of studies suggests that endogenous Epo–EpoR signaling contributes to the angiogenic aspect of wound healing, a feature that is inhibited by neutralizing anti-Epo antibodies and recombinant soluble EpoR.[63] In the central nervous system, where Epo is produced by astrocytes and EpoR is expressed by neurons, administration of soluble EpoR is associated with enhancement of ischemic brain injury in rats, demonstrating that Epo plays an important role in the brain's response to neuronal injury.[64] Epo and its novel derivatives have emerged as major tissue-protective cytokines that are being investigated in human studies involving both neurological and cardiovascular diseases.[65]

Although Epo is a survival factor for retinal photoreceptors,[66] significant upregulation of endogenous Epo in the vitreous of patients with diabetes was found to be associated with PDR.[67] Furthermore, Epo blockade was shown to inhibit retinal NV in the ischemic mouse retina, suggesting that Epo signaling may be a potential therapeutic target in the pathological angiogenesis of PDR.[67] In a meta-analysis of Epo treatment for prematurity-related anemia, early Epo administration was associated with a significantly increased risk of ROP,[68] an effect that may be associated with EpoR activation on endothelial cells and NV.[69] This finding, however, was contradicted by those of Shah et al.,[70] who found no significant difference in the onset or progression of ROP or the incidence of plus, prethreshold, or threshold disease between rhEPO-treated and nontreated groups of very low birth weight infants, all of whom received ROP treatment. In conclusion, although Epo-EpoR signaling has been implicated in various angiogenic processes, its precise role in ocular angiogenesis has yet to be elucidated.

INTERLEUKINS

The interleukins (IL) comprise a family of soluble proteins that mediate the interaction between immune cells and inflammatory cells. Today, at least 34 ILs and IL subtypes have been identified.

For some time, it has been known that the inflammatory response can solicit an angiogenic response. Because ILs induce the proliferation of immune cells, investigators hypothesized that some ILs might affect endothelial cells in the same way. In an early study, BenEzra et al.[71] tested IL-1α, IL-1β, and IL-2 in a model of corneal angiogenesis. IL-1α and IL-1β induced a consistent angiogenic response. In another study, corneal explants exposed to IL-1β demonstrated an upregulation of IL-8, which has been shown to be proangiogenic.[72]

There is evidence that IL-4 may exert both proangiogenic and antiangiogenic effects, depending on the experimental setting. In the eye, IL-4 induced NV in the rabbit corneal micropocket assay.[73]

In human cerebral endothelial cells, IL-6 stimulates endothelial cell proliferation and migration in a dose-dependent manner and stimulates a concurrent increase in VEGF expression.[74] Interestingly, experiments designed to test for possible signaling mechanisms revealed an IL-6–dependent activation of VEGFR-2 and MMP-9 overexpression. MMP-9 has been shown to be important in the development of retinal NV.[75] Of particular clinical relevance, circulating blood endothelial progenitor cells (EPC) have received considerable attention because they home to sites of angiogenesis. IL-6 stimulates EPC proliferation, migration, and tube formation.[76] These findings suggest that IL-6 has the potential to stimulate EPC involvement and incorporation into ocular neovasculature.

IL-8 has been shown to be proangiogenic. This effect may be due to the ability of IL-8 to inhibit apoptosis and upregulate MMP-2 and MMP-9.[77] Like MMP-9, MMP-2 is involved in retinal angiogenesis.[75]

Experimental evidence suggests that IL-10 may exert a proangiogenic effect in the context of ocular angiogenesis. In a mouse model of OIR, IL-10–deficient mice showed less NV than did wild type controls.[78] The authors attribute this response to the finding that wild type macrophages produced IL-10, which induced higher levels of retinal VEGF, contributing to the pathology. In another study of inflammation-induced corneal NV, IL-10–deficient mice demonstrated a delayed NV response.[79] These studies suggest that IL-10, in the context of retinal and corneal NV, contributes to the angiogenic phenotype. IL-10 has also been hypothesized to contribute to the angiogenic phenotype in AMD. It is believed that during the pathogenesis of AMD, macrophages can switch from an antiangiogenic to a proangiogenic phenotype.[80–82] Studies in mice have shown that low levels of IL-10 result in an antiangiogenic macrophage phenotype.[82] According to theory, young macrophages express low levels of IL-10, leading to increased levels of IL-6 and IL-12, which have antiangiogenic activities in this context. Furthermore, this phenotype is characterized by high levels of FasL and TNF-α, proteins that mediate an antiangiogenic effect by inducing apoptosis in angiogenic endothelial cells. Increasing age induces a polarized phenotype that is proangiogenic, characterized by increased levels of IL-10, which is functionally linked to decreased levels of IL-6, IL-12, FasL, and TNF-α.[81,82]

IL-13 and IL-17 are also known to be involved in the angiogenic cascade in nonocular contexts.[83–85] In the eye, however, their role(s) are not clear.

In summary, the ILs are a family of soluble factors with pleiotropic roles. In the eye, ILs have demonstrated both proangiogenic and antiangiogenic effects, which are dependent upon context and environment. This finding necessitates further research into the precise roles of specific ILs before they can be exploited as a targeted therapy for human use.

OTHER GROWTH FACTORS

Platelet-derived growth factor (PDGF) has been shown to promote cell survival, induce endothelial cell proliferation, and recruit pericytes to the retinal vasculature.[86,87] Rats that were exposed to a model of OIR and treated with an inhibitor of the PDGF receptor demonstrated increased VEGF, pericyte dropout, and exacerbated angiogenesis.[88] However, in another study, targeting PDGF-BB and VEGF in combination led to a greater reduction in corneal and choroidal NV than when either protein was targeted alone.[89] These studies suggest that PDGF mediates context-specific aspects of ocular NV, both alone and in combination with VEGF.

Hepatocyte growth factor (HGF) induces the proliferation of hepatic and renal cells. Recently, a potential role of HGF in retinal angiogenesis has been identified.[90,91] Levels of HGF are increased in the vitreous and subretinal space of patients with PDR and ROP.[90,92,93] Transcriptome data suggest a possible synergy between VEGF and HGF. A three-way transcriptome comparison of HUVEC treated with VEGF, HGF, or VEGF + HGF was performed. The combination treatment revealed altered expression of a nonoverlapping set of genes that were unperturbed when these cells were treated with VEGF or HGF alone.[94] These studies suggest that HGF promotes retinal NV, possibly demonstrating synergy with the proangiogenic effects of VEGF.

Placental growth factor (PlGF) is a structural and functional homologue of VEGF. However, in contrast to VEGF, PlGF only binds and activates VEGFR-1.[95,96] PlGF is a weak mitogen for some endothelial cell types.[95] Bovine retinal endothelial cells treated with PlGF and FGF-2 in combination demonstrated increased tube formation and secondary sprouting, suggesting a mechanism for its angiogenic influence.[97]

Transforming growth factor-beta (TGF-β) is generally an inhibitor of endothelial cell proliferation. Endothelial cells treated with TGF-β demonstrate increased expression of plasminogen activator inhibitor-1 (PAI-1), suggesting a possible mechanism for the antiangiogenic capacity of TGF-β.[98,99]

Tumor necrosis factor-alpha (TNF-α) inhibits endothelial cell proliferation, and administering high doses of TNF-α selectively destroys tumor vasculature.[100,101] However, several in vivo studies indicate that TNF-α demonstrates a proangiogenic role.[101] These studies indicate that TNF-α induces proangiogenic VEGF expression in various cell types, which may explain a mechanism for its angiogenic activity.[102] In the eye, wild type and TNF-α–deficient mice were exposed to OIR. The TNF-α–deficient mice demonstrated increased intraretinal vascular development and significantly reduced preretinal NV in response to OIR exposure, suggesting that TNF-α is involved in promoting ocular angiogenesis.[103]

KEY POINTS

VEGF is the principal growth factor responsible for the pathological angiogenesis characterizing a number of ocular diseases. However, recent evidence suggests that several other factors play pivotal roles in the angiogenic cascade in the eye. Exploiting the therapeutic potential of these factors, alone or in combination with VEGF-directed therapies, may enhance the current standard of treatment for ocular angiogenic diseases.

- FGF-2 is thought to act in synergy with VEGF, promoting angiogenesis.
- COX-2 and its PG products are thought to play a proangiogenic role in ocular NV. Inhibiting COX activity with NSAIDs significantly reduces pathological angiogenesis in the eye.
- Ang2 acts in concert with VEGF to promote vessel destabilization and the angiogenic phenotype. Preclinical tests of Ang2 inhibition are currently underway.
- Epo-EpoR signaling has been implicated in a number of angiogenic processes and diseases. There are conflicting findings about the precise role of Epo in the eye.
- IL-1, IL-4, IL-6, IL-8, and IL-10 appear to promote ocular angiogenesis. Other members of the IL family, for example, IL-12, appear to be antiangiogenic. The literature suggests that the specific roles of each of the ILs are disease and context dependent. This may complicate development of IL-targeted treatment, but once developed, these drugs may provide a more directed therapeutic with fewer undesirable side effects.

REFERENCES

1. Aiello LP, Avery RL, Arrigg PG, et al. Vascular endothelial growth factor in ocular fluid of patients with diabetic retinopathy and other retinal disorders. *N Engl J Med.* 1994;331: 1480–1487.
2. Grisanti S, Tatar O. The role of vascular endothelial growth factor and other endogenous interplayers in age-related macular degeneration. *Prog Retin Eye Res.* 2008;27: 372–390.
3. van Wijngaarden P, Qureshi SH. Inhibitors of vascular endothelial growth factor (VEGF) in the management of neovascular age-related macular degeneration: a review of current practice. *Clin Exp Optom.* 2008;91:427–437.
4. Cook HL, Patel PJ, Tufail A. Age-related macular degeneration: diagnosis and management. *Br Med Bull.* 2008;85: 127–149.
5. Lynch SS, Cheng CM. Bevacizumab for neovascular ocular diseases. *Ann Pharmacother.* 2007;41:614–625.
6. Jonas JB, Spandau UH, Rensch F, et al. Infectious and non-infectious endophthalmitis after intravitreal bevacizumab. *J Ocul Pharmacol Ther.* 2007;23:240–242.
7. Galzie Z, Kinsella AR, Smith JA. Fibroblast growth factors and their receptors. *Biochem Cell Biol.* 1997;75:669–685.
8. D'Amore PA. Mechanisms of retinal and choroidal neovascularization. *Invest Ophthalmol Vis Sci.* 1994;35:3974–3979.
9. Bikfalvi A, Klein S, Pintucci G, et al. Biological roles of fibroblast growth factor-2, *Endocr Rev.* 1997;18:26–45.
10. Malek AM, Connors S, Robertson RL, et al. Elevation of cerebrospinal fluid levels of basic fibroblast growth factor in moyamoya and central nervous system disorders. *Pediatr Neurosurg.* 1997;27:182–189.
11. Gao H, Hollyfield JG. Basic fibroblast growth factor (bFGF) immunolocalization in the rodent outer retina demonstrated with an anti-rodent bFGF antibody. *Brain Res.* 1992;585: 355–360.
12. Kostyk SK, D'Amore PA, Herman IM, et al. Optic nerve injury alters basic fibroblast growth factor localization in the retina and optic tract. *Neurosci.* 1994;14:1441–1449.
13. Sivalingam A, Kenney J, Brown GC, et al. Basic fibroblast growth factor levels in the vitreous of patients with proliferative diabetic retinopathy. *Arch Ophthalmol.* 1990;108: 869–872.
14. Nyberg F, Hahnenberer R, Jakobson AM, et al. Enhancement of FGF-like polypeptides in the retinae of newborn mice exposed to hyperoxia. *FEBS Lett.* 1990;267:75–77.
15. Zhang NL, Samadani EE, Frank RN. Mitogenesis and Recent Developments 3979 retinal pigment epithelial cell antigen expression in the rat after krypton laser photocoagulation. *Invest Ophthalmol Vis Sci.* 1993;34:2412–2424.
16. Jain RK, Schlenger K, Höckel M, et al. Quantitative angiogenesis assays: progress and problems. *Nat Med.* 1997;3: 1203–1208.
17. Ozaki H, Okamoto N, Ortega S, et al. Basic fibroblast growth factor is neither necessary nor sufficient for the development of retinal neovascularization. *Am J Pathol.* 1998;153:757–765.
18. Tobe T, Ortega S, Luna JD, et al. Targeted disruption of the FGF2 gene does not prevent choroidal neovascularization in a murine model. *Am J Pathol.* 1998;153:1641–1646.
19. Ljubimov AJ. Growth factor synergy in angiogenesis. In: Penn JS, ed. *Retinal and Choroidal Angiogenesis*, 1st ed. The Netherlands: Springer; 2008:289–310.
20. Stahl A, Paschek L, Martin G, et al. Combinatory inhibition of VEGF and FGF2 is superior to solitary VEGF inhibition in an in vitro model of RPE-induced angiogenesis. *Graefes Arch Clin Exp Ophthalmol.* 2009;247:767–773.
21. DuBois RN, Abramson SB, Crofford L, et al. Cyclooxygenase in biology and disease. *FASEB J.* 1998;12:1063–1073.
22. Smith WL, DeWitt DL, Garavito RM. Cyclooxygenases: structural, cellular, and molecular biology. *Annu Rev Biochem.* 2000;69:145–182.
23. Kawamori T, Rao CV, Seibert K, et al. Chemopreventive activity of celecoxib, a specific cyclooxygenase-2 inhibitor, against colon carcinogenesis. *Cancer Res.* 1998;58:409–412.
24. Williams CS, Mann M, DuBois RN. The role of cyclooxygenases in inflammation, cancer and development. *Oncogene.* 1999;18:7908–7916.
25. Form DM, Auerbach R. PGE2 and angiogenesis. *Proc Soc Exp Biol Med.* 1983;172:214–218.
26. Ziche M, Jones J, Gullino PM. Role of prostaglandin E1 and copper in angiogenesis. *J Natl Cancer Inst.* 1982;69: 475–482.
27. Diaz-Flores L, Gutierrez R, Varela H. Angiogenesis: an update. *Histol Histopathol.* 1994;9:807–843.
28. Yamada M, Kawai M, Kawai Y, et al. The effect of selective cyclooxygenase-2 inhibitor on corneal angiogenesis in the rat. *Curr Eye Res.* 1999;19:300–304.
29. Castro MR, Lutz D, Edelman JL. Effect of COX inhibitors on VEGF-induced retinal vascular leakage and experimental corneal and choroidal neovascularization. *Exp Eye Res.* 2004;79:275–285.
30. Ayalasomayajula SP, Kompella UB. Celecoxib, a selective cyclooxygenase-2 inhibitor, inhibits retinal vascular endothelial growth factor expression and vascular leakage in a streptozotocin-induced diabetic rat model. *Eur J Pharmacol.* 2003;458:283–289.
31. Ayalasomayajula SP, Amrite AC, Kompella UB. Inhibition of cyclooxygenase -2, but not cyclooxygenase-1, reduces prostaglandin E2 secretion from diabetic rat retinas. *Eur J Pharmacol.* 2004;498:275–278.
32. Amrite AC, Ayalasomayajula SP, Cheruvu NPS, et al. Single periocular injection of celecoxib-PLGA microparticles inhibits diabetes-induced elevations in retinal PGE_2, VEGF, and vascular leakage. *Invest Ophthalmol Vis Sci.* 2006;47: 1149–1160.
33. Kern TS, Miller CM, Du Y, et al. Topical administration of nepafenac inhibits diabetes-induced retinal microvascular disease and underlying abnormalities of retinal metabolism and physiology. *Diabetes.* 2007;56:373–379.
34. Wilkinson-Berka JL, Alousis NS, Kelly DJ, et al. COX-2 inhibition and retinal angiogenesis in a mouse model of retinopathy of prematurity. *Invest Ophthalmol Vis Sci.* 2003;44:974–979.
35. Sennlaub F, Valamanesh F, Vazquez-Tello A, et al. Cyclooxygenase-2 in human and experimental ischemic proliferative retinopathy. *Circulation.* 2003;108:198–204.
36. Takahashi K, Saishin Y, Saishin Y, et al. Topical nepafenac inhibits ocular neovascularization. *Invest Ophthalmol Vis Sci.* 2003;44:409–415.

37. Yanni SE, Barnett JM, Clark ML, et al. The role of PGE2 receptor EP4 in pathologic ocular angiogenesis. *Invest Ophthalmol Vis* Sci 2009;50:5479-5486.
38. Takahashi H, Yanagi Y, Tamaki Y, et al. COX-2-selective inhibitor, etodolac, suppresses choroidal neovascularization in a mice model. *Biochem Biophys Res Commun.* 2004;325:461–466.
39. Hu W, Criswell MH, Ottlecz A, et al. Oral administration of lumiracoxib reduces choroidal neovascular membrane development in the rat laser-trauma model. *Retina.* 2005;25: 1054–1064.
40. Shim WS, Ho IA, Wong PE. Angiopoietin: a TIE(d) balance in tumor angiogenesis. *Mol Cancer Res.* 2007;5:655–665.
41. Carmeliet P, Jain RK. Angiogenesis in cancer and other diseases. *Nature.* 2000;407:249–257.
42. Davis S, Aldrich TH, Jones PF, et al. Isolation of angiopoietin-1, a ligand for the TIE2 receptor, by secretion-trap expression cloning. *Cell.* 1996;87:1161–1169.
43. Suri C, Jones PF, Patan S, et al. Requisite role of angiopoietin-1, a ligand for the TIE2 receptor, during embryonic angiogenesis. *Cell.* 1996;87:1171–1180.
44. Maisonpierre PC, Suri C, Jones PF, et al. Angiopoietin-2, a natural antagonist for Tie2 that disrupts in vivo angiogenesis. *Science.* 1997;277:55–60.
45. Holash J, Maisonpierre PC, Compton D, et al. Vessel cooption, regression, and growth in tumors mediated by angiopoietins and VEGF. *Science.* 1999;284:1994–1998.
46. Lobov IB, Brooks PC, Lang RA. Angiopoietin-2 displays VEGF-dependent modulation of capillary structure and endothelial cell survival in vivo. *Proc Natl Acad Sci U S A.* 2002;99:11205–11210.
47. Kontos CD, Cha EH, York JD, et al. The endothelial receptor tyrosine kinase Tie1 activates phosphatidylinositol 3-kinase and Akt to inhibit apoptosis. *Mol Cell Biol.* 2002;22: 1704–1713.
48. Chen-Konak L, Guetta-Shubin Y, Yahav H, et al. Transcriptional and post-translation regulation of the Tie1 receptor by fluid shear stress changes in vascular endothelial cells. *FASEB J.* 2003;17:2121–2123.
49. Yabkowitz R, Meyer S, Black T, et al. Inflammatory cytokines and vascular endothelial growth factor stimulate the release of soluble tie receptor from human endothelial cells via metalloprotease activation. *Blood.* 1999;93:1969–1979.
50. Oh H, Takagi H, Suzuma K, et al. Hypoxia and vascular endothelial growth factor selectively up-regulate angiopoietin-2 in bovine microvascular endothelial cells. *J Biol Chem.* 1999;274:15732–15739.
51. Mandriota SJ, Pepper MS. Regulation of angiopoietin-2 mRNA levels in bovine microvascular endothelial cells by cytokines and hypoxia. *Circ Res.* 1998;83:852–859.
52. Mandriota SJ, Pyke C, Di Sanza C, et al. Hypoxia-inducible angiopoietin-2 expression is mimicked by iodonium compounds and occurs in the rat brain and skin in response to systemic hypoxia and tissue ischemia. *J Pathol.* 2000;156:2077–2089.
53. Huang YQ, Li JJ, Hu L, et al. Thrombin induces increased expression and secretion of angiopoietin-2 from human umbilical vein endothelial cells. *Blood.* 2002;99:1646–1650.
54. Yao D, Taguchi T, Matsumura T, et al. High glucose increases angiopoietin-2 transcription in microvascular endothelial cells through methylglyoxal modification of mSin3A. *J Biol Chem.* 2007;282:31038–31045.
55. Zadeh G, Qian B, Okhowat A, et al. Targeting the Tie2/Tek Receptor in Astrocytomas. *A J Path.* 2004;164:467–476.
56. Stratmann A, Acker T, Burger AM, et al. Differential inhibition of tumor angiogenesis by tie2 and vascular endothelial growth factor receptor-2 dominant-negative receptor mutants. *Int J Cancer.* 2001;91:273–282.
57. Anagnostou A, Lee ES, Kessimian N, et al. Erythropoietin has a mitogenic and positive chemotactic effect on endothelial cells. *Proc Natl Acad Sci U S A.* 1990;87:5978–5982.
58. Anagnostou A, Liu Z, Steiner M, et al. Erythropoietin receptor mRNA expression in human endothelial cells. *Proc Natl Acad Sci U S A.* 1994;91:3974–3978.
59. Carlini RG, Reyes AA, Rothstein M. Recombinant human erythropoietin stimulates angiogenesis in vitro. *Kidney Int.* 1995:47:740–745.
60. Jaquet K, Krause K, Tawakol-Khodai M, et al. Erythropoietin and VEGF exhibit equal angiogenic potential. *Microvasc Res.* 2002;64:326–333.
61. Kertesz N, Wu J, Chen TH, et al. The role of erythropoietin in regulating angiogenesis. *Dev Biol.* 2004;276:101–110.
62. Wu H, Lee SH, Gao J, et al. Inactivation of erythropoietin leads to defects in cardiac morphogenesis. *Development.* 1999;126:3597–3605.
63. Haroon ZA, Amin K, Jiang X, et al. A novel role for erythropoietin during fibrin-induced wound-healing response. *Am J Pathol.* 2003;163:993–1000.
64. Sakanaka M, Wen TC, Matsuda S, et al. In vivo evidence that erythropoietin protects neurons from ischemic damage. *Proc Natl Acad Sci U S A.* 1998;95:4635–4640.
65. Ohori K, Miura T, Tanno M, et al. Ser9 phosphorylation of mitochondrial GSK-3beta is a primary mechanism of cardiomyocyte protection by erythropoietin against oxidant-induced apoptosis. *Am J Physiol Heart Circ Physiol.* 2008;295:H2079–H2086.
66. Grimm C, Wenzel A, Groszer M, et al. HIF-1-induced erythropoietin in the hypoxic retina protects against light-induced retinal degeneration. *Nat Med.* 2002;8:718–724.
67. Watanabe D, Suzuma K, Matsui S, et al. Erythropoietin as a retinal angiogenic factor in proliferative diabetic retinopathy. *N Engl J Med.* 2005;353:782–792.
68. Ohlsson A, Aher SM. Early erythropoietin for preventing red blood cell transfusion in preterm and/or low birth weight infants. *Cochrane Database Syst Rev.* 2006;3:CD004863.
69. Morita M, Ohneda O, Yamashita T, et al. HLF/HIF-2alpha is a key factor in retinopathy of prematurity in association with erythropoietin. *EMBO J.* 2003;22:1134–1146.
70. Shah N, Jadav P, Jean-Baptiste D, et al. The effect of recombinant human erythropoietin on the development of retinopathy of prematurity. *Am J Perinatol.* 2010;271:67–71.
71. BenEzra D, Hemo I, Maftzir G. In vivo angiogenic activity of interleukins. *Arch Ophthalmol.* 1990;108:573–576.
72. Elner VM, Strieter RM, Pavilack MA, et al. Human corneal interleukin-8 IL-1 and TNF-induced gene expression and secretion. *Am J Pathol.* 1991;139:977–988.
73. Fukushi J, Morisaki T, Shono T, et al. Novel biological functions of interleukin-4: formation of tube-like structures by vascular endothelial cells in vitro and angiogenesis in vivo. *Biochem Biophys Res Commun.* 1998;250:444–448.

74. Yao JS, Young WL, Zhai W, et al. Interleukin-6 triggers human cerebral endothelial cells proliferation and migration: The role for KDR and MMP-9. *Biochem Biophys Res Commun.* 2006;342:1396–1404.
75. Barnett JM, McCollum GW, Fowler JA, et al. Pharmacologic and Genetic Manipulation of MMP-2 and -9 Affects Retinal Neovascularization in Rodent Model of OIR. *Invest Ophthalmol Vis Sci.* 2007;48:907–915.
76. Yongfeng F, Jianqin Y, Fanzia S, et al. Interleukin-6 stimulates circulating blood-derived endothelial progenitor cell angiogenesis in vitro. *J Cereb Blood Flow Metab.* 2008;28:90–98.
77. Li A, Dubey S, Varney ML, et al. IL-8 Directly enhanced endothelial cell survival, proliferation, and matrix metalloproteinases production and regulated angiogenesis. *J Immunol.* 2003;170:3369–3376.
78. Sarman S, Aronsson M, Kvanta A, et al. Decrease pathologic retinal neovascularization in IL-10-deficient mice. *Invest Ophthalmol Vis Sci.* 2006;47:E-Abstract 1757.
79. Samolov B, Kvanta A, van der Ploeg I. Delayed neovascularization in inflammation-induced corneal neovascularization in interleukin-10-deficient mice. *Act Ophthalmol.* 2008;1:1755–1760.
80. Dace DS, Khan AA, Kelly J, et al. Interleukin-10 promotes pathological angiogenesis by regulating macrophage response to hypoxia during development. *PLoS ONE.* 2008;3:e3381.
81. Ferguson TA, Apte RS. Angiogenesis in eye disease: immunity gained or immunity lost? *Semin Immunopathol.* 2008;30: 111–119.
82. Kelly J, Khan AA, Yin J, et al. Senescence regulates macrophage activation and angiogenic fate at sites of tissue injury in mice. *J Clin Investig.* 2007;117:3421–3426.
83. Hallorran MM, Haskell CJ, Woods JM, et al. Interleukin-12 is an Endothelial Chemotaxin. *Pathobiology.* 1997;65:287–292.
84. Hass CS, Amin MA, Ruth JH, et al. In vivo inhibition of angiogenesis by interleukin-13 gene therapy in a rat model of rheumatoid arthritis. *Arthritis Rheum.* 2007;56:2535–2548.
85. Numasaki M, Watanabe M, Suzuki T, et al. IL-17 Enhances the net angiogenic activity and in vivo growth of human non-small cell lung cancer in SCID mice through promoting CXCR-2-dependent angiogenesis. *J Immunol.* 2005;175:6177–6189.
86. Saint-Geniez M, D'Amore PA. Development and pathology of the hyaloid, choroidal and retinal vasculature. *Int J Dev Biol.* 2004;48:1045–1058.
87. Ishikawa F, Miyazono K, Hellman U, et al. Identification of angiogenic activity and the cloning and expression of platelet-derived endothelial cell growth factor. *Nature.* 1989;338:557–562.
88. Wilkinson-Berka JL, Babic S, de Gooyer T, et al. Inhibition of platelet-derived growth factor promotes pericyte loss and angiogenesis in ischemic retinopathy. *Am J Pathol.* 2004;164:1263–1273.
89. Jo N, Mailhos C, Ju M, et al. Inhibition of platelet-derived growth factor B signaling enhances the efficacy of anti-vascular endothelial growth factor therapy in multiple models of ocular neovascularization. *Am J Pathol.* 2006;168: 2036–2053.
90. Kvanta A. Ocular angiogenesis: the role of growth factors. *Acta Ophthalmol.* 2006;84:282–288.
91. Cai W, Rook SL, Jiang ZY, et al. Mechanisms of hepatocyte growth factor-induced retinal endothelial cell migration and growth. *Invest Ophthalmol Vis Sci.* 2000;41:1885–1893.
92. Shinoda K, Ishida S, Kawashima S, et al. Comparison of the levels of hepatocyte growth factor and vascular endothelial growth factor in aqueous fluid and serum with grades of retinopathy in patients with diabetes mellitus. *Br J Ophthalmol.* 1999;83:763–764.
93. Lashkari K, Hirose T, Yazdany J, et al. Vascular endothelial growth factor and hepatocyte growth factor levels are differentially elevated in patients with advanced retinopathy of prematurity. *Am J Pathol.* 2000;156:1337–1344.
94. Gerritsen ME, Tomlinson JE, Zlot C, et al. Using gene expression profiling to identify the molecular basis of the synergistic actions of hepatocyte growth factor and vascular endothelial growth factor in human endothelial cells. *Br J Pharmacol.* 2003;140:595–610.
95. Mitamura Y, Tashimo A, Nakamura Y, et al. Vitreous levels of placenta growth factor and vascular endothelial growth factor in patients with proliferative diabetic retinopathy. *Diabetes Care.* 2002;25:2352.
96. Luttun A, Tjwa M, Carmeliet P. Placental growth factor (PlGF) and its receptor Flt-1 (VEGFR-1). Novel therapeutic targets for angiogenic disorders. *N Y Acad Sci.* 2002;979:80–93.
97. Castellon R, Hamdi HK, Sacerio I, et al. Effects of angiogenic growth factor combinations on retinal endothelial cells. *Exp Eye Res.* 2002;74:523–535.
98. Huang SS, Huang JS. TGF-β Control of Cell Proliferation. *J Cell Biochem.* 2005;96:447–462.
99. Goumans MJ, Liu Z, ten Dijke P. TGF-β signaling in vascular biology and dysfunction. *Cell Res.* 2009;19:116–127.
100. Frater-Schroder M, Risau W, Hallaman R, et al. Tumor–Necrosis Factor Type α, a Potent Inhibitor of Endothelial Cell Growth *in vitro*, is angiogenic *in vivo*. *PNAS.* 1987;84: 5277–5281.
101. Lejeune FJ, Ruegg C, Lienard D. Clinical Applications of TNF α in Cancer. *Curr Opin Immunol.* 1998;10:573–580.
102. Yin Y, Wang S, Sun Y, et al. JNK/AP-1 pathway is involved in tumor necrosis factor-α induced expression of vascular endothelial growth factor in MCF7 cells. *Biomed Pharmacother.* 2009;63:429–435.
103. Gardiner TA, Gibson DS, de Gooyer TE, et al. Inhibition of tumor necrosis factor-α improves physiological angiogenesis and reduces pathological neovascularization in ischemic retinopathy. *Am J Pathol.* 2005;166:637–644.

CHAPTER

7

Proteinases and Integrins in Ocular Angiogenesis

Sampathkumar Rangasamy • Alexander Ljubimov • Sayon Roy • Paul McGuire • Arup Das

Ocular angiogenesis involves two important key steps: endothelial cell proliferation and migration. Hypoxia upregulates growth factors most of which cause cell proliferation. Increased growth factors also cause increased expression of proteinases and integrins that are important for cell migration. The proteinases facilitate the breakdown of the basement membrane and extracellular matrix (ECM), allowing cells to migrate. This chapter focuses on the structure and function of the basement membrane first, then the roles of proteinases and integrins in ocular angiogenesis, and how inhibitors of these molecules can be utilized to inhibit angiogenesis in the eye.

BASEMENT MEMBRANE COMPONENTS: STRUCTURE AND FUNCTION

Basement membranes are complex, multicomponent structures with diverse functions. Studies investigating ultrastructural changes in diabetic retinopathy (DR) have established thickened vascular basement membrane as one of the earliest structural abnormalities. Evidence suggests that this fundamental structural lesion develops, at least in part, from excess accumulation of basement membrane material. Increased syntheses of several vascular basement membrane components have been identified in diabetes. While the composition of basement membranes is still incompletely known, some of the major components, including fibronectin, collagen type IV, and laminin,[1] are known (Table 7.1). These components attach to each other in a highly organized manner and form a continuous sheet beneath the endothelial cell layer. The sheet-like membranous structure provides support for attachment, spreading, migration, growth, repair, and differentiation of the overlying cells.[2–4]

Fibronectin is a glycoprotein that binds to integrins, collagen, fibrin, and heparan sulfate proteoglycans. It is a critical component of the basement membrane and is upregulated in diabetes. It consists of two similar monomers that are linked by disulfide bonds at their c-termini.[38] Considered as molecular glue, it facilitates the attachment of basement membrane components into an organized scaffold. Collagen type IV is another major component of all basement membranes that is overexpressed in diabetes. The triple helical collagen fibrils attach to each other in a head-to-head orientation and form a network-like arrangement with over 20 breaks in the (Gly-X-Y)n pattern.[39] The breaks contribute to the looseness with kinks that causes the collagen fibrils to form into a sheet. The collagen fibrils are reinforced through cross-links catalyzed by lysyl oxidase. Laminin is another major basement membrane component like fibronectin, and collagen is overexpressed in high glucose and diabetic conditions.[40–42] It is comprised of three chains, and through specific binding sites

Table 7.1.

ECM components in basement membrane

ECM Components	Effect of Diabetes or High Glucose (References)
Fibronectin	Increased (5–13)
Laminin	Increased (14–16)
Vitronectin	Increased (14,17,18)
Entactin	Unknown (19)
Bamin	Unknown (20)
Dystroglycan	Unknown (21)
Collagen I	Increased (13)
Collagen II	Unknown (22,23)
Collagen III	Increased (6,13)
Collagen IV	Increased (5,15,16,24–28)
Collagen V	Increased (13)
Collagen VI	Increased (14,29–31)
Elastin	Unknown (32)
Tenascin	Increased (7,11,13)
Chondroitin sulfate	Increased (33)
Hyaluronic acid	Increased (34)
Heparan sulfate	Increased (35)
Decorin	Increased (8,36)
Biglycan	Increased (8,37)

attaches to other ECM components such as collagen type IV and proteoglycans. These ECM components with their specialized repeat sequences facilitate cell-cell attachment and cell-matrix interactions. Importantly, many of these basement membrane proteins consist of a series of independently folded polypeptide repeats, which may have relevance to basement membrane structure and function.

SPROUTING ANGIOGENESIS

Sprouting angiogenesis is a multistep process involving degradation of the basement membrane, invasion into stroma, endothelial cell proliferation, and formation of sprout and tubular structures. It is initiated when angiogenic growth factors activate receptors present on endothelial cells in preexisting vessels. The activated endothelial cells release proteinases (matrix metalloproteinases [MMPs] and urokinase) that locally degrade the basement membrane, allowing endothelial cells to escape and proliferate. Cells destined to migrate out through the degraded basement membrane form solid sprouts. As sprouts extend, endothelial cells migrate in tandem and this process is facilitated by integrins. The endothelial cells at the tips of vascular sprouts extended long filopodia. The sprouts then form loops and encircle to become a full-fledged vessel lumen (Fig. 7.1).

The nascent vessels continue to lengthen as cells migrating to the site of angiogenesis facilitate the extension and formation of the vessels. These cells lay collagen fibers into the core to provide an ECM for growth of the vessel lumen. Much attention in sprouting angiogenesis has focused on distinct cellular responses by specific endothelial cells present at the tip of the sprout. The tip cells sense and respond to guidance cues provided by growth factors such as vascular endothelial growth factor (VEGF)[43] as they form filopodial extensions. Studies have shown that directed extension of endothelial filopodia is mediated by VEGFR2, which are highly expressed in endothelial tip cells.[44,45] Importantly, studies indicate that the Dll4-Notch1 pathway, a downstream event in VEGF signaling, regulates tip cell activity and facilitates proper vascular patterning in the retina.[46–48] The growth of new vessels from preexisting vessels involves complex interactions of several factors in which basement membrane plays a key role.

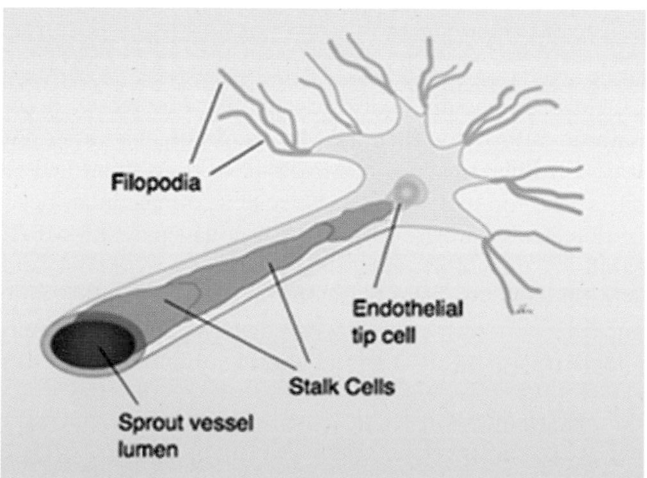

FIGURE 7.1. Sprouting angiogenesis exhibited by endothelial tip cells and their filopodia. Filopodia are highly enriched in actin filaments and respond to growth factor stimuli.

Proteinases in Ocular Angiogenesis

The process of angiogenesis in the retina and other tissues is characterized by distinct phases or activities including an initial response to locally produced angiogenic factors and signals.[49] This event is followed by a rapid upregulation of matrix-degrading enzymes or extracellular proteinases that facilitate the breakdown of the capillary basal lamina and migration and subsequent invasion of activated endothelial cells into the surrounding extracellular tissues. Extracellular proteinases (matrix-degrading enzymes) not only help in the degradation of interstitial ECM and basement membranes but they also help in the recruitment of progenitor cells into the ECM during tissue remodeling.[50] Proteinases are expressed by normal cells in tissue-remodeling events (wound healing) and also during pathological events such as cancer, DR, and age-related macular degeneration (AMD) (Fig. 7.2).

Extracellular Proteinases

Two families of proteinases that have been well studied in this process include the serine proteinase, urokinase plasminogen activator (uPA), and members of a family of zinc-dependent endopeptidases called matrix metalloproteinases (MMPs).

The Urokinase Plasminogen Activator System (uPA/uPAR System)

The roles of this serine protease urokinase-type plasminogen activator (uPA) and its receptor (uPAR) in retinal choroidal neovascularization have been well documented in recent studies. uPA is produced as an inactive single-chain protein known as pro-uPA, which binds to uPAR and is activated by plasmin. Receptor-bound pro-uPA is more rapidly cleaved by plasmin than the unbound form. The uPA is present in cells in two molecular forms, a 54-kDa high molecular weight form and a 32-kDa low molecular weight form, which lacks the amino terminal fragment (ATF) of the protein.[51,52] The ATF contains the growth factor and kringle domains of the protein that mediate binding to uPAR and play an important role in cell proliferation.[53] The main function of the uPA is to convert the inactive zymogen form of the enzyme plasminogen to plasmin, a broad spectrum of proteinase, which can cleave variety of ECM components including collagen IV, fibronectin, and elastin including uPA. The invasive and migratory potential of endothelial cells is largely determined upon the pool of active urokinase available on the cell surface. uPA has

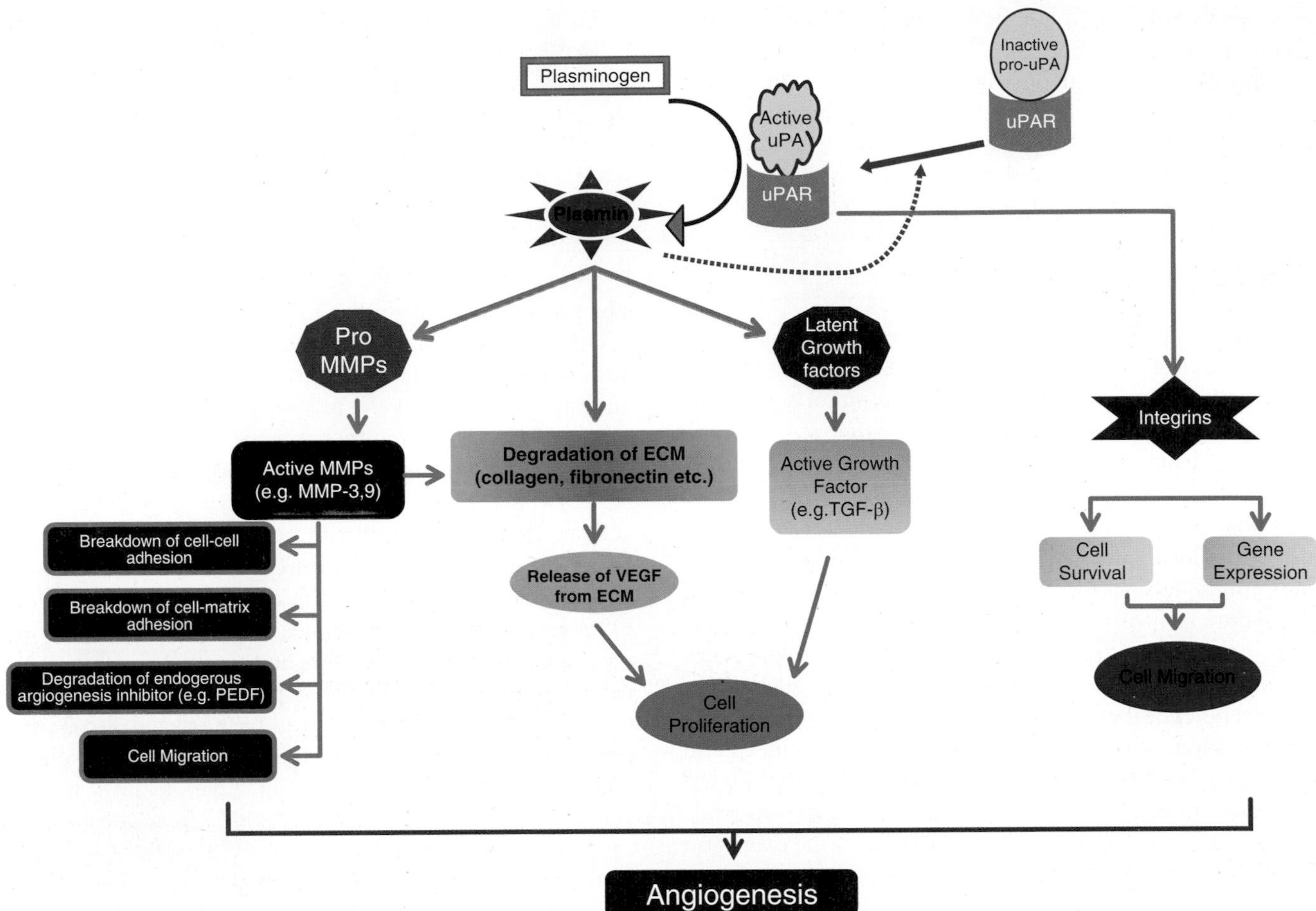

FIGURE 7.2. Role of proteinases in angiogenesis. Binding of urokinase receptor (uPAR) to inactive urokinase (pro-uPA) promotes the formation of active uPA. Active uPA then proteolytically converts the inactive zymogen plasminogen to active plasmin, which then breaks down ECM components or activates latent growth factors such as transforming growth factor-1 (TGF-1). Also, the active uPA-uPAR complex can integrate with integrins molecules and activate multiple signaling pathways, leading to cell migration. Plasmin activation also leads to the activation of pro–matrix metalloproteinases (pro-MMPs) leading to the formation of active MMPs, which can promote further ECM degradation and cell migration by its proteolytic activity. Activation of these proteases from the activated endothelial cells through the interaction between uPA and uPAR culminates in the angiogenesis process through the above-mentioned mechanisms.

also shown to directly activate the prohepatocyte growth factor/scatter factor (HGF/SF), and it also cleaves fibronectin and its own inhibitor, plasminogen activator inhibitor-1 (PAI-1), in a plasminogen-independent manner. The uPA/uPAR interaction represents a sensitive and flexible system to regulate proteolytic potential in endothelial cells. uPAR is a cell-surface molecule that interacts with many potential ligands.[54] uPAR has also shown to be associated with several members of the INTEGRIN family, which plays an important role in cell adhesion and migration.[55] This process is mediated through the low-density lipoprotein receptor–related protein (LRP), a multiligand receptor that can interact with both PAI-1 and uPAR. The uPA system also plays an important role in the activation of several MMPs and in the release and activation of growth factors stored in the ECM. The contribution of the uPA/uPAR system to angiogenesis has been studied in several animal models of tumor angiogenesis, choroidal and retinal angiogenesis (Box 7.1).

Matrix Metalloproteinases

The MMPs are a family of zinc-dependent proteases, originally identified for their ECM-degrading capabilities. At least 25 different types of MMPs have been identified to date. Based on their substrate specificity and cellular localization, MMPs are grouped into the collagenases (MMP-1, MMP-8, and MMP-13), the gelatinases (MMP-2 and MMP-9), the stromelysins (MMP-3, MMP-10, MMP-11), and the nontraditional MMPs (matrilysin/MMP-7, metalloelastase or MMP-12) and the membrane type MMPs (MT-MMPs) (Box 7.2).[50,56]

There are at least five distinct types of MT-MMPs (MMP-12, MMP-15, MMP-16, MMP-17, and MMP-21), and MT1-MMP has been studied in relation to its ability to regulate focused matrix lysis and the activation of MMP-2. In addition to their capacity to degrade a large variety of ECM molecules, MMPs are known to process a number of bioactive molecules. MMPs regulate a variety

BOX 7.1 Urokinase in Retinal and Choroidal Angiogenesis

uPA is a protein that regulates the activation of plasminogen to the serine protease plasmin at the leading edge of cells. Binding of pro-uPA to uPAR allows activation of pro-uPA into the active enzymatic form (uPA) (Fig. 7.3), which then mediates the plasmin generation. UPA-mediated conversion of plasminogen to plasmin regulates many functions including the degradation of extracellular matrix (ECM) components and other extracellular membrane proteins. This activity also regulates cell proliferation, migration, and physiological and pathological tissue remodeling. uPAR has been implicated in various pathological angiogenesis such as in tumor, retinal and choroidal neovascularization (CNV). A newly designed peptide inhibitor of the urokinase system, A6 (an octapeptide that inhibits the interaction of uPA with uPAR), was shown to reduce the extent of retinal neovascularization and uPAR expression in the experimental animals.[64] Also, systemic administration of the uPA/uPAR inhibitor, A6, dose dependently reduces laser-induced CNV. Also, in another study, it was found that the intravitreal injection of an adenoviral vector carrying the murine amino-terminal fragment (ATF) (targeting urokinase system) has been shown to inhibit retinal neovascularization in the OIR level.[68]

BOX 7.2 Matrix Metalloproteinases in Retinal and Choroidal Angiogenesis

MMPs are a family of highly homologous protein-degrading zinc-dependent enzymes endopeptidases, collectively referred to as metzincins. This family currently includes more than 25 members that can be divided into collagenases (MMP-1, MMP-8, and MMP-13), gelatinases (MMP-2 and MMP-9), stromelysins (MMP-3 and MMP-10), matrilysins (MMP-7 and MMP-26), and the membrane-type MMPs (MMP-14 to MMP-17 and MMP-24). MMPs are important in normal biological processes including wound healing, angiogenesis, and embryonic development. MMPs also play a major role in pathological processes such as inflammation, cancer, and eye diseases. The most important functional activity of MMPs is its ability to degrade virtually all extracellular matrix (ECM) components. Activation of MMPs will lead to degradation of matrix and cell-cell adhesion, there by promoting cell migration and angiogenesis. In retinal angiogenesis studies, use of broad-spectrum MMP inhibitor, BB-94 (1 mg/kg), has been shown to suppress retinal neovascularization.[64] An orally administered MMP-inhibitor *N*-BPHA has been shown to reduce the CNV in an animal model.[69] Also, the use of a small molecular weight synthetic MMP inhibitor, AG3340 (Prinomastat), was found to inhibit CNV in the rat model, when injected at the time of induction (prevention study).[70]

of cell behaviors such as cell proliferation, migration, differentiation, apoptosis, and host defense. In relation to retinal neovascularization, MMPs are implicated in the angiogenic process for their involvement in endothelial cell migration and invasion and posttranslational modification of antiangiogenic growth factor receptors (Fig. 7.3).

ENDOGENOUS INHIBITORS OF PROTEINASES

Tissue Inhibitors of Metalloproteinases

MMP activity is in part regulated by the Tissue Inhibitors of Metalloproteinases (TIMPs), which bind MMPs and inhibit their activity. Four TIMPs have been identified, which have overlapping activities with respect to their inhibition of most soluble MMPs.[50,57] More specificity exists regarding MT-MMPs, MMP-19, and proteolytically active ADAMs (proteins containing A Disintegrin and A Metalloproteinase domain) and ADAMTSs (proteins containing A Disintegrin and A Metalloproteinase domain *with a Thrombospondin type 1 motif*). TIMP-2 and TIMP-3 are good inhibitors of MT1-MMP, MMP-19, and ADAM-17, while TIMP-1 is poor in this respect. TIMPs also have biological effects unrelated to metalloproteinase inhibition. TIMP-3, but neither TIMP-1 nor TIMP-2, is involved in binding to the VEGF receptor-2 (Kinase insert Domain Receptor [KDR]) and competes for the binding of VEGF to this receptor. Overexpression of TIMP-3 can induce apoptosis. TIMP-1 and TIMP-2 display antiapoptotic properties and indirectly induce cell signaling. A point mutation of the TIMP-3 gene has been implicated in Sorsby's fundus dystrophy, an autosomal dominant macular disease similar to wet macular degeneration, but with earlier onset of symptoms.[58,59]

Plasminogen Activator Inhibitors

The proteolytic activity of uPA is regulated by PAIs, which are members of the serine proteinase inhibitor (SERPIN) family. PAI-1 and PAI-2 have been found to interact with urokinase in 1:1 ratio to inhibit enzyme activity and cause enzyme/inhibitor internalization and turnover.[60] PAI-1 has been shown to be a strong prognostic marker for several cancer types.[61]

Proteinases in Retinal Neovascularization

Significant upregulation of uPA (both the 54 and 32 kDa isoforms) along with increases in secretion and activation

I.B. Principles Molecular Mechanisms

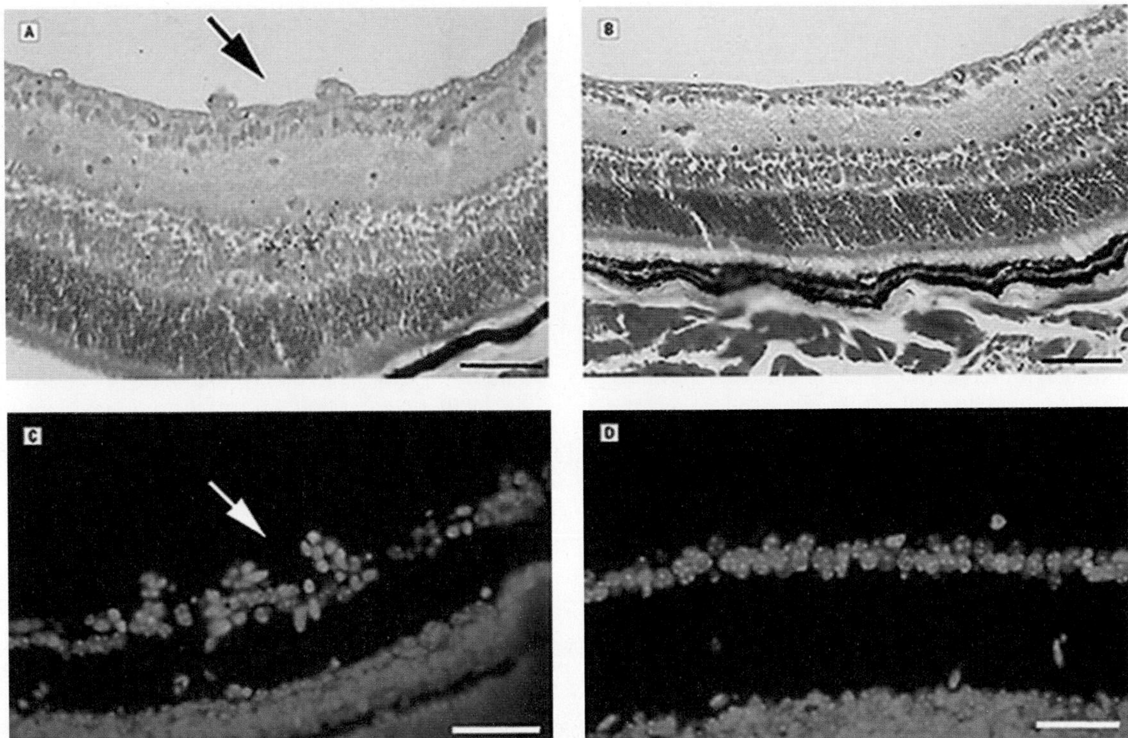

FIGURE 7.3. Use of a MMP inhibitor suppresses the development of retinal neovascularization. **A:** Hematoxylin-eosin–stained cross section from the retina of a mouse exposed to 75% oxygen for 5 days followed by room air for an additional 5 days. Capillary tufts are present on the vitreal side of the inner limiting membrane, characteristic of the angiogenic response in this tissue (*arrow*). **B:** Representative hematoxylin and eosin–stained section from the retina of an experimental mouse treated with BB-94m 1 mg/kg, on postnatal days 12, 14, and 16. **C:** Similar section from an experimental animal stained with diamidinophenylindole showing individual endothelial cell nuclei that belongs to new vessels (*arrow*). **D:** Similar section from the retina of a BB-94–treated mouse stained with diamidoniphenylindole showing a significant reduction in the number of neovascular nuclei. Only a single endothelial cell nucleus is present on the vitreal side of the inner limiting membrane. Scale bars: **A** and **B**, 166 µm; **C** and **D**, 113 µm. (Reproduced from Das et al. *Arch Ophthalmol.* 1999;117:498–503, with permission.)

of MMP-2 and MMP-9 were observed in the retinas of animals with neovascularization.[62] These results suggest that proteolytic activity and its regulatory mechanisms might play an important role in the angiogenic process. Examination of proteinases in epiretinal neovascular membranes removed surgically from humans with proliferative diabetic retinopathy (PDR) showed a similar increase in the levels of uPA and pro and active forms of MMP-2 and MMP-9 as compared to normal retinas.[63]

In an animal model of hypoxia-induced retinal neovascularization, it was found that the expression of the urokinase receptor (uPAR) was required to mediate an angiogenic response. uPAR$^{-/-}$ mice demonstrated normal retinal vascularity but showed a significant reduction (by 73%) in the extent of pathological neovascularization as compared to wild-type controls (Fig. 7.4).[64] Also the expression of uPAR mRNA was upregulated in experimental animals during the active phase of angiogenesis and uPAR protein was localized to endothelial cells in the superficial layers of the retina.

In the retinas of normal mice, TIMP-2 mRNA and protein levels have been found to increase steadily between postnatal days 13 to 17. This was in contrast to retinas of mice with hypoxia-induced retinal angiogenesis, in which TIMP-2 mRNA and protein remained low and significantly less than in retinas of "room air" controls.[65] Thus, a temporal correlation between proteinases (MMP-2 and MMP-9 and MT1-MMP) and TIMP-2 was seen in retinas with neovascularization as compared to controls.[65]

Proteinases in Choroidal Neovascularization

Real-time PCR studies have shown the upregulation of uPA and uPAR in the choroidal tissues of mice with laser-induced choroidal neovascularization (CNV) as well as in CNV membranes from patients with AMD.[66,67] The uPAR localized to endothelial cells of fibrovascular tissue within the CNV complex in the laser-induced NV model. Studies in single-gene-deficient mice have shown that the absence of uPA, tPA (tissue plasminogen activator), or

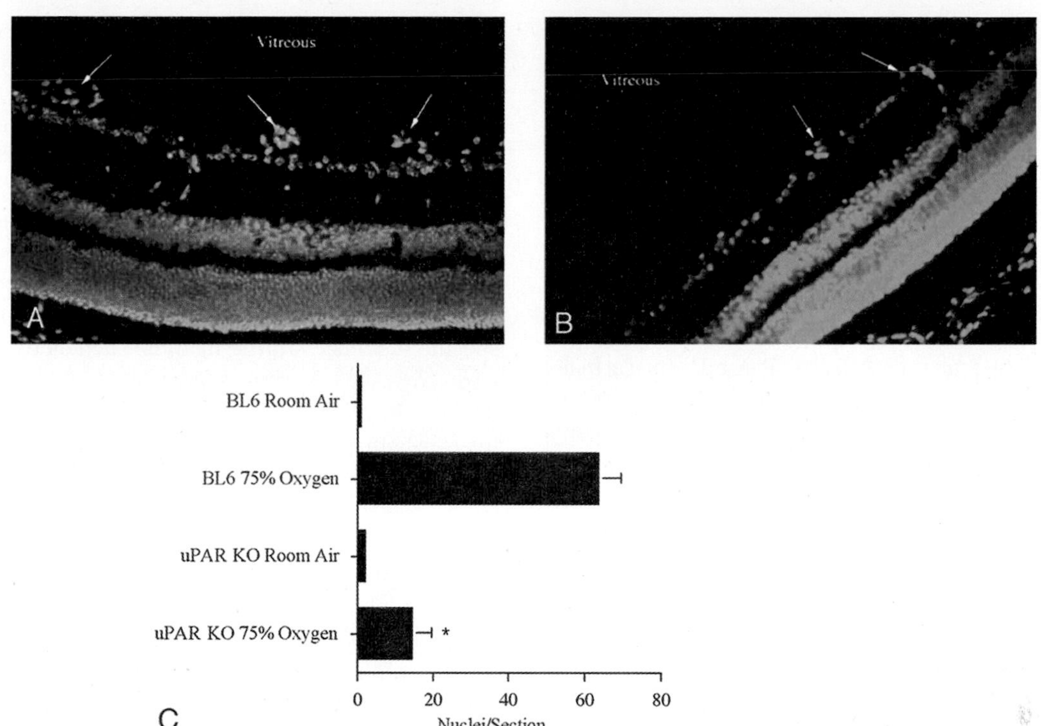

FIGURE 7.4. Absence of the urokinase receptor uPAR reduced the extent of retinal neovascularization in the mouse. **A:** Representative section of the retina from an experimental oxygen-treated P17 C57BL6 mouse demonstrating numerous neovascular tufts on the surface of the retina (*arrows.*). **B:** A similar section from an experimental oxygen-treated P17 uPAR$^{-/-}$ mouse with many fewer vascular tufts (*arrows*). **C:** Quantitation of neovascularization in C57BL6 and uPAR$^{-/-}$ mice. The uPAR$^{-/-}$ mice demonstrated 73% less neovascularization compared with the normal C57BL6 mice. Values are the mean ± SEM for $n = 4$ mice in each group (eight eyes, 15–20 sections/eye). *Significantly less than in C57BL6 mice, $p < 0.01$. (Reproduced from McGuire et al. *Invest Ophthalmol Vis Sci.* 2003;44:2736–2742, with permission.)

plasminogen significantly decreased the development of experimental CNV and that this effect could be explained by a modulation of MMP activity in the laser-induced wounds.

INHIBITION OF RETINAL AND CHOROIDAL NEOVASCULARIZATION

Inhibition of Retinal Angiogenesis by MMP Inhibitors

Systemic injection of a broad-spectrum MMP inhibitor, BB-94 (1 mg/kg), in the murine model has been shown to suppress retinal neovascularization by 72%[64] (see Fig. 7.3). The retinas of BB-94-treated animals demonstrated a significant decrease in the levels of active forms of MMP-2 and MMP-9 compared to controls. In a mouse model of oxygen-induced retinopathy (OIR), the extent of preretinal neovascularization was drastically reduced in MMP-2$^{-/-}$ (75%) and MMP-9$^{-/-}$ mice (44%) at postnatal day 19, compared to wild-type control mice. The functional association of MMP-2 and $\alpha v\beta 3$ on the cell surface of angiogenic blood vessels points to the ability of MMPs to regulate cell adhesion- and integrin-mediated behavior.

Inhibition of Retinal Angiogenesis by Inhibitors of the uPA/uPAR System

A peptide inhibitor of the urokinase system, A6 (an octapeptide that inhibits the interaction of uPA with uPAR), was able to reduce the extent of retinal neovascularization and uPAR expression in the experimental animals[64] (Fig. 7.4). Intravitreal injection of an adenoviral vector carrying the murine amino-terminal fragment (ATF) has been shown to inhibit retinal neovascularization by 78% in the OIR level.[68] These results suggest that inhibition of the urokinase receptor might be a promising target for antiangiogenic therapy in the retina.

Inhibition of Choroidal Neovascularization by MMP Inhibitors

In an animal model of laser-induced CNV, an orally administered MMP-inhibitor, *N*-biphenyl sulfonyl-phenylalanine hydroxamic acid (BPHA), has been shown to reduce neovascularization.[69] Similarly, intravitreal injection of a nonpeptide small molecular weight synthetic MMP inhibitor, AG3340 (Prinomastat), was found to inhibit CNV in the rat model, when injected at the time of induction (prevention study).[70] However, once the new vessels are formed, the drug did not

BOX 7.3 Proteinase Inhibitors in Clinical trials

MMP Inhibitors

AG 3340, a MMP inhibitor (Agouron, La Jolla, CA), was tested in patients with wet ARMD patients and was found to be ineffective.

Urokinase Inhibitors

A6, an octapeptide that inhibits interaction of urokinase with its receptor, is being currently tested in a Phase 2/3 clinical trial in patients with ovarian carcinoma. The drug has shown to be effective in animal models of both retinal neovascularization and CNV and thus appears to be of promising interest.

help in reducing the CNV (regression study). A clinical trial, an oral MMP inhibitor, AG 3340 (Agouron Pharmaceuticals), in wet ARMD (Age Related Macular Degeneration) patients did not show any effective results.

Inhibition of Choroidal Neovascularization by Inhibitors of the uPA/uPAR System

Systemic administration of the uPA/uPAR inhibitor, A6, in mice has been shown to significantly reduce laser-induced CNV by 94%, and the response was found to be dose dependent[67] (Fig. 7.5). Thus, studies in both retinal neovascularization and CNV show that the uPA/uPAR system plays an important role in this process, and the uPA/uPAR system may represent a novel therapeutic target in development of the antiangiogenic therapy for ocular angiogenesis (Box 7.3).

INTEGRINS IN OCULAR ANGIOGENESIS

Integrins: Structure, Functions, and Signaling

Integrins comprise a class of structurally related proteins that serve as cell-surface receptors to the ECM and immunoglobulin superfamily molecules.[71,72] They have been postulated and then discovered in the early 1980s.[73–81] Currently, the number of published papers dealing with integrins is over 43,000, as compared to over 60,000 for ECM, which has been studied much longer. This huge interest may be due to the fact that integrins convey signals from the outside of the cell to its inside and actively participate in intracellular signaling and various aspects of cell behavior during development and in the adult life.[71,82] Integrins are divalent cation-dependent transmembrane heterodimers of one α chain and one β chain, with each chain spanning the plasma membrane. To date, 18 α subunits and 8 β subunits have been described in mammals; they give rise to 24 different integrins (Fig. 7.6).[71,72,83,84] Some subunits, like β1, can form dimers with several α subunits, and many integrins can specifically bind to more than one ECM component, which makes the integrin family and its interactions with ECM more complex.[83,84] Invertebrates also have integrin analogs, such as PS proteins in *Drosophila*.[84]

Although different integrins have similar structure, a half of mammalian α subunits has an additional von Willebrand factor–like insert domain, or I domain.[84] It has been shown that αI-containing integrins (examples are leukocyte-specific receptors) bind to their ligands in this same region; those that do not contain I domain rely on cooperation of both subunits for ligand binding.[83] Integrins may recognize specific sequences in the ligands, such as the famous RGD (Arg–Gly–Asp containing *peptide*), first discovered as the fibronectin cell-binding sequence that has a strong affinity for α5β1 integrin.[72,81] Other receptors, like α4β1, can recognize different short sequences, REDV or EILDV.[71,72]

Signaling

Integrins are normally in an inactive state on the cell surface. Because their major function is to ensure adhesion of tissue cells, integrins are different from many receptors in their ability to mediate bidirectional signaling and to couple the external (ECM or surface of another cell) and internal (cytoskeleton) forces.[82,83,85] Consistent with this notion, outside-in and inside-out signaling modes of integrin action are recognized.[82] Outside-in signaling involves transmission of signal inside the cell after integrin binding to its ligand, change in integrin conformation, and integrin clustering on the cell surface to form nascent adhesions.[82] This signaling further entails phosphorylation of many proteins linking integrins to the cytoskeleton, adhesive structure formation, and cell-substratum adhesion.[83,86,87]

Initial integrin binding to the ligand appears to be weak. However, it triggers outside-in signaling, resulting in integrin cytoplasmic tail phosphorylation among other events. This activates the integrin, in turn promoting clustering, and strengthening integrin binding to the ligand. Integrin activation necessary to form stable interaction with the extracellular ligand represents inside-out signaling. Activated integrin clusters become associated with rigid lipid rafts in the membrane that attract intracellular and transmembrane proteins including kinases, other receptors, and cytoskeletal elements.[82,84]

Integrins interact with the growth factor receptors and regulate their functions.[88] Integrin clustering can stimulate receptors of several major angiogenic growth factors even in the absence of these factors (reviewed in ref. [87]). It is worth mentioning here that β3 integrin can complex with and modulate phosphorylation and hence activity of VEGF receptor 2 (VEGFR2/KDR/flk-1) by VEGF.[89,90] This cross talk is dependent upon the activity of Src kinase.[90] Lack of β3 integrin results in increased VEGFR2 expression and enhanced VEGF-mediated vessel permeability.[91] Another integrin, α5β1, can bind soluble VEGFR1, promoting endothelial cell adhesion and spreading.[87]

Integrin interaction with proteinases is another important mediator of angiogenesis. Integrin αVβ3 functionally

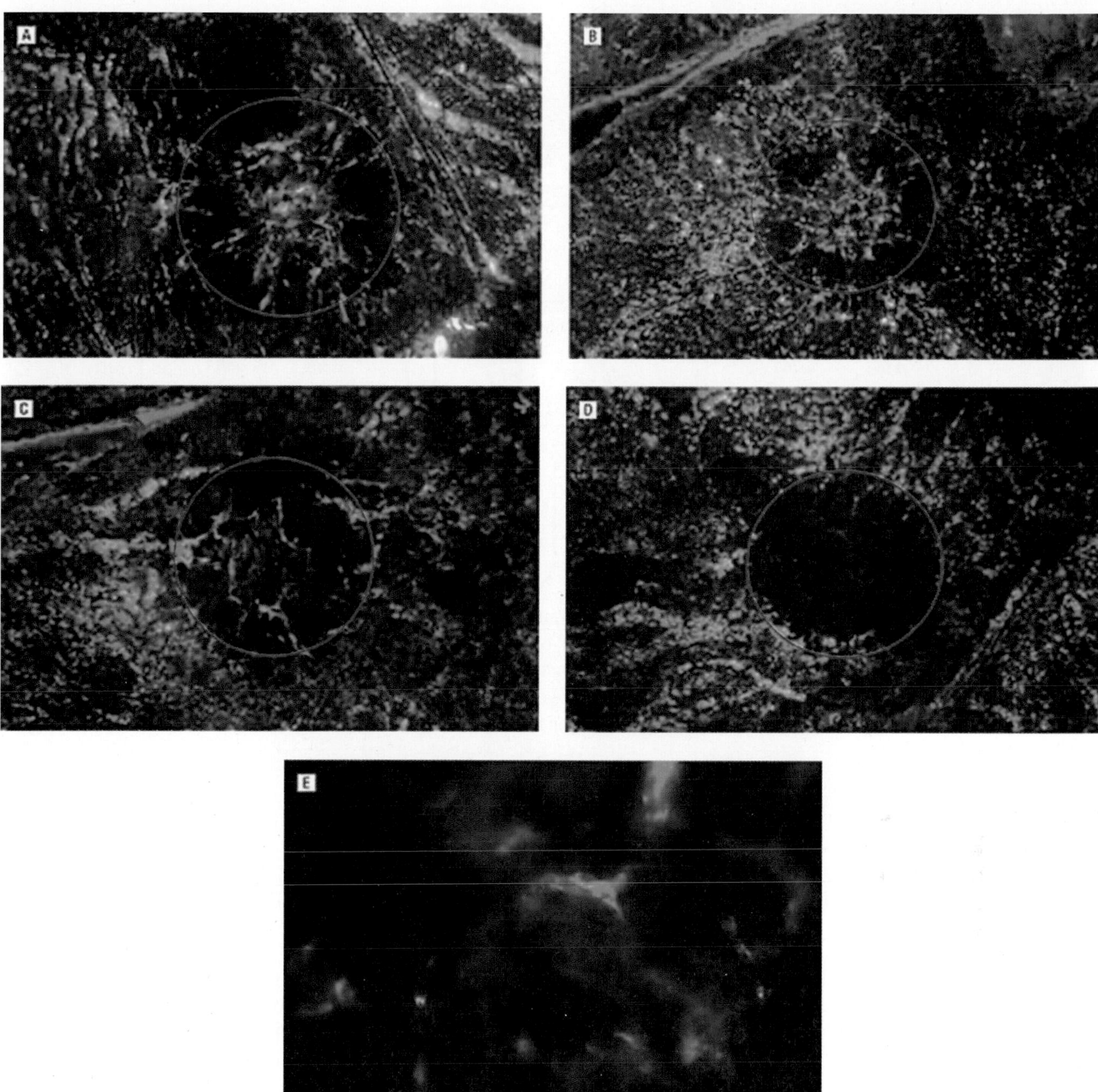

FIGURE 7.5. Treatment prevents neovascularization in the laser-induced model of CNV. Representative images of RPE–choroid whole mounts infused with fluorescein isothiocyanate–conjugated dextran 14 days after laser induction of CNV. Images are from mice treated with phosphate-buffered saline or Å6 peptide dosed at differing frequencies. The red circle roughly outlines the area of the laser burn. The fluorescence in the center of the burn area demonstrates the extent of the new vessel formation under the retina. The surrounding fluorescence represents the normal choroidal vasculature. **A:** Mouse treated with phosphate-buffered saline twice a day for 14 days. **B:** Mouse treated with the Å6 peptide, 100 mg/kg twice a day once a week. **C:** Mouse treated with Å6, 100 mg/kg twice a day every 3rd day. **D:** Mouse treated with Å6, 100 mg/kg twice a day every day. **E:** A higher magnification image of the central region in section **D**. Only a few fluorescein isothiocyanate–conjugated dextran-labeled blood vessels could be seen in this area. (Reproduced from Das et al. *Arch Ophthalmol.* 2004:122:1844–1849, with permission.)

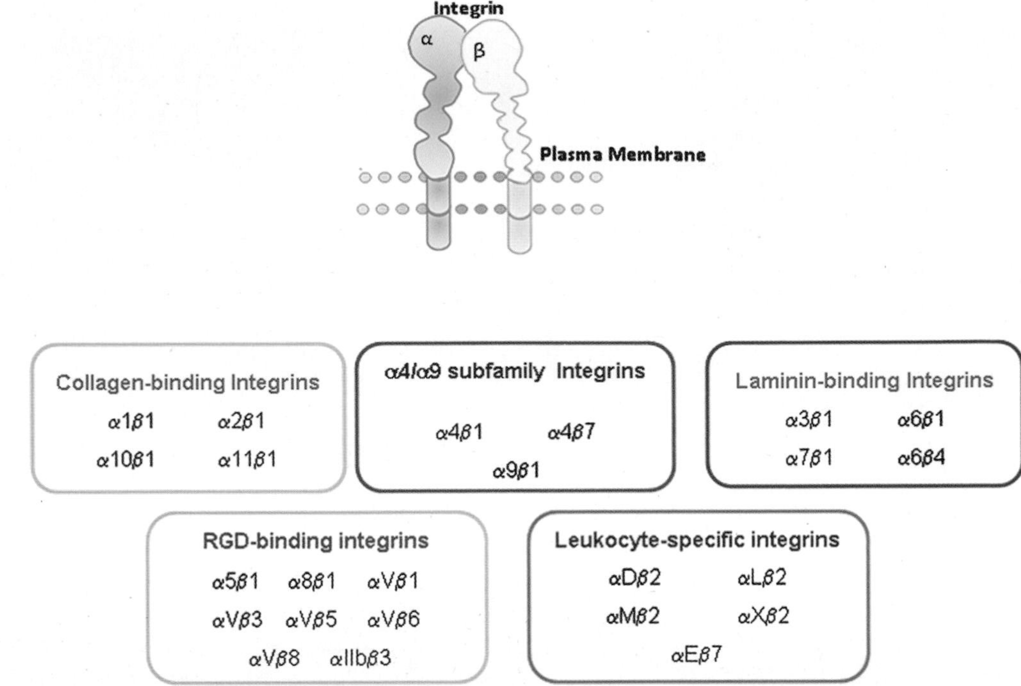

FIGURE 7.6. A: General backbone structure of Integrin is shown. Integrins are heterodimers that contains two distinct, the α (alpha) and β (beta) subunits. More than 18 α and 8 β subunits have been characterized in mammalian system. **B:** Different combinations of the alpha and beta subunits result in the generation of unique Integrins, which have different functional properties. Integrins couple the extracellular matrix (ECM) outside the cell to the intracellular actin filamentous system. Various ECM proteins such as collagen and laminin are ligands to the integrin in this process.

associates with MMP-2 on angiogenic blood vessels, and this association is needed for tumor angiogenesis.[92] A fragment of this proteinase (PEX) binding to the integrin blocks MMP-2 activity and can suppress angiogenesis and tumor growth.[93] Cell-surface MMP-14 can process pro-αV and enhance outside-in signaling through αVβ3 integrin.[94] This integrin can be also regulated by PAI-1 to promote migration of retinal endothelial cells (RECs).[95]

Overall, integrins comprise a big family of transmembrane receptors capable of bidirectional signaling, interaction with proteinases and growth factor receptors, and cytoskeleton organization. They are important for many vital cellular processes including angiogenesis and may be important targets for suppression in retinopathies and cancer.

INTEGRINS IN RETINAL ANGIOGENESIS AND DIABETIC RETINOPATHY

Normal Retina

At least nine integrin chains have been identified in the retina, and seven are strongly expressed in retinal vessels.[96] Most of these vascular integrins appear to have a β1 subunit. Although functions of many integrins in the normal retina remain unknown, some of them have been studied in more detail. β1-containing integrins are important for early retinogenesis and are also needed for neuroblast migration during retinal development.[97,98] Collagen-binding integrin α2β1 mediates tractional force generation by retinal Müller cells.[99] In the retinal pigment epithelium (RPE), the fibronectin receptor α5β1 integrin is localized to the apical cell membrane and promotes RPE migration and proliferation.[100] Knockout mouse experiments showed that integrin α1β1 expressed on the basal aspect of RPE appears to play a role in cell-basement membrane interactions and transducin translocation in photoreceptors.[101] Another integrin, αVβ5, plays an interesting role in the phagocytosis of photoreceptor outer segments by RPE. Although it is not required for phagocytosis per se,[102] it participates in photoreceptor binding to RPE[103] and is important for circadian synchronization of phagocytosis.[104]

Diabetic Retinopathy

In pathological conditions affecting the retina, most of the work on integrins has been conducted in widespread vasoproliferative disorders, primarily, in DR and its proliferative stage (PDR). REC culture studies used high glucose treatment to mimic diabetic conditions. High glucose induced an increased expression of α5β1 and α3β1 integrins in cultured macrovascular endothelium, which agreed well with an upregulation of β1-containing integrins in diabetic retinal vessels.[105] However, upregulation of fibronectin-binding α5β1 integrin could be an early event in diabetes. This may be inferred from a recent study showing that it is decreased when the cells are incubated with fibronectin modified by advanced glycation end (AGE) products, which accumulate during long-term diabetes.[106] In mouse REC, high glucose upregulates vitronectin receptor αVβ3 integrin.[107]

Analysis of retinas from PDR patients has revealed the expression of endothelial αVβ3[108] and αVβ5[109] integrins in areas of retinal neovascularization. These integrins were not found in adjacent areas or in normal human retinas. In vascularized epiretinal membranes removed from PDR patients during pars plana vitrectomy, overexpression of either αVβ3 and αVβ5 vascular integrins[110] or only αVβ3[111,112] was observed. Earlier studies described overexpression of fibronectin receptors, α4β1[113] and α5β1,[114] that are poorly or not at all expressed on quiescent endothelial cells.[71] In proliferative vitreoretinopathy, overexpression of fibronectin (α5β1) and vitronectin (αVβ3/β5) receptors was also noted.[114]

Leukocyte adhesion to vessels, leukostasis, and ensuing vaso-obliteration and Fas ligand-mediated endothelial death are also common in DR. The process of neutrophil adhesion enhanced in diabetes and reproduced in OIR model is largely dependent on integrins containing the β2 chain, namely, Mac-1 and LFA-1, which can bind endothelial intercellular adhesion molecule-1.[115–117] Antibodies to integrin β2 chain prevented these processes. Another integrin, α4β1, has been implicated in red blood cell retention in sickle cell retinopathy and vascular leakage in diabetes.[118,119]

Retinal Neovascularization in Oxygen-Induced Retinopathy

Because no animal can develop PDR, a model of OIR is widely considered and used as a PDR model, although it develops on normoglycemic background and represents developmental rather than pathological neovascularization.[120] Using this model, it was shown that αV integrins are upregulated in neovascular retinas early after release from hyperoxia (day P12) and decline after day P15, which is similar to VEGF expression patterns.[121] In another study,[52] αV mRNA showed a later increase starting from day P14; the reasons for this discrepancy are unknown. By immunostaining αV[122] and, more specifically, αVβ3[112], integrin was observed in neovascular retinal endothelium but not in normal retina. These data show that endothelial vitronectin receptors, αVβ3 and/or αVβ5, may be important modulators of retinal neovascularization. Paradoxical results on enhanced pathological angiogenesis in mice lacking these integrins may be explained by the concomitant upregulation of VEGF in these mice.[123,124]

INTEGRINS IN CHOROIDAL ANGIOGENESIS AND WET MACULAR DEGENERATION

Normal choriocapillaris vessels express essentially the same integrins as retinal vasculature.[96] Endothelial cells of experimental rat CNV induced by laser photocoagulation become positive for αVβ3 and α5β1 integrins.[125,126] Interestingly, CNV development is associated with leukocyte adhesion and vascular leakage that appear to be dependent on β2 integrins.[127] In choroidal neovascular membranes from patients with neovascular ("wet") form of AMD, distinct expressions of αVβ3 and α5β1 integrins were also found.[110,128] Additionally, and to a lesser extent, α1β1 and α2β1 integrins were observed in association with endothelial cells in these membranes.[128] Overall, integrins αVβ3 and α5β1 appear to be consistent markers of CNV in both animal models and human AMD, making them attractive targets for possible inhibitor therapy.

ANTI-INTEGRIN APPROACHES: ANIMAL AND CLINICAL STUDIES

Integrin Antagonists in Animal Models of Retinal Neovascularization

The data on specific integrin upregulation in neovascular diseases and animal models prompted investigations of integrin antagonists as antiangiogenic agents. Several compounds and routes of administration were tested in the mouse OIR preclinical model. The antagonists included RGD-based synthetic peptides specific for αV-containing integrins,[110,112,121,128,129] small molecule non–peptide inhibitors or peptidomimetic signaling inhibitors of αV or α5β1 integrins,[130–132] blocking antibody, and naturally occurring neutrophil α-defensin HNP-1 that binds α5β1 integrin.[133] In these studies, the inhibitors were administered either intraperitoneally, or subcutaneously, or subconjunctivally, or intravitreally, or even orally. Most reports showed only partial inhibition in the vicinity of 50% but not higher than 60%. This modest outcome could be the result of multifactorial nature of retinal neovascularization that necessitated combination therapy.[134] In fact, when an integrin signaling antagonist was combined with a VEGF aptamer and a fragment of tRNA synthetase blocking VE-cadherin-mediated adhesion, the effect on retinal neovascularization was dramatically augmented.[130] Therefore, in relation to retinal neovascularization and PDR, integrin antagonists may be considered only as parts of a combination therapy targeting several players of angiogenic cascade together. It should be noted that low doses of antagonists may actually promote angiogenesis by activating rather than blocking integrins.[135] These new data imply that doses of integrin inhibitors should be kept rather high even in combination therapy formulations.

Preclinical Anti-integrin Studies for Blocking Choroidal Neovascularization

Several integrin inhibitors have been tested so far in an animal model of laser-induced CNV using mice and rats. The results have been overall more promising than in the OIR model. An αV antagonist EMD478761 was able to inhibit CNV by more than 60% with sustained release from intravitreal implants.[136] A similar effect was observed for αVβ3-specific antagonist BS-1417 with intraperitoneal administration.[137] A weaker dose-dependent inhibition was achieved with a cyclic RGD peptide targeting αV integrins using intravitreal administration.[138]

Administration of a small molecule α5β1 integrin inhibitor JSM6427 using a subcutaneous pump also resulted in a modest CNV inhibition.[125] However, in a recent follow-up of this study with weekly intravitreal injections using rabbit and monkey models,[139] it was possible to achieve a much stronger CNV inhibition (around 70%). Importantly, in both models, no adverse effects were observed. A chimeric humanized antibody to α5β1 (M200, Volociximab) showed significant reduction of CNV.[140] Another potent integrin inhibitor, C16Y peptide, which blocks both αVβ3 and α5β1 integrins and can reduce tumor growth, was recently applied to a rat CNV model. When encapsulated into polylactate/polylactate-polyethylene oxide nanoparticles, intravitreally injected C16Y was able to reduce CNV by 65% to 70%.[141] This combination therapy inhibitor also appears promising for future clinical interventions.

Emerging Human Studies with Integrin Antagonists for Ocular Diseases

Due to a considerable success in preclinical studies, some integrin inhibitors have entered clinical trials. Many of them are being tested in Phases 1–3 for inhibiting various forms of cancer. To mention just a few blockers relevant to eye disease,[142] these include antibodies to αVβ3 (LM609/MEDI-522/Vitaxin), αV (CNTO 95), and α5β1 (Volociximab); peptide inhibitors of αV (EMD121974/Cilengitide) and α5β1 (ATN-161); and peptidomimetics, in particular those that block both αV and α5β1 integrins (BCH-15046).

For α5β1 antagonist JSM6427, a phase 1 trial has been initiated in ARMD by Jerini Ophthalmic (clinicaltrials.gov identifier NCT00536016). This is a safety trial for single-dose and repeated-dose intravitreal injections.[139] Another Phase 1 open-label multicenter trial of an antibody to α5β1 integrin (Volociximab) in combination with anti-VEGF drug Lucentis is being conducted (clinicaltrials.gov identifier NCT00536016) by Ophthotech Corporation; the antibody appears to be safe (Box 7.4).[143] In light of the apparent complexity of neovascular response in PDR and modest results in animal models, no clinical trials for PDR using integrin inhibition are being currently conducted. Overall, the clinical application of integrin blockers for vasoproliferative eye diseases is still in its infancy. Its future may depend on the outcomes of more advanced clinical trials in the field of oncology.

BOX 7.4 Integrin Inhibitors in Clinical trials

JSM 6427

An inhibitor of integrin a5b1, JSM 6427 (Jerini AG, New York, NY), is being tested in a Phase 1 clinical trial in patients with wet ARMD. This intravitreal drug addresses angiogenesis, inflammation, and fibrosis.

Volociximab

A monoclonal antibody against integrin a5b1 (Ophthotech, New York, NY) is also being tested in a clinical trial in patients with wet ARMD. Volociximab inhibits endothelial cell proliferation downstream of growth factor stimulation, irrespective of the upstream proangiogenic stimulating factors.

COMBINATION THERAPY

Currently, the majority of the clinical trials in retinal diseases have targeted the VEGF molecule. As the angiogenic cascade has been explored with more potential molecules involved, other therapeutic options using inhibitors other than VEGF inhibitors are being explored. At least in preclinical studies as pointed out in this chapter, many of these molecules have proved to be attractive targets for intervention in PDR. The rationale for searching other novel pathways is twofold. First, in macular degeneration patients, clinical experience shows that the drugs, ranibizumab or bevacizumab, have to be administered every 4 weeks as complete regression is not possible with just a few injections. Repeated intravitreal injections have potential side effects of infection, vitreous hemorrhage, and retinal detachment, and also there may be unknown potential side effects from continuous VEGF inhibition as VEGF has been shown to be a neuroprotective agent. Secondly, a combination therapy using more than one antiangiogenic agent seems to be more attractive as one can attack different steps of the angiogenesis cascade rather than one. Such a combination therapy is common in glaucoma management where intraocular pressure–lowering agents are added one after another until the optimal therapeutic level is achieved. Also, the other scenario is possible where one can combine the current panretinal photocoagulation therapy with anti-VEGF or anti-VEGF treatment with other antiangiogenic agents. The urokinase inhibitor, A6 (Angstrom Pharmaceuticals, San Diego, California), which is currently in a Phase 2 clinical trial in ovarian carcinoma patients, has been shown to be a promising agent in both retinal and choroidal angiogenesis in preclinical studies. Several MMP inhibitors and integrin inhibitors are currently in clinical trials for different types of cancer, and many of these agents have been shown to be effective in retinal angiogenesis as well. As we develop new drugs for antiangiogenic effects, one needs to consider the fact that factors other than VEGF are also critical in the angiogenesis cascade, and one should target against these "other" molecules as well. A combination therapy with proteinase or integrin inhibitors with

KEY POINTS

- Basement membranes are complex, multicomponent structures with diverse functions. They provide support for attachment, spreading, migration, growth, repair, and differentiation of the overlying cells.
- The angiogenesis cascade consists of several phases including upregulation of angiogenic factors and increased expression of extracellular proteinases and integrins.
- Proteinases facilitate the breakdown of the basement membrane and ECM, allowing endothelial cells to migrate.
- Proteinases include the serine proteinase, urokinase (uPA), and members of the MMPs.
- Increased expressions of proteinases have been shown in animal models of both retinal neovascularization and CNV.
- Preclinical studies have shown proteinases may serve as important therapeutic targets in retinal neovascularization and CNV.
- Integrins are transmembrane heterodimeric receptors for ECM present on all tissue and circulating cells.
- Integrins interact with and modulate the activity of various growth factor receptors.
- Pathological ocular neovascularization as exemplified by PDR and wet form of AMD are accompanied by increased expression of specific vascular integrins, in particular $\alpha V\beta 3$, $\alpha V\beta 5$, and $\alpha 5\beta 1$.
- Antagonists of integrins overexpressed in PDR and wet AMD can suppress retinal neovascularization and CNV, respectively, in animal models.
- Clinical trials using integrin antagonists in wet macular degeneration are currently in progress.

the currently used anti-VEGF agents may be an effective treatment for ocular neovascularization that needs to be explored. Such an option may reduce the number of intravitreal injections that is often needed to control the extent of neovascularization.

REFERENCES

1. Das A, Frank RN, Zhang NL, et al. Ultrastructural localization of extracellular matrix components in human retinal vessels and Bruch's membrane. *Arch Ophthalmol*. 1990;108(3):421–429.
2. Ffrench-Constant C, Van de Water L, Dvorak HF, et al. Reappearance of an embryonic pattern of fibronectin splicing during wound healing in the adult rat. *J Cell Biol*. 1989;109:903–914.
3. Furcht LT, McCarthy JB, Palm SL, et al. *Peptide Fragments of Laminin and Fibronectin Promote Migration (Haptotaxis and Chemotaxis) of Metastatic Cells*. In: Ciba Foundation Symposia. London, UK: Pitman Publishing Ltd; 1984.
4. Podestá F, Roth T, Ferrara F, et al. Cytoskeletal changes induced by excess extracellular matrix impair endothelial cell replication. *Diabetologia*. 1997;40(8):879–886.
5. Ljubimov AV, Burgeson RE, Butkowski RJ, et al. Basement membrane abnormalities in human eyes with diabetic retinopathy. *J Histochem Cytochem*. 1996;44(12):1469–1479.
6. Ljubimov AV, Huang ZS, Huang GH, et al. Human corneal epithelial basement membrane and integrin alterations in diabetes and diabetic retinopathy. *J Histochem Cytochem*. 1998;46(9):1033–1041.
7. Monnier VM, Bautista O, Kenny D, et al. Skin collagen glycation, glycoxidation, and crosslinking are lower in subjects with long-term intensive versus conventional therapy of type 1 diabetes: relevance of glycated collagen products versus HbA1c as markers of diabetic complications. DCCT Skin Collagen Ancillary Study Group. Diabetes Control and Complications Trial. *Diabetes*. 1999;48(4):870–880.
8. Monnier VM, Vishwanath V, Frank KE, et al. Relation between complications of type I diabetes mellitus and collagen-linked fluorescence. *N Engl J Med*. 1986;314(7):403–408.
9. Nwomeh BC, Yager DR, Cohen IK. Physiology of the chronic wound. *Clin Plast Surg*. 1998;25(3):341–356.
10. Risteli L, Puistola U, Hohtari H, et al. Collagen metabolism in normal and complicated pregnancy: changes in the aminoterminal propeptide of type III procollagen in serum. *Eur J Clin Invest*. 1987;17(1):81–86.
11. Roux E, Cherbit G, Regnault F. Collagen-induced platelet aggregation and collagen glycosyltransferase activity in diabetic patients. *Thromb Res*. 1977;11(6):847–858.
12. Roy S, Cagliero E, Lorenzi M. Fibronectin overexpression in retinal microvessels of patients with diabetes. *Invest Ophthalmol Vis Sci*. 1996;37(2):258–266.
13. Salmela PI, Oikarinen A, Pirttiaho H, et al. Increased nonenzymatic glycosylation and reduced solubility of skin collagen in insulin-dependent diabetic patients. *Diabetes Res*. 1989;11(3):115–120.
14. Bek T, Ledet T. Glycoprotein deposition in vascular walls of diabetic retinopathy. A histopathological and immunohistochemical study. *Acta Ophthalmol Scand*. 1996;74(4):385–390.
15. Das A, Frank RN, Zhang NL, et al. Increases in collagen type IV and laminin in galactose-induced retinal capillary basement membrane thickening–prevention by an aldose reductase inhibitor. *Exp Eye Res*. 1990;50(3):269–280.
16. Sank A, Wei D, Reid J, et al. Human endothelial cells are defective in diabetic vascular disease. *J Surg Res*. 1994;57(6):647–653.
17. Hannan KM, Little PJ. Mechanisms regulating the vascular smooth muscle Na/H exchanger (NHE-1) in diabetes. *Biochem Cell Biol*. 1998;76(5):751–759.
18. Weller M, Wiedemann P, Bresgen M, et al. Vitronectin and proliferative intraocular disorders. II. Expression of cell surface receptors for fibronectin and vitronectin in periretinal membranes. *Int Ophthalmol*. 1991;15(2):103–108.
19. Carlin B, Jaffe R, Bender B, et al. Entactin, a novel basal lamina-associated sulfated glycoprotein. *J Biol Chem*. 1981;256(10):5209–5214.
20. Rohrbach DH, Robinson LK, Murrah VA. Loss of the basement membrane matrix molecule, bamin, in diphenylamine-treated mice. *Matrix*. 1993;13(5):341–350.

21. Henry MD, Campbell KP. A role for dystroglycan in basement membrane assembly. *Cell*. 1998;95(6):859–870.
22. Klues HG, Radke PW, Hoffmann R, et al. Pathophysiology and therapeutic concepts in coronary restenosis. *Herz*. 1997;22(6):322–334.
23. Spirin KS, Saghizadeh M, Lewin SL, et al. Basement membrane and growth factor gene expression in normal and diabetic human retinas. *Curr Eye Res*. 1999;18(6):490–499.
24. Cooper ME, Cao Z, Rumble JR, et al. Attenuation of diabetes-associated mesenteric vascular hypertrophy with perindopril: morphological and molecular biological studies. *Metabolism*. 1998;47:24–27.
25. Rasmussen LM, Ledet T. Aortic collagen alterations in human diabetes mellitus. Changes in basement membrane collagen content and in the susceptibility of total collagen to cyanogen bromide solubilisation. *Diabetologia*. 1993;36(5):445–453.
26. Roy S, Maiello M, Lorenzi M. Increased expression of basement membrane collagen in human diabetic retinopathy. *J Clin Invest*. 1994;93(1):438–442.
27. Rumble JR, Gilbert RE, Cox A, et al. Angiotensin converting enzyme inhibition reduces the expression of transforming growth factor-beta1 and type IV collagen in diabetic vasculopathy. *J Hypertens*. 1998;16(11):1603–1609.
28. Yokoyama H, Deckert T. Central role of TGF-beta in the pathogenesis of diabetic nephropathy and macrovascular complications: a hypothesis. *Diabet Med*. 1996;13(4):313–320.
29. Bakillah A, Grigorova-Borsos AM, Guillot R, et al. Effect of an aldose reductase inhibitor on type IV collagen production by human endothelial cells cultured in high glucose. *Diabetologia*. 1996;39(6):641–648.
30. Shinoda Y. Immunohistochemical localization of type IV collagen and laminin in the gingival capillary basement membrane of the diabetic rat. *J Osaka Dent Univ*. 1992; 26(2):49–66.
31. Spiro MJ, Crowley TJ. Increased rat myocardial type VI collagen in diabetes mellitus and hypertension. *Diabetologia*. 1993;36(2):93–98.
32. Grant MB, Ellis EA, Caballero S, et al. Plasminogen activator inhibitor-1 overexpression in nonproliferative diabetic retinopathy. *Exp Eye Res*. 1996;63(3):233–244.
33. Hagedorn M, Esser P, Wiedemann P, et al. Tenascin and decorin in epiretinal membranes of proliferative vitreoretinopathy and proliferative diabetic retinopathy. *Ger J Ophthalmol*. 1993;2(1):28–31.
34. Brenner MA. Tracking the diabetic foot: adjunctive treatment with collagen material. *Adv Wound Care*. 1994;7(6):44, 46, 48–52.
35. Chowdhury TA, Kumar S, Barnett AH, et al. Nephropathy in type 1 diabetes: the role of genetic factors. *Diabet Med*. 1995;12(12):1059–1067.
36. Pfeiffer A, Schatz H. Diabetic microvascular complications and growth factors. *Exp Clin Endocrinol Diabetes*. 1995;103(1):7–14.
37. Hesse L, Chofflet J, Kroll P. Tissue plasminogen activator as a biochemical adjuvant in vitrectomy for proliferative diabetic vitreoretinopathy. *Ger J Ophthalmol*. 1995;4(6):323–327.
38. Pankov R, Yamada KM. Fibronectin at a glance. *J Cell Sci*. 2002;115(Pt 20):3861–3863.
39. Mohs A, Popiel M, Li Y, et al. Conformational features of a natural break in the type IV collagen Gly-X-Y repeat. *J Biol Chem*. 2006;281(25):17197–17202.
40. Oshitari T, Polewski P, Chadda M, et al. Effect of combined antisense oligonucleotides against high-glucose- and diabetes-induced overexpression of extracellular matrix components and increased vascular permeability. *Diabetes*. 2006;55(1):86–92.
41. Oshitari T, Brown D, Roy S. SiRNA strategy against overexpression of extracellular matrix in diabetic retinopathy. *Exp Eye Res*. 2005;81(1):32–37.
42. Sato T, Paryani G, Kao RS, et al. Antisense oligonucleotides modulate high glucose-induced laminin overexpression and cell proliferation: a potential for therapeutic application in diabetic microangiopathy. *Antisense Nucleic Acid Drug Dev*. 2001;11(6):387–394.
43. Ruhrberg C, Gerhardt H, Golding M, et al. Spatially restricted patterning cues provided by heparin-binding VEGF-A control blood vessel branching morphogenesis. *Genes Dev*. 2002;16(20):2684–2698.
44. Fruttiger M. Development of the mouse retinal vasculature: angiogenesis versus vasculogenesis. *Invest Ophthalmol Vis Sci*. 2002;43(2):522–527.
45. Gerhardt H, Golding M, Fruttiger M, et al. VEGF guides angiogenic sprouting utilizing endothelial tip cell filopodia. *J Cell Biol*. 2003;161(6):1163–1177.
46. Hellström M, Phng LK, Hofmann JJ, et al. Dll4 signalling through Notch1 regulates formation of tip cells during angiogenesis. *Nature*. 2007;445(7129):776–780.
47. Lobov IB, Renard RA, Papadopoulos N, et al. Delta-like ligand 4 (Dll4) is induced by VEGF as a negative regulator of angiogenic sprouting. *Proc Natl Acad Sci U S A*. 2007;104(9):3219–3224.
48. Suchting S, et al. The Notch ligand Delta-like 4 negatively regulates endothelial tip cell formation and vessel branching. *Proc Natl Acad Sci U S A*. 2007;104(9):3225–3230.
49. Das A, McGuire PG. Retinal and choroidal angiogenesis: pathophysiology and strategies for inhibition. *Progr Retinal Eye Res*. 2003;22:721–748.
50. Pepper MS. Role of the matrix metalloproteinase and plasminogen activator-plasmin systems in angiogenesis. *Arterioscler Thromb Vasc Biol*. 2001;21:1104–1117.
51. Quax P, van Muijen G, Weening-Verhoeff E, et al. Metastatic behavior of human melanoma cell lines in nude mice correlates with urokinase type plasminogen activator, its type inhibitor, urokinase-mediated matrix degradation. *J Cell Biol*. 1991;115:191–199.
52. Manchanda N, Schwartz BS. Single chain urokinase: augmentation of enzymatic activity upon binding to monocytes. *J Biol Chem*. 1991;266:14580–14584.
53. Blasi R. Urokinase and urokinase receptor: a paracrine/autocrine system regulating cell migration and invasiveness. *Bioassays*. 1993;15:105–111.
54. Rabbani SA, Desjardins J, Bell AW, et al. An amino terminal fragment of urokinase isolated from a prostate cancer cell line is mitogenic for osteoblast-like cells. *Biochem Biophys Res Commun*. 1990;173:1058–1064.
55. Blasi F, Carmeliet P. uPA: a versatile signaling orchestrator. *Nat Rev Mol Cell Biol*. 2002;3:931–943.
56. Stetler-Stevenson WG. The role of matrix metalloproteinases in tumor invasion, metastasis and angiogenesis. *Surg Oncol Clin N Am*. 2001;10:383–392.
57. Baramova E, Foidart JM. Matrix metalloproteinase family. *Cell Biol Int*. 1995;19:239–242.

58. Weber BHF, Vogt G, Pruett RC, et al. Mutations in the tissue inhibitor of metalloproteinases-3 (TIMP-3) in patients with Sorsby's fundus dystrophy. *Nat Genet*. 1994;8:352–356.
59. Farris RN, Apte SS, Luhert PJ, et al. Accumulations of tissue inhibitor metalloproteinases-3 in human eyes with Sorsby's fundus dystrophy or retinitis pigmentosa. *Br J Ophthalmol*. 1998;82:1329–1334.
60. Andreasen PA, Georg B, Lund LR, et al. Plasminogen activator inhibitors: hormonally regulated serpins. *Mol Cell Endocrinol*. 1990;68:1–19.
61. Thorgeirson UP, Linsay CK, Cottam DW, et al. Tumor invasion, proteolysis, angiogenesis. *J Neuro-Oncology*. 1994; 18: 89–103.
62. Das A, McLamore A, Song W, et al. Retinal neovascularization is suppressed with a MMP inhibitor. *Arch Ophthalmol*. 1999;117:498–503.
63. Das A, McGuire PG, Eriqat C, et al. Human diabetic neovascular membranes contain high levels of urokinase and metalloproteinase enzymes. *Invest Ophthalmol Vis Sci*. 1999; 40:809–813.
64. McGuire PG, Jones TR, Talarico, et al. The urokinase/urokinase receptor system in retinal neovascularization: inhibition by A6 suggests a new therapeutic target. *Invest Ophthalmol Vis Sci*. 2003;44:2736–2742.
65. Majka S, McGuire PG, Colombo S, et al. The balance between proteinases and inhibitors in a murine model of proliferative retinopathy. *Invest Ophthalmol Vis Sci*. 2001;42:210–215.
66. Lambert V, Munaut P, Carmeliet P, et al. Dose-dependent modulation of choroidal neovascularization by plasminogen activator type 1: Implications for clinical trials. *Invest Ophthalmol Vis Sci*. 2003;44:2791–2797.
67. Das A, Boyd TR, Jones TR, et al. Inhibition of choroidal neovascularization by a peptide inhibitor of the urokinase plasminogen activator and receptor system in a mouse model. *Arch Ophthalmol*. 2004;45:635–640.
68. Le Gat L, Gogat K, Bouquet C, et al. In vivo adenovirus-mediated delivery of a uPA/uPAR antagonist reduces retinal neovascularization in a mouse model of retinopathy. *Gene Ther*. 2003;10:2098–2103.
69. Kohri T, Moriwaki M, Nakajima H, et al. Reduction of experimental laser-induced choroidal neovascularization by orally administered BPHA, a selective metalloproteinase inhibitor. *Graefes Arch Clin Exp Ophthalmol*. 2003;241;943–952.
70. Bradey ME, Cheng L, Bartsch DU, et al. Prevention vs treatment effect of AG3340, a potent matrix metalloproteinase inhibitor in a rat model of choroidal neovascularization. *J Ocul Pharmacol Ther*. 2004;20:217–236.
71. Avraamides CJ, Garmy-Susini B, Varner JA. Integrins in angiogenesis and lymphangiogenesis. *Nat Rev Cancer*. 2008;8:604–617.
72. Barczyk M, Carracedo S, Gullberg D. Integrins. *Cell Tissue Res*. 2010;339:269–280.
73. Bevilacqua MP, Amrani D, Mosesson MW, et al. Receptors for cold-insoluble globulin (plasma fibronectin) on human monocytes. *J Exp Med*. 1981;153:42–60.
74. Davignon D, Martz E, Reynolds T, et al. Lymphocyte function-associated antigen 1 (LFA-1): a surface antigen distinct from Lyt-2,3 that participates in T lymphocyte-mediated killing. *Proc Natl Acad Sci U S A*. 1981;78:4535–4539.
75. Plow EF, Ginsberg MH. Specific and saturable binding of plasma fibronectin to thrombin-stimulated human platelets. *J Biol Chem*. 1981;256:9477–9482.
76. Hansen MS, Clemmensen I. A fibronectin-binding glycoprotein from human platelet membranes. *Biochem J*. 1982;201:629–633.
77. Ljubimov AV, Vasiliev JM. Distribution of fibronectin-containing structures on the surface of lamelloplasm and endoplasm of fibroblasts; hypothesis of receptor-mediated assembly of fibronectin structures. *Cell Biol Int Repts*. 1982;6:105–112.
78. Zinkevich OD, Litvinov RI, Kuravskaia MS. Fibronectin and fibronectin receptors on the surfaces of polymorphonuclear leukocytes. *Biull Eksp Biol Med*. 1982;94:86–88. Russian.
79. Sanchez-Madrid F, Krensky AM, Ware CF, et al. Three distinct antigens associated with human T-lymphocyte-mediated cytolysis: LFA-1, LFA-2, and LFA-3. *Proc Natl Acad Sci U S A*. 1982;79:7489–7493.
80. McKeown-Longo PJ, Mosher DF. Binding of plasma fibronectin to cell layers of human skin fibroblasts. *J Cell Biol*. 1983;97:466–472.
81. Pytela R, Pierschbacher MD, Ruoslahti E. A 125/115-kDa cell surface receptor specific for vitronectin interacts with the arginine-glycine-aspartic acid adhesion sequence derived from fibronectin. *Proc Natl Acad Sci U S A*. 1985;82: 5766–5770.
82. Legate KR, Wickström SA, Fässler R. Genetic and cell biological analysis of integrin outside-in signaling. *Genes Dev*. 2009;23:397–418.
83. Gahmberg CG, Fagerholm SC, Nurmi SM, et al. Regulation of integrin activity and signalling. *Biochim Biophys Acta*. 2009;1790:431–444.
84. Johnson MS, Lu N, Denessiouk K, et al. Integrins during evolution: Evolutionary trees and model organisms. *Biochim Biophys Acta*. 2009;1788:779–789.
85. Huveneers S, Danen EHJ. Adhesion signaling – crosstalk between integrins, Src and Rho. J Cell Sci. 2009;122: 1059–1069.
86. Contois L, Akalu A, Brooks PC. Integrins as "functional hubs" in the regulation of pathological angiogenesis. Semin Cancer Biol. 2009;19:318–328.
87. Streuli CH, Akhtar N. Signal co-operation between integrins and other receptor systems. Biochem J. 2009;418:491–506.
88. Ricono JM, Huang M, Barnes LA, et al. Specific cross-talk between epidermal growth factor receptor and integrin aVb5 promotes carcinoma cell invasion and metastasis. Cancer Res. 2009;69:1383–1391.
89. Soldi R, Mitola S, Strasly M, et al. Role of aVb3 integrin in the activation of vascular endothelial growth factor receptor-2. EMBO J. 1999;18:882–892.
90. Somanath PR, Malinin NL, Byzova TV. Cooperation between integrin aVb3 and VEGFR2 in angiogenesis. Angiogenesis. 2009;12:177–185.
91. Robinson SD, Reynolds LE, Wyder L, et al. b3-integrin regulates vascular endothelial growth factor-A-dependent permeability. Arterioscler Thromb Vasc Biol. 2004;24:2108–2114.
92. Silletti S, Kessler T, Goldberg J, et al. Disruption of matrix metalloproteinase 2 binding to integrin aVb3 by an organic molecule inhibits angiogenesis and tumor growth in vivo. Proc Natl Acad Sci U S A. 2001;98;119–124.
93. Brooks PC, Silletti S, von Schalscha TL, et al. Disruption of angiogenesis by PEX, a noncatalytic metalloproteinase fragment with integrin binding activity. Cell. 1998;92: 391–400.

94. Deryugina EI, Ratnikov BI, Postnova TI, et al. Processing of integrin aV subunit by membrane type 1 matrix metalloproteinase stimulates migration of breast carcinoma cells on vitronectin and enhances tyrosine phosphorylation of focal adhesion kinase. J Biol Chem. 2002;277:9749–9756.
95. Basu A, Menicucci G, Maestas J, et al. Plasminogen activator inhibitor-1 (PAI-1) facilitates retinal angiogenesis in a model of oxygen-induced retinopathy. Invest Ophthalmol Vis Sci. 2009;50:4974–4981.
96. Brem RB, Robbins SG, Wilson DJ, et al. Immunolocalization of integrins in the human retina. Invest Ophthalmol Vis Sci. 1994;35;3466–3474.
97. Cann GM, Bradshaw AD, Gervin DB, et al. Widespread occurrence of β1 integrins in the developing chick retina: evidence for a role in migration of retinal ganglion cells. *Dev Biol.* 1996;180:82–96.
98. Skeith A, Dunlop L, Galileo DS, et al. Inhibition of β1-integrin expression reduces clone size during early retinogenesis. *Brain Res Dev Brain Res.* 1999;116:123–126.
99. Guidry C, Bradley KM, King JL. Tractional force generation by human Müller cells: growth factor responsiveness and integrin receptor involvement. *Invest Ophthalmol Vis Sci.* 2003;44:1355–1363.
100. Li R, Maminishkis A, Zahn G, et al. Integrin α5β1 mediates attachment, migration, and proliferation in human retinal pigment epithelium: relevance for proliferative retinal disease. *Invest Ophthalmol Vis Sci.* 2009;50:5988–5996.
101. Peng YW, Zalocchi M, Meehan DT, et al. Progressive morphological and functional defects in retinas from α1 integrin-null mice. *Invest Ophthalmol Vis Sci.* 2008;49: 4647–4654.
102. Hall MO, Abrams TA, Burgess BL. Integrin αVβ5 is not required for the phagocytosis of photoreceptor outer segments by cultured retinal pigment epithelial cells. *Exp Eye Res.* 2003;77:281–286.
103. Lin H, Clegg DO. Integrin αVβ5 participates in the binding of photoreceptor rod outer segments during phagocytosis by cultured human retinal pigment epithelium. *Invest Ophthalmol Vis Sci.* 1998;39:1703–1712.
104. Nandrot EF, Finnemann SC. Lack of αVβ5 integrin receptor or its ligand MFG-E8: distinct effects on retinal function. *Ophthalmic Res.* 2008;40:120–123.
105. Roth T, Podestá F, Stepp MA, et al. Integrin overexpression induced by high glucose and by human diabetes: potential pathway to cell dysfunction in diabetic microangiopathy. *Proc Natl Acad Sci U S A.* 1993;90:9640–9644.
106. McDonald DM, Coleman G, Bhatwadekar A, et al. Advanced glycation of the Arg-Gly-Asp (RGD) tripeptide motif modulates retinal microvascular endothelial cell dysfunction. *Mol Vis.* 2009;15:1509–1520.
107. Huang Q, Sheibani N. High glucose promotes retinal endothelial cell migration through activation of Src, PI3K/Akt1/eNOS, and ERKs. *Am J Physiol Cell Physiol.* 2008;295:C1647–C1657.
108. Casaroli Marano RP, Preissner KT, Vilaró S. Fibronectin, laminin, vitronectin and their receptors at newly-formed capillaries in proliferative diabetic retinopathy. *Exp Eye Res.* 1995;60:5–17.
109. Ljubimov AV, Burgeson RE, Butkowski RJ, et al. Basement membrane abnormalities in human eyes with diabetic retinopathy. *J Histochem Cytochem.* 1996;44:1469–1479.
110. Friedlander M, Theesfeld CL, Sugita M, et al. Involvement of integrins $\alpha_V\beta_3$ and $\alpha_V\beta_5$ in ocular neovascular diseases. *Proc Natl Acad Sci U S A.* 1996;93:9764–9769.
111. Ning A, Cui J, Maberley D, et al. Expression of integrins in human proliferative diabetic retinopathy membranes. *Can J Ophthalmol.* 2008;43:683–688.
112. Luna J, Tobe T, Mousa SA, et al. Antagonists of integrin αVβ3 inhibit retinal neovascularization in a murine model. *Lab Invest.* 1996;75:563–573.
113. Robbins SG, Brem RB, Wilson DJ, et al. Immunolocalization of integrins in proliferative retinal membranes. *Invest Ophthalmol Vis Sci.* 1994;35:3475–3485.
114. Weller M, Wiedemann P, Bresgen M, et al. Vitronectin and proliferative intraocular disorders. II. Expression of cell surface receptors for fibronectin and vitronectin in periretinal membranes. *Int Ophthalmol.* 1991;15:103–108.
115. Barouch FC, Miyamoto K, Allport JR, et al. Integrin-mediated neutrophil adhesion and retinal leukostasis in diabetes. *Invest Ophthalmol Vis Sci.* 2000;41:1153–1158.
116. Joussen AM, Murata T, Tsujikawa A, et al. Leukocyte-mediated endothelial injury and death in the diabetic retina. *Am J Pathol.* 2001;158:147–152.
117. Ishida S, Yamashiro K, Usui T, et al. Leukocytes mediate retinal vascular remodeling during development and vaso-obliteration in disease. *Nat Med.* 2003;9:781–788.
118. Lutty GA, Taomoto M, Cao J, et al. Inhibition of TNF-α-induced sickle RBC retention in retina by a VLA-4 antagonist. *Invest Ophthalmol Vis Sci.* 2001;42:1349–1355.
119. Iliaki E, Poulaki V, Mitsiades N, et al. Role of α4 integrin (CD49d) in the pathogenesis of diabetic retinopathy. *Invest Ophthalmol Vis Sci.* 2009;50:4898–4904.
120. Smith LE, Wesolowski E, McLellan A, et al. Oxygen-induced retinopathy in the mouse. *Invest Ophthalmol Vis Sci.* 1994;35:101–111.
121. Chavakis E, Riecke B, Lin J, et al. Kinetics of integrin expression in the mouse model of proliferative retinopathy and success of secondary intervention with cyclic RGD peptides. *Diabetologia.* 2002;45:262–267.
122. Takagi H, Suzuma K, Otani A, et al. Role of vitronectin receptor-type integrins and osteopontin in ischemia-induced retinal neovascularization. *Jpn J Ophthalmol.* 2002;46:270–278.
123. Reynolds LE, Wyder L, Lively JC, et al. Enhanced pathological angiogenesis in mice lacking β_3 integrin or β_3 and β_5 integrins. *Nat Med.* 2002;8:27–34.
124. Mahabeleshwar GH, Feng W, Phillips DR, et al. Integrin signaling is critical for pathological angiogenesis. *J Exp Med.* 2006;203:2495–2507.
125. Umeda N, Kachi S, Akiyama H, et al. Suppression and regression of choroidal neovascularization by systemic administration of an $\alpha_5\beta_1$ integrin antagonist. *Mol Pharmacol.* 2006;69:1820–1828.
126. Tang R, Long J, Chen B. Expression of integrin alphavbeta3, tissue factor, and vascular endothelial growth factor in experimental choroidal neovascularization. *Zhong Nan Da Xue Xue Bao Yi Xue Ban.* 2009;34:762–767. Chinese.
127. Sakurai E, Taguchi H, Anand A, et al. Targeted disruption of the CD18 or ICAM-1 gene inhibits choroidal neovascularization. *Invest Ophthalmol Vis Sci.* 2003;44:2743–2749.
128. Cui J, Maberley D, Samad A, et al. Expression of integrins on human choroidal neovascular membranes. *J Ocul Biol Dis Inform.* 2009;2:12–19.

129. Riecke B, Chavakis E, Bretzel RG, et al. Topical application of integrin antagonists inhibits proliferative retinopathy. *Horm Metab Res.* 2001;33:307–311.
130. Dorrell MI, Aguilar E, Scheppke L, et al. Combination angiostatic therapy completely inhibits ocular and tumor angiogenesis. *Proc Natl Acad Sci U S A.* 2007;104:967–972.
131. Santulli RJ, Kinney WA, Ghosh S, et al. Studies with an orally bioavailable alpha V integrin antagonist in animal models of ocular vasculopathy: retinal neovascularization in mice and retinal vascular permeability in diabetic rats. *J Pharmacol Exp Ther.* 2008;324:894–901.
132. Maier AK, Kociok N, Zahn G, et al. Modulation of hypoxia-induced neovascularization by JSM6427, an integrin alpha5beta1 inhibiting molecule. *Curr Eye Res.* 2007;32:801–812.
133. Economopoulou M, Bdeir K, Cines DB, et al. Inhibition of pathologic retinal neovascularization by α-defensins. *Blood.* 2005;106:3831–3838.
134. Afzal A, Shaw LC, Ljubimov AV, et al. Retinal and choroidal microangiopathies: therapeutic opportunities. *Microvasc Res.* 2007;74:131–144.
135. Reynolds AR, Hart IR, Watson AR, et al. Stimulation of tumor growth and angiogenesis by low concentrations of RGD-mimetic integrin inhibitors. *Nat Med.* 2009;15:392–400.
136. Fu Y, Ponce ML, Thill M, et al. Angiogenesis inhibition and choroidal neovascularization suppression by sustained delivery of an integrin antagonist, EMD478761. *Invest Ophthalmol Vis Sci.* 2007;48:5184–5190.
137. Honda S, Nagai T, Negi A. Anti-angiogenic effects of non-peptide integrin αvβ3 specific antagonist on laser-induced choroidal neovascularization in mice. *Graefes Arch Clin Exp Ophthalmol.* 2009;247:515–522.
138. Yasukawa T, Hoffmann S, Eichler W, et al. Inhibition of experimental choroidal neovascularization in rats by an α_V-integrin antagonist. *Curr Eye Res.* 2004;28:359–366.
139. Zahn G, Vossmeyer D, Stragies R, et al. Preclinical evaluation of the novel small-molecule integrin α5β1 inhibitor JSM6427 in monkey and rabbit models of choroidal neovascularization. *Arch Ophthalmol.* 2009;127:1329–1335.
140. Ramakrishnan V, Bhaskar V, Law DA, et al. Preclinical evaluation of an anti-α5β1 integrin antibody as a novel anti-angiogenic agent. *J Exp Ther Oncol.* 2006;5:273–286.
141. Kim H, Csaky KG. Nanoparticle-integrin antagonist C16Y peptide treatment of choroidal neovascularization in rats. *J Control Release.* 2010;142:286–293.
142. Rüegg C, Alghisi GC. Vascular integrins: therapeutic and imaging targets of tumor angiogenesis. In: Liersch R, et al., eds. *Angiogenesis Inhibition,* Recent Results in Cancer Research. Berlin Heidelberg, Germany: Springer Verlag; 2010:180:83–101.
143. Kuppermann BD, Patel S. Beyond Anti-VEGF in wet AMD: intereference of cell survival signals by targeting α5β1 integrin (Volociximab) in subjects with wet AMD. *Invest Ophthalmol Vis Sci.* 2009;50:E-Abstract 964.

CHAPTER

8

Endogenous Inhibitors of Ocular Angiogenesis

Shozo Sonoda • Parameswaran G. Sreekumar • Ram Kannan • David R. Hinton

INTRODUCTION

Physiologic angiogenesis is carefully regulated by a critical balance between endogenous stimulators and inhibitors. However, this balance can be tipped toward a more angiogenic phenotype under pathological conditions such as inflammation, ischemia, oxidant injury, and tumor growth. While most attention in studies of ocular angiogenesis has been focused on angiogenic stimulators, the focus of this chapter is on endogenous inhibitors of angiogenesis and how they may be regulated or utilized to prevent or treat ocular angiogenic disorders. The emphasis of this chapter is on those endogenous inhibitors of angiogenesis that have been shown to modulate angiogenesis in preclinical ocular models of disease and those that have the greatest potential for clinical application.

The number and variety of endogenous inhibitors of angiogenesis, which have been identified over the past 2 decades, are surprisingly large. An unusual feature of many of these endogenous inhibitors of angiogenesis is that they are cleavage products of larger proteins without any activity related to angiogenesis or are antiangiogenic splice variants of proteins involved in proangiogenic pathways. Endogenous inhibitors of angiogenesis can be classified into several defined categories based on their derivation and activity. These include extracellular matrix (ECM)–derived angiogenesis inhibitors (Table 8.1); growth factors, soluble growth factor receptors, and cytokines (Table 8.2); fragments of blood coagulation factors (Table 8.3); and a fourth category of other molecules having potent antiangiogenic activity (Table 8.4). The matrix-derived factors include those derived from larger ECM proteins such as collagens (arresten, canstatin, endostatin, tumstatin), fibronectin (anastellin), and perlecan (endorepellin) or are found as intact ECM molecules such as Fibulin 3 and 5, and thrombospondin (TSP). The prominent members of the second category encompassing growth factors, soluble receptors, and cytokines are pigment epithelium–derived factor (PEDF), a splice variant of vascular endothelial growth factor (VEGF165b), transforming growth factor beta (TGF-β), and soluble extracellular domains of the receptors for VEGF (sFlt1) and the angiopoietins (sTie2). The third category includes fragments of blood coagulation, namely angiostatin, antithrombin III, and prothrombin kringle-2 and platelet factor-4. The fourth category includes a diverse group of angiogenesis inhibitors including apoptosis signal-regulating kinase-1 interacting protein-1 (AIP1), cleavage products of prolactin (PRL) (vasoinhibins), a fragment of matrix metalloproteinase-2 (PEX), troponin I, vasostatin, 2-methoxyestradiol, chondromodulin-1, tissue inhibitors of metalloproteinases, and tryptophan tRNA synthetase.

ENDOGENOUS INHIBITORS OF ANGIOGENESIS AS MEDIATORS OF AVASCULARITY IN THE EYE

A unique feature of the eye is that there are naturally avascular structures, which require a lack of vascularity in order to attain normal function with optical clarity; these include the cornea and the fovea. Interestingly, it is the high expression of endogenous antiangiogenic inhibitors that is thought to generate and maintain this avascular environment. For the cornea, high expression of sFlt-1 is thought to maintain avascularity,[33] while for the fovea, high expression of PEDF in the ganglion cell layer is thought to generate the avascular area.[91]

INHIBITION OF ANGIOGENESIS IN DIFFERENT OCULAR MODELS

Pathological ocular angiogenesis is a key component of many blinding ocular diseases such as age-related macular degeneration (AMD), diabetic retinopathy, retinopathy of prematurity (ROP), and corneal angiogenesis. Animal models of ocular angiogenesis are among the most frequently utilized in the evaluation of antiangiogenic agents because of their ease of analysis and reproducibility. In fact, many of the endogenous inhibitors of angiogenesis were first studied or were evaluated in most detail in ocular models of angiogenesis. Our laboratory has shown

Table 8.1.

Matrix-derived endogenous angiogenesis inhibitors

Endogenous Inhibitor	Size in kDa	Production Site	Mechanism of Action
Arresten	26	Derived from the COOH-terminal of NC1 domain of the α1 chain of type IV collagen.[1]	Inhibition of endothelial cell proliferation, migration, tube formation, blood vessel formation.[1] Inhibition of FAK/c-Raf/MEK/ERK1/2/p38 MAPK activation in ECs. Inhibit HIF1α expression.[2,3]
Canstatin	24	Derived from the COOH-terminal of NC1 domain of the α2 chain of type IV collagen.[4]	Inhibition of endothelial cell migration, tube formation, proliferation, and induction of apoptosis.[4–6] Canstatin inhibits the phosphorylation of multiple signaling molecules in endothelial cells.[3] It binds to integrins $\alpha_v\beta_3$ and αvβ5, which initiates apoptotic pathways.[4,5,7]
Endorepellin	85	A basement membrane heparin sulfate proteoglycan C-terminal domain V of human perlecan[8]	Inhibition of endothelial cell migration, collagen-induced endothelial tube morphogenesis, and vessel growth in the chorioallantoic membrane, and Matrigel plug assays. Endorepellin binds endostatin and counteracts its antiangiogenic effects.[8] Angiostatic effects in vivo are mediated by a specific interaction of endorepellin with the α2β1 integrin receptor.[9] Endorepellin triggers a signaling cascade, leading to disruption of the actin cytoskeleton.[10]
Endostatin	20	Conditioned media of murine hemangioendothelioma cells.[11] NC1 domains of Basement membrane collagens.[12,13]	Inhibition of migration of endothelial cells by blocking downstream signaling of α5β1 integrin (Src kinase, RhoA GTPase, Ras, Raf).[2] Endostatin also binds to HSPGs that are involved in growth factor signaling.[14] These events promote disassembly of the actin cytoskeleton, disorders in cell-matrix interactions, and decrease in endothelial mobility.[15] Endostatin inhibits proliferation of endothelial cells, inducing their apoptosis through inhibition of cyclin D1. Endostatin induces autophagy by upregulating and complexing Beclin 1, Bcl-2, and Bcl-x (L).[16]
Anastellin	29	Derived from the first type III repeat of fibronectin	Anastellin blocks serum-dependent proliferation of endothelial cells by suppressing Ras activation and preventing ERK activation and subsequent cell proliferation.[17] Inhibits endothelial cell migration.[18]
Fibulin 3 and 5	50–60	Vascular smooth muscle, endothelial cells	Fibulin inhibits endothelial cell tubulogenesis, proliferation, and migration.[19] It reduces angiogenic sprouting stimulated by bFGF, inhibits matrix metalloproteinase expression and activity, and stimulates tissue inhibitor of metalloproteinase expression. It prevents angiogenesis and vessel infiltration into bFGF-supplemented Matrigel plugs implanted in mice.[20]
TSP	145	ECM glycoprotein synthesized by endothelial cells, epithelial cells, smooth muscle cells, and macrophages.	TSP-1 inhibits endothelial cell migration, adhesion, and proliferation and induces apoptosis. TSP-1 activates TGF-β. TSP-1 antagonizes VEGF-mediated survival signaling, inhibits VEGF mobilization by MMP9, and directly binds VEGF. TSP-1 antagonizes VEGF-driven Akt survival, signaling in part through the recruitment of Fyn to membrane domains containing CD36.[21]
Tumstatin	28	Purified from MMP-degraded basement membrane preparations from kidney, placenta, and testis.[22]	Inhibits formation of new blood vessels in Matrigel plug assay by inducing apoptosis.[22] It inhibits endothelial proliferation. Through the interaction with $\alpha_v\beta_3$integrin, tumstatin inhibits activation of FAK, P13K, protein kinase B/Akt, and prevents dissociation of eukaryotic initiation factor 4E protein from 4E-BP1, leading to inhibition of Cap-dependent protein synthesis.[23] Binding of tumstatin to integrin $\alpha_v\beta_3$ is dependent on the PTEN/Akt pathway.[24]

Table 8.2.

Growth factors, soluble receptors, and cytokines as endogenous angiogenesis inhibitors

Endogenous Inhibitor	Size in kDa	Origin	Mechanism of Action
PEDF	50	Ocular sites of synthesis include RPE, endothelial cells, corneal epithelial cells, lens epithelial cells, ciliary epithelial cells, and retinal ganglion cells.	Inhibits angiogenesis by induction of FasL and apoptosis of endothelial cells.[25] Inhibits vascular permeability and vascular leakage by preventing blood retinal breakdown through tight junction restoration. Inhibits inflammatory molecules. MAPK, JNK, and p38 influence endothelial cell apoptosis by modulating c-FLIP or caspase activity in the presence of PEDF.[26–28]
VEGF165b	38 (nonglycosylated)	Distal splice variant of VEGF165. In primary RPE cultures, VEGF165b is major form of VEGF.	Inhibits VEGF- and hypoxia-induced angiogenesis, and VEGF-induced cell migration and proliferation in vitro. Inhibits oxygen-induced ROP. IGF1 and TNFα treatment favors proximal splice site selection (increasing VEGF165), whereas TGF-β1 favored distal splice site selection (DSS), increasing VEGFb levels. TGF-β1-induced DSS selection was prevented by inhibition of p38 MAPK and the CLK/sty (CDC-like kinase, CLK1) splicing factor kinase family, but not ERK1/2.[29]
TGF-β	25	Widely expressed in epithelial, endothelial, hematopoietic, neural, and certain mesenchymal cells.[30]	Contact with pericytes and endothelial cells activate TGF-β to inhibit endothelial cell migration, proliferation and differentiation of pericytes. TGF-β treatment switches VEGF splicing toward antiangiogenic isoforms.[29]
Soluble Flt-1	180	Extracellular domain of Flt1 receptor. Expressed in endothelial cells, monocytes, and corneal epithelial cells.[31–33]	It includes the extracellular ligand-binding domain but not the transmembrane and intracellular domains; it is secreted (hence "soluble") and antagonizes VEGF and PlGF by binding and preventing their interaction with endothelial VEGF receptors.[31] sFlt-1 blocks VEGF-induced cell proliferation and migration.
Soluble Tie2	160	Extracellular domain of Tie2. Expressed by vascular endothelial cells	Angiopoietins, the natural ligands of Tie2, modulate Tie2-dependent signaling, which in turn regulates the survival and apoptosis of endothelial cells, controls vascular permeability, and regulates the capillary sprouting that occurs during normal angiogenesis.[34] sTie2 binds angiopoietins to prevent binding to receptor.

Table 8.3.

Fragments of blood coagulation as endogenous angiogenesis inhibitors

Endogenous Inhibitor	Size in kDa	Origin	Mechanism of Action
Angiostatin	38 kDa	Internal fragment of plasminogen	Inhibits endothelial cell proliferation.[35,36] Inhibits the F(1)-F(0) ATP synthase expressed on endothelial cell surface, allowing the intracellular pH to drop, triggering apoptotic events in the endothelial cells.[37,38] Angiostatin induces apoptosis by downregulating mitochondrial Bcl-2.[39]
Antithrombin III	53–55	Cleaved form of antithrombin III	Inhibits endothelial cell proliferation.[40]
Prothrombin kringle-2	22		
Platelet factor-4	70 amino-acid	Released from alpha-granules of activated platelets.[41]	Inhibits blood vessel proliferation in chicken chorioallantoic membrane. Inhibits angiogenesis by associating directly with FGF-2, inhibiting its dimerization and blocking FGF-2 binding to endothelial cells.[42]

that endogenous angiogenesis inhibitors such as PEDF and TSP-1 are differentially regulated in the murine ROP model in a strain-dependent manner,[92] suggesting that strain must be carefully considered when evaluating angiogenesis inhibition in animal models. A detailed table listing the preclinical assessment of endogenous angiogenic inhibitors in various models of ocular angiogenesis is provided (Table 8.5). In most preclinical animal studies, the endogenous angiogenic inhibitors are delivered as recombinant proteins/peptides by various routes (intraperitoneal, intravenous, subconjunctival, intravitreous, subretinal), by overexpression using viral vectors (adenovirus, adenoassociated virus, lentivirus) delivered systemically, intravitreally, or subretinally, or by use of nanoparticles (Fig. 8.1).

Endostatin

Endostatin is a 20-kDa fragment of the carboxy terminus of collagen XVIII, first identified and purified from the conditioned media of murine hemangioendothelioma cells[11] and later characterized in human.[93] Despite the common primary and secondary structures between endostatin and collagen XVIII, they do not share the same biological functions because of differences in their tertiary structures.[94,95] The NH_2-terminal zinc-binding domain of endostatin is reported to have antitumor and antimigration activities.[96] Collagen XVIII is the core protein of a heparan sulfate proteoglycan in vascular and epithelial basement membranes,[97] and in the eye, it is a major constituent of Bruch membrane and the basement membranes of the choroidal vessels.[12] Some proteases, such as matrix metalloproteinases, can cleave a proteinase-sensitive hinge so that endostatin can be released from collagen XVIII and become available.[98,99] While the mechanisms of endostatin's action as an angiogenesis inhibitor have been well characterized in tumors, its function in the retina is less well known. However, studies suggest that endostatin has a critical role in the eye since ocular abnormalities have been described in mice and humans that either lack or have reduced expression of collagen XVIII.[12,13,100–102] For instance, mice lacking collagen XVIII/endostatin show delayed regression of blood vessels in the vitreous along the surface of the retina after birth and also show lack of or abnormal outgrowth of retinal vessels.[101]

The expression pattern of collagen XVIII and the endostatin in the retina and choroid of human age-matched control and AMD eyes shows its predominant localization in the choroidal stroma, intercapillary septa, Bruch membrane, and inner limiting membrane.[103] Endostatin immunoreactivity was higher in the inner limiting membrane of AMD retina and significantly less in the choriocapillaris, Bruch membrane, and retinal pigment epithelium (RPE) basal lamina of AMD choroids.[103] Decreased levels of angiogenic inhibitors at the RPE–Bruch membrane–choriocapillaris complex in eyes with AMD could make Bruch membrane vulnerable to choroidal neovascularization (CNV). Mice lacking the basement membrane component collagen XVIII/endostatin have accumulation of sub-RPE deposits with striking similarities to basal laminar deposits, abnormal RPE, and age-dependent loss of vision[104] that is similar in appearance and composition to basal laminar deposits in early AMD[105] and contains excess basement membrane material. This suggests that the absence of collagen XVIII or endostatin leads to altered properties

Table 8.4.

Other endogenous angiogenesis inhibitors

Endogenous Inhibitor	Size in kDa	Origin	Mechanism of Action
AIP1	70–75	vascular endothelial cells, epithelial cells	AIP1 through its Ras GTPase-activating protein activity inhibits Ras-mediated cell survival signaling, causing cell growth inhibition.[43] AIP1 regulates apoptosis by mediating activation of ASK1.[44] AIP1 binds to VEGFR2-P13K complex and inhibits the VEGFR2-dependent angiogenesis.[45] Inhibits VEGF-induced migration and tube formation.
Vasoinhibins (PRL)	16	Generated by proteolytic cleavage of PRL, growth hormone, and placental lactogen in pituitary gland. Vasoinhibins occur naturally in the eye.[46]	Vasoinhibins interfere with ocular angiogenesis by blocking several endothelial functions and their actions mediated by the inactivation of endothelial nitric oxide synthase. They inhibit endothelial cell attachment to laminin and reduce endothelial growth induced by FGF-2.[47]
PEX	210 amino acid fragment	Noncatalytic COOH-terminal hemopexin-like domain of MMP2.	PEX prevents binding of MMP-2 to integrin $\alpha_v\beta_3$, inhibiting proteolytic activity on the cell surface and disrupting angiogenesis. Inhibits cell invasion, formation of capillary-like structures.[48]
Troponin I	21	Cartilage-derived	Inhibits endothelial cell proliferation and angiogenesis.[49]
Vasostatin	aa 1–180	NH2-domain of calreticulin inclusive of aa 1–180	Inhibits angiogenesis by inhibiting endothelial cells' proliferation and inducing apoptosis.[50,51]
2-Methoxyestradiol	0.28	Endogenous 2ME2 is synthesized by the hydroxylation at the 2-position of estradiol and subsequent O-methylation by catechol-O-methyltransferase	Destabilization of microtubules with a block in nuclear accumulation and activity of HIF-1α, leading to a significant reduction in VEGF. It has ability to bind to the colchicine-binding site of tubulin and the inhibition of superoxide dismutase enzymatic activity.[52] 2ME2 inhibits growth and sprouting of endothelial tubular formations. Inhibits angiogenesis induced by bFGF.[53]
Chondromodulin-1	25	Cartilage-specific NC1 matrix protein	Inhibits tube morphogenesis of retinal endothelial cells and DNA synthesis.[54,55]
Tissue inhibitors of metalloproteinases	21–28	Astrocytes, endothelial cells, epithelial cells, fibroblasts	Suppress MMP activity and ECM turnover. TIMP-2 inhibits cell proliferation and angiogenesis.[56,57]
Tryptophan tRNA synthetase (T2-TrpRS)	43–48	Proteolysis or alternative splicing of TrpRS.[58]	T1-TrpRS and T2-TrpRS block VEGF-induced migration of human umbilical vein endothelial cells. TrpRS blocks VEGF-stimulated angiogenesis in in vivo murine matrigel assay.[59] A recombinant form of a COOH-terminal fragment of TrpRS is a potent antagonist of VEGF-induced retinal angiogenesis.[58] T2-TrpRS inhibits pathologic neovascularization and facilitates physiological revascularization of ischemic tissue.[60]

Table 8.5.

Inhibition of angiogenesis in ocular models of neovascularization

Species	Pharmacologic Approach	Route of Administration	Ocular Condition/ Disease	Outcome
		Endostatin		
Mouse	rh endostatin	Intra peritoneal	Laser-induced CNV	CNV lesions were almost undetectable in endostatin-injected animals. Endostatin at physiological levels inhibited induced angiogenesis in vivo and reduced vascular leakage.[61]
Mouse	AAV-endostatin	Subconjunctival	Corneal neovascularization	AAV-endostatin significantly inhibited corneal neovascularization induced by silver nitrate.[62]
Mouse	AAV-endostatin	Subretinal	Retinal neovascularization	AAV-endostatin reduced retinal neovascularization, vascular permeability, and retinal detachment in VEGF transgenic mouse.[63]
Mouse	AAV-endostatin	Subretinal	ROP	Significantly inhibited ischemia-induced neovascularization.[64]
Mouse	AAV-endostatin	Intravenous	Laser-induced CNV	~10-fold higher endostatin serum levels and nearly complete prevention of CNV. A strong inverse correlation between endostatin serum level and area of CNV was observed.[65]
		VEGF 165b		
Mouse	rhVEGF165b peptide	Intravitreous	ROP	Inhibited the percentage area of retinal neovascularization from 23% to 12% and increased normal vascular areas from 62% to 74%.[66]
		PEDF		
Mouse	Ad5-PEDF/ Ad35-PEDF	Intravitreous	Laser-induced CNV	Ad35 better than Ad5 vector with respect to durability and level of transgene expression. PEDF expression from an Ad35.PEDF vector was able to inhibit CNV lesion growth by greater than 80% at Day 42 as compared to the no-injection control.[67]
RCS rat	SIV-hPEDF/SIV-hFGF2	Subretinal	Retinitis pigmentosa	SIV-hPEDF or SIV-hFGF-2 significantly delayed the histological degeneration. Delays were synergistically and significantly pronounced by combined injection of SIV-hPEDF and SIV-hFGF-2.[68]

(Continued)

Table 8.5.

Inhibition of angiogenesis in ocular models of neovascularization (*Continued*)

Species	Pharmacologic Approach	Route of Administration	Ocular Condition/ Disease	Outcome
Mouse	Recombinant PEDF/PEDF peptide/ PEDF-nanospheres	Intravitreous	Retinal ischemia-reperfusion	PEDF prevented approx. 44% of the cell death in the RGC layer. $PEDF_{82-121}$ peptide was as effective as full-length PEDF when injected as either a free peptide or delivered in PLGA nanospheres.[69]
Mouse	Recombinant PEDF	Intravitreous	AGE-induced diabetes	50% decrease in blood retinal breakdown and vascular permeability in PEDF-treated diabetic groups.[70]
Rat	Recombinant PEDF	Intravitreous	OIR	Most potent effect of PEDF was observed at 48 h after injection, with the retinal vascular permeability in PEDF-treated eyes decreasing to 56% of the PBS control (downregulation of VEGF, VEGF receptor-2, MCP-1, TNF-α, and ICAM-1).[28]
Rat	rPEDF	Intravitreous	STZ-diabetes	PEDF prevented VEGF-induced endothelial permeability and blood-retina-barrier breakdown, at least partially by blocking the disorganization of tight junction proteins.[28]
Mouse	PEDF peptide	Intravitreous	Nonproliferative diabetic retinopathy	Reduced VEGF-induced vascular permeability by 84%.[71]
Mouse	Recombinant PEDF	Intravitreous	Nonproliferative diabetic retinopathy	Inhibited VEGF-induced vascular permeability by 96%.[71]
Mouse	AAV-PEDF	Intravitreous	Retinal ischemia –reperfusion injury	Significantly increased cell survival after ischemia-reperfusion injury of the retina.[72]
RCS rat/ rds mice	Simian lentiviral vector-PEDF	Subretinal	Retinitis pigmentosa	Significant protection of loss of photoreceptor cells in regions of gene transfer with fewer TUNEL-positive cells. PEDF-treated eyes retained sensitivity to light flash.[73]
Mouse	rAAV2-PEDF	Intravitreous	ROP	Decrease in number of neovascular tufts; overall vasculature pattern appeared similar to that in the normal animal. Endothelial cell counts in PEDF-treated eyes were reduced by 74% compared with controls.[74]
Mouse	AdrPEDF	Intravitreous	CNV	Prominent immunoreactivity for PEDF in RPE with strong inhibition of CNV.[75]

Species	Pharmacologic Approach	Route of Administration	Ocular Condition/ Disease	Outcome
Mouse	Recombinant PEDF	Intravenous	ROP	Vascular tufts were reduced or not observed. At highest dose (22.4 μg/d) of PEDF, there was 67% inhibition of neovascularization.[76]
Rat	Recombinant PEDF/ peptide	Hydron pellets implanted into the avascular rat cornea	Corneal neovascularization	Significantly inhibited corneal neovascularization.[77]
Mouse	AdPEDF.11	Periocular	Laser-induced CNV	Periocular injection of AdPEDF.11 strongly suppressed CNV.[78]
Mouse	AdPEDF.11	Periocular	ROP	Periocular injection of AdPEDF.11 did not inhibit retinal neovascularization because retinal PEDF levels were 10-fold lower than levels of PEDF in the choroid.[78]
Mouse	AAV-PEDF	Intravitreal PEDF transfection	Inherited glaucoma	Potent reduction of retinal ganglion cell loss and vision decline with decrease in TNF, IL-18, and gliosis.[79]
RCS Rat	SIV-hPEDF	subretinal	Retinitis pigmentosa	Protected photoreceptors from cell death by inhibiting the nuclear translocation of apoptosis-inducing factor with upregulation of Bcl-2.[80]
Rat	AdPEDF.11	Intravitreous	Light-induced photoreceptor cell death	Increased photoreceptor cell survival by inhibition of light-induced apoptotic processes.[81]
			TSP-1	
Mouse	Wispostatin-1 (TSP-1 peptide repeat)	Intravitreous	Corneal micropocket (bFGF) and laser induced CNV	Abolished bFGF-induced neovascularization in corneal micropocket assay. Significant inhibition of CNV was also found with peptide treatment.[82]
Rat	rhTSP-1 and TSP-1 peptide	Intravitreous	ROP	Decrease in retinal neovascularization with platelet-derived TSP-1 or rh-TSP-1.[83]
			Soluble Flt-1	
Rat	Ad-sFlt-1	Intramuscular	Laser-induced CNV	Increased serum levels of sFlt-1. Less prominent vessel formation with decreased fibroblast proliferation and decreased inflammatory cell infiltration.[84]
Rat	Ad-HD-sFlt-1	Intravitreous	OIR	60% inhibition in retinal neovascularization. Average endothelial cell count was reduced by 80%.[85]
Rat (Torii SDT)	Ad-sFlt-1	Subretinal	Spontaneous Diabetes	Decrease in avascular area, hyperfluorescence, and arterial narrowing 30 weeks after vector administration. No adverse effects were observed.[86]

(Continued)

Table 8.5.

Inhibition of angiogenesis in ocular models of neovascularization (*Continued*)

Species	Pharmacologic Approach	Route of Administration	Ocular Condition/ Disease	Outcome
Rat	Ad-sFlt-1	Intravitreous	ROP	98% decrease in peak retinal neovascularization. No significant difference in retinal vessel number detected in oxygen-injured and normoxic groups at p28.[87]
Mouse	sFlt-1-Fc (recombinant fusion protein)	Intravitreous	ROP	37% inhibition of retinal neovascularization. Retinal vasculature appeared relatively intact.[88]
Mouse	AAV-sFlt-1/ AdsFlt-1	Intravitreous	ROP	Reduction in the number of neovascular endothelial cells by 56% and 52% for adenovirus and AAV vectors, respectively.[89]
		Tryptophanyl-tRNA synthetases		
Mouse	rh mini TrpRS/ T2-TrpRS	Intravitreous	Physiological angiogenesis in the neonatal retina	Complete inhibition of the outer network was observed in 28% of mini TrpRS (5 pmol)-treated eyes. The smaller T2-TrpRS variant was far more potent, with dose-dependent activity; 14% were completely inhibited after treatment with 1 pmol of T2-TrpRS, 40% after treatment with 2.5 pmol and 69% after 5 pmol.[58]
Mouse	T2-TrpRS	Intravitreous	OIR	A strong, dose-dependent angiostatic effect of T2-TrpRS on pathologic neovascularization in the OIR model was observed. Injection of 1.25 μg/eye T2-TrpRS resulted in nearly complete inhibition of neovascular tuft formation. T2-TrpRS also inhibited pathologic neovascularization and reduced tuft formation by more than 75%.[60]
		Soluble Tie2		
Mouse	AAV-Tie2 receptor	Intramuscular	ROP	Treatment inhibited retinal neovascularization by 47%.[90]
Mouse	AAV-Tie2 receptor	Intramuscular	Laser-induced CNV	Treatment significantly reduced the incidence and extent of fluorescein leakage from CNV lesions by 52% and 36%, with 45% reduction in CNV area.[90]
Mouse	sTie2-Fc (recombinant fusion proteins)	Intravitreous	ROP	Retinal neovascularization at P17 reduced in 92% of animals. The average magnitude of inhibition compared with IgG control was 23%.[88]

Supported by: The Arnold and Mabel Beckman Foundation, National Institutes for Health Grants (EY01545, EY03040), and a grant to the Department of Ophthalmology by Research to Prevent Blindness.

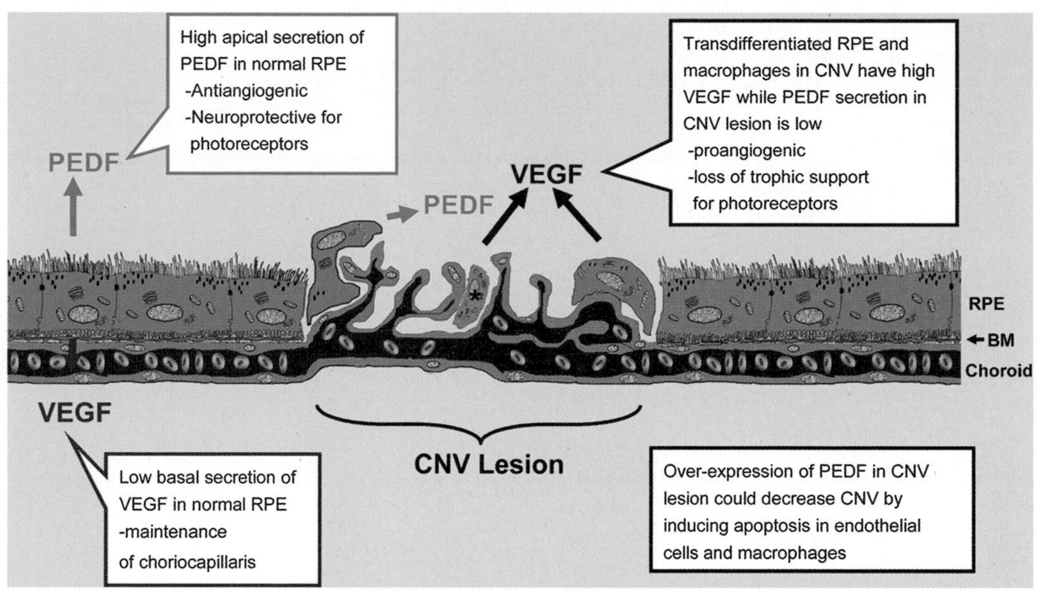

FIGURE 8.1. Diagram illustrating the balance between PEDF and VEGF in the normal RPE monolayer and in CNV. The left side of the diagram shows that RPE cells normally secrete high levels of PEDF from their apical surface, which may provide photoreceptor neuroprotection. Normal RPE cells also secrete low levels of VEGF from their basal surface, which may allow for maintenance of the choriocapillaris. Under conditions of neovascularization (CNV), choroidal endothelial cells break through Bruch membrane and form subretinal neovascular channels. Transdifferentiated RPE and macrophages (indicated with an *asterisk*) within the lesion secrete significantly higher amounts of VEGF and much less PEDF, thereby altering the VEGF/PEDF ratio and creating a proangiogenic microenvironment.

of Bruch membrane that either cause the RPE to produce excess basement membrane material or interfere with the clearance of such basement membrane material, eventually resulting in a progressive accumulation of basal laminar deposit–like material under the RPE with age. Inactivating mutations in the human gene for collagen XVIII, *COL18A1*, have been identified in patients with Knobloch syndrome[100]; these patients have progressive retinal degeneration, high myopia, and occipital encephalocele.

The molecular mechanisms associated with endostatin's ability to inhibit angiogenesis are emerging; however, most of these are in the field of tumor angiogenesis. Different studies have reported that endostatin (a) interferes with FGF-2-induced signal transduction, blocking endothelial motility[106]; (b) blocks cell-cycle progression at the G1/S transition by downregulating the transcriptional activity of the cyclin-D1 promoter via the lymphoid enhancer-binding factor 1 site; (c) interferes with VEGF-R2 (Kinase insert domain receptor [KDR], also known as VEGFR2/FLK1) leading to reduced cell motility, proliferation, and survival[107]; (d) affects cell-matrix interaction by inducing tyrosine phosphorylation of focal adhesion kinase (FAK) and paxillin[106]; (e) activates proapoptotic pathways through induction of caspase-9 activation by reducing the level of the antiapoptotic proteins Bcl-2, Bcl-XL, and Bad[108]; (f) induces autophagy by upregulating and complexing Beclin 1, Bcl-2, and Bcl-x (L)[16]; and (g) interferes with proliferation by reducing the mRNA level of several proliferative genes including MAPK1, MAPK2, or c-myc.[109] Endostatin also affects signaling events that are not related with angiogenesis, revealing the significance of interpathway communication in intricate cellular signaling networks.[110]

Endostatin was the first endogenous angiogenic inhibitor to enter clinical trials. These trials were based on animal studies showing that recombinant endostatin efficiently blocked angiogenesis and suppresses primary tumor growth and metastasis in experimental animal models without any apparent side effects, toxicity, or development of drug resistance.[11,111] Endostatin shows linear pharmacokinetics in which an increasing dose results in proportionally increased bioavailability in plasma, with a mean half-life of 10.7 ± 4.1 hours.[112] Some endogenous antiangiogenic agents (e.g., Interferon α2a) that inhibit tumor angiogenesis have no effect on models of ocular angiogenesis such as laser-induced CNV. However, in multiple models of ocular angiogenesis, endostatin significantly reduced vascular leakage and neovascular complications (Table 8.5). For example, mice injected with a construct in which *sig-mEndo* was driven by the simian cytomegalovirus promoter had significantly higher endostatin serum levels and had nearly complete prevention of laser-induced CNV.[65] Similarly, recombinant endostatin potently inhibited vascular leakage and laser-induced CNV.[61] In a mouse model of ROP, adeno-associated viral–mediated delivery of endostatin inhibited ischemia-induced neovascularization.[64] In transgenic mice overexpressing VEGF in the retina, subretinal injection of adenovirus expressing endostatin significantly reduced retinal vascular hyperpermeability and VEGF-induced neovascularization and retinal detachment[63] (Fig. 8.2).

sVEGFR-1 (sFlt-1)

The VEGFR-1 gene was originally isolated from a human placenta cDNA library and its product was designated as Fms-like tyrosine kinase-1 (Flt-1) because of structural similarity to the Fms family.[113] The nascent polypeptide is 150 kDa without modifications; however, after synthesis, Flt-1 is glycosylated to an intermediate form (170 kDa), then further glycosylated and expressed on the cell surface as a mature protein of 180 to 185 kDa.[113,114] Only this mature form is autophosphorylated in response to VEGF and to other VEGFR-1-specific ligands. Alternative splicing of Flt pre-mRNA generates two distinct products encoding the full-length membrane-spanning receptor (receptor form of VEGFR-1) that mediates VEGF mitogenic activity and a truncated soluble form (soluble form of VEGFR-1) that inhibits angiogenic activity.[115] sVEGFR-1 is also produced as a consequence of ectodomain shedding.[116]

Since soluble VEGFR-1 has a strong affinity for VEGF and since this molecule is an endogenously expressed protein, several research groups have attempted to use it as a VEGF-blocking reagent in experimental models of ocular angiogenesis (Table 8.5). sVEGFR-1 at doses of 100 to 1,000 ng/mL reduced VEGF-induced tube formation in vitro in human endothelial cells,[117] without causing cell death even with the highest dose. In experimental subretinal neovascularization, injection of adenovirus expressing the entire ectodomain of the human VEGF receptor/flt-1 in pigmented rats resulted in a significant reduction in neovascularization.[84] The serum concentration of this soluble receptor increased for 7 days and, thereafter, gradually decreased. Further, this study showed that fibroblast cell proliferation and inflammatory cell infiltration were reduced in the photocoagulation spot of Adflt-ExR-treated rats. In mouse models of ROP, intravitreal injection with an adenoviral vector expressing sFlt-1 resulted in up to 97.5% decrease in retinal neovascularization without affecting preexisting retinal vessels.[87] Intravitreous injection of HD-Ad vectors expressing sFlt-1 inhibited retinal neovascularization by more than 60% in a rat model of ROP.[85] In the spontaneously diabetic nonobese Torii (SDT) rats, an adeno-associated viral vector (AAV-sFlt-1) was injected into the subretinal space, and the progression of diabetic retinopathy was assessed 30 weeks later for the presence of an avascular area, hyperfluorescence, and arterial narrowing.[86] These pathologic diabetic changes were insignificant in the AAV-sFlt-1 treated group with no adverse side effects, suggesting the potential for this endogenous inhibitor for preventing retinal neovascularization as well as CNV. sFlt-1's angiostatic effects are exerted via 2 inhibitory mechanisms; (a) it sequestrates VEGF, which it binds with high affinity, and (b) it forms inactive heterodimers with membrane-spanning isoforms of the VEGF receptors, VEGFR-1 and VEGFR-2.[115,118,119]

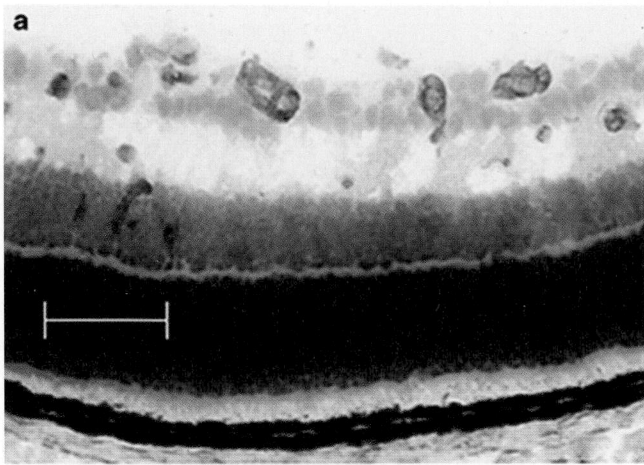

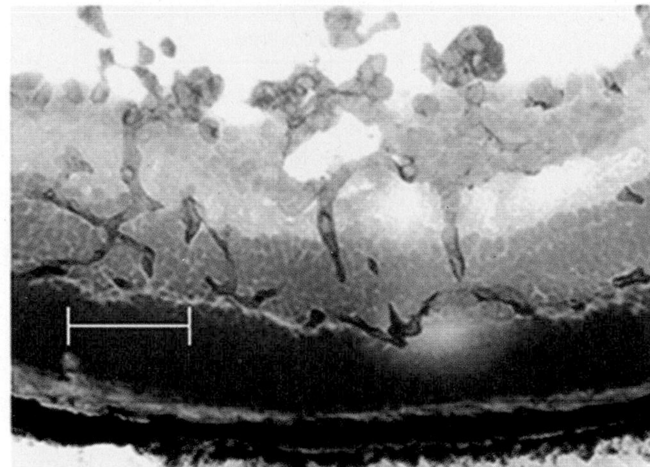

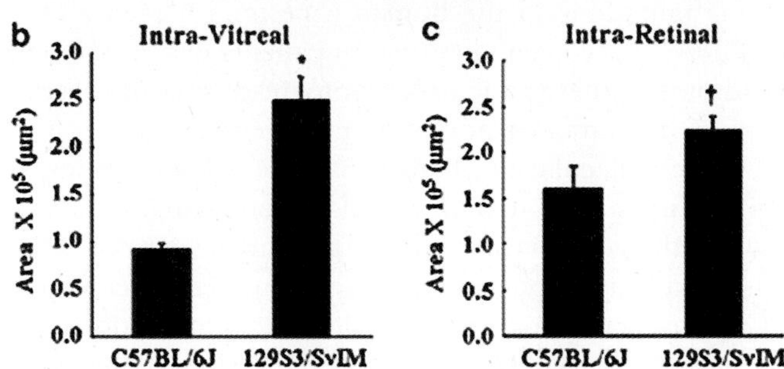

FIGURE 8.2. Differential expression of angiogenesis in mouse strain–dependent hypoxia-induced retinal neovascularization. Intraretinal and intravitreal angiogenesis are increased in 129S3/SvIM. **A:** Retinal neovascularization at P17 in C57BL/6J (n = 12) and 129S3/SvIM (n = 10) strains. Endothelial cells were identified with *G. simplicifolia* lectin I-B_4 (*red*) and sections counterstained with hematoxylin (*blue*). **B:** Quantification of total neovascular surface area from serial sections. Intravitreal neovascularization was increased 2.7-fold in 129S3/SvIM (n = 10) compared to C57BL/6J (n = 12) mouse strain ($^*p < 0.0001$). **C:** Intraretinal neovascularization was increased nearly 40% in 129S3/Sv (n = 10) compared to C57BL/6J (n = 12) ($^\dagger p < 0.0009$). Bar = 100 μm. (Reproduced from Chan, et al. *Lab Invest.* 2005;85:721–733, with permission.)

Pigment Epithelium–Derived Factor

Pigment epithelium–derived factor (PEDF), also known as SERPIN F1 and EPC1, a 418-amino acid 50-kDa glycoprotein, was first identified in 1987 by Tombran-Tink and Johnson in conditioned medium from fetal human RPE cell culture and characterized as a neurotrophic factor able to promote neuronal differentiation of Y79 retinoblastoma tumor cells.[120] Subsequently, the PEDF gene was cloned and sequenced.[121] The gene spans approximately 16 kb, is divided among eight exons and seven introns, and is conserved in higher vertebrates.[122] It maps to chromosome 17p13.1, a region that also contains a cluster of cancer-related genes.[121,123] The 1.5-kb transcript has been widely detected in many fetal and adult tissues such as adult liver, testis, stomach, ovaries, prostate, eye, heart, colon, brain, and spinal cord.[124–126] The crystal structure of PEDF shows a unique serpin protease inhibitor motif and heparin- and collagen-binding domains, all of which might be important to its antiangiogenic function.[124,127]

PEDF is a non–inhibitory member of the serpin superfamily and it has pleiotropic effects including antiangiogenic, antivasopermeability, antitumorigenic, anti-inflammatory, antioxidative, neurotrophic, and neuroprotective activities.[28,71,128–131] PEDF binds at least two receptors: an 80-kDa PLA2/nutrin/patatin-like phospholipase domain-containing two[132] receptor and the non–integrin 37/67-kDa laminin receptor.[133] An appealing aspect of PEDF's activity is its selectivity since it induces apoptosis of endothelial cells in newly forming vessels and spares preestablished vasculature.[128] PEDF discriminates between endothelial cells forming new vessels and those that are a part of preexisting vessels by making use of the Fas ligand (FasL)–Fas receptor system.[25] This selective induction of endothelial cell death is dependent on the dual induction of Fas and FasL.[25] MAPK JNK and p38 influence endothelial cell apoptosis by modulating c-FLIP or caspase activity in the presence of PEDF.[26,27] PEDF inhibits VEGF-induced angiogenesis in retinal microvascular endothelial cells by enhancing γ-secretase-dependent cleavage of the C terminus of VEGF receptor-1, thus blocking VEGF receptor-2 –induced angiogenesis.[134] PEDF specifically inhibits both the migration and proliferation of endothelial cells in several cell culture and animal models[77] and also permeability induced by VEGF by interacting with specific cell surface receptors[135,136] and by upregulating tight junction proteins.[28] PEDF inhibited endothelial cell migration in a dose-dependent manner with a median effective dose (ED_{50}) of 0.4 nM, and this places PEDF above other endogenous angiogenesis inhibitors such as endostatin (ED_{50} of 3 nM) and TSP-1 (ED_{50} 0.5 nM).[137] In cerebellar granule cells, PEDF stimulates phosphorylation of IκB, which leads to activation and nuclear translocation of NF-κB, which in turn leads to transcription of antiapoptotic and neuroprotective genes.[138,139]

The advantages of PEDF as a therapeutic endogenous inhibitor include (a) the antiangiogenic activity of PEDF is selective and reversible, (b) it is not expected to activate drug-resistance genes and offers the potential for effective long-term antiangiogenic therapy, (c) it is unlikely to produce the toxic side effects of synthetic inhibitors, and (d) given its neurotrophic activity, PEDF has the additional advantage of preserving neurons from the damage often caused by vascular disease.

Stitt et al.[140] reported that penetrating ocular injury suppresses retinal neovascularization and modulates expression of PEDF. These findings have implications for intravitreal delivery of angiostatic agents since ocular perforation may provoke an acute, endogenous antiangiogenic response. A similar study in the oxygen-induced retinopathy (OIR) model revealed that penetrating ocular injury resulted in a 30% decrease in neovascular area in the retina.[141] Argon laser photocoagulation can upregulate the expression of PEDF protein in the vitreous and retina of diabetic rats and inhibit neovascularization.[142]

In the retina, RPE cells are a major source of PEDF. Polarized RPE monolayers secrete PEDF significantly more toward the neural retina where it may serve as a neuroprotective molecule. Work in our laboratory established that in highly polarized human RPE cells, the apical secretion of PEDF is significantly higher than basolateral secretion.[143] However, in contrast to PEDF, proangiogenic VEGF secretion (which is more than two orders of magnitude lower than the PEDF) is predominantly secreted from the basolateral side (toward the choroid) where it may function in normal circumstances for the maintenance of the choriocapillaris. In normal RPE, the balance between proangiogenic VEGF and antiangiogenic PEDF favors an antiangiogenic environment. However, under pathological conditions (e.g., CNV) with the disruption of blood-retinal barrier, breaks in Bruch membrane, and inflammation, PEDF secretion is significantly reduced in RPE and VEGF secretion is upregulated in transdifferentiated RPE and macrophages, altering the equilibrium and promoting a proangiogenic environment (see Fig. 8.1).

PEDF is an endogenous angiogenesis inhibitor that has characteristics that make it suitable for development into a drug for pharmacological inhibition of ocular angiogenesis because of its dual roles as an angiogenesis inhibitor as well as a neuroprotective molecule. PEDF is effective against multiple angiogenesis inducers,[77] and it has been tested in multiple animal models using both systemic and local deliveries (Table 8.5). Systemic delivery of recombinant protein prevented neovascularization in a mouse model of ischemia-induced retinal angiogenesis[76] and in a model of advanced glycation end products (AGE)–induced retinal vascular permeability.[70] Intravitreal administration of rhPEDF significantly inhibited retinal neovascularization.[144] The most widely used vectors for ocular gene delivery are based on adeno-associated virus (AAV) because they elicit minimal immune responses and mediate long-term transgene expression.[145] In multiple animal models, viral-mediated PEDF gene delivery significantly or completely inhibited retinal[28,64,72,74–76,144] or choroidal[28,67,75,78,146,147] neovascularization in mice or rats. A phase 1 clinical trial of adenoviral PEDF (AdGVPEDF.11D; NCT00109499) in neovascular AMD has been completed.[148]

Thrombospondin

(TSP-1), a high molecular weight calcium-binding extracellular trimeric glycoprotein originally identified in α-granules of platelets stimulated with thrombin, was later described as a major secretory product of vascular smooth muscle cells and endothelial cells.[149] It was the first protein shown to play a critical role as a naturally occurring angiogenesis inhibitor.[150] The TSP family consists of five members (TSP-1–TSP-4, and cartilage oligomeric matrix protein COMP or TSP-5). TSP-1 and TSP-2 have been the most extensively studied members of this family, and they share similar domains and overall structure and contain three type 1 repeat domains.[151] Many other molecules contain a TSP-1 repeat domain; however, only a subset of these molecules have been shown to have antiangiogenic activity. TSP-1 and TSP-2 contain an amino-terminal heparin-binding domain, a procollagen-like domain, three type 1 repeats, three type 2 or EGF-like repeats, seven type 3 or calcium-binding repeats, and a globular carboxyl-terminal domain.[151] TSP-1 interacts with at least 9 receptors on endothelial cells including integrins (α3β1, α4β1, α6β1, α9β1, and αvβ3), the LDL receptor-related protein in association with calreticulin, heparan sulfate proteoglycans, CD36, and CD47.[152] TSP regulates various biological events, such as cell adhesion, angiogenesis, cell proliferation and survival, TGF-β activation, and protease activation.[153] Possible mechanisms for this antiangiogenic activity are inhibition of VEGF-induced endothelial cell migration, tube formation, and increased endothelial cell–specific apoptosis.[150] It should be noted that TSP-1 may act as a proangiogenic or a antiangiogenic factor, depending on the proteases that cleave fragments of TSP-1.[154,155]

In vivo, TSP-1 suppresses FGF-2-mediated angiogenesis and inhibits growth of blood vessels.[156] TSP-1 suppressed the neovascular response mediated by bFGF in the rat cornea.[157] The specific mechanism that results in angiogenic suppression is complex and complicated by the interaction of TSP-1with a variety of extracellular macromolecules and growth factors. TSP-1 inhibits corneal neovascularization through the induction of apoptosis, which involves the sequential activation of CD36, p59*fyn*, caspase-3 like proteases, and p38 mitogen-activated protein kinases.[158] In the ischemic retina, retinal neovascular cells increase TSP-1 expression, and VEGF may stimulate endogenous TSP-1 induction, which inhibits endothelial cell growth through a negative feedback mechanism.[159]The antiangiogenic activity of TSP-1 has been mapped to the type 1 repeats and TSP-1 and peptides from the type 1 repeat region (tryptophan-rich, heparin-binding sequences and TGF-β1 activation sequences) in two models of retinal angiogenesis: a retinal explant assay and a rat model of ROP. TSP-1 inhibited angiogenesis in both models, but peptides from the native TSP-1 sequence containing both the tryptophan-rich repeat and the TGF-β1 activation sequence or containing only the tryptophan-rich, heparin-binding sequence had distinct efficiencies in the two models. These results suggest that the type 1 repeats of TSP-1 contain two subdomains that might independently influence the process of neovascularization.[83] The existence of two subdomains also explains how TSP-1 may block FGF-2 and VEGF angiogenic signals by two independent pathways.[160] TSP-1 is able to distinguish pathologic neovascularization from preexisting vasculature due to the dependence of proliferating endothelial cells on Fas/FasL-mediated apoptosis. TSP-1 upregulates FasL expression on endothelial cells. Expression of the receptor of FasL was low on quiescent endothelial cells but greatly enhanced by inducers of angiogenesis, thereby specifically sensitizing the stimulated cells to apoptosis by inhibitor-generated FasL.[25] A set of 18 peptides of 17 to 20 amino acids has been identified from the type I TSP repeats; all are antiangiogenic, inhibiting the proliferation and migration of human umbilical vein endothelial cells in vitro.[161] To reflect the origin, peptides are named as adamtsostatin-4, adamtsostatin-16, adamtsostatin-18, cartilostatin-1, cartilostatin-2, fibulostatin-6.2, fibulostatin-6.3, papilostatin-1, papilostatin-2, properdistatin, scospondistatin, semastatin-5A.1, semastatin-5A.2, semastatin-5B, thrombostatin containing-1, thrombostatin containing-3, thrombostatin containing-6, and wispostatin-1.[161] In a mouse CNV model, intravitreous injection of wispostatin-1 (human sequence) exhibited an approximately 28% reduction and a 43% inhibition on the area of CNV.[82] Wispostatin-1 completely abolished bFGF-induced neovascularization in the corneal micropocket assay.[82]

TSP plays an important role in maintaining vascular homeostasis in the eye. The aqueous humor and vitreous from normal human eyes contain elevated levels of the TSP-1 protein.[162] However, TSP-1 levels in the aqueous humor and vitreous are downregulated in some diabetic animal models.[163] TSP-1 is also implicated in the pathogenesis of CNV, and the expression of antiangiogenic TSP-1 is significantly decreased in Bruch membrane and choriocapillaris in AMD eyes; TSP-1 levels correlate inversely with severity of disease.[164,165] In aged control eyes, in the macular region, TSP-1 expression was observed intensely in Bruch membrane and weakly in RPE basement membrane, choriocapillaris, and the wall of large choroidal blood vessels. In eyes with AMD, TSP-1 immunoreactivity was significantly lower in all structures except RPE basement membrane. There was significantly lower TSP-1 in the far periphery than the equator and submacular regions in all eyes.[164,165] Decreased levels of angiogenic inhibitors at the RPE-Bruch membrane-choriocapillaris complex in eyes with AMD may make Bruch membrane vulnerable to CNV.[165] The therapeutic efficiency of TSP-1 has been tested in two models of angiogenesis including CNV and ROP using recombinant as well as TSP-1 type 1 repeat peptide (Table 8.5).

VEGF-165b

VEGF-A is a major angiogenesis promoter and is known to be upregulated in diabetic retinopathy, CNV, and retinal neovascularization. Conventional VEGF exists in multiple isoforms resulting from alternative pre-mRNA splicing of eight exons encoding at least six proteins[166] that act as proangiogenic and propermeability vasodilator peptides. However, in 2002, Bates et al.[167] identified an alternative isoform, VEGF165b, which contained part of the 3'UTR within exon 8 of the VEGF gene, resulting in two subexons, namely, exon 8a and exon 8b. VEGF165b differs from VEGF-A 165 only in the carboxy-terminal six amino acids. Exons 8a and 8b both encode six amino acids, exon 8a for Cys-Asp-Lys-Pro-Arg-A and exon 8b for Ser-Leu-Thr-Arg-Lys-Asp, respectively, and the unique C'-terminal six amino acid encoded by exon 8b code for VEGF 165b. These differences have considerable implications in the structure as well as function of the protein; VEGF165 is proangiogenic, and VEGF165b is antiangiogenic.

VEGFxxxb isoforms are expressed in human retina, vitreous, and iris, being abundant in normal vitreous.[168] Human RPE cells in culture express more VEGF165b (74% of the total VEGF secreted) than the angiogenic VEGF165.[29] These isoforms are downregulated in diabetic vitreous, suggesting a switch to an angiogenic phenotype. However, the pattern of expression of these isoforms in retinal layers is not clearly established at present. In a mouse model of ROP, a single injection of VEGF165b significantly reduced preretinal neovascularization without inhibiting physiological intraretinal angiogenesis.[66] Quantitatively, VEGF165b inhibition of retinal neovascularization resulted in the recovery of a morphologically normal intraretinal vasculature. Intravitreal injection of 10 ng/mL human recombinant VEGF165b or enhancing distal splicing of exon 8 with SRPIN340 significantly inhibited laser-induced CNV in a mouse model.[169]

The mechanism through which VEGF165b inhibits angiogenesis is not fully elucidated. However, studies have revealed that VEGF165b is able to bind with VEGFR1 and VEGFR2[170,171] but initiates only weak signaling of the

BOX 8.1 Approaches for Increasing Intraocular Levels of Endogenous Antiangiogenic Inhibitors

A. Increased expression of endogenous inhibitors or derived peptides with antiangiogenic activity
- intravitreal human recombinant inhibitors in slow release form
- subretinal or intravitreal injection of viral vectors expressing inhibitors
- intravitreal nanoparticle encapsulated inhibitors
- cell replacement therapy
  - encapsulated cells secreting inhibitors
  - subretinal transplantation of RPE (or stem cell–derived RPE) secreting endogenous inhibitors
  - subretinal transplantation of RPE transduced to overexpress endogenous inhibitors

B. Increased expression of endogenous inhibitors from existing retinal cells
- drugs that promote alternate splicing of growth factors to form antiangiogenic forms (e.g., VEGF165b)

KEY POINTS

- A wide range of naturally occurring angiogenesis inhibitors have been identified. They fall into four categories: (a) matrix derived (e.g., endostatin, TSP-1); (b) growth factors, soluble growth factor receptors, and cytokines (e.g., PEDF, sFlt-1); (c) fragments of blood coagulation factors; and (d) other endogenous antiangiogenic molecules.
- Many of the endogenous angiogenesis inhibitors are cleavage products, or alternative splicing products, of larger proteins with diverse functions.
- Endogenous inhibitors act in general by inhibiting endothelial cell proliferation, and cell migration, and activating apoptotic or autophagic pathways in activated endothelial cells mediated through multiple signaling mechanisms.
- Endogenous angiogenesis inhibitors play important normal developmental roles in the generation of avascularity in cornea and fovea.
- Endogenous angiogenesis inhibitors are regulated during the course of ocular angiogenic disorders and may play an important role in the pathogenesis of these diseases.
- Pharmacologic preparations of endogenous angiogenesis inhibitors have been evaluated in animal models of ocular angiogenesis and many have been shown to effectively inhibit angiogenesis.
- Because these inhibitors are endogenous in origin, their side effects and toxicity in therapeutic applications may be minimal.
- Endogenous angiogenic inhibitors may be increased in the eye through use of recombinant products, viral expression vectors, cell replacement therapy, or alternative splicing of endogenous genes in existing cells.

receptor to induce tyrosine phosphorylation[170,171] and is also unable to make phenotypic proangiogenic changes in endothelial cells. Overexpression of VEGF165b in tumor cells inhibits the growth of different types of carcinomas in xenografted mouse tumor models. Further, overexpression of VEGF165b also inhibited tumor-mediated endothelial cell migration and proliferation by preventing tumor-secreted endothelial growth factors such as VEGF165 or other VEGFxxx forms.[172] These effects are specific for VEGF because VEGF165b does not affect FGF-induced endothelial proliferation.[167] Thus, VEGF165b is an endogenous antiangiogenic factor, which inhibits angiogenesis-dependent conditions such as tumor growth,[172,173] experimental proliferative retinopathy,[66] and diabetic retinopathy.[168] The ability to use a pharmacological approach to promote distal splice-site selection (exon 8b) may be a promising future therapy for angiogenic ocular disorders.

SUMMARY

This chapter has provided an overview of the wide range of known endogenous angiogenesis inhibitors with focus on those that have been evaluated in ocular models of angiogenesis and that may have the greatest promise for therapy of ocular angiogenic disorders. Future use of these inhibitors as therapeutic agents will require development of appropriate drug delivery systems.

ACKNOWLEDGMENT

We thank Christine Spee and Ernesto Barron for their excellent technical support.

REFERENCES

1. Colorado PC, Torre A, Kamphaus G, et al. Anti-angiogenic cues from vascular basement membrane collagen. *Cancer Res.* 2000;60:2520–2526.
2. Sudhakar A, Sugimoto H, Yang C, et al. Human tumstatin and human endostatin exhibit distinct antiangiogenic activities mediated by alpha v beta 3 and alpha 5 beta 1 integrins. *Proc Natl Acad Sci U S A.* 2003;100:4766–4771.
3. Mundel TM, Kalluri R. Type IV collagen-derived angiogenesis inhibitors. *Microvasc Res.* 2007;74:85–89.
4. Kamphaus GD, Colorado PC, Panka DJ, et al. Canstatin, a Novel Matrix-derived Inhibitor of Angiogenesis and Tumor Growth. *J Biol Chem.* 2000;275:1209–1215.
5. Panka DJ, Mier JW. Canstatin inhibits Akt activation and induces Fas-dependent apoptosis in endothelial cells. *J Biol Chem.* 2003;278:37632–37636.
6. He GA, Luo JX, Zhang TY et al. The C-terminal domain of canstatin suppresses in vivo tumor growth associated with proliferation of endothelial cells. *Biochem Biophys Res Commun.* 2004;318:354–360.
7. Magnon C, Galaup A, Mullan B, et al. Canstatin acts on endothelial and tumor cells via mitochondrial damage initiated through interaction with alphavbeta3 and alphavbeta5 integrins. *Cancer Res.* 2005;65:4353–4361.
8. Mongiat M, Sweeney SM, San Antonio JD, et al. Endorepellin, a novel inhibitor of angiogenesis derived from the C terminus of perlecan. *J Biol Chem.* 2003;278:4238–4249.
9. Woodall BP, Nyström A, Iozzo RA, et al. Integrin alpha2beta1 is the required receptor for endorepellin angiostatic activity. *J Biol Chem.* 2008;283:2335–2343.
10. Iozzo RV. Basement membrane proteoglycans: from cellar to ceiling. *Nat Rev Mol Cell Biol.* 2005;6:646–656.
11. O'Reilly MS, Boehm T, Shing Y, et al. Endostatin: an endogenous inhibitor of angiogenesis and tumor growth. *Cell.* 1997;88:277–85.
12. Marneros AG, Keene DR, Hansen U, et al. Collagen XVIII/endostatin is essential for vision and retinal pigment epithelial function. *EMBO J.* 2004;23:89–99.
13. Marneros AG, Olsen BR. Physiological role of collagen XVIII and endostatin. *FASEB J.* 2005;19:716–728.
14. Sasaki T, Larsson H, Kreuger J, et al. Structural basis and potential role of heparin/heparan sulfate binding to the angiogenesis inhibitor endostatin. *EMBO J.* 1999;18:6240–6248.
15. Digtyar AV, Pozdnyakova NV, Feldman NB, et al. Endostatin: current concepts about its biological role and mechanisms of action. *Biochemistry (Mosc).* 2007;72:235–246.
16. Nguyen TM, Subramanian IV, Xiao X et al. Endostatin induces autophagy in endothelial cells by modulating Beclin 1 and beta-catenin levels. *J Cell Mol Med.* 2009;13:3687–3698.
17. Ambesi A, McKeown-Longo PJ. Anastellin, the angiostatic fibronectin peptide, is a selective inhibitor of lysophospholipid signaling. *Mol Cancer Res.* 2009;7:255–265.
18. Neskey DM, Ambesi A, Pumiglia KM, et al. Endostatin and anastellin inhibit distinct aspects of the angiogenic process. *J Exp Clin Cancer Res.* 2008;27:61.
19. Albig AR, Schiemann WP. Fibulin-5 antagonizes vascular endothelial growth factor (VEGF) signaling and angiogenic sprouting by endothelial cells. *DNA Cell Biol.* 2004;23:367–379.
20. Albig AR, Neil JR, Schiemann WP. Fibulins 3 and 5 antagonize tumor angiogenesis in vivo. *Cancer Res.* 2006;66:2621–2629.
21. Sun J, Hopkins BD, Tsujikawa K, et al. Thrombospondin-1 modulates VEGF-A-mediated Akt signaling and capillary survival in the developing retina. *Am J Physiol Heart Circ Physiol.* 2009;296:H1344–H1351.
22. Maeshima Y, Colorado PC, Torre A, et al. Distinct antitumor properties of a type IV collagen domain derived from basement membrane. *J Biol Chem.* 2000;275:21340–21348.
23. Maeshima Y, Sudhakar A, Lively JC et al. Tumstatin, an endothelial cell-specific inhibitor of protein synthesis. *Science.* 2002;295:140–143.
24. Kawaguchi T, Yamashita Y, Kanamori M, et al. The PTEN/Akt pathway dictates the direct alphaVbeta3-dependent growth-inhibitory action of an active fragment of tumstatin in glioma cells in vitro and in vivo. *Cancer Res.* 2006;66:11331–11340.
25. Volpert OV, Zaichuk T, Zhou W et al. Inducer-stimulated Fas targets activated endothelium for destruction by anti-angiogenic thrombospondin-1 and pigment epithelium-derived factor. *Nat Med.* 2002;8:349–357.

26. Zaichuk TA, Shroff EH, Emmanuel R, et al. Nuclear Factor of Activated T Cells Balances Angiogenesis Activation and Inhibition. *J Exp Med*. 2004;199:1513–1522.
27. Chen L, Zhang SS, Barnstable CJ, et al. PEDF induces apoptosis in human endothelial cells by activating p38 MAP kinase dependent cleavage of multiple caspases *Biochem Biophys Res Commun*. 2006;348:1288–1295.
28. Zhang SX, Wang JJ, Gao G, et al. Pigment epithelium-derived factor (PEDF) is an endogenous antiinflammatory factor. *FASEB J*. 2006;20:323–325.
29. Nowak DG, Woolard J, Amin EM, et al. Expression of pro- and anti-angiogenic isoforms of VEGF is differentially regulated by splicing and growth factors. *J Cell Sci*. 2008;121: 3487–3495.
30. Duenker N. Transforming growth factor-beta (TGF-beta) and programmed cell death in the vertebrate retina. *Int Rev Cytol*. 2005;245:17–43.
31. Maynard SE, Min JY, Merchan J, et al. Excess placental soluble fms-like tyrosine kinase 1 (sFlt1) may contribute to endothelial dysfunction, hypertension, and proteinuria in preeclampsia. *J Clin Invest*. 2003;111:649–658.
32. Ito TK, Ishii G, Saito S, et al. Degradation of soluble VEGF receptor-1 by MMP-7 allows VEGF access to endothelial cells. *Blood*. 2009;113:2363–2369.
33. Ambati BK, Nozaki M, Singh N, et al. Corneal avascularity is due to soluble VEGF receptor-1. *Nature*. 2006;443: 993–997.
34. Peters KG, Kontos CD, Lin PC, et al. Functional significance of Tie2 signaling in the adult vasculature. *Recent Prog Horm Res*. 2004;59:51–71.
35. Tarui T, Majumdar M, Miles LA, et al. Plasmin-induced migration of endothelial cells. A potential target for the anti-angiogenic action of angiostatin. *J Biol Chem*. 2002; 277:33564–33570.
36. Cao Y. Endogenous angiogenesis inhibitors and their therapeutic implications. Int *J Biochem Cell Biol*. 2001;33: 357–369.
37. Moser TL, Stack MS, Asplin I, et al. Angiostatin binds ATP synthase on the surface of human endothelial cells. *Proc Natl Acad Sci U S A*. 1999;96:2811–2816.
38. Moser TL, Stack MS, Wahl ML, et al. The mechanism of action of angiostatin: can you teach an old dog new tricks? *Thromb Haemost*. 2002;87:394–401.
39. Lee TY, Muschal S, Pravda EA, et al. Angiostatin regulates the expression of antiangiogenic and pro-apoptotic pathways via targeted inhibition of mitochondrial proteins. *Blood*. 2009;114:1987–1998.
40. Lee TH, Rhim T, Kim SS. Prothrombin kringle-2 domain has a growth inhibitory activity against basic fibroblast growth factor-stimulated capillary endothelial cells. *J Biol Chem*. 1998;273:28805–28812.
41. Maione TE, Gray GS, Petro J, et al. Inhibition of angiogenesis by recombinant human platelet factor-4 and related peptides. *Science*. 1990;247:77–79.
42. Hagedorn M, Zilberberg L, Lozano RM, et al. A short peptide domain of platelet factor 4 blocks angiogenic key events induced by FGF-2. *FASEB J*. 2001;15:550–552.
43. Wang Z, Tseng CP, Pong RC, et al. The mechanism of growth-inhibitory effect of DOC-2/DAB2 in prostate cancer. Characterization of a novel GTPase-activating protein associated with N-terminal domain of DOC-2/DAB2. *J Biol Chem*. 2002;277:12622–12631.
44. Zhang R, He X, Liu W, et al. AIP1 mediates TNF-alpha-induced ASK1 activation by facilitating dissociation of ASK1 from its inhibitor 14–3–3. *J Clin Invest*. 2003;111:1933–1943.
45. Zhang H, He Y, Dai S, et al. AIP1 functions as an endogenous inhibitor of VEGFR2-mediated signaling and inflammatory angiogenesis in mice. *J Clin Invest*. 2008;118:3904–3916.
46. Clapp C, Thebault S, Arnold E, et al. Vasoinhibins: novel inhibitors of ocular angiogenesis. *Am J Physiol Endocrinol Metab*. 2008;295:E772–E778.
47. Garcia C, Aranda J, Arnold E, et al. Vasoinhibins prevent retinal vasopermeability associated with diabetic retinopathy in rats via protein phosphatase 2A-dependent eNOS inactivation. *J Clin Invest*. 2008;118:2291–2300.
48. Brooks PC, Silletti S, von Schalscha TL, et al. Disruption of angiogenesis by PEX, a noncatalytic metalloproteinase fragment with integrin binding activity. *Cell*. 1998;92:391–400.
49. Moses MA, Wiederschain D, Wu I, et al. Troponin I is present in human cartilage and inhibits angiogenesis. *Proc Natl Acad Sci U S A*. 1999;96:2645–2650.
50. Pike SE, Yao L, Jones KD, et al. Vasostatin, a calreticulin fragment, inhibits angiogenesis and suppresses tumor growth. *J Exp Med*. 1998;188:2349–2356.
51. Xiao F, Wei Y, Yang L, et al. A gene therapy for cancer based on the angiogenesis inhibitor, vasostatin. *Gene Ther*. 2002;9:1207–1213.
52. Cushman M, He HM, Katzenellenbogen JA, et al. Synthesis, antitubulin and antimitotic activity, and cytotoxicity of analogs of 2-methoxyestradiol, an endogenous mammalian metabolite of estradiol that inhibits tubulin polymerization by binding to the colchicine binding site. *J Med Chem*. 1995;38:2041–2049.
53. Mooberry SL. New insights into 2-methoxyestradiol, a promising antiangiogenic and antitumor agent. *Curr Opin Oncol*. 2003;15:425–430.
54. Hiraki Y, Inoue H, Iyama K, et al. Identification of chondromodulin I as a novel endothelial cell growth inhibitor. Purification and its localization in the avascular zone of epiphyseal cartilage. *J Biol Chem*. 1997;272:32419–32426.
55. Funaki H, Sawaguchi S, Yaoeda K, et al. Expression and localization of angiogenic inhibitory factor, chondromodulin-I, in adult rat eye. *Invest Ophthalmol Vis Sci*. 2001;42: 1193–2000.
56. Brew K, Dinakarpandian D, Nagase H. Tissue inhibitors of metalloproteinases: evolution, structure and function. *Biochim Biophys Acta*. 2000;1477:267–283.
57. Baker AH, Edwards DR, Murphy G. Metalloproteinase inhibitors: biological actions and therapeutic opportunities. *J Cell Sci*. 2002;115(pt 19):3719–3727.
58. Otani A, Slike BM, Dorrell MI, et al. A fragment of human TrpRS as a potent antagonist of ocular angiogenesis. *Proc Natl Acad Sci U S A*. 2002;99:178–183.
59. Wakasugi K, Slike BM, Hood J, et al. A human aminoacyl-tRNA synthetase as a regulator of angiogenesis. *Proc Natl Acad Sci U S A*. 2002;99:173–177.
60. Banin E, Dorrell MI, Aguilar E, et al. T2-TrpRS inhibits preretinal neovascularization and enhances physiological vascular regrowth in OIR as assessed by a new method of quantification. *Invest Ophthalmol Vis Sci*. 2006;47:2125–2134.

61. Marneros AG, She H, Zambarakji H, et al. Endogenous endostatin inhibits choroidal neovascularization. *FASEB J.* 2007;21:3809–3818.
62. Lai LJ, Xiao X, Wu JH. Inhibition of corneal neovascularization with endostatin delivered by adeno-associated viral (AAV) vector in a mouse corneal injury model. *J Biomed Sci.* 2007;14:313–322.
63. Takahashi K, Saishin Y, Saishin Y, et al. Intraocular expression of endostatin reduces VEGF-induced retinal vascular permeability, neovascularization, and retinal detachment. *FASEB J.* 2003;17:896–898.
64. Auricchio A, Behling KC, Maguire AM, et al. Inhibition of retinal neovascularization by intraocular viral-mediated delivery of anti-angiogenic agents. *Mol Ther.* 2002;6:490–494.
65. Mori K, Ando A, Gehlbach P, Nesbitt D, et al. Inhibition of choroidal neovascularization by intravenous injection of adenoviral vectors expressing secretable endostatin. *Am J Pathol.* 2001;159:313–320.
66. Konopatskaya O, Churchill AJ, Harper SJ, Bates DO, Gardiner TA. VEGF165b, an endogenous C-terminal splice variant of VEGF, inhibits retinal neovascularization in mice. *Mol Vis.* 2006;12:626–632.
67. Hamilton MM, Byrnes GA, Gall JG, et al. Alternate serotype adenovector provides long-term therapeutic gene expression in the eye. *Mol Vis.* 2008;14:2535–2546.
68. Miyazaki M, Ikeda Y, Yonemitsu Y, et al. Synergistic neuroprotective effect via simian lentiviral vector-mediated simultaneous gene transfer of human pigment epithelium-derived factor and human fibroblast growth factor-2 in rodent models of retinitis pigmentosa. *J Gene Med.* 2008;10:1273–1281.
69. Li H, Tran VV, Hu Y, et al. A PEDF N-terminal peptide protects the retina from ischemic injury when delivered in PLGA nanospheres. *Exp Eye Res.* 2006;83:824–833.
70. Yamagishi S, Nakamura K, Matsui T, et al. Pigment epithelium-derived factor inhibits advanced glycation end product-induced retinal vascular hyperpermeability by blocking reactive oxygen species-mediated vascular endothelial growth factor expression. *J Biol Chem.* 2006;281:20213–20220.
71. Liu H, Ren JG, Cooper WL, et al. Identification of the antivasopermeability effect of pigment epithelium-derived factor and its active site. *Proc Natl Acad Sci U S A.* 2004;101: 6605–6610.
72. Takita H, Yoneya S, Gehlbach PL, et al. Retinal neuroprotection against ischemic injury mediated by intraocular gene transfer of pigment epithelium-derived factor. *Invest Ophthalmol Vis Sci.* 2003;44:4497–4504.
73. Miyazaki M, Ikeda Y, Yonemitsu Y, et al. Simian lentiviral vector-mediated retinal gene transfer of pigment epithelium-derived factor protects retinal degeneration and electrical defect in Royal College of Surgeons rats. *Gene Ther.* 2003;10:1503–1511.
74. Raisler BJ, Berns KI, Grant MB, et al. Adeno-associated virus type-2 expression of pigmented epithelium-derived factor or Kringles 1–3 of angiostatin reduce retinal neovascularization. *Proc Natl Acad Sci U S A.* 2002;99:8909–8914.
75. Mori K, Duh E, Gehlbach P, et al. Pigment epithelium-derived factor inhibits retinal and choroidal neovascularization. *J Cell Physiol.* 2001;188:253–263.
76. Stellmach V, Crawford SE, Zhou W, et al. Prevention of ischemia-induced retinopathy by the natural ocular antiangiogenic agent pigment epithelium-derived factor. *Proc Natl Acad Sci U S A.* 2001;98:2593–2597.
77. Dawson DW, Volpert OV, Gillis P, et al. Pigment epithelium-derived factor: a potent inhibitor of angiogenesis, *Science.* 1999;285:245–248.
78. Gehlbach P, Demetriades AM, Yamamoto S, et al. Periocular injection of an adenoviral vector encoding pigment epithelium-derived factor inhibits choroidal neovascularization. *Gene Ther.* 2003;10:637–646.
79. Zhou X, Li F, Kong L, Chodosh J, Cao W. Anti-inflammatory effect of pigment epithelium-derived factor in DBA/2J mice. *Mol Vis.* 2009;15:438–450.
80. Murakami Y, Ikeda Y, Yonemitsu Y, et al. Inhibition of nuclear translocation of apoptosis-inducing factor is an essential mechanism of the neuroprotective activity of pigment epithelium-derived factor in a rat model of retinal degeneration. *Am J Pathol.* 2008;173:1326–1338.
81. Imai D, Yoneya S, Gehlbach PL, et al. Intraocular gene transfer of pigment epithelium-derived factor rescues photoreceptors from light-induced cell death. *J Cell Physiol.* 2005;202:570–578.
82. Cano MD, Karagiannis E, Soliman M, et al. Peptide derived from type 1 thrombospondin repeat-containing protein WISP-1 inhibits corneal and choroidal neovascularization. *Invest Ophthalmol Vis Sci.* 2009;50:3840–3845.
83. Shafiee A, Penn JS, Krutzsch HC, et al. Inhibition of retinal angiogenesis by peptides derived from thrombospondin-1. *Invest Ophthalmol Vis Sci.* 2000;41:2378–2388.
84. Honda M, Sakamoto T, Ishibashi T, et al. Experimental subretinal neovascularization is inhibited by adenovirus-mediated soluble VEGF/flt-1 receptor gene transfection: a role of VEGF and possible treatment for SRN in age-related macular degeneration. *Gene Ther.* 2000;7:978–985.
85. Lamartina S, Cimino M, Roscilli G, et al. Helper-dependent adenovirus for the gene therapy of proliferative retinopathies: stable gene transfer, regulated gene expression and therapeutic efficacy. *J Gene Med.* 2007;9:862–874.
86. Ideno J, Mizukami H, Kakehashi A, et al. Prevention of diabetic retinopathy by intraocular soluble flt-1 gene transfer in a spontaneously diabetic rat model. *Int J Mol Med.* 2007;19:75–79.
87. Rota R, Riccioni T, Zaccarini M, et al. Marked inhibition of retinal neovascularization in rats following soluble-flt-1 gene transfer. *J Gene Med.* 2004;6:992–1002.
88. Takagi H, Koyama S, Seike H, et al. Potential role of the angiopoietin/tie2 system in ischemia-induced retinal neovascularization. *Invest Ophthalmol Vis Sci.* 2003;44:393–402.
89. Bainbridge JW, Mistry A, De Alwis M, et al. Inhibition of retinal neovascularisation by gene transfer of soluble VEGF receptor sFlt-1. *Gene Ther.* 2002;9:320–326.
90. Hangai M, Moon YS, Kitaya N, et al. Systemically expressed soluble Tie2 inhibits intraocular neovascularization. *Hum Gene Ther.* 2001;12:1311–1321.
91. Kozulin P, Natoli R, O'Brien KM, et al. Differential expression of anti-angiogenic factors and guidance genes in the developing macula. *Mol Vis.* 2009;15:45–59.
92. Chan CK, Pham LN, Zhou J, et al. Differential expression of pro-and antiangiogenic factors in mouse strain-dependent hypoxia-induced retinal neovascularization. *Lab Invest.* 2005; 85:721–733.

93. Ständker L, Schrader M, Kanse SM, et al. Isolation and characterization of the circulating form of human endostatin. *FEBS Lett.* 1997;420:129–133.
94. Sim BK, MacDonald NJ, Gubish ER. Angiostatin and endostatin: endogenous inhibitors of tumor growth. *Cancer Metastasis Rev.* 2000;19:181–190.
95. Ruegg C, Hasmim M, Lejeune FJ, et al. Antiangiogenic peptides and proteins: from experimental tools to clinical drugs. *Biochim Biophys Acta.* 2006;1765:155–177.
96. Tjin Tham Sjin RM, Satchi-Fainaro R, Birsner AE, et al. A 27-amino-acid synthetic peptide corresponding to the NH2-terminal zinc-binding domain of endostatin is responsible for its antitumor activity. *Cancer Res.* 2005;65:3656–3663.
97. Zatterstrom UK, Felbor U, Fukai N, et al. Collagen XVIII/helper-dependent adenovirus endostatin structure and functional role in angiogenesis. *Cell Struct Funct.* 2000;25:97–101.
98. Sasaki T, Fukai N, Mann K, et al. Structure, function and tissue forms of the C-terminal globular domain of collagen XVIII containing the angiogenesis inhibitor endostatin. *EMBO J.* 1998;17:4249–4256.
99. Ferreras M, Felbor U, Lenhard T, et al. Generation and degradation of human endostatin proteins by various proteinases. *FEBS Lett.* 2000;486:247–251.
100. Sertie AL, Sossi V, Camargo AA, et al. Collagen XVIII, containing an endogenous inhibitor of angiogenesis and tumor growth, plays a critical role in the maintenance of retinal structure and in neural tube closure (Knobloch syndrome). *Hum Mol Genet.* 2000;9:2051–2058.
101. Fukai N, Eklund L, Marneros AG, et al. Lack of collagen XVIII/endostatin results in eye abnormalities. *EMBO J.* 2002;21:1535–1544.
102. Suzuki OT, Sertie AL, Der Kaloustian VM, et al. Molecular analysis of collagen XVIII reveals novel mutations, presence of a third isoform, and possible genetic heterogeneity in Knobloch syndrome. *Am J Hum Genet.* 2002;71:1320–1329.
103. Bhutto IA, Kim SY, McLeod DS, et al. Localization of collagen XVIII and the endostatin portion of collagen XVIII in aged human control eyes and eyes with age-related macular degeneration. *Invest Ophthalmol Vis Sci.* 2004;45:1544–1552.
104. Marneros AG, Olsen BR. Age-dependent iris abnormalities in collagen XVIII/endostatin deficient mice with similarities to human pigment dispersion syndrome. *Invest Ophthalmol. Vis Sci.* 2003;44:2367–2372.
105. van der Schaft TL, Mooy CM, de Bruijn WC, et al. Immunohistochemical light and electron microscopy of basal laminar deposit. *Graefes Arch Clin Exp Ophthalmol.* 1994;232:40–46.
106. Dixelius J, Cross M, Matsumoto T, et al. Endostatin regulates endothelial cell adhesion and cytoskeletal organization. *Cancer Res.* 2002;62:1944–1947.
107. Kim YM, Hwang S, Kim YM, et al. Endostatin blocks vascular endothelial growth factor-mediated signaling via direct interaction with KDR/Flk-1. *J Biol Chem.* 2002;277:27872–27879.
108. Dhanabal M, Ramchandran R, Waterman MJ, et al. Endostatin induces endothelial cell apoptosis. *J Biol Chem.* 1999;274:11721–11726.
109. Shichiri M, Hirata Y. Antiangiogenesis signals by endostatin. *FASEB J.* 2001;15:1044–1053.
110. Abdollahi A, Hahnfeldt P, Maercker C, et al. Endostatin's antiangiogenic signaling network. *Mol Cell.* 2004;13:649–663.
111. Boehm T, Folkman J, Browder T, et al. Antiangiogenic therapy of experimental cancer does not induce acquired drug resistance. *Nature.* 1997;390:404–407.
112. Herbst RS, Mullani NA, Davis DW, et al. Development of biologic markers of response and assessment of antiangiogenic activity in a clinical trial of human recombinant endostatin. *J Clin Oncol.* 2002;20:3804–3814.
113. Shibuya M, Yamaguchi, S, Yamane A, et al. Nucleotide sequence and expression of a novel human receptor-type tyrosine kinase gene (flt) closely related to the fms family. *Oncogene.* 1990;5:519–524.
114. De Vries C, Escobedo JA, Ueno H, et al. The fms-like tyrosine kinase, a receptor for vascular endothelial growth factor. *Science.* 1992;255:989–991.
115. Kendall RL, Thomas KA. Inhibition of vascular endothelial cell growth factor activity by an endogenously encoded soluble receptor. *Proc Natl Acad Sci U S A.* 1993;90 10705–10709.
116. Rahimi N, Golde TE, Meyer RD. Identification of ligand-induced proteolytic cleavage and ectodomain shedding of VEGFR-1/FLT1 in leukemic cancer cells. *Cancer Res.* 2009;69:2607–2614.
117. Matsunaga N, Chikaraishi Y, Izuta H, et al. Role of soluble vascular endothelial growth factor receptor-1 in the vitreous in proliferative diabetic retinopathy. *Ophthalmology.* 2008;115:1916–1922.
118. Aiello LP, Pierce EA, Foley ED, et al. Suppression of retinal neovascularization in vivo by inhibition of vascular endothelial growth factor (VEGF) using soluble VEGF-receptor chimeric proteins, *Proc Natl Acad Sci U S A.* 1995;92:10457–10461.
119. Kendall RL, Wang G, Thomas KA. Identification of a natural soluble form of the vascular endothelial growth factor receptor, FLT-1, and its heterodimerization with KDR, *Biochem Biophys Res Commun.* 1996;226:324–328.
120. Tombran-Tink J, Johnson LV. Neuronal differentiation of retinoblastoma cells induced by medium conditioned by human RPE cells. *Invest Ophthalmol Vis Sci.* 1989;30:1700–1707.
121. Steele FR, Chader GJ, Johnson LV, et al. Pigment epithelium-derived factor: neurotrophic activity and identification as a member of the serine protease inhibitor gene family. *Proc Natl Acad Sci U S A.* 1993;90:1526–1530.
122. Xu X, Zhang SS, Barnstable CJ, Tombran-Tink J. Molecular phylogeny of the antiangiogenic and neurotrophic serpin, pigment epithelium derived factor in vertebrates. *BMC Genomics.* 2006;7:248.
123. Tombran-Tink J, Pawar H, Swaroop A, et al. Localization of the gene for pigment epithelium-derived factor (PEDF) to chromosome 17p13.1 and expression in cultured human retinoblastoma cells. *Genomics.* 1994;19:266–272.
124. Tombran-Tink J, Mazuruk K, Rodriguez IR, et al. Organization, evolutionary conservation, expression and unusual Alu density of the human gene for pigment epithelium-derived factor, a unique neurotrophic serpin. *Mol Vis.* 1996;2:11.

125. Bilak MM, Corse AM, Bilak SR, et al. Pigment epithelium-derived factor (PEDF) protects motor neurons from chronic glutamate-mediated neurodegeneration. *J Neuropathol Exp Neurol.* 1999;58:719–728.
126. Cheung LW, Au SC, Cheung AN, et al. Pigment epithelium-derived factor is estrogen sensitive and inhibits the growth of human ovarian cancer and ovarian surface epithelial cells. *Endocrinology.* 2006;147:4179–4191.
127. Simonovic M, Gettins PGW, Volz K. Crystal structure of human PEDF, a potent anti-angiogenic and neurite growth-promoting factor. *Proc Natl Acad Sci U S A.* 2001;98: 11131–11135.
128. Bouck, N. PEDF: anti-angiogenic guardian of ocular function. *Trends Mol Med.* 2002;8:330–334.
129. Tombran-Tink J, Barnstable CJ. PEDF: a multifaceted neurotrophic factor. *Nat Rev Neurosci.* 2003;4:628–636.
130. Becerra SP. Focus on Molecules: Pigment epithelium-derived factor (PEDF). *Exp Eye Res.* 2006;82:739–740.
131. Ek ET, Dass CR, Choong PF. PEDF: a potential molecular therapeutic target with multiple anti-cancer activities. *Trends Mol Med.* 2006;12:497–502.
132. Notari L, Baladron V, Aroca-Aguilar JD, et al. Identification of a lipase-linked cell membrane receptor for pigment epithelium-derived factor. *J Biol Chem.* 2006;281: 38022–38037.
133. Bernard A, Gao-Li J, Franco CA, et al. Laminin receptor involvement in the anti-angiogenic activity of pigment epithelium-derived factor. *J Biol Chem.* 2009;284:10480–10490.
134. Cai J, Jiang WG, Grant MB, et al. Pigment epithelium-derived factor inhibits angiogenesis via regulated intracellular proteolysis of vascular endothelial growth factor receptor 1. *J Biol Chem.* 2006;281:3604–3613.
135. Alberdi E, Aymerich MS, Becerra SP. Binding of pigment epithelium-derived factor (PEDF) to retinoblastoma cells and cerebellar granule neurons. Evidence for a PEDF receptor. *J Biol Chem.* 1999;274:31605–31612.
136. Aymerich MS, Alberdi EM, Martinez A, et al. Evidence for pigment epithelium-derived factor receptors in the neural retina. *Invest Ophthalmol Vis Sci.* 2001;42:3287–3293.
137. Filleur S, Nelius T, de Riese W, et al. Characterization of PEDF: a multi-functional serpin family protein. *J Cell Biochem.* 2009;106:769–775.
138. Yabe T, Wilson D, Schwartz JP. NF-κB activation is required for the neuroprotective effects of pigment epithelium-derived factor (PEDF) on cerebellar granule neurons. *J Biol Chem.* 2001;276:43313–43319.
139. Smith ND, Schulze-Hoepfner FT, Veliceasa D, et al. Pigment epithelium-derived factor and interleukin-6 control prostate neuroendocrine differentiation via feed-forward mechanism. *J Urol.* 2008;179:2427–2434.
140. Stitt AW, Graham D, Gardiner TA. Ocular wounding prevents pre-retinal neovascularization and upregulates PEDF expression in the inner retina. *Mol Vis.* 2004;10:432–438.
141. Penn JS, McCollum GW, Barnett JM, et al. Angiostatic effect of penetrating ocular injury: role of pigment epithelium-derived factor. *Invest Ophthalmol Vis Sci.* 2006;47:405–414.
142. Li Z, Wang HY, Rong A. The expression of PEDF in intraocular tissue of diabetic rats after argon laser photocoagulation. *Int J Ophthalmol.* 2008;8:261–264.
143. Sreekumar PG, Zhou J, Sohn J, et al. N-(4-hydroxyphenyl) retinamide augments laser-induced choroidal neovascularization in mice. *Invest Ophthalmol Vis Sci.* 2008;49:1210–1220.
144. Duh EJ, Yang HS, Suzuma I, et al. Pigment epithelium-derived factor suppresses ischemia-induced retinal neovascularization and VEGF-induced migration and growth. *Invest Ophthalmol Vis Sci.* 2002;43:821–829.
145. Stieger K, Lhériteau E, Moullier P, et al. AAV-mediated gene therapy for retinal disorders in large animal models. *ILAR J.* 2009;50:206–224.
146. Mori K, Gehlbach P, Yamamoto S, et al. AAV-mediated gene transfer of pigment epithelium-derived factor inhibits choroidal neovascularization. *Invest Ophthalmol Vis Sci.* 2002;43:1994–2000.
147. Saishin Y, Silva RL, Saishin Y, et al. Periocular gene transfer of pigment epithelium-derived factor inhibits choroidal neovascularization in a human-sized eye. *Hum Gene Ther.* 2005;16:473–478.
148. Rassmussen H, Chu KW, Campochiaro P, et al. Clinical protocol: an open-label, phase 1, single administration, dose-escalation study of ADGVPEDF.11D (ADPEDF) in neovascular age-related macular degeneration (AMD). *Hum Gene Ther.* 2001;12:2029–2032.
149. Mosher DF. Physiology of thrombospondin. *Annu Rev Med.* 1990;41:85–97.
150. Good DJ, Polverini PJ, Rastinejad F, et al. A tumor suppressor-dependent inhibitor of angiogenesis is immunologically and functionally indistinguishable from a fragment of thrombospondin. *Proc Natl Acad Sci U S A.* 1990;87: 6624–6628.
151. Adams JC, Lawler J. The thrombospondins. *Int J Biochem Cell Biol.* 2004;36:961–968.
152. Isenberg JS, Frazier WA, Roberts DD. Thrombospondin-1: a physiological regulator of nitric oxide signaling. *Cell Mol Life Sci.* 2008;65:728–742.
153. Chen H, Herndon ME, Lawler J. The cell biology of thrombospondin-1. *Matrix Biol.* 2000;19:597–614.
154. Agah A, Kyriakides TR, Lawler J, et al. The lack of thrombospondin-1 (TSP1) dictates the course of wound healing in double-TSP1/TSP2-null mice. *Am J Pathol.* 2002;161: 831–839.
155. Iruela-Arispe ML, Luque A, Lee N. Thrombospondin modules and angiogenesis. *Int J Biochem Cell Biol.* 2004; 36:1070–1078.
156. Armstrong LC, Bornstein P. Thrombospondins 1 and 2 function as inhibitors of angiogenesis. *Matrix Biology.* 2003;22:63–71.
157. Rastinejad F, Polverini PJ, Bouck NP. Regulation of the activity of a new inhibitor of angiogenesis by a cancer suppressor gene. *Cell.* 1989;56:345–355.
158. Jiménez B, Volpert OV, Crawford SE, et al. Signals leading to apoptosis-dependent inhibition of neovascularization by thrombospondin-1. *Nat Med.* 2000;6:41–48.
159. Suzuma K, Takagi H, Otani A, et al. Expression of thrombospondin-1 in ischemia-induced retinal neovascularization. *Am J Pathol.* 1999;154:343–354.
160. Iruela-Arispe ML, Lombardo M, Krutzsch HC, et al. Inhibition of angiogenesis by thrombospondin-1 is mediated by 2 independent regions within the type 1 repeats. *Circulation.* 1999;100:1423–1431.

161. Karagiannis ED, Popel AS. Anti-angiogenic peptides identified in thrombospondin type I domains. *Biochem Biophys Res Commun.* 2007;359:63–69.
162. Hiscott P, Paraoan L, Choudhary A, et al. Thrombospondin 1, thrombospondin 2 and the eye. *Prog Retin Eye Res.* 2006;25:1–18.
163. Sheibani N, Sorenson CM, Cornelius LA, et al. Thrombospondin-1, a natural inhibitor of angiogenesis, is present in vitreous and aqueous humor and is modulated by hyperglycemia. *Biochem Biophys Res Commun.* 2000;267: 257–261.
164. Uno K, Bhutto IA, McLeod DS, et al. Impaired expression of thrombospondin-1 in eyes with age related macular degeneration. *Br J Ophthalmol.* 2006;90:48–54.
165. Bhutto IA, Uno K, Merges C, et al. Reduction of endogenous angiogenesis inhibitors in Bruch's membrane of the submacular region in eyes with age-related macular degeneration. *Arch Ophthalmol.* 2008;126:670–678.
166. Neufeld G, Cohen T, Gengrinovitch S, et al. Vascular endothelial growth factor (VEGF) and its receptors. *FASEB J.* 1999;13:9–22.
167. Bates DO, Cui TG, Doughty JM, et al. VEGF165b, an inhibitory splice variant of vascular endothelial growth factor, is down-regulated in renal cell carcinoma. *Cancer Res.* 2002;62:4123–31.
168. Perrin RM, Konopatskaya O, Qiu Y, et al. Diabetic retinopathy is associated with a switch in splicing from anti- to proangiogenic isoforms of vascular endothelial growth factor. *Diabetologia.* 2005;48:2422–2427.
169. Hua J, Spee C, Barron E, et al. Therapeutic Potential of Small Molecule Splicing Factor-inhibitor Srpin340 in Treatment of Choroidal Neovascularization (CNV). *Invest Ophthalmol Vis Sci.* 2009;50:E-Abstract 2333.
170. Woolard J, Wang WY, Bevan HS, et al. VEGF165b, an inhibitory vascular endothelial growth factor splice variant: mechanism of action, in vivo effect on angiogenesis and endogenous protein expression. *Cancer Res.* 2004;4:7822–7835.
171. Cebe Suarez S, Pieren M, Cariolato L, et al. VEGF-A splice variant defective for heparan sulfate and neuropilin-1 binding shows attenuated signaling through VEGFR-2. *Cell Mo Life Sci.* 2006;63:2067–2077.
172. Rennel ES, Hamdollah-Zadeh MA, Wheatley ER, et al. Recombinant human VEGF165b protein is an effective anticancer agent in mice. *Eur J Cancer.* 2008;44:1883–1894.
173. Varey AH, Rennel ES, Qiu Y, et al. VEGF 165 b, an antiangiogenic VEGF-A isoform, binds and inhibits bevacizumab treatment in experimental colorectal carcinoma: balance of pro- and antiangiogenic VEGF-A isoforms has implications for therapy. *Br J Cancer.* 2008;98:1366–1379.

CHAPTER

9

Diabetic Macular Edema: Molecular Mechanisms

Sampathkumar Rangasamy • Ramprasad Srinivasan • Paul McGuire • Arup Das

INTRODUCTION

Diabetic retinopathy is the leading cause of blindness in working-age populations (20–64 years old) of developed countries and is responsible for 12% of new cases of blindness each year.[2,3] Diabetic macular edema (DME) is the leading cause of any degree of visual impairment in diabetic subjects.[4–6] The presence of DME can be found at any stage of diabetes, and it is widely seen in patients with longer diabetes duration. Many studies have indicated the important role of DME in the loss of visual acuity. In the Early Treatment Diabetic Retinopathy Study (ETDRS), macular edema was the second most common cause of severe visual loss.[7] The U.S. Wisconsin Epidemiologic Study of Diabetic Retinopathy has indicated that 13% to 25% of patients with diabetes mellitus develop DME in 10 years, with a point prevalence ranging from 2% to 6%. It has also been indicated that over a 10-year period, non–clinically significant DME and clinically significant DME will develop in 14% and 10% of Americans with known diabetes, respectively.[8] Studies have also concluded that approximately half of patients with DME will lose two or more lines of visual acuity within 2 years of the diagnosis.[9]

At the global level, World Health Organization (WHO) estimates that about 50% of the 8 million subjects diagnosed annually with diabetes do not receive appropriate eye care. It has estimated that if they are untreated, there is a 25% to 30% risk of developing clinically significant macular edema (CSME) with moderate visual loss. Furthermore, it has been predicted that the diabetes-related blindness and visual impairment place a significant burden on society with increased cost and declined quality of life.[10,11] The clinical significance of macular edema highlights the importance of investigating the basic mechanism and the potentially modifiable risk factors for this condition for the development of effective treatment and prevention.[10,12]

RISK FACTORS FOR DME

The presence of macular edema was associated with longer duration of diabetes, higher systolic blood pressure, insulin use, HbA1c, and presence of proteinuria. Hyperglycemia, assessed by glycated hemoglobin (HbA1c), results in significantly greater rates of macular edema. In the Diabetes Control and Complications Trial (DCCT) as well as in other epidemiological studies, HbA1c was a strong predictor of DME.[13,14] The rate of DME in late-onset, long-term (>15 years) diabetes increased from 18.1% in the lowest quartile HgbA1c level (6.8%–9.7%) to 36.4% in the highest quartile HbA1c level (13.2%–19.2%).[15] The relative risk for DME was shown as 1.44 for each 1% increase in HbA1c level.[16] Importantly, the DCCT shown that intensive treatment of diabetes to achieve near-normal blood glucose levels resulted in a 23% risk reduction in clinically significant DME.[17]

Studies such as WESDR and ETDRS reported a clear relationship between cholesterol levels and the presence of retinal hard exudates.[18,19] A large prospective study in type 1 diabetes indicates that elevated serum lipids, particularly total-to-HDL cholesterol ratio and triglycerides, are independent risk factors for both CSME and retinal hard exudates.[20] In another progressive study, it has been also shown that there was no association of lipids with macular edema after controlling for HbA1c and other risk factors.[21] Existing evidence indicates that the relationship between lipid levels and macular edema appears to be biologically plausible. Also, elevated levels of LDL and triglycerides in type 1 diabetes have been linked with higher levels of fluorescent advanced glycation end (AGE) products, which are hypothesized to play an important role in the pathogenesis of diabetes complications.[22]

Systolic and diastolic hypertension has also shown to markedly increase the risk for DME from three- to fivefold. Diabetic renal disease evidenced by proteinuria increases the risk for DME up to five fold in early-onset and late-onset diabetes. The duration of diabetes also has shown to increase the prevalence of macular edema. The rate of DME increased from 3% in subjects with diabetes for <5 years to 28% in those with diabetes duration of more than 20 years.[15,23,24] Pregnancy has shown to increase the progression of diabetic retinopathy, and studies has shown that in the presence of hypertension and proteinuria, pregnancy can lead to macular edema with marked capillary nonperfusion. Most often DME progression will be contained in the late third trimester or after delivery, but in rare cases, it might also lead to visual loss.[25–27]

PATHOPHYSIOLOGY OF DME

The pathogenesis of DME is still not completely understood in spite of intensive studies. The pathophysiological characterization of macular edema is the retinal thickening from leaky blood vessels due to alteration of the blood-retinal barrier (BRB), and it can develop at all stages of retinopathy. The events that lead to the macular edema in diabetic patients involve the changes in the structure and cellular composition of retinal microvasculature over a time period. It has been observed that the thickening of the basement membrane and damage to retinal microvascular endothelial cells lead to increased permeability and incompetence of retinal vasculature. This compromise of BRB leads to the leakage of plasma constituents in the surrounding retina, resulting in retinal edema. The loss of pericytes is considered to be an important hallmark of DME.[28] Early in the development of diabetic retinopathy, functional loss of pericytes surrounding the retinal capillaries leads to the altered regulation of retinal capillary perfusion and retinal hemodynamic, including abnormal blood flow.[29] These events are shown to correlate with microaneurysm formation, thickening of capillary basement membrane, and increased deposition of extracellular matrix (ECM) components that aid in the development of DME.[5]

Studies have demonstrated that chronic hyperglycemia as well as the associated metabolic entities such as hyperlipidemia and hypertension contributes to the pathogenesis of DR/DME.[15–24] The current understanding of hyperglycemia as the strongest known risk factor for DR/DME is clear, but the exact mechanism by which the elevated glucose levels in diabetes condition initiate the vascular disruption in retinopathy remains unclear, and several pathways have been implicated. The hyperglycemia-induced pathogenesis of diabetic retinopathy is linked to four main biochemical alterations such as (a) increased polyol pathway flux, (b) increased AGE-product formation, (c) activation of protein kinase C (PKC) isoforms, and (d) increased hexosamine pathway flux.[30] All these pathways culminate in increased oxidative stress, inflammation, and vascular dysfunction. Vascular dysfunction ensues with eventual vascular occlusion and local ischemia. The resulting hypoxia upregulates a variety of growth factors such as insulin-like growth factor (IGF), angiopoietins, stromal-derived factor-1, fibroblast growth factor-2 (FGF-2), tumor necrosis factor (TNF), interleukin-6 (IL-6), and vascular endothelial growth factor (VEGF), which contribute to the development of DME (Fig. 9.1).

The key pathological event that occurs in macular edema is increased vascular permeability. Vascular permeability has shown to be initiated by various vaso-permeable

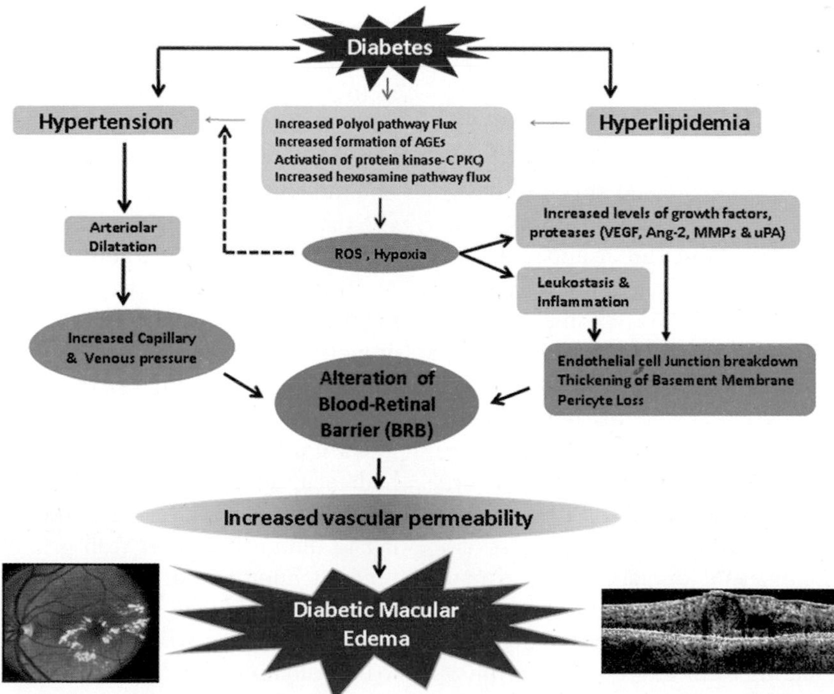

FIGURE 9.1. Schematic diagram showing how diabetes in conjunction with hypertension and hyperlipidemia causes alteration of the BRB, leading to DME. Both increased levels of growth factors and proteinases, as well as leukostasis/inflammation result in endothelial cell junction breakdown. Several steps of this cascade can be used as therapeutic targets to inhibit DME.

agents such as VEGF, TNF, Interleukin, and Ang2 that are upregulated in DME.[31,32] The other important and nascent area of research in terms of DME is inflammation. TNF, interleukins, and adhesion molecules such as Inter cellular adhesion molecule (ICAM) and Vascular cell adhesion molecule (VCAM) can attract inflammatory cells to the retina. This phenomenon is called retinal leukostasis. These activated inflammatory cells can release various soluble chemokines that can induce vasopermeability. Alternatively, these inflammatory cells can breach the endothelial barrier through the process called diapedesis leading to the pathogenesis of DME.[33–36] The detailed information of the importance of BRB, inflammation, growth factors, and the potential therapeutic targets of DME is discussed further below.

Composition of the Blood-Retinal Barrier

The blood-retinal barrier is one of most important ocular architectures, which is involved in the tight regulation and maintenance of the fluid electrolyte balance in the retina. Basically, the BRB partition the neural retina from the circulation by acting as a barrier for the molecules that can enter. Breakdown of this barrier contributes to the fluid accumulation in the retinal disorders including DME. The inner BRB is made of the endothelial cells in the inner retina, and the outer BRB by retinal pigment epithelial (RPE) cells on the Bruch membrane between the fenestrated choroidal vessels and the outer retina.[28,29]

The endothelial cells form a very tight monolayer, which is helped by the adherens and the tight junction proteins. Adherens junctions are formed through the interactions between cadherins, a family of functionally related transmembrane glycoproteins, which mediate calcium-dependent, cell-cell adhesion.[37] The important adherent junctional protein is the VE-cadherin (cadherin-5). VE-cadherin proteins are expressed specifically by the endothelial cells, which are implicated in a number of endothelial cell functions. The most important function of VE-cadherin is the maintenance of the endothelial cell barrier function.[38] Endothelial monolayer permeability is regulated by VE-cadherin through the interaction of its cytoplasmic tail with cytoplasmic proteins called catenins. β-Catenin, plakoglobin (γ-catenin), and α-catenin bring out the attachment of the cadherin complex with the actin cytoskeleton. The attachment of cadherin to the actin cytoskeleton is required for the formation of a restrictive endothelial monolayer.[39,40] A fourth catenin, p120, associates with the cadherin cytoplasmic domain just proximal to the membrane, a region termed the juxtamembrane domain (JMD).[41,42] The phosphorylation state of p120 plays an important role in regulating cadherin function. Studies have indicated that molecules such as thrombin, histamine, and importantly VEGF decrease endothelial barrier function mediated through the phosphorylation mechanism of catenins. Also, the retinal endothelial cells and the pigmented epithelial cells are tightly connected through a network of intercellular tight junctional proteins that regulate fluid flux. It has been estimated that around 40 tight junctional proteins in the peripheral cytoplasm and apical plasma membrane provide a fine control of influx of water and solutes.[43] The principal proteins found in endothelial tight junctions are occludin, claudin-5, and JAMs, which create a tight seal so that water-soluble molecules cannot easily penetrate between the cells. These transmembrane proteins have linkages to the actin cytoskeletal proteins such as zona occludin-1 (ZO-1) and zona occludin-2 (ZO-2). 1 details the function of some important junctional proteins involved in the maintenance of BRB.

Also the BRB integrity is maintained tightly by the presence of pericytes in the endothelium. Pericytes cover the apical side of the lumen and are separated by the matrix from the endothelial cells. Brain microvascular pericytes have been shown to send out processes through the lamina, which help to communicate with endothelial cells. It is estimated that the endothelial: pericyte ratio is 1:1 in the retina, and any decrease in the pericyte cell number leads to increased vascular permeability. In diabetes, there is an increased pericyte loss, which leads to an increased leakage of the retinal capillaries.[44] Also, the ECM acts as a foundation for the endothelial cells to form a monolayer. The basement membrane is mainly composed of collagen IV, fibronectin, and laminin that interact with endothelial cells and aid in adhesiveness to the matrix.[45] Degradation of the matrix results in endothelial cells migration and also in the loss of barrier function.

Alteration of Blood-Retinal Barrier in Diabetes

The disruption of BRB in diabetes involves numerous factors and events within the vascular lumen and in the retinal parenchyma. Prominent among them is the VEGF, which was initially called as vascular permeability factor. The inflammatory factors such as tumor necrosis factor-α (TNF-α) and interleukin-1β (IL-1β) have also shown to alter the vascular permeability through various molecular mechanisms. Other growth factors and cytokines including hepatocyte growth factor (HGF), FGF, insulin-like growth factor-1 (IGF-1), and histamine have shown to alter the retinal vascular permeability.[46–48]

It has been proposed that the factors that contribute to DME alter the starling equilibrium in the retina (role of hydrostatic and oncotic forces (the so-called Starling forces) in the movement of fluid across capillary membranes), leading to diminished fluid reabsorption capacity resulting in fluid retention within the microvessel lumens. One important example is that the diabetic patients associated with macroalbuminuria will have decreased oncotic pressure due to hypoalbuminemia, which will diminish the fluid retention capacity of the vessel lumens.[49] Those diabetic patients with persistent macroalbuminuria due to poorly controlled diabetes will have severe macular edema. Also, diabetes drugs such as glitazones have been implicated in the aggravation of macular edema due to its fluid retention property.[50]

The important mechanism that leads to vision loss in DME due to altered BRB involves (a) light scattering, (b) disruption of retinal ionic balances, and (c) impaired cell-cell communication that involves not only the retinal microvascular cells but also the retinal neuronal cells.[46] The details on the physical aspects of the visual-optometric functional impairment and its molecular details are still not known but the association of vascular leakage with the vision impairment has been well established.[51] The importance of the fluid accumulation or the edema involves multiple and/or prolonged insult to the macula. Importantly, the RPE cells act as the major fluid-absorbing sponge in the retina, but in prolonged insults, they lose their ability, thus leading to the progression of macular edema and subsequent vision loss.[52] These final events include the dysfunction of retinal glial and neuronal cells, and therefore the functional restoration of those vascular and neuronal cells may provide a better therapy for maintaining vision.

PROTEINASES IN DME

The vitreous level of MMP9 was higher in diabetic subjects with DR than with the diabetic subjects without DR. This study shows that MMPs must have a potential role in the pathogenesis of DR.[53] Furthermore, in animal model of diabetes, both MMP2 and MMP9 are elevated, which are involved in the alteration of blood-retinal barrier.[54] Another form of MMP called MT1-MMP, which is a membrane-bound MMP, is also increased along with MMP2 in the diabetic animals, and concomitant to this, there is an increased apoptosis of pericytes in the diabetic retina when compared to the normal retina. This may further accelerate BRB alteration in the diabetic state. We have shown that retinal vascular permeability was significantly increased in rats following 2 weeks of diabetes, coincident with a decrease of VE-cadherin expression. This increased vascular permeability could be inhibited with an MMP inhibitor (Figs. 9.2–9.6). AGE increases a loss of VE-Cadherin, which is prevented by MMP inhibitor, suggesting that MMP has a direct role in the alteration of endothelial monolayer.[55] These observations suggest a possible mechanism by which diabetes contributes to BRB breakdown through proteolytic degradation of VE-cadherin. This may indicate a role for extracellular proteinases in alteration of the BRB seen in diabetic retinopathy.[55] High glucose can activate many soluble mediators such as AGE, ROS, inflammatory cytokines, which can increase MMP expression and activity in the diabetic state. In a recent work, the oxidative stress has been implicated to have an influence in the MMP2 and MT1-MMP expressions and activities.[56] The role of MMP-9 is implicated in the alteration of barrier function, which is shown to be mediated by TGF-β.[57] Studies have hinted that diabetes causes retinal inflammation, which unleashes a sequelae of events resulting in the vascular leakage. Retinal inflammation attracts increased leukocytes to the retina, which then bind to the vascular endothelium.

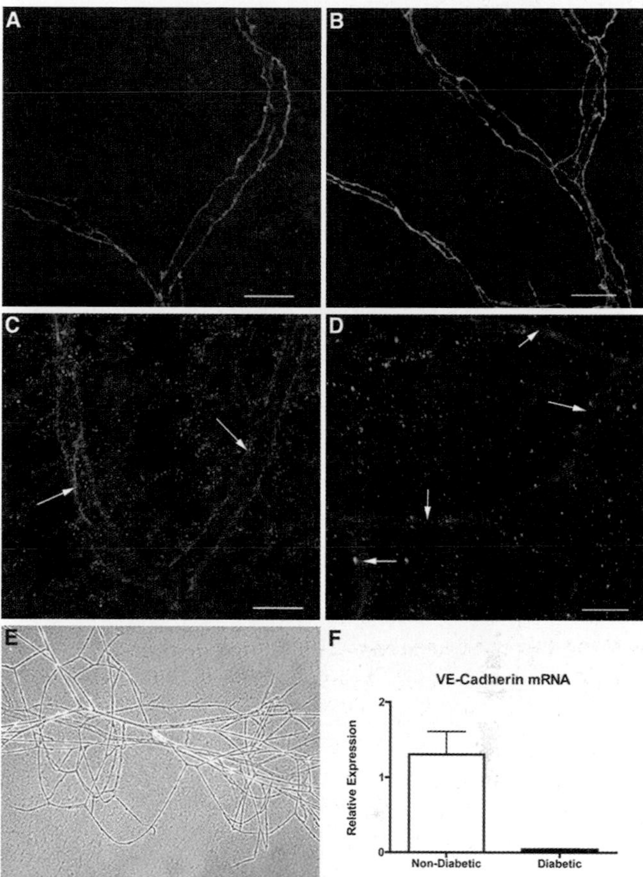

FIGURE 9.2. VE-cadherin protein and mRNA are decreased in the retinal vessels of diabetic rats. Representative retinal whole mounts from control and diabetic rats stained with anti–VE-cadherin antibody and examined by confocal microscopy. VE-cadherin expression was evident at the interfaces between adjacent endothelial cells in control nondiabetic animals (**A,B**), while it was mostly obliterated from the microvessels in the diabetic retina at 2 weeks (**C**) and 8 weeks (**D**) of diabetes. Images shown are reconstructions of a series of Z-stacks of retinal blood vessel segments. Vascular networks were isolated from whole retinas of diabetic and nondiabetic animals, as described in research design and methods. A phase-contrast image of such a network is shown in (**E**). Total RNA was isolated, and semiquantitative real-time RT-PCR was performed. Vessels from diabetic animals demonstrated less VE-cadherin mRNA than vessels from non–diabetic controls (**F**). *Significantly less than nondiabetic controls ($p = 0.0002$). $n = 3$ animals for staining and PCR analysis. Bar = 25 μm. (Reproduced from Navaratna, et al. *Diabetes.* 2007;56:2380–2387, with permission.)

The binding of leukocyte to the endothelial cells activates cellular proteases such as elastase, which may clip off VE-cadherin and its associated protein from the cell surface, resulting in endothelial monolayer alteration.[58]

ROLE OF INFLAMMATION IN DME

Recent studies reveal that inflammatory cytokines play a major role in the pathogenesis of DME. Many cytokines

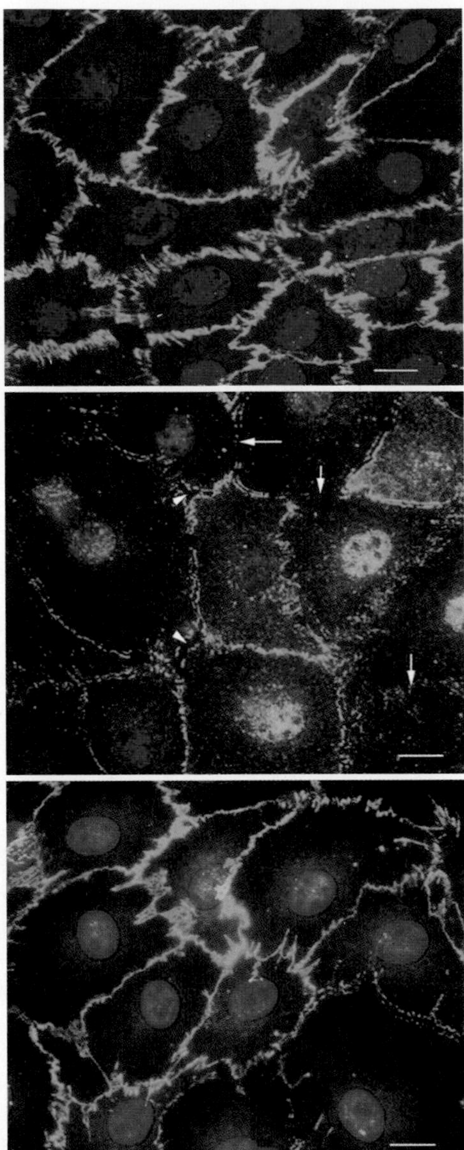

FIGURE 9.3. AGE stimulation alters endothelial cell morphology and cell surface expression of VE-cadherin. Representative images of bovine retinal endothelial cells cultured in serum-free media for 48 hours under various treatment conditions, fixed, and stained for VE-cadherin. The treatment conditions were serum-free media alone (**A**), AGE-BSA (50 μg/mL) (**B**), and AGE-BSA (50 μg/mL) with BB-94 (2 μmol/L) (**C**). Disruption of the continuous pattern of VE-cadherin staining (*arrows*) and the presence of open gaps between adjacent cells (*arrowheads*) are seen in cultures treated with AGE-BSA. n = 3 cultures from two separate experiments. Bar = 10 μm. (Reproduced from Navaratna, et al. *Diabetes.* 2007;56:2380–2387, with permission.)

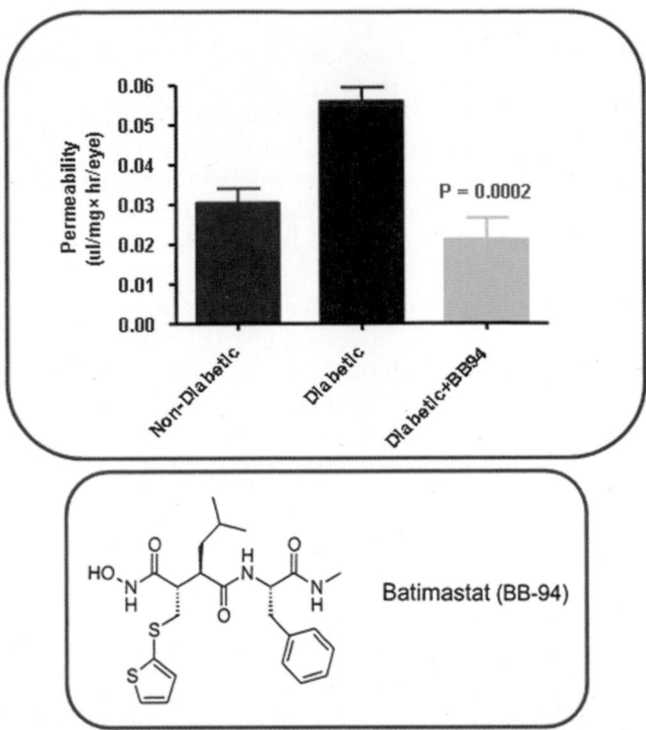

FIGURE 9.4. MMP inhibitor blocks retinal vascular permeability in the diabetic rat. Diabetic rats received an intraperitoneal injection of the MMP inhibitor BB-94 (1 mg/kg) daily for 2 weeks. Retinal vascular permeability was quantitated using the Evans blue assay. The permeability of the retinal vasculature was nearly twofold lower in BB-94–injected diabetic rats compared with vehicle-injected diabetic rats, Diabetic versus nondiabetic, $p < 0.01$; diabetic + MMP inhibitor versus diabetic, $p < 0.01$; nondiabetic versus diabetic + MMP inhibitor, $p > 0.05$. (Reproduced by permission from Navaratna, et al. *Diabetes.* 2007;56:2380–2387.).

such as VEGF, ICAM-1, IL-6, and MCP-1 are increased in the vitreous of DME patients when compared with diabetic patients without any form of diabetic retinopathy or nondiabetic subjects. Among those inflammatory mediators, VEGF and ICAM-1 had a stronger influence on the severity of DME.[32] IL-1β is a potential inflammatory cytokine, which causes severe alteration to the retinal permeability, the effects of which are inhibited by TGF-β.[59] TNF-α is an important cytokine that is increased in diabetes. IL-β and TNF-α have shown to alter the retinal barrier after exposure. TNF-α and IL-1β induced changes in the tight junctional protein adhesion property of endothelial cells, leading to extensive cellular infiltration leading to inflammation and hemorrhage.[60–62] The adhesion molecules such as ICAM-1 can also attract leukocytes to the diabetic retina, and these leukocytes penetrate the retinal barrier through a process called diapedesis and thus cause a BRB breakdown. In the hyperglycemic state, the increased formation of AGE mediates increased retinal leukostasis and upregulation of integrins, which are involved in the leukocyte adhesion.[63]

In an animal model of experimental diabetes, retinal leukostasis was increased within a few weeks of diabetes and the retina displayed classical signs of diabetic retinopathy including increased capillary permeability and loss of endothelial cells and pericytes, resulting in acellular capillaries. Diabetic mice lacking CD18 and ICAM-1

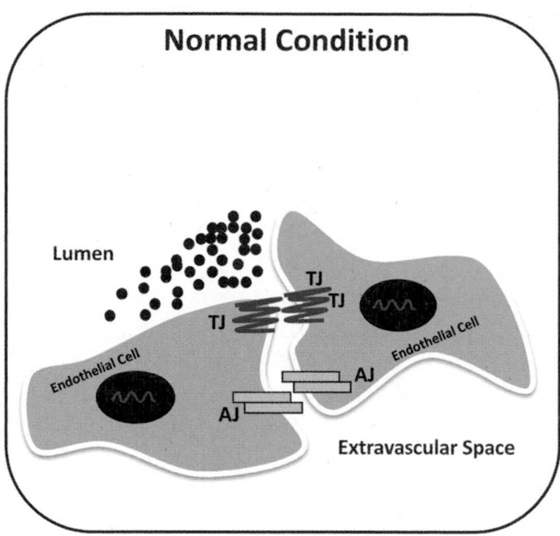

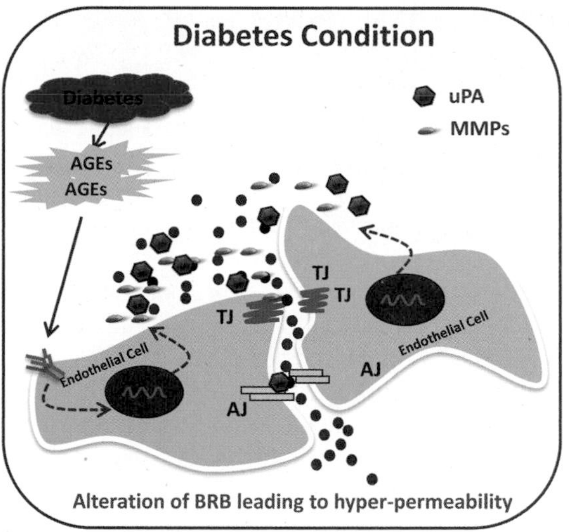

FIGURE 9.5. Alteration of the BRB in diabetes. Under normal conditions, the inner BRB is maintained by the cell junctional proteins (tight and adherens junctions) between the endothelial cells. In diabetes, hyperglycemia increases expression of proteinases (matrix metalloproteinases and urokinase) that proteolytically degrade cell junctional proteins, thus allowing molecules to come out of the lumen to the extracellular space.

had very few adherent leukocytes in the retina and did not display the sign and symptoms of DR, indicating that the inflammatory markers ICAM-1 and CD18 are crucial for retinal leukostasis.[64] TNF-α is one of the crucial mediators of retinal leukostasis, and studies have shown that mice lacking TNF-α had 80% reduction in retinal leukostasis even in the presence of VEGF (Box 9.1)[65].

VEGF

Among all those factors, VEGF has been the most important factor that has been studied extensively in relation to the alteration of BRB. Since the seminal discovery of VEGF accumulation in eyes with diabetic retinal neovascularization, it is considered as an important therapeutic target for the treatment of proliferative diabetic retinopathy and DME.[66–69] Various studies have shown that in patients with DME, VEGF levels are significantly elevated when compared with nondiabetic ocular disease states.[70,71] Since then, VEGF has been the focus of potential therapies for DME as

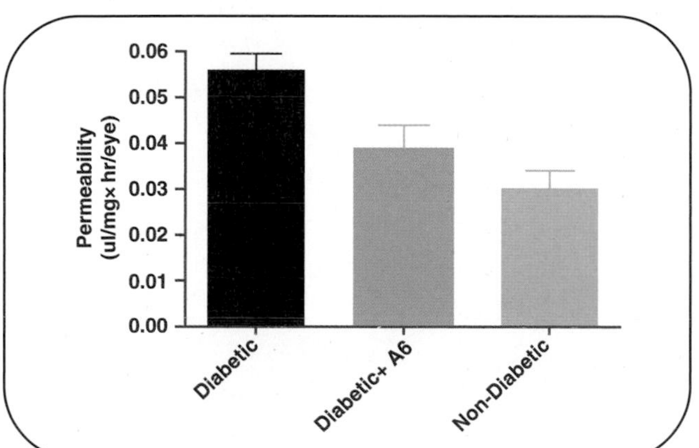

FIGURE 9.6. Å6 treatment prevents microvascular permeability and loss of VE-cadherin in the diabetic retina. Retinal vascular permeability was assessed using the Evans blue dye technique. The permeability of the retinal vasculature in Å6-injected diabetic rats is comparable to that of noninjected nondiabetic controls. Diabetic versus diabetic + Å6 or nondiabetic, $p < 0.001$; diabetic + Å6 versus nondiabetic, $p > 0.05$. (Reproduced by permission from *FASEB J.* 2008;22:3310–3317).

BOX 9.1 Inflammation and DME

Increased retinal leukostasis has shown to alter the retinal endothelial function, resulting in increased vascular permeability in diabetes. This process might lead to the development of capillary nonperfusion, endothelial cell damage, and vascular leakage leading to DME. Leukostasis has also been indicated in the increased secretion of Tumor necrosis factor-α (TNF-α) and Interleukin-1 β (IL-1β), which are proinflammatory cytokines. Intravitreous injection of TNF-α and IL-1β causes BRB breakdown and inflammation. It has been proposed that high glucose levels induce leukocyte-endothelial cell (EC) adhesion by upregulating cell surface adhesion molecules. Inflammatory mediators such as PKC, TNF-α, and nuclear factor-κB (NF-κB) have been linked to glucose-mediated leukocyte-EC adhesion. Leukocytes in the diabetic environment release a higher amount of reactive oxygen species as compared with cells in a physiologic environment. This results in generation of toxic superoxide radicals and proteolytic enzymes. The release of these reactive metabolites and the trapped leukocytes in the endothelium will damage the vessel wall and cause leakage of intravascular contents into the surrounding tissue, leading to the development of DME. Currently various steroids and nonsteroidal anti-inflammatory drugs are being tested in clinical trials for the treatment of DME.

BOX 9.2 VEGF and DME

Currently, VEGF is considered as a potential therapeutic target and anti-VEGF therapies are focused to be potential therapies for DME. Studies have clearly established the role of VEGF in DME pathogenesis. VEGF has been associated with the breakdown of the BRB, with increased vascular permeability by affecting endothelial tight junction proteins, resulting in retinal edema and accumulation of extracellular fluid. VEGF-A level is elevated in vitreous of patients with DME, and VEGF levels in the vitreous fluid of subjects with extensive DME have been shown to be higher than the levels in subjects with minimal DME. However, in transgenic mice overexpressing VEGF, retinal vascular leakage dissipates over time in spite of elevated VEGF levels in tissues. Many anti-VEGF drugs are currently available in the treatment of tumor and are also being used and studied for the management of DME. Different isoforms (nine isoform identified) of human VEGF have been recognized, which arise from alternate exon splicing of the VEGF gene. Drugs that act on the VEGF protein directly as an inhibitor include (a) Pegaptanib, a ribonucleic acid aptamer that selectively binds only to the VEGF165 isoform (Macugen; OSI Pharmaceuticals, Melville, New York); (b) Ranibizumab, a monoclonal antibody fragment that is directed toward human VEGF (Lucentis; Genentech Inc, South San Francisco, California); (c) Bevacizumab, a full-length recombinant humanized antibody, active against all isoforms of VEGF-A (Avastin; Genentech Inc.,); and (d) VEGF Trap (Regeneron Inc., Tarrytown, New York). Other approaches to inhibit VEGF RNA such as bevasiranib (Opko Health Inc., Miami, Florida) or to inhibit molecules further upstream of VEGF such as rapamycin (Sirolimus; MacuSight Inc, Union City, California) are being explored in clinical trials.

VEGF may play a central role in DME pathogenesis. VEGF is a potent vasoactive cytokine that acts as a critical stimulator of angiogenesis and inducer of vascular permeability. Of the many VEGF isoforms, VEGF 165 is considered the major isoform that is involved in the pathogenesis of DME.[70] VEGF binds to its receptors in the endothelial cells, namely, the VEGF-R1 and the VEGF-R2. Signaling through VEGF-R2 alters many proteins involved in the barrier function and, thus, leads to its functional loss. VEGF has been associated with the breakdown of the BRB, with increased vascular permeability by affecting endothelial tight junction proteins, resulting in retinal edema and accumulation of extracellular fluid. VEGF may cause the retinal vascular permeability in multiple ways. VEGF induces the phosphorylation of VE-cadherin, occludin, and ZO-1, which loses its function owing to change in structural confirmation (due to phosphorylation status) and thus causes a disruption in the barrier integrity.[72] VEGF also stimulates increased leukostasis in the microvessels of the retina, and sticky leukocytes release cytokines or may migrate via the transendothelial route, which causes BRB breakdown (Box 9.2).[69]

Angiopoietin-2

Angiopoietins represent a group of growth factors that bind to the receptor tyrosine kinase Tie2 and are important modulators of angiogenesis. The vitreous levels of angiopoietin-2 were significantly elevated in patients with CSME,[31] indicating the role of Ang-2 in the alteration of BRB. In a recent study, our laboratory has shown increased expression of Ang-2 mRNA and proteins in the retinas of diabetic animals. Furthermore, the hyperglycemic condition induces a high level of Ang-2 secretion by the human retinal microvascular endothelial cells. Intravitreal injection of Ang-2 in nondiabetic rats showed a threefold increase in retinal vascular permeability. Also, Ang-2 caused increased permeability of the endothelial monolayer. Ang-2 induces loss of VE-cadherin, mediated through the phosphorylation mechanism (Fig. 9.7) [ARVO abstract, 2009]. Further, studies have indicated that ang-2 induces pericyte "migration" and loss from the endothelium, which might be another important cause for the loss of vascular integrity.[73]

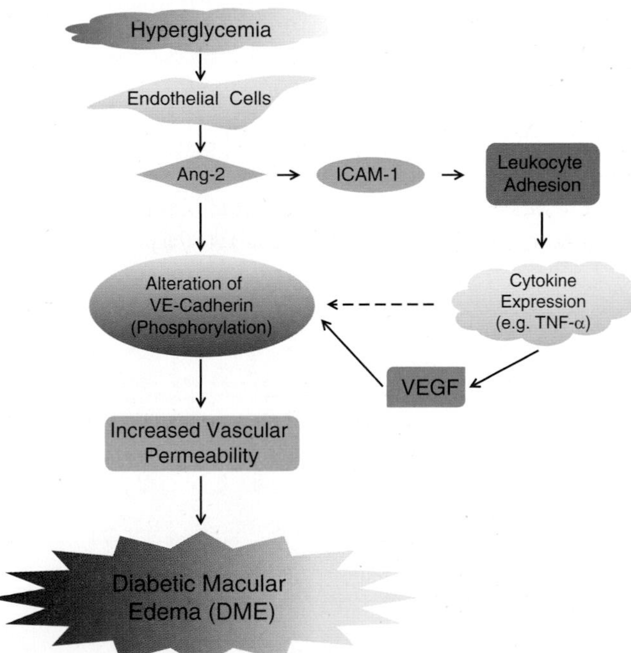

FIGURE 9.7. Diagram describing how diabetes alters cell junctional proteins like VE-cadherin, leading to alteration of the BRB. Hyperglycemia causes increased Angiopoietin-2 expression in endothelial cells, which then either directly alters cell junction proteins between endothelial cells (through phosphorylation of VE-cadherin), or increases leukocyte adhesion to the retinal capillaries, resulting in increased cytokine expression (TNFα, IL). These cytokines then cause increased VEGF expression, leading to alteration of the cell junctional proteins. Cytokines can also directly alter this barrier.

PKC AND DME

PKC is a serine threonine class of enzyme, which has 12 different isoenzymes generated through alternate splicing. The predominant isoform that is expressed in the diabetic retina is the PKC-βII, which is activated by diacylglyceol and mediates its action by gene regulation and also by activating other growth factors.[74–76] In the hyperglycemic state, DAG synthesis is increased, which results in the activation of the PKC pathway. PKC has been shown to augment the expression of VEGF.[77] A large multicenter phase 3 clinical trial called The PKC-Diabetic macular edema study (DMES) was carried out to test the efficacy of the PKC inhibitor Ruboxistaurin. Although the trial failed to achieve the primary outcome, which is a significant improvement in the macular edema condition, thereby preventing the progression of DME to a sight-threatening stage and also reduction in laser treatment, there was a significant reduction in the secondary endpoint of the progression of DME within 100 μm from the fovea (Box 9.3).[78]

MANAGEMENT OF DME

CSME has a significant contribution to the incidence of new blindness due to diabetes. It has been estimated that if left untreated, 25% to 30% of patients with CSME exhibit doubling of visual angle within 3 years and treatment of CSME leads to 50% drop in the risk.[1] The important risk factors that are associated with the development of DME include (a) type of diabetes (type 1 or type 2), (b) duration of diabetes, (c) hypertension, (d) hyperlipidemia, and (e) pregnancy. Among the important risk factors, hyperglycemia is established as the most important determinant in the progression of diabetic retinopathy. The DCCT clearly demonstrated that tighter control of blood glucose is strongly associated with the reduced incidence of diabetic retinopathy and DCCT guidelines have established that the level of glycated hemoglobin (HbA1c) is important predictor of disease progression.[13] Hence the important medical treatment in the management of DME is mainly focused on normalizing hyperglycemia, hypertension, and hyperlipidemia. Various molecular agents such as intravitreal anti-VEGF agents such as pegaptanib sodium, ranibizumab and bevacizumab, and intravitreal triamcinolone acetonide (IVTA) are currently explored in the treatment of DME. These trials will be discussed in detail in two other later chapters. The use of various pharmacological interventions and their multiple biochemical/molecular targets in clinical trials has been detailed in Table 9.1.

BOX 9.3 Approaches to Treatment of DME

The primary objective of the treatment modality in DME is to improve the visual acuity through the reduction in the amount of macular edema. Important factors that are considered for the improvement of the clinical condition include i) improving metabolic control through tight glycemic control, ii) normalization of blood pressure, and iii) serum lipid control. Focal/grid laser photocoagulation is still the gold standard treatment of DME to prevent vision loss. Pharmacological therapies that are currently considered are corticosteroids and VEGF antagonists. In patients with DME and taut hyaloid face with traction, vitrectomy can be performed to prevent vision loss. Although the anti-VEGF treatment is beneficial in wet macular degeneration, the effect seems to be much less robust in DME. It is possible that "other molecules" like Ang-2, proteinases, TNF may be involved in the etiology of DME, and VEGF inhibition does not achieve neutralization of other vasopermeability factors. A combination therapy with inhibitors of these molecules combined with laser or anti-VEGF agents may be effective in slowing the progression of DME.

Table 9.1.

Important junctional protein and its function

	Junctional Proteins	Function
1	VE-Cadherin (Cad-5, CD144)	Forms a Homophilic interaction and stabilizes the endothelial barrier
2	Claudin-5	Junctional protein anchored to the actin cytoskeleton and tightly regulates the barrier integrity
3	Occludin	A 65-kDa tight junction protein that interacts with other proteins such as p120, rab-13, c-src to form a tight barrier
4	ZO-1	Helps anchoring the tight junction proteins
5	JAM	Expressed in RPE cells and helps in maintaining cellular polarity

I.B. Principles Molecular Mechanisms

Even though much therapeutics is being tested, laser photocoagulation is still the proven therapy to reduce the risk of vision loss in DME. Focal /grid laser photocoagulation has been shown to be more effective with fewer side effects than the intravitreal triamcinolone in most patients with DME. The photocoagulation reduced the risk of moderate visual loss from DME from 24% to 12% (50%), 3 years after initiation of treatment. Laser treatment is most effective when initiated before visual acuity is lost from DME.[79] Also, the biologic plausibility of vitrectomy for DME has been suggested by clinical observations. It has been found that the posterior vitreous detachment (PVD) is associated with a lower incidence of DME.[80] Pars plana vitrectomy (PPV) is also considered as an important treatment option and has been shown to have significant reduction in the edema associated with posterior hyaloidal traction. Studies have also indicated that removal of vitreous gel could decrease the concentration of DME-promoting factors and also improve the fluid currents and thus oxygenation of the inner retina.

BOX 9.4 Potential Therapeutic Targets for DME

The molecular mechanisms underlying the development of DME are not well understood. Current studies are focusing on identifying novel molecular targets and therapeutics that could be used to treat DME. Various clinical trials are being evaluated to test the efficacy of new drugs aiming specific molecular mechanisms. Steroids including (a) Triamcinolone, (b) Dexamethasone, and (c) Flucinolone that target the inflammatory pathways are being evaluated in clinical trials in DME. Diclofenac is also being evaluated as a nonsteroidal anti-inflammatory drug in DME. Development of ICAM-1 antibodies and leukostasis inhibitors such as aprotinin is being considered as a potential therapeutic target to block the inflammatory pathway that leads to the alteration of BRB. Also Infliximab, a TNF-α inhibitor, is currently considered in the clinical trial studies. Mecamylamine, an inhibitor of A3β4 nicotinic receptors; Choline Fenofibrate, inhibitor of PPAR-α; Microplasmin, inhibitor of blood clotting proteins; and dietary supplement adjuvants (AREDS minerals & antioxidant vitamins) are potential therapeutic agents targeting inflammation and oxidative stress. Various molecular targets in the vessel wall such as adherens (VE-cadherin) and tight junctional proteins have been recently identified as therapeutic targets. Molecules such as TGF-β, peroxisome proliferator-activated receptor-γ (PPAR-γ), TNF-α, p38 MAP kinase, receptor for advanced glycation end products (RAGE), carbonic anhydrase-1, prostaglandins, matrix metalloproteinases, and uPAR are considered to be potential drug targets. These signaling molecules have been implicated in the alteration of barrier function. Targeting these molecules might yield a potential therapy to treat DME.

MOLECULAR TARGETS AND THE PROSPECTIVE TREATMENT

The limitation of the current treatments and the clinical outcomes demand development of new pharmacological therapies, targeting the underlying biochemical and molecular mechanism that cause DME. Various agents are being developed with the goal of preventing the damage of retinal microvasculature. The biochemical mechanisms that contribute to cellular damage in the retina have been proposed as unifying mechanism that included increased flux through the polyol pathway, leading to sorbitol accumulation, production of AGE products (AGEs), increased oxidative stress, and activation of the protein kinase C-β (PKC-β) pathway. These biochemical mechanisms have yielded multiple targets that lead to development of specific inhibitory compounds. Importantly, the molecular mechanism underlying the development of DME is the loss of BRB integrity that has been studied for many years. The disruption of retinal barrier involves multifactorial processes and events within the vascular luminal site. Various growth factors and inflammatory cytokines have been implicated in the loss of BRB integrity, and these molecular targets yielded multiple inhibitors that are either under clinical trials or currently being developed. Also the mechanism that causes the stabilization of the adherent and tight junctional proteins is of pertinent interest to cell biologists that could yield new drug targets (Box 9.4).

CONCLUSION

DME results from a series of biochemical and cellular changes that leads to the breakdown of BRB. The complete understanding of the molecular and cellular mechanisms that cause leakage and exudation in retina will help the efforts to prevent the vision impairment in diabetes. Studies such as DCCT have pinpointed the importance of metabolic risk factors and also help in the accurate prediction of future DME in the patients, which could help in devising new intervention and life style modification therapies that could save their vision. A number of pharmacological agents are now being tested to slow the progression of DME in earlier stages. Recently, new treatment options targeting a single molecule, VEGF, are in clinical trials (RIDE/RISE and READ-2 study) for DME. This treatment option appears to have limitations as the improvement in retinal thickening, as measured by OCT, is transient, and the edema tends to recur in many patients.[81] In a recent study by the DRCR that compared focal laser with intravitreal bevacizumab, only half of the eyes showed an initial positive response to intravitreal bevacizumab (only 11% reduction in retinal thickness) compared with the baseline at 3- or 6-weeks.[82] This transient response was similar to that observed in the laser group, and the magnitude of the response was not large for most subjects.

KEY POINTS

- The pathophysiology of DME involves retinal thickening from leaky blood vessels due to alteration of the BRB.
- Chronic hyperglycemia, as well as the associated metabolic entities such as hyperlipidemia and hypertension, contribute to the pathogenesis of DME.
- The hyperglycemia-induced pathogenesis of diabetic retinopathy is linked to four main biochemical alterations such as (a) increased polyol pathway flux, (b) increased AGE-product formation, (c) activation of PKC isoforms, and (d) increased hexosamine pathway flux.
- All these pathways culminate in increased oxidative stress, inflammation, and vascular dysfunction. Vascular dysfunction ensues with eventual vascular occlusion and local ischemia. The resulting hypoxia upregulates a variety of growth factors.
- One of the possible mechanisms by which diabetes contributes to BRB breakdown is through proteolytic degradation of cell junctional proteins (VE-cadherin).
- Inflammatory cytokines (VEGF, ICAM-1, IL-6, and MCP-1) play a major role in the pathogenesis of DME.
- VEGF is one of the most important factors that has been studied extensively in relation to the alteration of BRB.
- Another important growth factor, angiopoietin-2 (Ang-2), causes increased permeability of the endothelial monolayer. Ang-2 induces loss of VE-cadherin mediated through the phosphorylation mechanism.
- Although the anti-VEGF treatment is beneficial in wet macular degeneration, the effect seems to be much less robust in DME. It is possible that "other molecules" like Ang-2, proteinases, TNF may be involved in the etiology of DME, and VEGF inhibition does not achieve neutralization of other vaso-permeability factors. A combination therapy with inhibitors of these molecules combined with laser or anti-VEGF agents may be effective in slowing the progression of DME.

Although the anti-VEGF treatment is beneficial in wet macular degeneration, as evidenced by the MARINA and ANCHOR trials, the effect seems to be much less robust in DME.[83] It has been suggested that the mechanism of increased permeability in wet ARMD is different from that in DME. In wet ARMD, the new vessels grow from fenestrated choriocapillaris (which lack typical pericyte association and have incomplete basement membrane), whereas in DME, the leakage occurs in retinal vessels probably due to breakdown of cell-cell junctions.[83] It is possible that "other molecules" like Ang-2, proteinases, TNF may be involved in the etiology of DME, and VEGF inhibition does not achieve neutralization of other vaso-permeability factors. It is being considered that one or more of these pharmacological agents, or a combination therapy may be effective in slowing the progression of DME.

REFERENCES

1. Early Treatment Diabetic Retinopathy Study Research Group. Treatment techniques and clinical guidelines for photocoagulation of diabetic macular edema. Early Treatment Diabetic Retinopathy Study Report Number 2. *Ophthalmology*. 1987;94(7):761–774.
2. Centers for Disease Control and Prevention. Blindness caused by diabetes: Massachusetts, 1987–1994. *MMWR*. 1996;45:937–941.
3. Aiello LM. Perspectives on diabetic retinopathy. *Am J Ophthalmol*. 2003;136:122–135.
4. Riordan-Eva P. Eye. In: *Current Medical Diagnosis and Treatment*. Tierney LM, McPhee SJ, Papadakis MA, eds. 42nd ed. New York: Lange Medical Books/McGraw-Hill; 2003: 146–177.
5. Ciulla TA, Amador AG, Zinman B. Diabetic retinopathy and diabetic macular edema: pathophysiology, screening, and novel therapies. *Diabetes Care*. 2003;26(9):2653–2664.
6. Frank RN. Diabetic retinopathy. *N Engl J Med*. 2004;350: 48–58.
7. Fong DS, Ferris FL III, Davis MD, et al. Causes of severe visual loss in the early treatment diabetic retinopathy study: ETDRS report no. 24: Early Treatment Diabetic Retinopathy Study Research Group. *Am J Ophthalmol*. 1999;127: 137–141.
8. Klein R, Klein BE, Moss SE, et al. The Wisconsin Epidemiologic Study of Diabetic Retinopathy: XVII. The 14-year incidence and progression of diabetic retinopathy and associated risk factors in type 1 diabetes. *Ophthalmology*. 1998;105:1801–1815.
9. Ferris FL III, Patz A. Macular edema: a complication of diabetic retinopathy. *Surv Ophthalmol*. 1984;28(Suppl.): 452–461.
10. Chiang YP, Bassi LJ, Javitt JC. Federal budgetary costs of blindness. *Milbank Q*. 1992;70:319–340.
11. Brown MM, Brown GC, Sharma S, et al. Utility values and diabetic retinopathy. *Am J Ophthalmol*. 1999;128:324–330.
12. White NH, Cleary PA, Dahms W, et al. Beneficial effects of intensive therapy of diabetes during adolescence: outcomes after the conclusion of the Diabetes Control and Complications Trial (DCCT). *J Pediatr*. 2001;139:804–812.
13. The Diabetes Control and Complications Trial/Epidemiology of Diabetes Interventions and Complications Research Group. Retinopathy and nephropathy in patients with type 1 diabetes four years after a trial of intensive insulin therapy. *N Engl J Med*. 2000;342:381–389.
14. Klein R, Klein BE, Moss SE. The Wisconsin Epidemiologic Study of Diabetic Retinopathy. XVI. The relationship of C-peptide to the incidence and progression of diabetic retinopathy. *Diabetes*. 1995;44(7):796–801.
15. Klein R, Klein BE, Moss SE, et al. The Wisconsin Epidemiologic Study of Diabetic Retinopathy, IV: diabetic macular edema. *Ophthalmology*. 1984;91:1464–1474.

16. Klein R, Klein BE, Moss SE, et al. Association of ocular disease and mortality in a diabetic population. *Arch Ophthalmol.* 1999;117:1487–1495.
17. DCCT Research Group. Progression of retinopathy with intensive versus conventional treatment in the Diabetes Control and Complications Trial. *Ophthalmology.* 1995;102: 647–661.
18. Moss SE, Klein R, Klein B. The 14-year incidence of visual loss in a diabetic population. *Ophthalmology.* 1998;105: 998–1003.
19. ETDRS Research Group. Photocoagulation for diabetic macular edema: ETDRS Report 1. *Arch Ophthalmol.* 1985;103:1796–1806.
20. Miljanovic B, Glynn RJ, Nathan DM, et al. A prospective study of serum lipids and risk of diabetic macular edema in type 1 diabetes.*Diabetes.* 2004;53(11):2883–2892.
21. Klein BE, Klein R, Moss SE. Is serum cholesterol associated with progression of diabetic retinopathy or macular edema in persons with younger-onset diabetes of long duration? *Am J Ophthalmol.* 1999;128:652–654.
22. Galler A, Muller G, Schinzel R, et al. Impact of metabolic control and serum lipids on the concentration of AGE products in the serum of children and adolescents with type 1 diabetes, as determined by fluorescence spectroscopy and Nε-(carboxymethyl)lysine ELISA. *Diabetes Care.* 2003;26:2609–2615.
23. Roy MS, Klein R. Macular edema and retinal hard exudates in African-Americans with type I diabetes: the New Jersey 725. *Arch Ophthalmol.* 2001;119:251–259.
24. Lopes de Faria JM, Jalkh AE, Trempe CL, et al. Diabetic macular edema: risk factors and concomitants. *Acta Ophthalmol Scand.* 1999;77:170–175.
25. Sinclair SH, Nesler C, Foxman B, et al. Macular edema and pregnancy in insulin-dependent diabetes. *Am J Ophthalmol.* 1984;97:154–167.
26. Best RM, Chakravarthy U. Diabetic retinopathy in pregnancy. *Br J Ophthalmol.* 1997;81:249–251.
27. Sunness JS. The pregnant woman's eye. *Surv Ophthalmol.* 1988;32:219–238.
28. Cunha-Vaz JG, Shakib M, Ashton N. Studies on the permeability of the blood–retinal barrier. I. On the existence, development and site of blood-retinal barrier. *Br J Ophthamol.* 1966;50:441–453.
29. Antcliff RJ, Marshall J. The pathogenesis of edema in diabetic maculopathy. *Semin Ophthalmol.* 1999;14:223–232.
30. Brownlee M. The pathobiology of diabetic complications: a unifying mechanism. *Diabetes.* 2005;54(6):1615–1625.
31. Patel JI, Hykin PG, Gregor ZJ, et al. Angiopoietin concentrations in diabetic retinopathy. *Br J Ophthalmol.* 2005;89(4): 480–483.
32. Funatsu H, Noma H, Mimura T, et al. Association of vitreous inflammatory factors with diabetic macular edema. *Ophthalmology.* 2009;116(1):73–79.
33. Joussen AM, Poulaki V, Qin W, et al. Retinal vascular endothelial growth factor induces intercellular adhesion molecule-1 and endothelial nitric oxide synthase expression and initiates early diabetic retinal leukocyte adhesion in vivo. *Am J Pathol.* 2002;160:501–509.
34. Chibber R, Ben-Mahmud BM, Chibber S, et al. Leukocytes in diabetic retinopathy. *Curr Diab Rev.* 2007;3:3–14.
35. Kaji Y, Usui T, Ishida S, et al. Inhibition of diabetic leukostasis and blood-retinal barrier breakdown with a soluble form of a receptor for advanced glycation end products. *Invest Ophthalmol Vis Sci.* 2007;48:858–865.
36. Joussen AM, Murata T, Tsujikawa A, et al. Leukocyte-mediated endothelial cell injury and death in the diabetic retina. *Am J Pathol.* 2001;158:147–152.
37. Angst BD, Marcozzi C, Magee AI. The cadherin superfamily: diversity in form and function. *J Cell Sci.* 2001;114:629–641.
38. Corada M, Liao F, Lindgren M, et al. Monoclonal antibodies directed to different regions of vascular endothelial cadherin extracellular domain affect adhesion and clustering of the protein and modulate endothelial permeability. *Blood.* 2001;97:1679–1684.
39. Lampugnani MG, Corada M, Caveda L, et al. The molecular organization of endothelial cell to cell junctions: differential association of plakoglobin, -catenin, and -catenin with vascular endothelial cadherin. *J Cell Biol.* 1995;129:203–217.
40. Navarro P, Caveda L, Breviario F, et al. Catenin-dependent and -independent functions of vascular endothelial cadherin. *J Biol Chem.* 1995;270:30965–30972.
41. Anastasiadis PZ, Reynolds AB. The p120 catenin family: complex roles in adhesion, signaling and cancer. *J Cell Sci.* 2000;113:1319–1334.
42. Ferber A, Yaen C, Sarmiento E, et al. An octapeptide in the juxtamembrane domain of VE-cadherin is important for p120ctn binding and cell proliferation. *Exp Cell Res.* 2002;274:35–44.
43. Erickson KK, Sundstrom JM, Antonetti DA. Vascular permeability in ocular disease and the role of tight junctions. *Angiogenesis.* 2007;10:103–117.
44. Hammes HP, Lin J, Renner O, et al. Pericytes and the pathogenesis of diabetic retinopathy. *Diabetes.* 2002;51(10):3107–3112.
45. Das A, Frank RN, Zhang NL, et al. Ultrastructural localization of extracellular matrix components in human retinal vessels and Bruch's membrane. *Arch Ophthalmol.* 1990;108(3):421–429.
46. Antonetti DA, Barber AJ, Bronson SK, et al. Diabetic retinopathy: seeing beyond glucose-induced microvascular disease. *Diabetes.* 2006;55:2401–2411.
47. Skondra D, Noda K, Almulki L, et al. Characterization of azurocidin as a permeability factor in the retina: involvement in VEGF-induced and early diabetic blood-retinal barrier breakdown. *Invest Ophthalmol Vis Sci.* 2008;49:726–731.
48. Vandenbroucke E, Mehta D, Minshall R, et al. Regulation of endothelial junctional permeability. *Ann NY Acad Sci.* 2008;1123:134–145.
49. Pournaras CJ, Rungger-Brändle E, Riva CE, et al. Regulation of retinal blood flow in health and disease. *Prog Retin Eye Res.* 2008;27(3):284–330.
50. Fong DS, Contreras R. Glitazone use associated with diabetic macular edema. *Am J Ophthalmol.* 2009;147(4):583–586.
51. Soliman W, Sander B, Soliman KA, et al. The predictive value of optical coherence tomography after grid laser photocoagulation for diffuse diabetic macular oedema. *Acta Ophthalmol.* 2008;86(3):284–291.
52. Gardner TW, Antonetti DA. Novel potential mechanisms for diabetic macular edema: leveraging new investigational approaches. *Curr Diab Rep.* 2008;8:263–269.

53. Jin M, Kashiwagi K, Iizuka Y, et al. Matrix metalloproteinases in human diabetic and nondiabetic vitreous. *Retina*. 2001; 21(1):28–33.
54. Giebel SJ, Menicucci G, McGuire PG, et al. Matrix metalloproteinases in early diabetic retinopathy and their role in alteration of the blood-retinal barrier. *Lab Invest*. 2005;85(5):597–607.
55. Navaratna D, McGuire PG, Menicucci G, et al. Proteolytic degradation of VE-cadherin alters the blood-retinal barrier in diabetes. *Diabetes*. 2007;56:2380–2387.
56. Kowluru RA, Kanwar M. Oxidative stress and the development of diabetic retinopathy: contributory role of matrix metalloproteinase-2. *Free Radic Biol Med*. 2009;46(12): 1677–1685.
57. Behzadian MA, Wang XL, Windsor LJ, et al. TGF-beta increases retinal endothelial cell permeability by increasing MMP-9: possible role of glial cells in endothelial barrier function. *Invest Ophthalmol Vis Sci*. 2001;42:853–859.
58. Allport JR, Muller WA, Luscinskas FW. Monocytes induce reversible focal changes in vascular endothelial cadherin complex during transendothelial migration under flow. *J Cell Biol*. 2000;148(1):203–216.
59. Cuff CA, Martiney JA, Berman JW, et al. Differential effects of transforming growth factor-beta 1 on interleukin-1-induced cellular inflammation and vascular permeability in the rabbit retina. *J Neuroimmunol*. 1996;70(1):21–28.
60. Claudio L, Martiney JA, Brosnan CF. Ultrastructural studies of the blood-retina barrier after exposure to interleukin-1 beta or tumor necrosis factor-alpha. *Lab Invest*. 1994;70(6): 850–861.
61. Luna JD, Chan CC, Derevjanik NL, et al. Blood-retinal barrier (BRB) breakdown in experimental autoimmune uveoretinitis: comparison with vascular endothelial growth factor, tumor necrosis factor alpha, and interleukin-1beta-mediated breakdown. *J Neurosci Res*. 1997;49(3):268–280.
62. Bamforth SD, Lightman SL, Greenwood J. Interleukin-1 beta-induced disruption of the retinal vascular barrier of the central nervous system is mediated through leukocyte recruitment and histamine. *Am J Pathol*. 1997;150(1): 329–340.
63. Moore TC, Moore JE, Kaji Y, et al. The role of advanced glycation end products in retinal microvascular leukostasis. *Invest Ophthalmol Vis Sci*. 2003;44(10):4457–4464.
64. Joussen AM, Poulaki V, Le ML, et al. A central role for inflammation in the pathogenesis of diabetic retinopathy. *FASEB J*. 2004;18(12):1450–1452.
65. Vinores SA, Xiao WH, Shen J, et al. TNF-alpha is critical for ischemia-induced leukostasis, but not retinal neovascularization nor VEGF-induced leakage. *J Neuroimmunol*. 2007;182(1–2):73–79.
66. Ishida S, Usui T, Yamashiro K, et al. VEGF164 is proinflammatory in the diabetic retina. *Invest Ophthalmol Vis Sci*. 2003;44:2155–2162.
67. Miller JW, Adamis AP, Aiello LP. Vascular endothelial growth factor in ocular neovascularization and proliferative diabetic retinopathy. *Diabetes Metab Rev*. 1997;13:37–50.
68. Aiello LP, Avery RL, Arrigg PG, et al. Vascular endothelial growth factor in ocular fluid of patients with diabetic retinopathy and other retinal disorders. *N Engl J Med*. 1994;331:1480–1487.
69. Aiello LP, Bursell S-E, Clermont A, et al. Vascular endothelial growth factor-induced retinal permeability is mediated by PKC in vivo and suppressed by an orally effective β-isoform-selective inhibitor. *Diabetes*. 1997;46:1473–1480.
70. Caldwell RB, Bartoli M, Behzadian MA, et al. Vascular endothelial growth factor and diabetic retinopathy:pathophysiological mechanisms and treatment perspectives. *Diabetes Metab Res Rev*. 2003;19(6):442–455.
71. Funatsu H, Yamashita H, Ikeda T, et al. Vitreous levels of interleukin-6 and vascular endothelial growth factor are related to diabetic macular edema. *Ophthalmology*. 2003;110(9):1690–1696.
72. Antonetti DA, Barber AJ, Hollinger LA, et al. Vascular endothelial growth factor induces rapid phosphorylation of tight junction proteins occludin and zonula occluden 1. A potential mechanism for vascular permeability in diabetic retinopathy and tumors. *J Biol Chem*. 1999;274: 23463–23467.
73. Pfister F, Feng Y, vom Hagen F, et al. Pericyte migration: a novel mechanism of pericyte loss in experimental diabetic retinopathy. *Diabetes*. 2008;57(9):2495–2502.
74. Shiba T, Inoguchi T, Sportsman JR, et al. Correlation of diacylglycerol level and protein kinase C activity in rat retina to retinal circulation. *Am J Physiol*. 1993;265:E783–E793.
75. Koya D, King GL. Protein kinase C activation and the development of diabetic complications. *Diabetes*. 1998;47: 859–866.
76. Aiello LP, Bursell SE, Clermont A, et al. Vascular endothelial growth factor-induced retinal permeability is mediated by protein kinase C in vivo and suppressed by an orally effective beta-isoform-selective inhibitor. *Diabetes*. 1997;46: 1473–1480.
77. Xia P, Aiello LP, Ishii H, et al. Characterization of vascular endothelial growth factors effect on the activation of protein kinase C, its isoforms, and endothelial cell growth. *J Clin Invest*. 1996;98:2018–2026.
78. PKC-DMES Study Group. Effect of ruboxistaurin in patients with diabetic macular edema: thirty-month results of the randomized PKC-DMES clinical trial. *Arch Ophthalmol*. 2007;125:318–324.
79. Scott IU, Danis RP, Bressler SB, et al. Diabetic Retinopathy Clinical Research Network. Effect of focal/grid photocoagulation onvisual acuity and retinal thickening in eyes with non-center-involved diabetic macular edema. *Retina*. 2009;29(5):613–617.
80. Recchia FM, Ruby AJ, Carvalho Recchia CA. Pars plana vitrectomy with removal of the internal limiting membrane in the treatment of persistent diabetic macular edema. *Am J Ophthalmol*. 2005;139(3):447–454.
81. Biester S, Ziemssen F, Ulrich Bartz-Schmidt K, et al. Is intravitreal bevacizumab treatment effective in diffuse diabetic macular edema? *Graefes Arch Clin Exp Ophthalmol*. 2009;247:1575–1577.
82. Diabetic Retinopathy Clinical Research Network, Scott IU, Edwards AR, et al. A phase 2 randomized clinical trial of intravitreal bevacizumab for diabetic macular edema. *Ophthalmology*. 2007;114:1860–1867.
83. Sang DN, D'Amore PA. Is blockade of vascular endothelial growth factor beneficial for all types of diabetic retinopathy? *Diabetologia*. 2008;51:1570–1573.

SECTION II
Practice

PART A
Clinical Trials and Current Strategies

CHAPTER

10

Anti-VEGF Therapies in ARMD in Practice

Grant P. Janzen • Jeffrey S. Heier

The advent of antivascular endothelial growth factor (anti-VEGF) therapy has greatly expanded the retina specialists' treatment armamentarium for vascular-mediated diseases of the eye, particularly the neovascular stage of age-related macular degeneration (wet ARMD). ARMD is the leading cause of irreversible blindness in the developed world in those older than 50 years of age,[1–3] and it is becoming an important public health issue as the life expectancy increases across the population in developed countries.[4–6] The importance of new treatment modalities for this disease is clear. This paradigm shift of specifically targeting portions of the pathologic neovascularization cascade, through inhibition of VEGF, in the management of wet macular degeneration has provided a mechanism for stabilizing the large majority of patients with recent onset of exudative disease and leading to significant visual recovery in upwards of 30% to 40%.[7–11] Prior to these advances, visual recovery was relatively uncommon, and success was measured by a treatment's ability to slow visual loss rather than prevent it.

CHOROIDAL NEOVASCULARIZATION

Choroidal neovascularization (CNV) in ARMD is stimulated, at least, in part, by VEGF-A. Studies examining surgically removed fibrovascular membranes from eyes with wet ARMD have demonstrated the presence of VEGF mRNA, particularly in areas of fibroblast-like cells.[12] Retinal neovascularization is dependent on the presence of VEGF in animal models.[13] Messenger RNA splicing and proteolytic cleavage result in many forms of VEGF-A that are theoretically biologically active,[14] and several isoforms have been detected and isolated from choroidal neovascular lesions.[15] While the evidence for VEGF's role in wet ARMD was building, other therapeutic options, such as verteporfin with photodynamic therapy (PDT) and macular laser, were being used in an attempt to improve treatment and visual outcomes of the disease.

Neovascularization in ARMD is categorized as classic or occult or a combination of the two, based upon the fluorescein angiography appearance.[16] Classification of the type of neovascularization was important prior to the introduction of anti-VEGF therapy, as certain types of neovascularization only responded to certain therapies. Laser ablation was shown to offer a treatment benefit over observation alone in a series of trials in the 1980s.[11] However, these patients had an immediate loss of vision in the area that was treated with the laser. Subfoveal treatment in these studies required that the lesions have well-demarcated boundaries throughout the lesion, some evidence of classic CNV, and smaller lesions usually had better outcomes. While the treatment did prove better than no treatment in visual acuity outcomes after 2 years, the drop in vision at time of treatment was often substantial, and the prognosis for vision gain was poor.[17] Almost no eyes with juxtafoveal lesions, regardless of laser treatment versus observation, had an improvement in vision over baseline visual acuity measurements, but slightly more of the treated eyes maintained baseline vision when compared to no treatment. Also of note, twice as many treated patients versus untreated patients retained 20/40 or better over 5 years in the eyes with juxtafoveal lesions.[18] Extrafoveal treatment, in contrast, substantially reduced the rate of large losses of visual acuity over the 5-year study term versus no treatment.[17] Regardless of lesion location, the risk for progression was present in all of the photocoagulation studies.

PHOTODYNAMIC THERAPY

The year 2000 marked the first pharmacologic treatment approved by the Food and Drug Administration (FDA) for the treatment of exudative ARMD, Verteporfin with PDT. PDT has U.S. FDA approval for wet ARMD lesions in which 50% or more of the lesion consists of classic CNV, termed "predominantly classic."[7–9,19] Approval by the European Agency for the Evaluation of Medicinal Products includes predominantly classic lesions and occult lesions without any classic component.[7–9,19] PDT has been proven to slow progression of vision loss due to wet ARMD, but a relatively small percentage of treated patients show meaningful improvement in visual acuity.[8,20] Both thermal laser and PDT still have a role in the management

BOX 10.1 VISION Trial: Vascular Endothelial Growth Factor Inhibition Study in Ocular Neovascularization

Purpose: Two Phase 3 randomized, prospective double-blind, clinical trials to examine the efficacy of intravitreal injection of Pegaptanib (Macugen) versus sham treatment every 6 weeks for 48 weeks in patients with subfoveal CNV secondary to ARMD. In two separate trials, one in United States and the other in Europe, patients received 0.3, 1.0, or 3.0 mg intravitreal pegaptanib or sham injection.

Results: In the group given pegaptanib at 0.3 mg, 70% of patients lost fewer than 15 letters of visual acuity, as compared with 55% among the controls. The risk of severe vision loss (30 letters or more) was reduced from 22% in the sham-injection group to 10% in the group receiving 0.3 mg of pegaptanib. More patients receiving pegaptanib (0.3 mg), as compared with sham injection, maintained their visual acuity or gained acuity (33% vs. 23%). Only 6% of patients receiving 0.3 mg of pegaptanib gained at least 15 letters of visual acuity.

Conclusions: Pegaptanib appears to be an effective therapy for neovascular ARMD, and its long-term safety is unknown. Compared with 2 years' usual care or cessation of therapy at year 1, patients on pegaptanib continued to improve visual acuity. (Gragoudas ES, Adamis AP, Cunningham ET, et al. Pegaptanib for neovascular age-related macular degeneration. *N Engl J Med.* 2004;351:2805–2816; VISION Trial Group, *Ophthalmology.* 2006;113:1508.)

of wet ARMD and other retinal diseases, but their niche is changing and being reevaluated in the era of the anti-VEGF pharmaceuticals.[21,22] Indeed, thermal laser is still used in some cases of small, classic, extrafoveal lesions, as discussed above, because it gives the opportunity to treat the lesion once and achieve quiescence of the lesion, rather than subjecting the patient to a series of injections (Box 10.1).

ANTI-VEGF THERAPY

The FDA approval of anti-VEGF therapy for the treatment of exudative ARMD has heralded a new era for the management of this devastating disease, offering patients and their families true hope for the maintenance of useful vision throughout their life. Currently, there are two FDA-approved anti-VEGF drugs available for intravitreal injection, and more are undergoing clinical trials. While a class of medications serving as antagonists to an "angiogenic factor" with a goal of treating disease was first proposed in *The New England Journal of Medicine* in 1971,[23] the year 2004 officially ushered in the era of intravitreal medications targeting VEGF.[24] Pegaptanib (Macugen; Eyetech Pharmaceuticals) was the first FDA-approved anti-VEGF medication for wet ARMD. This was shortly followed by the introduction of off-label use of bevacizumab (Avastin; Genentech)[25] and the approval of ranibizumab (Lucentis; Genentech).[26]

Pegaptanib

Pegaptanib is a 28-base ribonucleic acid aptamer, or an RNA ligand with high affinity for VEGF, that is covalently linked to two branched 20-kD polyethylene glycol moieties that primarily targets one isoform of VEGF (VEGF-165).[27] This drug is the product of a sugar structure with glycol additions to increase its half-life in the vitreous.[28] The VEGF Inhibition Study in Ocular Neovascularization (VISION) trials demonstrated that pegaptanib stabilized visual acuity in patients with wet ARMD, as compared to sham injection.[27,29,30] The injections were performed every 6 weeks in patients with any of the angiographic subtypes (classic, minimally classic, occult) of wet ARMD. Pegaptanib reduced the chance of loss of 15 letters (3 lines on the study chart) (Fig. 10.1), in addition to reducing the chance of severe visual loss (more than 30 letters, or 6 lines, on the study chart).[27] At the conclusion of 2 years of treatment in the VISION trials, ten percent of pegaptanib-treated patients gained at least three lines of vision (Fig. 10.2). This was greater than with only 1 year of treatment with pegaptanib or with usual care.[29] The benefit of the treatment appeared to be regardless of size or angiographic type of wet ARMD neovascularization, in contrast to older modalities of treatment.

Bevacizumab

While approval of pegaptanib for all forms of wet ARMD began the anti-VEGF revolution, the introduction of other intravitreal medications has offered additional, more promising options for patients with wet macular degeneration. In the summer of 2005, reports of improvement in wet ARMD with intravitreal administration of bevacizumab, an FDA-approved treatment for metastatic colon cancer, appeared in the medical literature.[31] This treatment arose between the introduction of pegaptanib and the FDA approval of ranibizumab for treatment of wet ARMD. While it is closely related to ranibizumab in its structure and function, differences in size, design, and cost do exist. Both bevacizumab and ranibizumab bind all biologically active forms of VEGF-A, whereas pegaptanib binds only 165 kD and, possibly, larger forms of VEGF-A.[27,32] Bevacizumab is a humanized monoclonal antibody against VEGF. It is larger than ranibizumab, which is an antigen-binding fragment against VEGF. One of the appealing qualities of

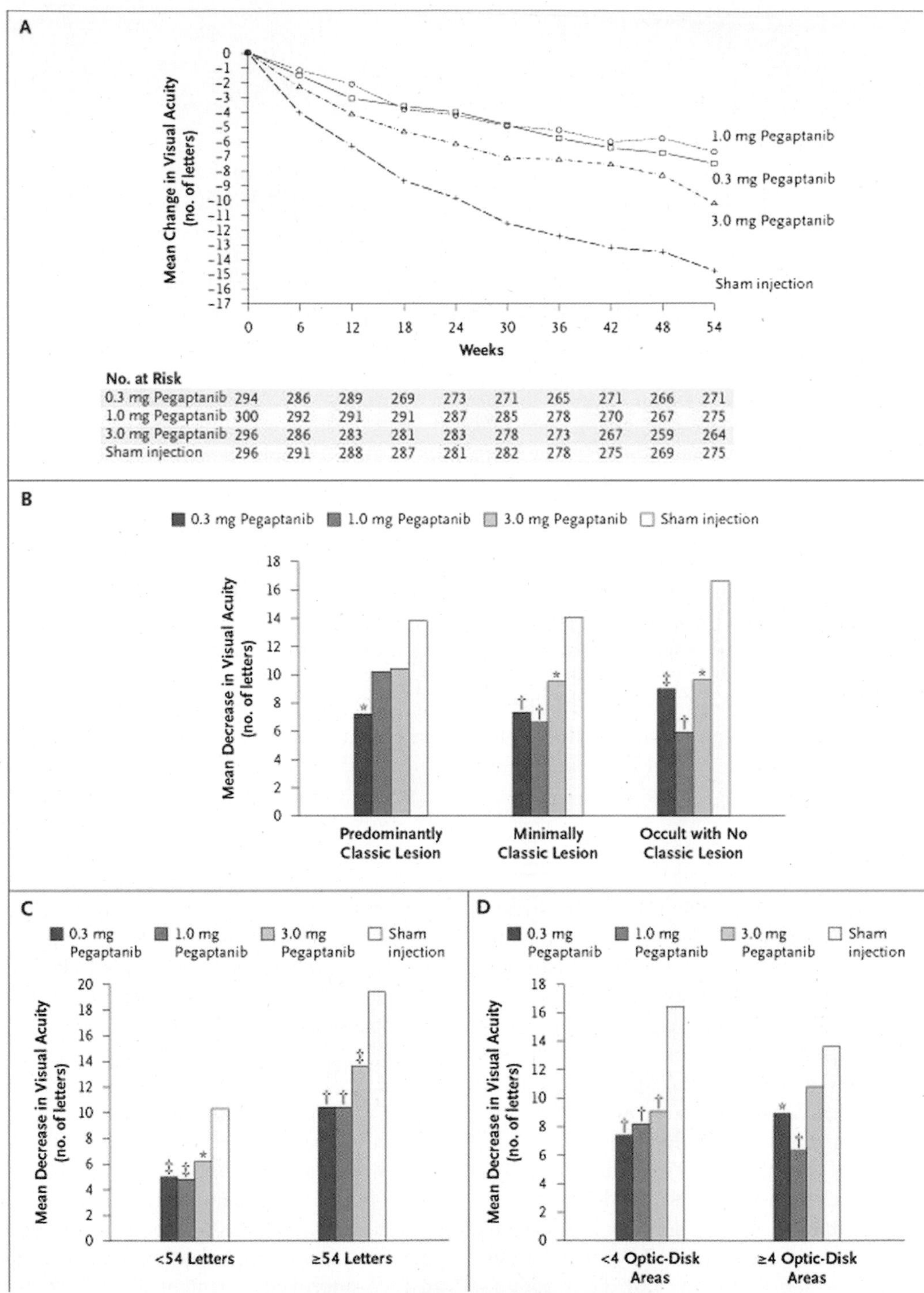

FIGURE 10.1. Mean change in scores for visual acuity. **Panel A** shows the mean changes in visual acuity from baseline to week 54 ($p < 0.002$ at every point for the comparison of 0.3 or 1.0 mg of pegaptanib with sham injection at week 54, and $p < 0.05$ at every point for the comparison of 3.0 mg of pegaptanib with sham injection at all other points after baseline). **Panels B, C,** and **D** show the mean changes in visual acuity according to the angiographic subtype, visual acuity, and lesion size at baseline, respectively. In relation to the visualization of choroidal new vessels (classic) in the fluorescein angiogram, a predominantly classic lesion includes 50% or more classic CNV, a minimally classic lesion includes <50% classic CNV, and an occult lesion includes no classic CNV. For lesion size, the unit of measurement was one optic-disc area, equal to 2.54 mm^2. For this analysis, lesions were categorized as less than four optic disc areas or four or more optic disc areas in size. In **Panels B, C,** and **D**, the *denotes $p < 0.05$ for the comparison of pegaptanib with sham injection, $^{\dagger}p < 0.001$ for the comparison of pegaptanib with sham injection, and the $^{\ddagger}p < 0.01$ for the comparison of pegaptanib with sham injection. Of a total of 1,186 patients, 294 received 0.3 mg of pegaptanib, 300 received 1.0 mg of pegaptanib, 296 received 3.0 mg pegaptanib, and 296 received sham injection. (Reprinted from Gragoudas, et al. Pegaptanib for neovascular age-related macular degeneration. *N Engl J Med.* 2004; 351:2805–2816, with permission.)

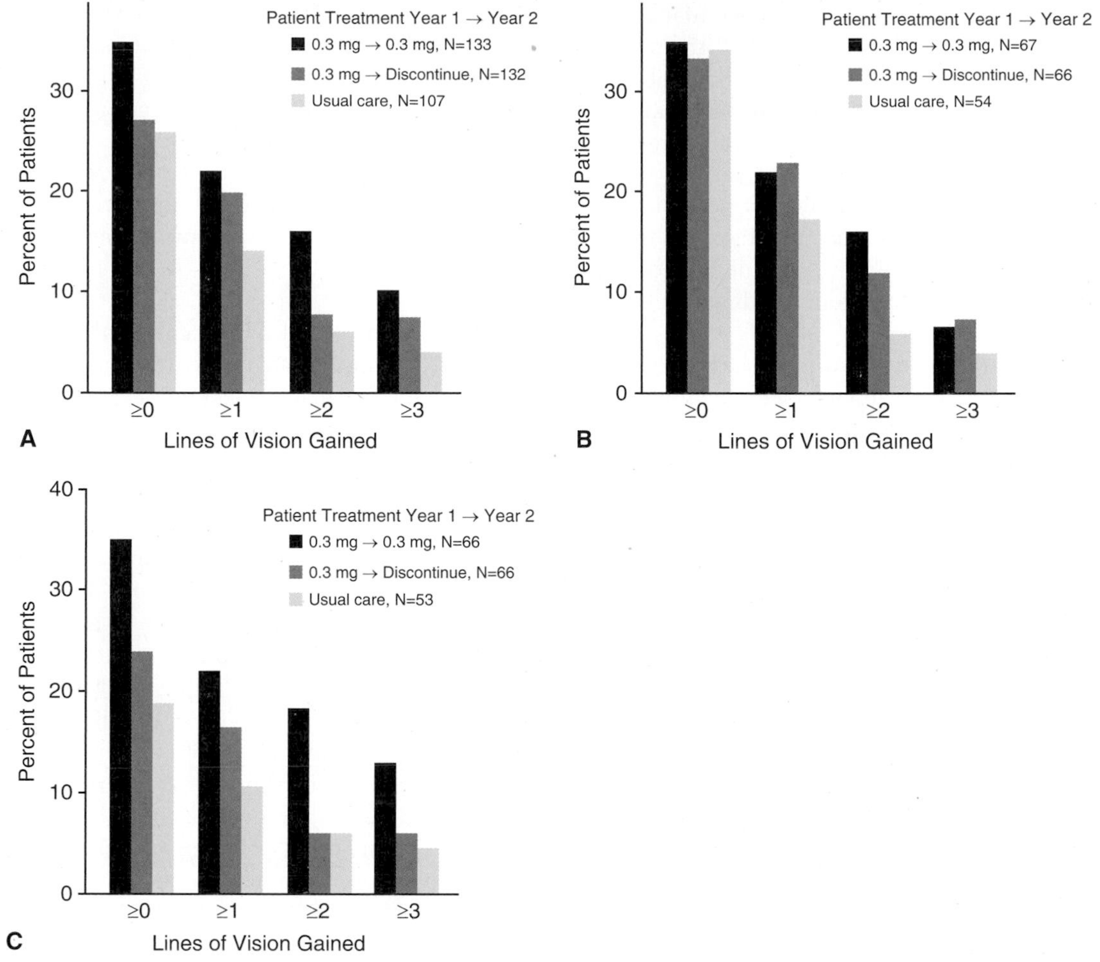

FIGURE 10.2. Vision gain. **A:** Studies 1003 and 1004 combined. **B:** Study 1003. **C:** Study 1004. (Reprinted from VEGF Inhibition Study in Ocular Neovascularization (V.I.S.I.O.N.) Clinical Trial Group. *Ophthalmology.* 2006;113:1508e.1–1508e.25, with permission.)

bevacizumab is its price, which has partially led to its widespread adoption for off-label treatment of wet ARMD.[33] A large portion of the pricing of the drug for cancer resides in the extensive cost related to the clinical trials necessary for FDA approval for cancer therapy; intravitreal doses are a portion of the cancer dose, so the intravitreal cost is dramatically less.

While price plays a role in bevacizumab's widespread use for wet ARMD therapy, numerous reports, small series, and small trials have demonstrated significant efficacy, suggesting similar results to those of ranibizumab.[34–36] However, it remains an off-label treatment. At the time of this publication, there is at least one large-scale clinical trial looking at the efficacy of bevacizumab in comparison to the FDA-approved ranibizumab, the Comparison of Age-Related Macular Degeneration Treatments Trial (CATT trial), which will be discussed in greater detail below. Of the completed randomized controlled trials for bevacizumab to date, all showed that bevacizumab is more effective than PDT. While these trials demonstrated an overall lack of masking, the results still show efficacy of bevacizumab.[34–36] Some reports include patients receiving systemic (intravenous) bevacizumab, which currently is much less common than intravitreal injection as a treatment for ARMD.[33,37] The adverse events reported in a recent meta-analysis of intravitreal bevacizumab consisted of postinjection inflammation, rare cases of endophthalmitis, pigment epithelial tears, submacular hemorrhage, cataract progression, and few systemic events, the majority of which were common to patients with advanced age or other cardiovascular risk factors.[33] Specific concern should be paid to arterial thromboembolic events since the data in ANCHOR,[46] discussed below, seemed to show a trend, though not statistically significant, of arterial thromboembolic events in the higher 0.5-mg ranibizumab dose cohort. These risks appear to be of approximately equal occurrences in the treatment versus nontreatment groups in a majority of studies listed above.

Of the trials for bevacizumab in wet ARMD analyzed in a recent review of the literature, the bevacizumab treatment arms demonstrated mean visual change of +8.6 ETDRS letters, and central retinal thickness decreased by a mean of 90 μm over a study population of 1,396 patients.[33] Three randomized controlled trials within this meta-analysis demonstrated that bevacizumab was superior to PDT, either with or without intravitreal triamcinolone.[33] While it is difficult to compare study results unless the study designs are identical, comparison is necessary to obtain an overall understanding of potential treatment benefits and pitfalls. The bevacizumab results in the literature appear to be of similar magnitude to those obtained with ranibizumab in the pivotal studies that will be discussed later.[36–38]

The standard of care, prior to the launch of anti-VEGF therapy, was PDT with verteporfin. Bevacizumab 2.5 mg has been compared to PDT for the treatment of predominantly classic wet ARMD in a randomized, prospective trial. This study found that all 32 eyes (100%) receiving bevacizumab lost <15 letters in visual acuity when compared with eyes that received PDT (73.3% lost <15 letters) at the 6-month endpoint ($p = 0.002$).[34] Recently, several small studies have indicated that there could be synergism between either pegaptanib or bevacizumab, in combination with PDT for the treatment of wet ARMD.[41–44] One such study demonstrated stability of lesions over 12 weeks with combination of PDT and bevacizumab treatment. This also correlated with improved or stabilized visual acuity. At the 24-week visit, 7 of the 11 treated eyes showed CNV leakage on fluorescein and were retreated with the combination therapy. It is important to note that these patients had CNV progression, despite PDT, prior to the study onset. It is reasonable to conclude that, in this small study, the combination of PDT and bevacizumab could possibly reduce the number of re-treatments and provide better visual acuity than would be provided by PDT alone.[41] Currently, the goal to reduce intervention frequency is driving combination trials of two or more therapies, ranibizumab or pegaptanib + PDT ± triamcinolone ± vitrectomy, attempting to decrease treatment burden of regular intravitreal injections.[45] This drive to reduce intervention frequency has also led clinicians to reduce the frequency of intravitreal injections, which is discussed further in the discussion of ranibizumab therapy below.

Ranibizumab

The most impressive results thus far in the anti-VEGF revolution have been provided in pivotal trials of the humanized monoclonal antibody fragment, ranibizumab. A new era in the treatment of exudative ARMD began with the release of the first phase 3 data evaluating ranibizumab (Miller, ASRS abstract, Montreal, 2005). Indeed, this single drug has revolutionized the concept of stabilizing and, in many cases, improving vision in wet ARMD. Ranibizumab is FDA approved for treatment of all angiographic subtypes of wet ARMD.[25] The pivotal phase 3 clinical trials, MARINA and ANCHOR, provide the evidence that led to ranibizumab being the first FDA-approved agent that truly prevents vision loss and significantly improves vision in many patients with wet ARMD.[40,46] Further studies, such as PrONTO and PIER, were aimed at determining less-frequent ranibizumab dosing regimens, since the prior studies utilized monthly injections.[39,47] The SAILOR trial was designed to evaluate the safety of two doses of intravitreal ranibizumab.[45] All of these will be discussed below, followed by a brief report on newer anti-VEGF drugs that are in development or clinical trials.

MARINA Trial

The Minimally Classic/Occult Trial of the Anti-VEGF Antibody Ranibizumab in the Treatment of Neovascular Age-Related Macular Degeneration (MARINA) was a 2-year, prospective, randomized, double-masked, sham-controlled study that evaluated the safety and efficacy of ranibizumab versus control in the treatment of minimally classic or occult CNV.[40] Intravitreal injection of 0.3 mg ranibizumab, 0.5 mg ranibizumab, or sham was administered once a month, for a total of 24 injections over 2-year period of the study. At both time-points of 12 and 24 months, 90% to 95% of the patients who were treated with one of the ranibizumab doses lost <15 letters (ETDRS) visual acuity. This was compared to 53% to 64% of the controls (sham). With regard to vision gains, 25% to 34% of the patients treated with ranibizumab gained 15 letters or more of visual acuity. Only 4% to 5% of the control patients achieved a 15-letter gain ($p < 0.001$) (Fig. 10.3). Serious ocular adverse events were uncommon and included uveitis (1.3%) and endophthalmitis (1%) (Box 10.2).[40]

ANCHOR Trial

The Anti-VEGF Antibody for the Treatment of Predominantly Classic Choroidal Neovascularization in Age-Related Macular Degeneration (ANCHOR) trial was the second pivotal, 2-year, prospective, randomized, double-masked, sham-controlled study in which treatment with ranibizumab was performed, and it was compared to treatment with PDT (photodynamic therapy with verteporfin).[46] Again, subjects were randomized to receive monthly intravitreal injections of 0.3 mg ranibizumab or 0.5 mg ranibizumab for 2 years. The control in this study was PDT every 3 months, as needed, according to the accepted, standardized guidelines. The findings were, again, similar to those presented in MARINA. Ninety to ninety-six percent of the ranibizumab-treated patients lost <15 letters of visual acuity at 12 and 24 months. This was compared to the control, PDT, in which 64% to 66% of the treated patients lost <15 letters of visual acuity. Regarding gains in vision, 34% to 41% of the ranibizumab-treated patients gained more than 15 letters versus approximately 6% of the PDT-treated patients[46] (Figs. 10.4 and 10.5). One important note from ANCHOR is in regard to safety. Arterial thromboembolic events, defined in the study as nonfatal myocardial infarction, nonfatal ischemic stroke, hemorrhagic stroke, or death due to vascular or unknown causes, were noted to be slightly higher in number in the

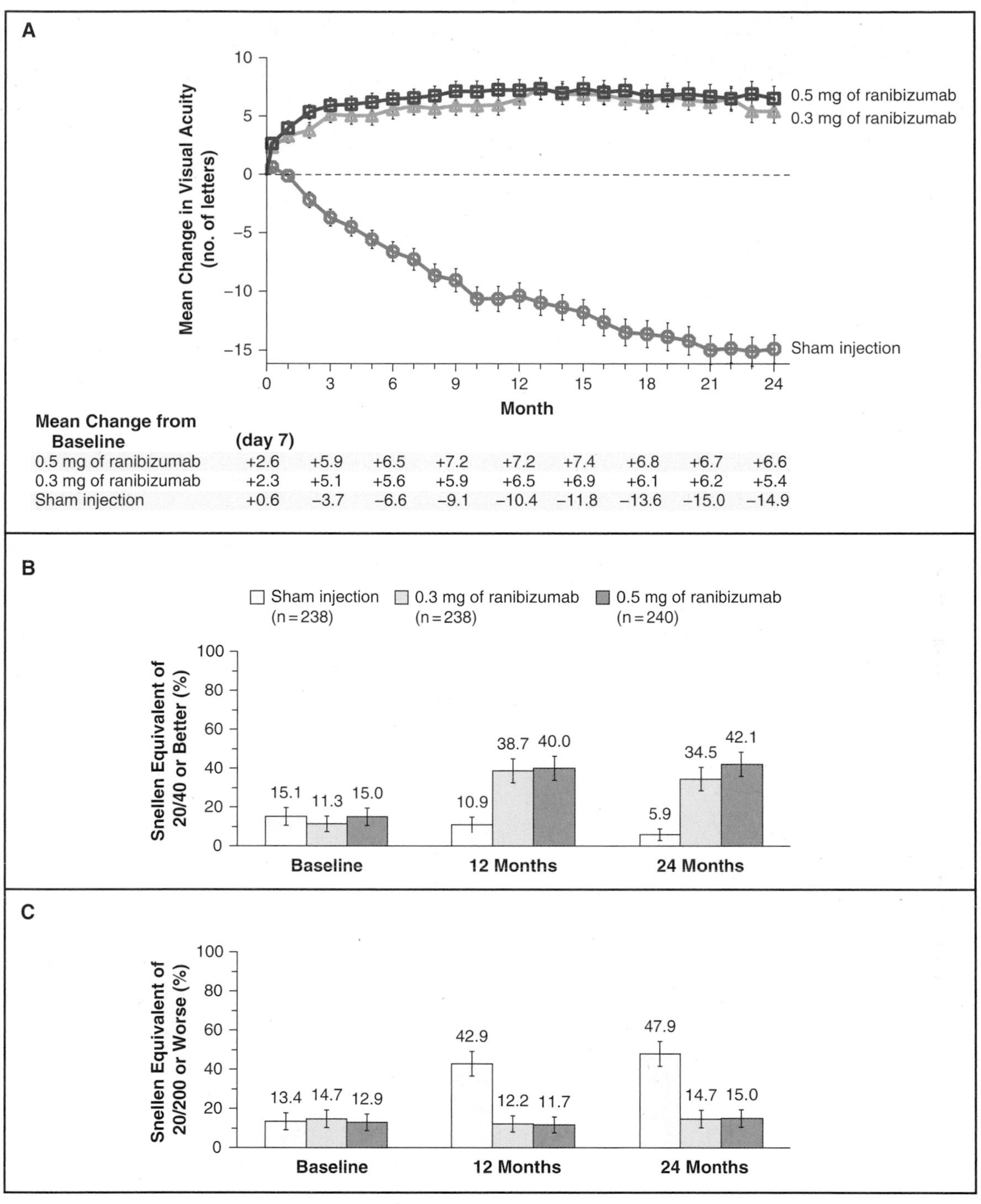

FIGURE 10.3. Mean changes from baseline in visual acuity and Snellen equivalents at 12 and 24 months. **Panel A** shows the mean changes from baseline in visual acuity during a 24-month period. At each monthly assessment, $p < 0.001$ for the comparison between each ranibizumab group and the sham-injection group. On day 7, $p = 0.006$ for patients receiving 0.3 mg of ranibizumab and $p = 0.003$ for those receiving 0.5 mg. **Panels B** and **C** show the change from baseline in the percentage of patients with a Snellen equivalent of 20/40 or better and the percentage of patients with 20/200 or worse, respectively, at 12 and 24 months ($p < 0.001$ for the comparison between each ranibizumab group and the sham-injection group at 12 and 24 months). Treatment comparisons use pair-wise models adjusted for visual acuity scores at day 0 (<55 letters vs. ≥55 letters) and for the type of CNV. Analysis of variance was used to assess the change in visual acuity from baseline at each monthly assessment. The Cochran χ^2 test was used for the comparison of percentages. The last-observation-carried-forward method was used to handle missing data. All statistical tests were two-sided. I bars represent SE in **Panel A** and 95% confidence intervals in **Panels B** and **C**. (Reprinted from Rosenfeld, et al, MARINA Study Group. *N Engl J Med.* 2006;355:1426, with permission.)

BOX 10.2 MARINA Trial: *M*inimally Classic/Occult Trial Of The *A*nti-VEGF Antibody *R*anibizumab *I*n The Treatment Of *N*eovascular *A*RMD

Purpose: To compare efficacy of Ranibizumab versus sham injections in neovascular ARMD.
Methods: In a multicenter, 2-year, double-blind, randomized, sham-controlled study, macular degeneration patients (716) with either minimally classic or occult CNV received 24 monthly intravitreal injections of ranibizumab (either 0.3 or 0.5 mg) or sham injections. The primary end point was the proportion of patients losing fewer than 15 letters from baseline visual acuity at 12 months.
Results: At 12 months, 94% patients treated with ranibizumab lost fewer than 15 letters, as compared with 62.2% of patients receiving sham injections. Visual acuity improved by 15 or more letters in 24% to 33% patients treated with ranbizumab as compared with 5.0% of the sham-injection group. The benefit in visual acuity was maintained at 24 months. During 24 months, presumed endophthalmitis was identified in five patients (1.0%) and serious uveitis in six patients (1.3%) given ranibizumab.
Conclusions: Intravitreal administration of ranibizumab for 2 years prevented vision loss and improved mean visual acuity, with low rates of serious adverse events. (Reprinted with permission from Rosenfeld PJ, Brown DM, Heier JS, et al, MARINA Study Group. Ranibizumab for neovascular age-related macular degeneration. *N Engl J Med.* 2006; 355:1419–1431.).

0.5-mg ranibizumab treatment group.[46] While this was not statistically significant, and it has not been duplicated in many studies following ANCHOR, many clinicians prefer not to treat with intravitreal anti-VEGF agents if a patient has had a recent stroke or heart attack (within 3–12 months of the injection) (Box 10.3).

FOCUS Trial

The RhuFab V2 Ocular Treatment Combining the Use of Visudyne to Evaluate Safety (FOCUS) trial had similar results to the above-mentioned ANCHOR trial.[48,49] This was a prospective, randomized, single-masked, phase 1/2 study that compared stand-alone PDT to ranibizumab plus PDT. PDT was performed on all patients upon entry to the study. Then, they were given monthly sham injections or monthly 0.5-mg ranibizumab for 2 years. PDT could be repeated every 3 months, as needed, according to the previously mentioned, accepted, standardized guidelines. The results reiterated prior study results, demonstrating that 68% of patients receiving PDT alone lost fewer than 15 ETDRS letters, and 90% of the patients in the combination treatment group lost fewer than 15 ETDRS

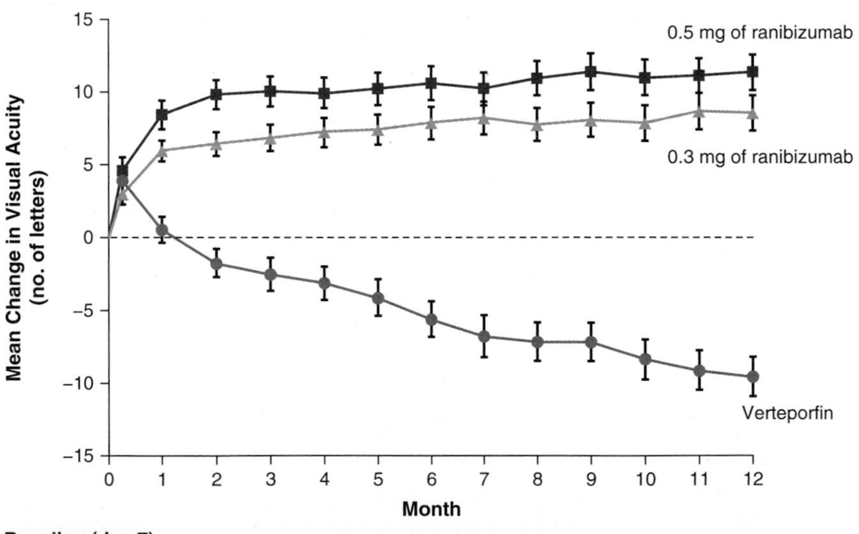

Mean Change from Baseline (day 7)													
0.5 mg of ranibizumab	+4.6	+8.4	+9.8	+10.0	+9.9	+10.2	+10.6	+10.2	+10.9	+11.4	+10.9	+11.1	+11.3
0.3 mg of ranibizumab	+2.9	+5.9	+6.4	+6.8	+7.2	+7.4	+7.9	+8.2	+7.7	+8.1	+7.8	+8.6	+8.5
Verteporfin	+3.9	+0.5	−1.8	−2.5	−3.1	−4.1	−5.6	−6.8	−7.1	−7.1	−8.3	−9.1	−9.5

FIGURE 10.4. Mean (±SE) changes in the number of letters read as a measure of visual acuity from baseline through 12 months. $p < 0.001$ for all monthly comparisons of each dose of ranibizumab with verteporfin. Pair-wise analysis of variance adjusting for the visual-acuity score on day 0 (<45 letters vs. ≥45 letters) was used to analyze the mean change in visual acuity from baseline at each monthly assessment. The last-observation-carried-forward method was used to impute missing data. All statistical tests were two-sided. (Reprinted from Brown, et al. *N Engl J Med.* 2006;355:1438, with permission.)

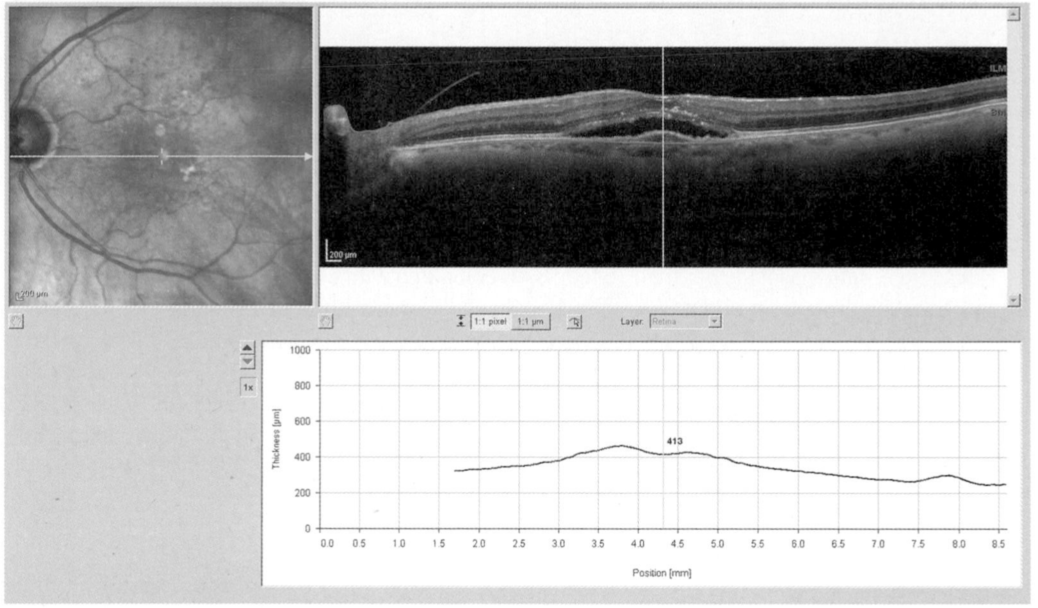

A

B

FIGURE 10.5. OCT pictures of wet ARMD. **A**: Before treatment with ranibizumab. **B**: After treatment with ranibizumab.

letters at 12 months. Regarding the gains in vision, 24% of subjects in the combination treatment group versus 5% of the PDT-alone treatment group gained at least 15 ETDRS letters.[48,49]

Less Frequent Dosing

The obvious benefit of monthly intravitreal injections of ranibizumab led the way to other studies that looked at less-frequent dosing regimens. The potential of monthly follow-ups and injections represents a major burden to patients, their families, and clinicians, alike. This is particularly the case when patients must travel long distances to reach their retina doctor's office or when both of the patients' eyes are being treated. The trials above were performed over 2-year periods, but there was no finite endpoint to the need for monthly treatment. Concerns abound regarding the cost of such treatment to the healthcare system, as well as the long-term drain on family resources to maintain regular follow-up. Current clinically applied treatment regimens for stand-alone intravitreal injections typically follow one of the following patterns: (a) regular treatments at a given interval, say

BOX 10.3 ANCHOR Trial: *AN*ti-VEGF Antibody for the Treatment of Predominantly Classic *CHOR*oidal Neovascularization in ARMD

Purpose: To compare ranibizumab with PDT with verteporfin in the treatment of predominantly classic neovascular ARMD.
Methods: In a 2-year, multicenter, randomized, double-blind study, patients (423) in a 1:1:1 ratio received monthly intravitreal injections of ranibizumab (0.3 or 0.5 mg) plus sham verteporfin therapy or monthly sham injections plus active verteporfin therapy. The primary end point was the proportion of patients losing fewer than 15 letters from baseline visual acuity at 12 months.
Results: About 94% to 96% patients lost fewer than 15 letters, as compared with 64.3% of those in the verteporfin group. Visual acuity improved by 15 letters or more in about 35% to 40% patients treated with ranibizumab as compared with 5.6% of the verteporfin group. Among 140 patients treated with 0.5 mg of ranibizumab, presumed endophthalmitis occurred in two patients (1.4%) and serious uveitis in 1 (0.7%).
Conclusions: Intravitreal Ranibizumab was superior to verteporfin with low rates of serious ocular adverse events. (Reprinted with permission from Brown DM, Kaiser PK, Michels M, et al. Ranibizumab versus verteporfin for neovascular age-related macular degeneration. *N Engl J Med.* 2006;355:1432–1444.)

monthly (as in the pivotal trials above) or every 6 weeks; (b) an initial loading dose (of one to four injections), followed by regular follow-up visits with re-treatment only at signs of recurrence (treat and follow); or (c) a loading dose followed by extension of the follow-up period, with re-treatment at each follow-up (referred to as "treat and extend").[33,39,50] Clearly, trying to decrease the treatment burden is an important factor.

An additional area of debate revolves around retinal imaging and the importance of various modalities in the management of new, persistent, and recurrent exudative disease. Until recently, fluorescein angiography had been the standard of care and the modality most relied upon for detecting disease and monitoring treatment response. The use of optical coherence tomography (OCT) has increased tremendously in recent years, largely due to the dramatic anatomic responses visualized with anti-VEGF therapy, anatomic responses that are easily measured with OCT. Anatomic responses were easily seen in ANCHOR and MARINA, yet very few sites had OCT capabilities at the time of study initiation. Today, few sites don't have this capability, and OCT has gained widespread acceptance as the modality of choice for following these patients.

PRONTO Trial

The Prospective OCT Imaging of Patients With Neovascular ARMD Treated with Intraocular Lucentis (PrONTO) trial was a 2-year open-label trial evaluating an OCT-guided, variable-dosing regimen of intravitreal ranibizumab.[39] Patients received monthly intravitreal 0.5 mg of ranibizumab for 3 months. This "loading dose" was followed by as-needed intravitreal injections of 0.5-mg ranibizumab, based on OCT-defined criteria for retreatment (Fig. 10.6). The study enrolled 40 patients with any of the angiographic subtypes of wet ARMD. 38/40, or 95%, of the treated patients had lost <15 ETDRS letters of vision at the end of year 1. Regarding vision gainers, 35% had gained at least 15 ETDRS letters of vision. The mean number of injections was 5.6 for the first year and ranged from 3 to 13 injections. In further evaluation of the year-1 results, the most common reason for retreatment with ranibizumab was the presence of macular fluid with a loss of at least five ETDRS letters. Twelve-month data for mean decrease in central retinal thickness on OCT were a decrease of 178 μm ($p < 0.001$).[39] Twenty four-month results were similar, with mean visual acuity improving by 11.1 ETDRS letters and OCT central retinal thickness decreasing by 212 μm ($p < 0.001$ for each statistic).[50]

PIER Trial

The PIER Study was a 2-year, randomized, double-masked, sham-controlled trial of ranibizumab designed to determine if a less frequent dosing schedule could also prevent loss

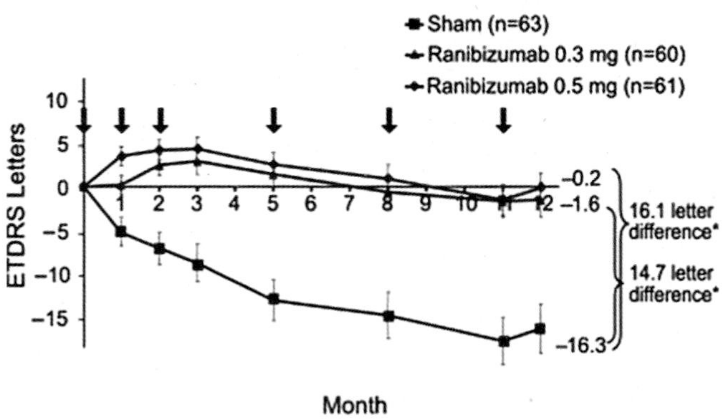

FIGURE 10.6. Ranibizumab for neovascular ARMD. Mean change from baseline visual acuity, measured as letters read on the Early Treatment of Diabetic Retinopathy Study (ETDRS) chart, at monthly intervals. At month 12, the 0.3 mg ranibizumab group and the 0.5 mg ranibizumab group differed from the sham group by 14.7 and 16.1 letters, respectively ($p <$ 0001). The *arrows* indicate that ranibizumab or sham injections occurred at day 0, months 1, 2, 5, 8, and 11. (Reprinted from Regillo CD PIER Study. *Am J Ophthalmol.* 2008;145:2, with permission.)

of visual acuity in patients with wet ARMD.[47] It was also designed to further study safety of 0.3- and 0.5-mg doses of ranibizumab. Patients were randomized to either the 0.3- or 0.5-mg dose of ranibizumab, which was administered monthly for 3 months, followed by quarterly administration of the randomized dose of ranibizumab. The data for year 1 showed that 49.2% of the patients receiving sham injections lost <15 ETDRS letters, versus 83% of those receiving 0.3-mg and 90.2% of those receiving 0.5-mg of intravitreal ranibizumab ($p < 0.0001$ for each dose level when compared to sham). When it came to vision gains of 15 or more ETDRS letters, however, the data failed to show significant differences between treatment groups and sham (11.7% for 0.3-mg and 13.1% for 0.5-mg ranibizumab vs. 9.5% of sham). While the vascular leakage area on fluorescein angiography enlarged in the sham group, it shrank in the treatment groups. The safety data confirmed that the intervention was safe: no cases of endophthalmitis, retinal detachment, vitreous hemorrhage, severe uveitis, or lens damage were reported. Intraocular pressure was elevated in the short term in many cases, but was usually <10 mm Hg higher than predosing values. There was no imbalance in systemic effects or associations in any of the groups, and, in particular, there were no cases of arterial thromboembolic events in any of the treatment groups. Development of hypertension was about equal in each of the treatment and sham groups. Even though treated patients in this study maintained their vision throughout the first year of dosing, on average, those gains were primarily lost during the quarterly injection phase. The results of the PIER treatment regimen are not as robust as those seen in MARINA and ANCHOR.[40,46,47] Further evaluation of PrONTO and PIER suggests that OCT-guided administration of ranibizumab injections less frequent than monthly but more frequent than quarterly may be beneficial to vision and result in fewer injections than described in prior studies (Fig. 10.7). However, whether or not a less than-monthly treatment regimen can be as robust with regard to visual

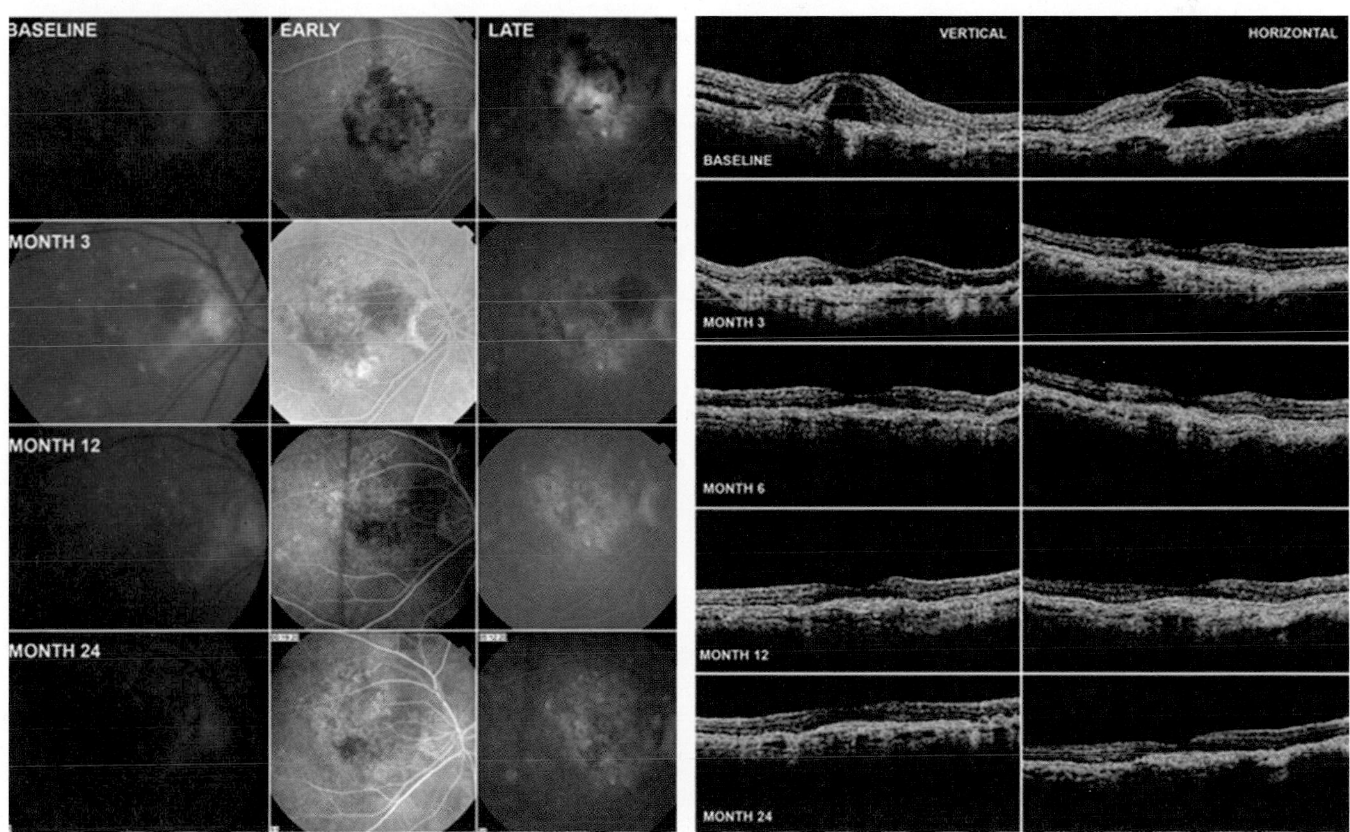

FIGURE 10.7. A variable-dosing regimen with intravitreal ranibizumab for neovascular ARMD: (PrONTO Study). (*Left*) Case 1: A 74-year-old woman with neovascular ARMD diagnosed with a minimally classic lesion in her right eye. She received only the first 3 required ranibizumab injections and then was followed up for 24 months. Color fundus images with early- and late-phase fluorescein angiographic images are shown at baseline, month 3 (1 month after the third injection), month 12, and month 24 without any additional injections of ranibizumab. (*Right*) Case 1: OCT response from baseline through month 24 in an eye with neovascular ARMD and a minimally classic lesion given a total of three injections through month 2, with no additional injections through month 24. (*Left column*) Vertical and (*Right column*) horizontal OCT scans, CRT measurements, and VA of the left eye are shown at baseline (526 μm; VA, 20/80), first ranibizumab injection; month 3 (188 μm; VA, 20/50), observed; month 6 (178 μm; VA, 20/25), observed; month 12 (198 μm; VA, 20/20), observed; month 24 (176 μm; VA, 20/16), observed. (Reproduced from Lalwani et al. *Am J Ophthalmol.* 2009;148:43–58 e1, with permission.)

BOX 10.4 PrONTO Trial: *Pr*ospective *O*CT Imaging of Patients with *N*eovascular ARMD *T*reated with intra*O*cular Ranibizumab

Purpose: To assess the long-term efficacy of an OCT-guided variable-dosing regimen with ranibizumab in wet ARMD, patients followed for 2 years. (Three consecutive monthly intravitreal injections of ranibizumab [0.5 mg] and re-treatment with ranibizumab at each monthly visit if an increase in OCT-CRT of at least 100 µm or a loss of five letters or more.) During the second year, the re-treatment criteria were amended to include re-treatment if any qualitative increase in the amount of fluid.

Conclusions: Mean visual acuity improved by 11.1 letters, and the OCT-CRT decreased by 212 micron. These Visual acuity (VA) and OCT outcomes were achieved with an average of 9.9 injections over 24 months. The PrONTO Study resulted in visual outcomes comparable with the outcomes from the phase 3 clinical studies, but fewer intravitreal injections were required.

PIER Trial: *P*hase 3b, Multicenter, Randomized, Double-Masked, Sham *I*njection-Controlled Study of the *E*fficacy and Safety of *R*anibizumab

Purpose: To evaluate the efficacy and safety of ranibizumab administered monthly for three months and then quarterly in patients with wet ARMD.

Conclusions: About 90% of ranibizumab-treated subjects maintained vision for 12 months. The effect declined in the ranibizumab groups during quarterly dosing (e.g., at 3 months, the mean changes from baseline VA had been gains of 4.3 letters for the 0.5-mg doses). Overall, it provided significant visual benefit to patients with wet ARMD and was well tolerated. However, the results of the PIER treatment regimen were not as robust as those seen in MARINA and ANCHOR.

gains as monthly injections has yet to be proven conclusively. The CATT trial may provide much needed data toward this question (Box 10.4).

SAILOR Trial

The Safety Assessment of Intravitreal Lucentis for Age-Related Macular Degeneration (SAILOR) trial is a single-masked, multicenter study to evaluate the safety of variable doses of ranibizumab for wet ARMD. Concerns for patient safety include ocular side effects, such as endophthalmitis, retinal tear or detachment, uveitis, or vitreous hemorrhage, and systemic effects. The primary systemic safety data focused on vascular events, including myocardial infarction, stroke, arterial thromboembolic events, and vascular or nonvascular death. The 1-year results, presented by Regillo et al. and Boyer, indicate that the systemic risks were <3%.[51,52] While there were trends toward greater risk of stroke or nonvascular death for the higher dosage (0.5-mg) of ranibizumab compared to the 0.3-mg dosage, this was not statistically significant. There were some subgroup analyses that seemed to show slightly increased stroke rates in those with known cardiovascular risk factors who received the 0.5-mg dosage when compared to the 0.3-mg dosage, but the number of patients in the subgroups was small, and this was not statistically significant.[51,52]

The disadvantage that the SAILOR data have when compared with the other pivotal trials (MARINA and ANCHOR) is that the dropout rates were high (between 18% and almost 50%) for SAILOR vs. 10% in MARINA and ANCHOR).[51,52] While it is possible that some patients or investigators decided to withdraw from SAILOR due to the desire to treat recurrent wet ARMD prior to 100µm of macular thickening (one of the criteria in SAILOR), the increased commercial availability of bevacizumab and ranibizumab outside of the study centers throughout the study course may have allowed patients to receive treatment elsewhere.[52] Regardless of the reason behind the dropout rates for SAILOR, a recent article evaluating the annual rates of arterial thromboembolic events in the Medicare population shows that patients with wet ARMD have about a 3.6% rate of Cardio-vascular accident (CVA), whereas controls have a similar rate, at 3.6%.[53] Also, patients with a previous event, classified as either myocardial infarction or ischemic stroke, definitely had a higher rate of subsequent events. The authors go on to state that the adverse events reported in major clinical trials of wet ARMD treatment fall within the range expected for the general public of the same age and risk factor status.[53]

Safety Data

Both systemic and ocular risks appear to be low with intravitreal ranibizumab injections. Boyer et al reported an overview of safety data from the following trials: MARINA and ANCHOR trials endophthalmitis rate of 0.05%, PIER with a rate of 0%, SAILOR cohort number one had an endophthalmitis rate of 0.06%.[54] The other ocular complications, which have been listed elsewhere in this chapter, appear to have relatively low occurrence rates, as well, indicating that intravitreal injections of ranibizumab are relatively safe and well tolerated.

While ranibizumab has been extensively studied in regard to safety, there is much less information regarding safety of the off-label intravitreal use of bevacizumab for wet ARMD. A recent retrospective, multicenter, open-label, uncontrolled interventional case series of 1,173 consecutive patients injected with bevacizumab for a variety of

BOX 10.5 Other Trials in Wet ARMD

SAILOR Trial

Purpose: A single-masked, multicenter study to evaluate the safety of variable doses of ranibizumab for wet ARMD.

Conclusions: Systemic risks were <3%. While there were trends toward greater risk of stroke or nonvascular death for the higher dosage (0.5-mg) of ranibizumab compared to the 0.3-mg dosage, this was not statistically significant. The disadvantage of this trial was that dropout rates were high (18%–50%) for SAILOR versus 10% in MARINA and ANCHOR.

SUSTAIN Trial: Study of Ranibizumab in Patients with Subfoveal CNV Secondary to ARMD

Purpose: A trial to evaluate safety of individualized, flexible treatment regimen on disease progression. Initially, three monthly injections of ranibizumab are given, and then additional injections are given based on clinical and OCT criteria, while following the patients on a monthly basis. From month 3 onward, doses were administered if VA decreased by greater than five letters or central retinal thickness was increased by more than 100 μm, with the option to withhold treatment if VA was better than 79 letters or if central retinal thickness was 225 μm or less.

Status: Ongoing.

EXCITE Trial: Efficacy and Safety of Ranibizumab in Patients with Subfoveal CNV Secondary to ARMD

Purpose: A Phase 3 randomized, double-masked, active-controlled, multicenter study to compare the efficacy and safety of Ranibizumab given as two dosing regimens in wet ARMD patients: (a) intravitreal ranibizumab for 3 monthly loading doses and re-treated on the basis of OCT or visual acuity criteria and (b) an initial intravitreal ranibizumab and re-treated at physician discretion.

Conclusions: Intravitreal ranibizumab was safe and well tolerated in a large population of subjects with neovascular ARMD. Ranibizumab had a beneficial effect on VA.

FOCUS Trial: RhuFab V2 Ocular Treatment Combining the Use of Visudyne to Evaluate Safety

Purpose: To compare the safety, tolerability, and efficacy of ranibizumab treatment in conjunction with PDT versus PDT alone in patients with subfoveal, predominantly classic CNV secondary to ARMD.

Conclusions: Through 2 years, ranibizumab + PDT patients exhibited less lesion growth and greater reduction of CNV leakage and subretinal fluid accumulation and required fewer PDT re-treatments than PDT-alone patients. Incidences of serious nonocular adverse events were similar in the two treatment groups.

ocular disorders was reported.[55] A total of 4,303 injections were administered, with a reported systemic adverse event in 1.5% of patients. These consisted of six strokes, five myocardial infarctions, two iliac artery aneurysms, seven cases of acute elevation of systemic blood pressure, five deaths, and two toe amputations. Keep in mind that these patients had a variety of ocular conditions being treated with bevacizumab, not just wet ARMD. The serious ocular complication rates in their study were as follows: 0.16% endophthalmitis, 0.16% traction retinal detachments, 0.09% uveitis, 0.02% vitreous hemorrhage, and 0.02% rhegmatogenous retinal detachment. Dosages used were either 1.25- or 2.5-mg of bevacizumab.[55] These results are similar to results from the safety data for the ranibizumab studies, presented earlier in this chapter, indicating that both medicines appear to be safe for the treatment of wet ARMD (Box 10.5).

SUSTAIN Trial

Several other clinical trials are ongoing and are looking at both the safety and dosing regimen issues with ranibizumab, bevacizumab, or both. The SUSTAIN study (the Study of Ranibizumab in Patients with Subfoveal CNV Secondary to ARMD) is similar to the SAILOR trial, in that it initiates therapy with three injections of ranibizumab spaced 1 month apart. Additional injections are given based upon similar clinical and OCT criteria, while following the patients on a monthly basis. The fact that patients are followed more closely than quarterly, after the induction of three monthly doses, is one major difference between SUSTAIN and SAILOR. The hope is that even though there are specific treatment criteria in SUSTAIN, similar to SAILOR, the ability to treat patients more frequently will lead to improved visual acuity throughout the term of the study.[56]

Despite the design of the SUSTAIN and SAILOR studies to have very stringent treatment guidelines, clinicians would often employ more liberal retreatment criteria. Many would treat with any degree of unexplained decrease in vision and/or even subtle evidence of macular fluid (with or without macular thickening). Other treatment protocols that have been suggested, in the wake of the promising data from the PrONTO Study, include something termed "inject and extend" (or treat and extend).[57] With this regimen, patients receive an induction, or a series of injections at monthly intervals for a set number of injections, usually 3, and then return in 5 or 6 weeks for another evaluation. At the visit that was "extended" beyond the normal 4-week visit, the patient undergoes regular examination and OCT testing. Regardless of whether they have evidence of new disease or signs of recurrence, such as macular fluid on exam and OCT, they are injected. If this exam showed that they had no signs of recurrent disease, their next visit, consisting of repeat exam and planned injection, would be extended two more weeks (a total of 8 weeks). However, if they had evidence of recurrent or persistent exudation on their initially extended visit, then they would be injected and instructed to return at the usual 4-week interval. This is done until the optimal treatment and examination interval would be established, with the hope that it would decrease the burden on the physician and the patient generated by automatic 4-week visits.[57] To date, no randomized, controlled clinical trial has demonstrated the efficacy of such an approach.

Bevacizumab Versus Ranibizumab?

The goal with treatment of wet ARMD is to achieve a balance. How can we best meet the needs of the patient by maximizing efficacy of treatment and visual outcome while, at the same time, decreasing cost and treatment burden to the patient, their family members, and the person or entity paying the bills? As alluded to earlier in the chapter, the two commercially available anti-VEGF treatments with the best efficacy and the most widespread use are ranibizumab and bevacizumab. Bevacizumab was first introduced as a drug for metastatic colon cancer, but, in 2005, it found its way into the retina armamentarium against wet ARMD with the report from Rosenfeld et al.[31] When the colon cancer dosage is split into smaller aliquots, as is done for intravitreal injection, the cost of the drug is much less than that for commercially available ranibizumab. Another factor playing into the potential role of bevacizumab is its longer half-life in the vitreous when compared to ranibizumab, 4.3 days versus 3 days, respectively, in the eyes of rabbits.[58,59] This debate over efficacy and cost, as well as frequency of dosing, is currently undergoing rigorous scrutiny in a nationwide clinical study, the CATT trial.

CATT Trial

The CATT trial is a randomized, double-blind, multicenter, interventional treatment trial that is designed to evaluate the safety and efficacy of the two most commonly used anti-VEGF drugs, namely, ranibizumab and bevacizumab.[60] The treatment arms are 0.5-mg ranibizumab every 4 weeks on a fixed schedule, 1.25-mg bevacizumab on a fixed schedule of every 4 weeks, 0.5-mg ranibizumab with variable dosing (as deemed necessary by the investigator) and evaluation at monthly intervals, and 1.25-mg bevacizumab with variable dosing and evaluation at monthly intervals. This trial will hopefully answer the questions that many people, both inside and outside of the retina community, believe are critical: is a variable schedule of dosing as effective as a fixed monthly dose, and is bevacizumab as effective as ranibizumab?[60] (Box 10.6)

NEW THERAPIES

The likelihood that ranibizumab and bevacizumab represent the ultimate "best" anti-VEGF agents at such an early stage in our research and development of therapies for exudative ARMD is low. New therapies in the family of anti-VEGF treatment for wet ARMD (and other ocular diseases) are likely to find their way into the retina specialists' hands over the next several years. As previously mentioned, much of the excitement and hope related to these newer treatments is because of a decrease in the treatment burden on the physician and the patient as well as improved vision gains and disease stability. VEGF Trap-Eye is a promising agent undergoing clinical trials for wet ARMD, as well as other VEGF-mediated eye diseases.[61] These newer agents will be discussed briefly here, and they will be discussed in greater detail elsewhere in the book.

VEGF Trap-Eye

VEGF Trap-Eye is a 110-kDa, soluble, recombinant fusion protein that consists of an immunoglobulin G fragment

BOX 10.6 Bevacizumab Versus Ranibizumab?

A comparative, retrospective case series on 452 patients of wet ARMD treated with anti-VEGF drugs showed that both bevacizumab and ranibizumab seem to be effective in stabilizing VA loss. There was no difference in VA outcome between the two treatment groups (Gong DS, Custis P, Howes J. *Ophthalmology.* 2009; Dec 5). A large, randomized clinical trial, CATT trial will examine this issue.

CATT Trial: Comparison of ARMD Treatments Trial

Purpose: A randomized, double-blind, multicenter, interventional treatment trial to compare the relative safety and effectiveness of bevacizumab versus ranibizumab with following treatment regimens in 1,200 wet ARMD patients: (a) 0.5-mg ranibizumab every 4 weeks on a fixed schedule, (b) 1.25-mg bevacizumab on a fixed schedule of every 4 weeks, (c) ranibizumab 0.5-mg with variable dosing (as determined by the investigator) and evaluation at monthly intervals, and iv) 1.25-mg bevacizumab with variable dosing and evaluation at monthly intervals.

Status: Ongoing.

with copies of the extracellular VEGF receptor domain from VEGF receptors 1 and 2 attached.[61] VEGF Trap is reported to have a very high affinity for all VEGF-A isoforms, as well as VEGF-B, -C, and -D, and placental growth factor 1 and 2.[62] The reported results of a randomized, double-masked, placebo-controlled phase 1 study of VEGF Trap, infused intravenously to patients with wet ARMD, showed a dose-related increase in mean blood pressure, but the 3 mg/kg dose (the highest infused) was the only dosage where severe hypertension and proteinuria occurred.[62] All of the adverse events resolved after discontinuation of the drug. The maximum tolerated dose of 1.0-mg/kg resulted in mean foveal thickness reduction, as measured by OCT at day 71, of 80%.[62]

Recent reports of the phase 2, randomized, double-blind, multicenter study for intravitreal VEGF Trap-Eye, which were presented at the 26th Annual Meeting of the American Society of Retina Specialists by Slakter, et al.[63] analyzed the data that were available for the 157 patients in the study. Patients with active wet ARMD were randomized to either 2.0 or 0.5 mg of VEGF Trap-Eye once a month or 4.0, 2.0, or 0.5 mg of VEGF Trap-Eye every 3 months for a study period of 12 months. Patients were induced and then treated as needed according to specific criteria. All treatment groups experienced a decrease in the mean central retinal thickness on OCT. The mean improvements were 5.4 ETDRS letters for the lowest treatment group and nine ETDRS letters for the 2.0-mg monthly induction group. Fluorescein angiography and OCT confirmed that the total lesion size and CNV area were markedly decreased in the treatment group. The most promising result was that only one to two additional injections were needed, on average, in the 2.0-mg induction group, yet similar visual and anatomic gains to the current anti-VEGF therapy were demonstrated. VEGF Trap-Eye shows promise in decreasing the treatment burden for wet ARMD.[63]

Sirolimus

Another possible anti-VEGF treatment for wet ARMD that is currently being studied is sirolimus. As the roots for bevacizumab were located in oncology and the treatment of cancer, so were the roots for sirolimus. It was initially developed for the treatment of renal cell carcinoma, and it was also used in the prevention of rejection of renal transplants.[64,65] Sirolimus' antiangiogenic and anti-VEGF properties come from actions at a different portion of the VEGF cascade, the formation of VEGF.[62] Sirolimus inhibits hypoxia-inducible factor-alpha, suppressing post-VEGF receptor signaling, thereby inhibiting VEGF synthesis.[66] Sirolimus also inhibits mTOR, a protein kinase regulating proliferation and protein synthesis, which is the mammalian target of rapamycin.[67] Rapamycin itself has been reported to reduce retinal pigment epithelium VEGF expression,[68] and studies have indicated that rapamycin can reduce the burden of neovascularization in mouse models of CNV and retinopathy of prematurity.[69]

Other Inhibitors

Other exciting possibilities exist for the treatment of wet ARMD by modification or inhibition of other molecular level targets, as they relate to VEGF formation or action. These signal transduction modifiers show promise for reducing the treatment burden by either extending the action of currently available anti-VEGF agents or by altering some portion of the CNV development cascade independently. Small interfering RNAs that target the VEGF gene and the VEGF receptor are undergoing further evaluation. Research suggests that these interfering RNAs inhibit vascular permeability, and possibly neovascularization, in animal models.[70,71] It remains to be seen how these innovative approaches will perform when compared to the current standard of care for wet ARMD. Also of interest is the recent report from Diago and colleagues suggesting that an orally administered tyrosine kinase inhibitor, called sorafenib, might provide some benefit in treatment of wet ARMD when combined with one of the currently available intravitreal anti-VEGF therapies (ranibizumab).[72] Again, this additional medicine, sorafenib, has its roots in oncology and cancer therapy. It is currently approved for the treatment of certain cancers.[73] The recurring theme is that many anti-VEGF agents that could be useful for wet ARMD therapy obtain their initial approval for oncology uses and treatment of cancer.

CONCLUSIONS

Wet ARMD is an already common disease that is becoming even more so as the population of the developed world ages. Indeed, it is the leading cause of irreversible blindness in the developed world in the population over 50 years of age.[1–5] Anti-VEGF agents have revolutionized the treatment of this disease. In many cases, visual acuity can be dramatically improved, not just stabilized, by the use of intravitreal administration of anti-VEGF agents. The frequency of dosing and choice of therapeutic agents continue to change as our clinical experience and knowledge of wet ARMD mature. Pivotal studies and ongoing clinical and preclinical research add to our understanding of this disease on a frequent basis. The use of anti-VEGF therapeutics has unquestionably improved our patients' quality of life by stabilizing and often improving vision. However, as is often the case with advancement, new problems arise. Treatment burdens to both patients and their support networks, as well as clinicians, coupled with spiraling costs, complicate our approach to this devastating disease. These issues are constantly evolving, and, while this chapter attempts to make the clinical side of anti-VEGF use more clear, the landscape is one that is changing rapidly. We continue to seek the best solutions to the constantly changing realm of treatment for wet ARMD, and anti-VEGF therapies continue in the quest to improve management of wet ARMD.

KEY POINTS

- CNV in ARMD is stimulated, at least, in part, by VEGF-A.
- The VISION trial demonstrated that intravitreal pegaptanib (Macugen) stabilized visual acuity in patients with wet ARMD, as compared to sham injection, but only 10% patients gained vision by three lines.
- Of the completed randomized controlled trials for bevacizumab (Avastin) to date, all showed that bevacizumab is more effective than PDT.
- The pivotal phase 3 clinical trials, MARINA and ANCHOR, showed that ranibizumab (Lucentis) truly prevents vision loss and significantly improves vision in many patients with wet ARMD.
- Both PrONTO and PIER suggest that OCT-guided administration of ranibizumab injections less frequent than monthly but more frequent than quarterly may be beneficial to vision and result in fewer injections than described in prior studies.
- Several new drugs (VEGF Trap, Sirolimus, VEGF siRNA) are in clinical trials in patients with wet ARMD.

REFERENCES

1. Bressler NM. Age-related macular degeneration is the leading cause of blindness. *JAMA*. 2004;291:1900–1901.
2. Friedman DS, O'Colmain BJ, Munoz B, et al. Prevalence of age-related macular degeneration in the United States. *Arch Ophthalmol*. 2004;122:564–572.
3. Resnikoff S, Pascolini D, Etya'ale D, et al. Global data on visual impairment in the year 2002. *Bull World Health Organ*. 2004;82:844–851.
4. Arias E. United States life tables, 2002. *Natl Vital Stat Rep*. 2004;53:1–38.
5. Brown GC, Brown MM, Brown HC, et al. A value-based medicine comparison of interventions for subfoveal neovascular macular degeneration. *Ophthalmology*. 2007;114(6):1170–1178.
6. Klein R, Klein BE, Tomany SC, et al. Ten-year incidence and progression of age-related maculopathy: the Beaver Dam Eye Study. *Ophthalmology*. 2002;109:1767–1779.
7. Photodynamic therapy of subfoveal choroidal neovascularization in age-related macular degeneration with verteporfin: one-year results of 2 randomized clinical trials—TAP report. *Arch Ophthalmol* 1999;117:1329–1345; [Erratum, *Arch Ophthalmol*. 2000;118:488.]
8. Bressler NM. Photodynamic therapy of subfoveal choroidal neovascularization in age-related macular degeneration with verteporfin: two-year results of 2 randomized clinical trials—TAP report 2. *Arch Ophthalmol*. 2001;119:198–207.
9. Verteporfin in Photodynamic Therapy Study Group. Verteporfin therapy of subfoveal choroidal neovascularization in age-related macular degeneration: two-year results of a randomized clinical trial including lesions with occult with no classic choroidal neovascularization—Verteporfin In Photodynamic Therapy (VIP) report 2. *Am J Ophthalmol*. 2001;131:541–560.
10. Giansanti F, Eandi CM, Virgili G. Submacular surgery for choroidal neovascularisation secondary to age-related macular degeneration. *Cochrane Database Syst Rev*. 2009;4(2):CD006931.
11. Macular Photocoagulation Study Group. Laser photocoagulation of subfoveal neovascular lesions of age-related macular degeneration: updated findings from two clinical trials. *Arch Ophthalmol*. 1993;111:1200–1209.
12. Kvanta A, Algvere PV, Berglin L, et al. Subfoveal fibrovascular membranes in age-related macular degeneration express vascular endothelial growth factor. *Invest Ophthalmol Vis Sci*. 1996;37(9):1929–1934.
13. Aiello LP, Pierce EA, Foley ED, et al. Suppression of retinal neovascularization in vivo by inhibition of vascular endothelial growth factor using soluble VEGF-receptor chimeric proteins. *Proc Natl Acad Sci U S A*. 1995;92:10457–10461.
14. Ferrara N. Vascular endothelial growth factor: basic science and clinical progress. *Endocr Rev*. 2004;25:581–611.
15. Wada, M, Ogata, N, Otsuji, T, et al. Expression of vascular endothelial growth factor and its receptor (KDR/flk-1) mRNA in experimental choroidal neovascularization. *Curr Eye Res*. 1999:18,203–213.
16. Barbazetto I, Burdan A, Bressler NM, et al. Photodynamic therapy of subfoveal choroidal neovascularization with verteporfin: fluorescein angiographic guidelines for evaluation and treatment—TAP and VIP report No. 2. *Arch Ophthalmol*. 2003;121:1253–1268.
17. Macular Photocoagulation Study Group. Argon laser photocoagulation for neovascular maculopathy: five-year results from randomized clinical trials. *Arch Ophthalmol*. 1991;109:1109–1114.
18. Macular Photocoagulation Study Group. Laser photocoagulation for juxtafoveal choroidal neovascularization: five-year results from randomized clinical trials. *Arch Ophthalmol*. 1994;112:500–509.
19. Verteporfin Roundtable Participants. Guidelines for using verteporfin (Visudyne) in photodynamic therapy for choroidal neovascularization due to age-related macular degeneration and other causes: update. *Retina*. 2005;25:119–134.
20. Treatment of Age-related Macular Degeneration with Photodynamic Therapy (TAP) Study Group. Verteporfin therapy for subfoveal choroidal neovascularization in age-related macular degeneration: three-year results of an open-label extension of 2 randomized clinical trials—TAP report no. 5. *Arch Ophthalmol*. 2002;120:1307–1314.
21. Dadgostar H, Waheed N. The evolving role of vascular endothelial growth factor inhibitors in the treatment of neovascular age-related macular degeneration. *Eye*. 2008;22(6):761–767.
22. Shah GK, Sang DN, Hughes MS. Verteporfin combination regimens in the treatment of neovascular age-related macular degeneration. *Retina*. 2009;29(2):133–148.
23. Folkman J. Tumor angiogenesis: therapeutic implications. *N Engl J Med*. 1971;285:1182–1186.
24. FDA approves new drug treatment for age-related macular degeneration. U.S. Food and Drug Administration press release in *FDA News* 12/20/2004:P04–110. Available at: http://www.fda.gov/bbs/topics/news/2004/new01146.html

25. Rosenfeld PJ. Intravitreal avastin: the low cost alternative to lucentis? *Am J Ophthalmol.* 2006;142(1):141–143.
26. FDA approves new biologic treatment for wet age-related macular degeneration. U.S. Food and Drug Administration press release in *FDA News*; 6/30/2006:P06–94. Available at: http://www.fda.gov/bbs/topics/NEWS/2006/NEW01405.html
27. Gragoudas ES, Adamis AP, Cunningham ET, et al. Pegaptanib for neovascular age-related macular degeneration. *N Engl J Med.* 2004;351:2805–2816.
28. Ruckman J, Green LS, Beeson J, et al. 2'-Fluoropyrimidine RNA-based aptamers to the 165-amino acid form of vascular endothelial growth factor (VEGF-165): inhibition of receptor binding and VEGF-induced vascular permeability through interactions requiring the exon 7-encoded domain. *J Biol Chem.* 1998;273:20556–20567.
29. Chakravarthy U, Adamis AP, Cunningham ET Jr, et al. Year 2 efficacy results of 2 randomized controlled clinical trials of pegaptanib for neovascular age-related macular degeneration. *Ophthalmology.* 2006;113:1508.e1–1525.e1.
30. D'Amico DJ, Masonson HN, Patel M, et al. Pegaptanib sodium for neovascular age-related macular degeneration: two-year safety results of the two prospective, multicenter, controlled clinical trials. *Ophthalmology.* 2006;113:992.e6–1001.e6.
31. Rosenfeld PJ, Moshfeghi AA, Puliafito CA. Optical coherence tomography findings after an intravitreal injection of bevacizumab (avastin) for neovascular age-related macular degeneration. *Ophthalmic Surg Lasers Imaging.* 2005;36(4):331–335.
32. Yang JC, Haworth L, Sherry RM, et al. A randomized trial of bevacizumab, an anti-vascular endothelial growth factor antibody, for metastatic renal cancer. *N Engl J Med.* 2003;349:427–434.
33. Schouten JSAG, La Heij EC, Webers CAB, et al. A Systematic review on the effect of bevacizumab in exudative age-related macular degeneration. *Graefes Arch Clin Exp Ophthalmol.* 2009;247:1–11.
34. Bashshur ZF, Schakal A, Hamam RN, et al. Intravitreal bevacizumab vs verteporfin photodynamic therapy for neovascular age-related macular degeneration. *Arch Ophthalmol.* 2007;125:1357–1361.
35. Hahn R, Sacu S, Michels S, et al. Intravitreal bevacizumab versus verteporfin and intravitreal triamcinolone acetonide in patients with neovascular age-related macula degeneration. *Ophthalmologe.* 2007;104(7):588–593.
36. Lazic R, Gabric N. Verteporfin therapy and intravitreal bevacizumab combined and alone in choroidal neovascularization due to age-related macular degeneration. *Ophthalmology.* 2007;114:1179–1185.
37. Geitzenauer W, Michels S, Prager F, et al. Early effects of systemic and intravitreal bevacizumab (AvastinR) therapy for neovascular age-related macular degeneration. *Klin Monatsblat Augenheilkund.* 2006;223:822–827.
38. Brown MM, Brown GC, Sharma S, et al. The burden of age-related macular degeneration: a value-based analysis. *Curr opin Ophthalmol.* 2006;17:257–266.
39. Fung AE, Lalwani GA, Rosenfeld PJ, et al. An optical coherence tomography-guided, variable dosing regimen with intravitreal ranibizumab (Lucentis) for neovascular age-related macular degeneration. *Am J Ophthalmol.* 2007;143: 566–583.
40. Rosenfeld PJ, Brown DM, Heier JS, et al, MARINA Study Group. Ranibizumab for neovascular age-related macular degeneration. *N Engl J Med.* 2006; 355:1419–1431.
41. Costa RA, Jorge R, Calucci D, et al. Intravitreal bevacizumab (Avastin) in combination with verteporfin photodynamic therapy for choroidal neovascularization associated with age-related macular degeneration (IbeVe Study). *Graefes Arch Clin Exp Ophthalmol.* 2007;245:1273–1280.
42. Dhalla MS, Shah GK, Blinder KJ, et al. Combined photodynamic therapy with verteporfin and intravitreal bevacizumab for choroidal neovascularization in age-related macular degeneration. *Retina.* 2006;26:988–993.
43. Ladewig MS, Karl SE, Hamelmann V, et al. Combined intravitreal bevacizumab and photodynamic therapy for neovascular age-related macular degeneration. *Graefes Arch Clin Exp Ophthalmol.* 2008; 246:17–25.
44. Hughes MS, Sang DN. Safety and efficacy of intravitreal bevacizumab followed by pegaptanib maintenance as a treatment regimen for age-related macular degeneration. *Ophthalmic Surg Lasers Imaging.* 2006;37:446–454.
45. Ciulla TA, Rosenfeld PJ. Antivascular endothelial growth factor therapy for neovascular age-related macular degeneration. *Curr Opin Ophthalmol.* 2009;20:158–165.
46. Brown DM, Kaiser PK, Michels M, et al. Ranibizumab versus verteporfin for neovascular age-related macular degeneration. *N Engl J Med.* 2006;355:1432–1444.
47. Regillo CD, Brown DM, Abraham P, et al. Randomized, double-masked, sham-controlled trial of ranibizumab for neovascular age-related macular degeneration: PIER Study year 1. *Am J Ophthalmol.* 2008;145:239–248.
48. Heier JS, Boyer DS, Ciulla TA, et al. Ranibizumab combined with verteporfin photodynamic therapy in neovascular age-related macular degeneration: year 1 results of the FOCUS study. *Arch Ophthalmol.* 2006;124:1532–1542.
49. Antoszyk AN, Tuomi L, Chung CY, et al. Ranibizumab combined with verteporfin photodynamic therapy in neovascular age-related macular degeneration (FOCUS): year 2 results. *Am J Ophthalmol.* 2008;145:862–874.
50. Lalwani GA, Rosenfeld PJ, Fung AE, et al. A variable-dosing regimen with intravitreal ranibizumab for neovascular age-related macular degeneration: year 2 of the PrONTO study. *Am J Ophthalmol.* 2009;148:43–58.
51. Dadgostar H. Ranibizumab in neovascular ARMD: comparing data from multiple clinical trials. *Ophthalmol Rep.* 2009;2:13–19. Reporting on Regillo CD, Francom S, Rubio R. Ranibizumab (Lucentis) safety in wet age-related macular degeneration: SAILOR study results. Presented at the 2008 Annual Meeting of the American Academy of Ophthalmology; November 8–11, 2008; Atlanta, Georgia.
52. Dadgostar H. Ranibizumab in neovascular ARMD: comparing data from multiple clinical trials. *Ophthalmol Rep.* 2009;2:13–19. Reporting on Boyer DS. SAILOR study results. Presented at the 2008 Annual Meeting of the American Academy of Ophthalmology: Retina Subspecialty Day; November 7–8, 2008; Atlanta, Georgia.
53. Alexander SL, Linde-Zwirble WT, Werther W, et al. Annual rates of arterial thromboembolic events in Medicare neovascular age-related macular degeneration patients. *Ophthalmology.* 2007;114:2174–2178.
54. Dadgostar H. Ranibizumab in neovascular ARMD: Comparing data from multiple clinical trials. *Ophthalmol Rep.*

2009;2:13–19. Reporting on Boyer DS, Chung CY, Rundle AC, Tuomi L. A safety overview of ranibizumab in patients with wet ARMD: ANCHOR, MARINA, PIER, and SAILOR studies. Presented at the 2008 Annual Meeting of the American Academy of Ophthalmology; November 8–11; Atlanta, Georgia.

55. Wu L, Martinez-Castellanos MA, Quiroz-Mercado H, et al. Twelve-month safety of intravitreal injections of bevacizumab (Avastin): results of the Pan-American Collaborative Retina Study Group (PACORES). *Graefes Arch Clin Exp Ophthalmol.* 2008;246:81–87.
56. Meyer C, Eter N, Hoz FG. Ranibizumab in patients with subfoveal choroidal neovascularization secondary to age-related macular degeneration: interim results from the SUSTAIN trial. SUSTAIN Study Group. *Invest Ophthalmol Vis Sci.* 2008;49:E-273.
57. Spaide R. Ranibizumab according to need: a treatment for age-related macular degeneration. *Am J Ophthalmol.* 2007;143:679–680.
58. Bakri SJ, Snyder MR, Reid JM, et al. Pharmacokinetics of intravitreal bevacizumab (Avastin). *Ophthalmology.* 2007;114:855–9.
59. Gaudreault J, Fei D, Rusit J, et al. Preclinical pharmacokinetics of ranibizumab (rhuFabV2) after a single intravitreal administration. *Invest Ophthalmol Vis Sci.* 2005;46:726–733.
60. Comparison of Age-Related Macular Degeneration Treatments Trials: Lucentis-Avastin Trial. ClinicalTrials.gov Web site. http://clinicaltrials.gov/ct2/show/NCT00593450. Accessed May 23, 2009.
61. Saishin Y, Saishin Y, Takahasi K, et al. VEGF-TRAP R1R2 suppresses choroidal neovascularization and VEGF-induced breakdown of the blood-retinal barrier. *J Cell Physiol.* 2003;195:241–248.
62. Nguyen QD, Shah SM, Hafiz G, et al. A phase 1 trial of an IV-administered vascular endothelial growth factor trap for treatment in patients with choroidal neovascularization due to age-related macular degeneration. *Ophthalmology.* 2006;113:1522.e1–1522.e14.
63. Parrott MB. The evolution of current and future treatments for neovascular ARMD. *Ophthalmol Rep.* 2009;2:16–20. Reporting on Slakter JS. Phase 2, randomized, controlled study of intravitreal VEGF Trap-eye in neovascular ARMD: one year OCT and fluorescein angiography outcomes. Presented at the 26th Annual Meeting of the American Society of Retina Specialists; October 11–15, 2008; Maui, Hawaii.
64. Vakkalanka BK, Rini B. Targeted therapy in renal cell carcinoma. *Curr Opin Urol.* 2008;18:481–487.
65. Thomson AW, Woo J. Immunosuppressive properties of FK-506 and rapamycin. *Lancet.* 1989; 2:443–444.
66. Sabatini DM. mTOR and cancer: insights into a complex relationship. *Nat Rev Cancer.* 2006;6:729–734.
67. Dumont FJ, Su Q. Mechanism of action of the immunosuppressant rapamycin. *Life Sci.* 1996;58:373–395.
68. Stahl A, Paschek L, Martin G, et al. Rapamycin reduces VEGF expression in retinal pigment epithelium (RPE) and inhibits RPE-induced sprouting angiogenesis in vitro. *FEBS Letters* 2008;582:3097–3102.
69. Dejneka NS, Kuroki AM, Fosnot J, et al. Systemic rapamycin inhibits retinal and choroidal neovascularization in mice. *Mol Vis.* 2004;10:964–972.
70. Reich SJ, Fosnot J, Kuroki A, et al. Small interfering RNA (siRNA) targeting VEGF effectively inhibits ocular neovascularization in a mouse model. *Mol Vis.* 2003;9:210–216.
71. Tolentino MJ, Brucker AJ, Fosnot J, et al. Intravitreal injection of vascular endothelial growth factor small interfering RNA inhibits growth and leakage in a nonhuman primate, laser-induced model of choroidal neovascularization. *Retina.* 2004;24:132–138.
72. Diago T, Pulido JS, Molina JR, et al. Ranibizumab combined with low-dose sorafenib for exudative age-related macular degeneration. *Mayo Clin Proc.* 2008;83:231–234.
73. Stein MN, Flaherty KT. Sorafenib and sutinib in renal cell carcinoma. *Clin Cancer Res.* 2007;13:3765–3770.

CHAPTER 11

Anti-angiogenesis Drugs for Neovascular-AMD Currently in Clinical Trials

Mohamed Ibrahim • Roomasa Channa • Diana V. Do • Quan Dong Nguyen

INTRODUCTION

The prevalence of advanced stages of age-related macular degeneration (AMD) in the United States is estimated to be 1.75 million in 2004 and projected to increase to 3 million by 2020.[1] Rein et al. developed a model that predicted substantial increases in the numbers of patients with early and advanced AMD by the year 2050. However, they also showed that currently available treatment options, if used fully, could reduce the vision loss associated with AMD by up to 35%.[2] Such encouraging prediction makes a strong case for developing more effective medications to combat vision loss due to AMD.

Among the different treatment modalities for neovascular AMD (NV-AMD), pharmacologic treatments with agents that target vascular endothelial growth factor (VEGF) have shown considerable efficacy in improving visual acuity in patients with AMD.

The VEGF pathway is initiated when VEGF binds to its receptors on endothelial cells. The two best-characterized VEGF receptors are termed VEGF receptor 1 (VEGFR1) and VEGF receptor 2 (VEGFR2). VEGFR1 and VEGFR2 are highly related transmembrane tyrosine kinases that use their ectodomains to bind VEGF; this binding activates the intrinsic tyrosine kinase activity of their cytodomains, initiating intracellular signaling. Interestingly, although VEGFR1 binds to VEGF with substantially higher affinity, most of the biologic effects of VEGF seem to be mediated via VEGFR2.[3]

In addition to VEGF-A, there are other proteins with similar homology and activities, and they can activate VEGFR1 or VEGFR2. The genes that code for VEGF-A, and the other proteins: VEGF-B, C, and D, and placental growth factors 1 and 2, constitute the VEGF gene family. The role of VEGF family members other than VEGF-A in ocular neovascularization (NV) has not been completely elucidated, but there is evidence to suggest that placental growth factor 1 participates.[4]

In animals, blockade of the VEGF pathway has been achieved by various means, including blocking antibodies targeted against VEGF[5–7] or its receptors[8], soluble decoy receptors that prevent VEGF from binding to its normal receptors[9–13], as well as small molecule inhibitors of the tyrosine kinase activity of the VEGFRs.[14–16] Currently, in clinical trials are several pharmacological agents (Table 11.1) that target various mechanisms of angiogenesis (Fig. 11.1).

Pegaptanib, bevacizumab, and ranibizumab are examples of blocking antibodies targeted against VEGFR. Ranibizumab is currently the gold standard for managing choroidal neovascularization (CNV). Some studies have found that one of the most effective ways to block the VEGF signaling pathway is to prevent VEGF from binding to its normal receptors by administering decoy VEGFRs.[9,11,17,18] VEGF-Trap is a VEGF-targeting agent that acts as a decoy VEGFR and is currently undergoing phase 3 clinical trials. Vatalanib, pazopanib, and TG108001 are tyrosine kinase inhibitors that target the post-receptor signaling cascade of the VEGFR. Volociximab and JSM6427 are integrin inhibitors that target the $\alpha5\beta1$ integrin, which indirectly inhibits the VEGF pathway through inhibition of the post-VEGFR tyrosine kinase cascade.

VEGF pathway is not the only pathway that induces angiogenesis (Fig. 11.1); the process of angiogenesis develops as a result of collaboration of several factors that use different and intertwining pathways. Targeting these angiogenic factors and/or their pathways may provide alternative ways to effectively manage NV-AMD. Alternative methods of blocking angiogenesis include pigment epithelium–derived factor, bioactive lipids, nicotine receptor antagonists, and mTOR inhibitors. Different agents that employ these alternative pathways are currently in different phases of clinical trials in patients with NV-AMD (Table 11.1).

VEGF PATHWAY INHIBITORS

VEGF Receptor Decoy—VEGF Trap (Regeneron Pharmaceuticals)

The parenteral VEGF Trap is a soluble decoy receptor created by fusing the first three Ig domains of VEGFR1 to the constant region (Fc portion) of human IgG1, resulting in a forced homodimer that has picomolar binding affinity.[9,11] In tumor experiments, this VEGFR1-Fc reagent is efficacious

Table 11.1.

Antiangiogenic agents currently in clinical trials

Class	Agent
I. VEGF Pathway Inhibitors	
A. Anti-VEGF antibodies	• Pegaptanib (*EyeTech, Inc.*)
	• Bevacizumab (*Genentech, Inc.*)
	• Ranibizumab (*Genentech, Inc.*)
B. VEGFR decoy	• VEGF Trap (*Regeneron Pharmaceuticals*)
C. Tyrosine kinase inhibitors	• Pazopanib (*GlaxoSmithKline Inc.*)
	• Vatalanib (*Novartis Inc.*)
	• T tg100801 (*TargeGen Inc.*)
D. Integrin inhibitors	• JSM6427 (*Jerini Ophthalmic Inc.*)
	• Volociximab (*Ophthotech Corporation*)
II. PEDF	• ADGVPEDF.11 (*GenVec Inc.*)
III. Bioactive lipids	• Sonepcizumab (*iSONEP, Lpath, Inc.*)
IV. Nicotine receptor antagonists	• Mecamylamine (*ATG003, CoMentis Inc.*),
V. mTOR pathway modulators	• Sirolimus (*MacuSight Inc.*)
	• PF-04523655 (*Quark/Pfizer*)

at approximately 500-fold lower concentration than a similar VEGFR-2 construct.[18] Despite this high affinity, the VEGFR1-Fc was not feasible for clinical use because of its poor pharmacokinetic profile. In rodent studies, this protein had to be administered frequently and at very high levels to achieve clinical efficacy.[9,11,17] In addition, the VEGFR1-Fc exhibited certain toxicological side effects that are not seen with the VEGFR2-Fc.[18]

In 2002, VEGF-Trap$_{R1R2}$ was developed by Holash and colleagues by fusing the second Ig domain of VEGFR1 with the third Ig domain of VEGFR2. VEGF-Trap$_{R1R2}$ has a very high affinity for VEGF, prolonged in vivo pharmacokinetics and pharmacodynamics, lacks nonspecific toxicities, and can effectively suppress the growth and vascularization of a number of different types of tumors in vivo.[3]

The receptor portion of the VEGF Trap molecule has a high affinity for all VEGF-A isoforms (K_d < 1 pmol/L), placental growth factors 1 and 2, and VEGF-B, VEGF-C, and VEGF-D.[19] Therefore, VEGF Trap is distinguished from ranibizumab by its higher-binding affinity for all VEGF-A isoforms and its ability to inhibit other VEGF family members.[19]

Intravitreal administration of VEGF Trap strongly suppressed laser-induced CNV in mice[20] and primates (Wiegand et al. ARVO abstract 1411, 2005). These findings led to the development of a formulation for intraocular delivery, VEGF Trap-Eye, a formulation using ultrapurified VEGF Trap with a combination and concentration of buffers compatible with ocular tissues. In primate toxicology studies, there were no systemic safety signals after intraocular injections of VEGF Trap-Eye, and there was an excellent ocular safety profile based on ocular examinations, color photography, fluorescein angiography (FA), electroretinography, and postmortem microscopic examination of ocular tissues (*unpublished data*). The only abnormality identified was mild, reversible inflammation in the anterior chamber and vitreous in some primates after intraocular injection.[21]

A phase 1 randomized, multicenter, placebo-controlled clinical trial investigating the effect of intravenous VEGF Trap in patients with NVAMD showed elimination of approximately 60% of excess retinal thickness after either single or multiple infusions.[19] The maximum tolerated dose of intravenous VEGF Trap in this study population was 1.0 mg/kg. At 3 mg/kg, hypertension and proteinuria, which are side effects associated with systemic anti-VEGF therapy, were noted. The potential risks associated with the intravenous injection of VEGF Trap led to investigation of alternative routes of delivery. VEGF Trap-Eye is an intravitreal formulation, designed to increase the therapeutic window and decrease the adverse events associated with VEGF Trap.

The intravitreal injection of VEGF Trap-Eye was investigated in a phase 1 dose-escalation multicenter clinical trial that was designed to determine the safety, tolerability, maximum tolerated dose, and bioactivity of a single intravitreal injection of VEGF Trap-Eye.[21]

Twenty-one patients with NV-AMD lesions ≤12 disc areas in size and ≥50% active CNV) with best-corrected visual acuity (BCVA) ≤20/40 received a single intraocular injection of one of the following dosages: 0.05 mg (n = 3), 0.15 mg (n = 3), 0.5 mg (n = 3), 1 mg (n = 6), 2 mg (n = 3), or 4 mg (n = 3) of VEGF Trap-Eye. There were no serious adverse events and no identifiable signs of intraocular inflammation. The mean decrease in excess foveal thickness for all patients was 104.5 μm at 6 weeks, and the mean increase in visual acuity was 4.43 letters. In the two highest dose groups combined (2 and 4 mg), the mean increase in BCVA was 13.5 letters, with three of six patients demonstrating improvement of ≥3 lines and three

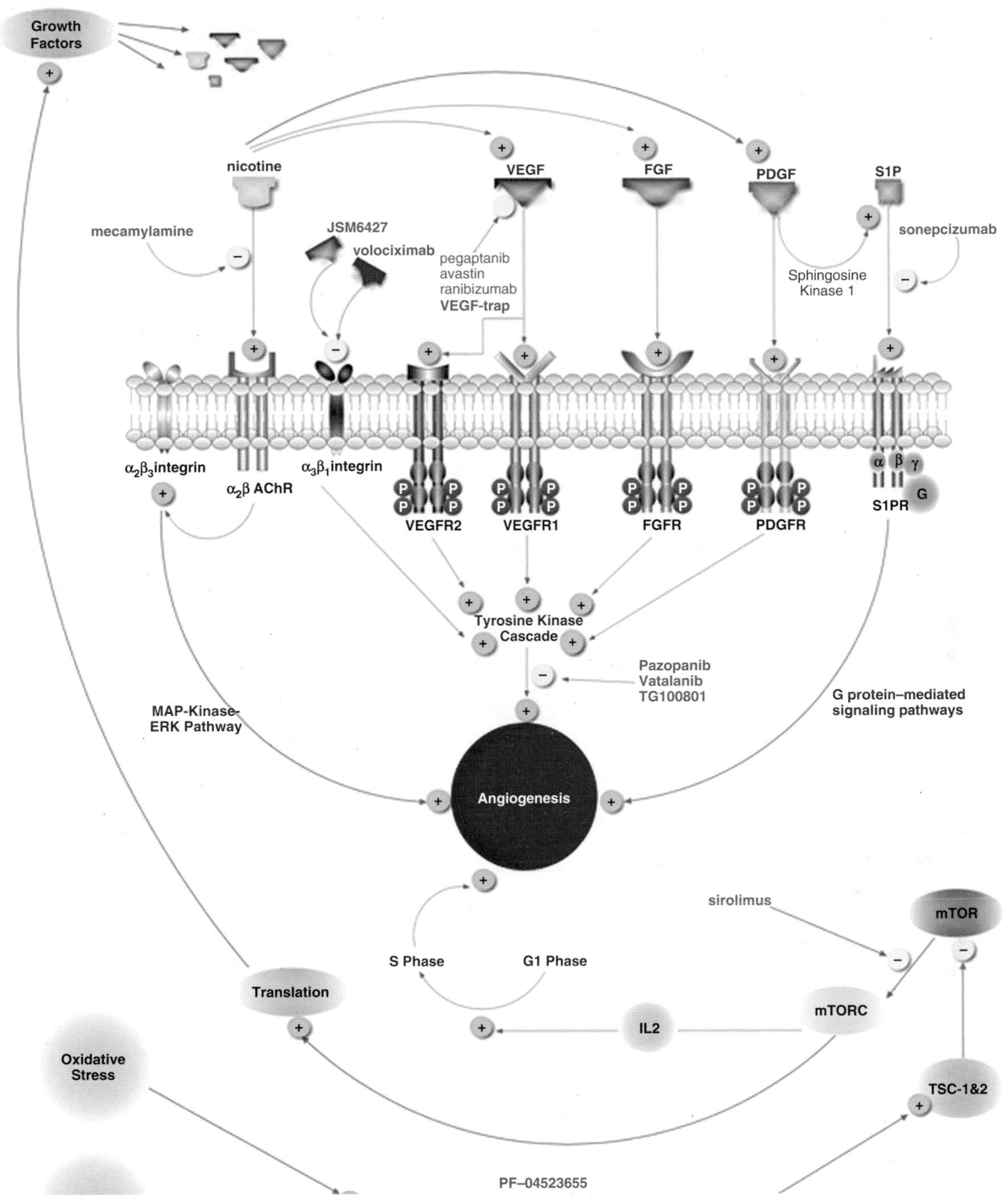

FIGURE 11.1. Pathways of angiogenesis and mechanisms of action of novel antiangiogenic agents currently in clinical trials for NV-AMD.

patients requiring no adjunctive treatment of any type to 12 weeks. Some showed elimination of fluorescein leakage and reduction in area of CNV (Fig. 11.2).[21]

In a phase 2 double-masked, prospective, randomized, multicenter clinical trial (CLEAR IT-2 Study), 157 patients were randomized to five dose groups and treated with VEGF Trap-Eye in one eye. Two groups initially received monthly doses of 0.5 or 2.0 mg of VEGF Trap-Eye (at weeks 0, 4, 8, and 12), and three groups received quarterly doses of 0.5, 2.0, or 4.0 mg of VEGF Trap-Eye (at baseline and week 12). Following the initial 12-week fixed-dosing phase of the trial, patients continued to receive therapy at the same dose on a PRN dosing schedule based upon the physician's assessment of the need for re-treatment in accordance with prespecified criteria. Patients were monitored for safety, retinal thickness, and visual acuity. The primary endpoint results of the CLEARIT-2 Study have been reported at various national and international meetings. In this study, VEGF Trap-Eye was generally well tolerated and there were no drug-related serious adverse events. There was

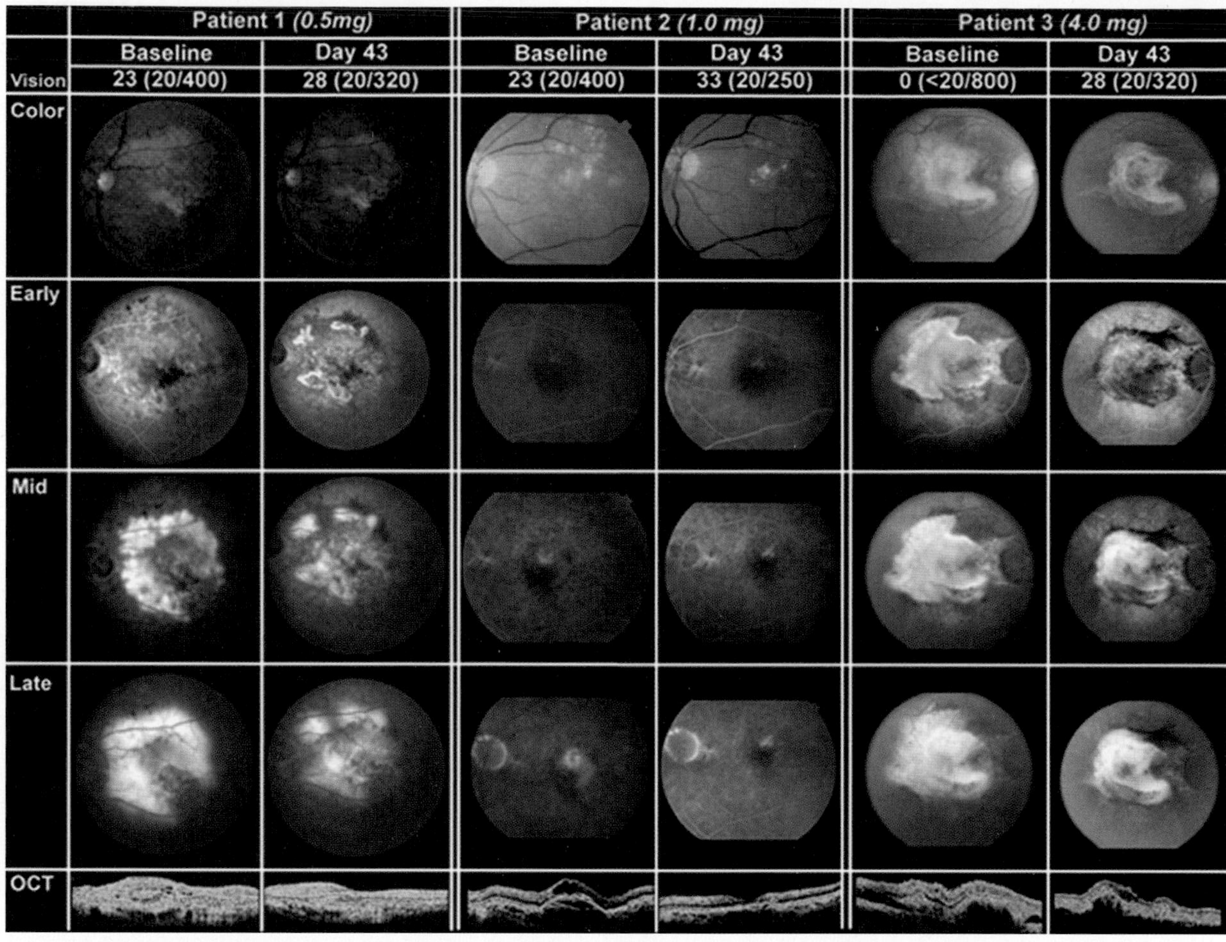

FIGURE 11.2. Changes on fundus photography, FA, and optical coherence tomography of three patients who were participating in the CLEAR-IT 1 Study of intravitreal VEGF Trap-Eye for NV-AMD. Each patient received a single intravitreal injection of VEGF Trap-Eye at baseline at one of several doses (as indicated). Changes were captured and noted at Day 43. (Reprinted with permission from Nguyen, et al. *Ophthalmology.* 2009;116:2141–2148 e1.)

one reported case of culture-negative endophthalmitis/uveitis in the study eye, which was deemed not to be drug related. The most common adverse events were those typically associated with intravitreal injections. Patients receiving monthly doses of VEGF Trap-Eye of either 2.0 or 0.5 mg for 12 weeks followed by PRN dosing achieved mean improvements in visual acuity versus baseline of 9 ($p < 0.0001$) and 5.4 letters ($p < 0.085$), respectively, at the end of 1 year. The proportion of patients with visual acuity of 20/40 or better increased from 23% at baseline to 45% at week 52 in patients initially treated with 2.0 mg monthly and from 16% at baseline to 47% at week 52 in patients initially treated with 0.5 mg monthly. During week 12 to week 52 PRN dosing period, patients initially dosed on a 2.0 mg monthly schedule received, on average, only 1.6 additional injections and those initially dosed on a 0.5 mg monthly schedule received, on average, 2.5 injections. Patients receiving monthly doses of VEGF Trap-Eye of either 2.0 or 0.5 mg for 12 weeks followed by PRN dosing also achieved mean decreases in retinal thickness versus baseline of 143 μm ($p < 0.0001$) and 125 μm ($p < 0.0001$) at week 52, respectively.

VEGF Trap-Eye was also associated with a reduction in the size of the total active CNV. Patients initially receiving either a 2 or 0.5 mg monthly fixed dose of VEGF Trap-Eye for 12 weeks followed by PRN dosing experienced statistically significant 3.41 and 1.42 mm^2 reductions in mean CNV size at 48 weeks (the final 1-year analysis from the independent reading center) versus baseline, respectively. Patients in the 2 mg monthly cohort also achieved a statistically significant 1.75 mm^2 reduction in total lesion size. A reduction in total lesion size was not seen in the cohort initially dosed with 0.5 mg monthly.

Patients receiving fixed dosing of VEGF Trap-Eye at baseline and week 12 of either 4.0, 2.0, or 0.5 mg followed by PRN dosing achieved mean improvements in visual acuity versus baseline of 4.2 letters ($p < 0.015$ vs. baseline), 5.2 letters ($p < 0.041$ vs. baseline), and 2.6 letters ($p < 0.344$ vs. baseline) respectively, at the end of 1 year. The proportion of patients with visual acuity of 20/40 or

BOX 11.1 VEGF Trap-Eye Trials in Wet Macular Degeneration

CLEAR-IT-2: A randomized, double-masked, active controlled phase 2 Study of the efficacy, safety, and tolerability of repeated doses of intravitreal VEGF trap in subjects with NV-AMD

Purpose: A phase 2 double-masked, prospective, randomized, multicenter clinical trial to study five different doses of VEGF Trap Eye in patients with neovascular ARMD.

Method: Two groups initially received monthly doses of 0.5 or 2.0 mg of VEGF Trap-Eye (at weeks 0, 4, 8, and 12) and three groups received quarterly doses of 0.5, 2.0, or 4.0 mg of VEGF Trap-Eye (at baseline and week 12). Following the initial fixed dose schedule, patients received PRN dosing as determined by the physicians.

Conclusions: Patients receiving monthly doses of VEGF Trap-Eye of either 2.0 or 0.5 mg for 12 weeks followed by PRN dosing achieved mean improvements in visual acuity versus baseline of 9 and 5.4 letters, respectively, at the end of 1 year, and achieved mean decreases in retinal thickness versus baseline of 143 and 125 μm at week 52, respectively.

CLEAR-IT Extension Study: The extension study showed that patients achieved and maintained significant improvement in visual acuity for 18 months with initial fixed dosing followed by 15 months of PRN. The extension study demonstrates that patients with NV-AMD achieved and maintained significant improvement in BCVA for 18 months with initial fixed dosing followed by 15 months of as-needed administration. On average, only 3.5 injections were given during the PRN dosing phase. Patients continue to be seen and treated in the extension stage of the CLEAR-IT 2 study dosing. On average, only 3.5 injections were given during the PRN dosing phase.

CLEAR-IT-3: A phase 3 trial is ongoing.

VIEW Study: VEGF Trap-Eye: Investigation of Efficacy and Safety in Wet AMD

Purpose: Two parallel phase 3 trials are evaluating VEGF Trap-Eye administered in neovascular ARMD patients at the following dosages: 0.5 mg every 4 weeks, 2 mg every 4 weeks, or 2 mg every 8 weeks (following three monthly doses) in direct comparison with ranibizumab administered 0.5 mg every 4 weeks during the first year. In the studies, PRN dosing will be evaluated during the second year of each study. The **VIEW1** study enrolled patients in the United States and Canada, and the **VIEW2** study enrolled patients in Europe, Asia Pacific, Japan, and Latin America.

Status: Ongoing study.

better increased from 16% at baseline to 36% at week 52, from 10% at baseline to 45% at week 52, and from 22% at baseline to 34% at week 52, in patients initially treated with 4, 2, and 0.5 mg, respectively. While PRN dosing following a fixed dosing at baseline and week 12 also yielded improvements in visual acuity and retinal thickness versus baseline at week 52, the results generally were not as robust as those obtained with initial fixed monthly dosing.

In an extension to the CLEAR IT-2 study, 117 patients from all groups have been enrolled into one group receiving PRN 2 mg of VEGF Trap-Eye every 2 months. In this extension study, the reported systemic serious adverse events included three deaths, a case of hemorrhagic stroke, and a case of myocardial infarction; all deemed not to be related to the study drug. Compared to baseline, there was an average gain of 7.1 letters at month 18 ($p < 0.0001$), compared to an average gain of 8.4 letters at month 12. Only 7% showed loss of ≥ 15 letters, 74% either gained vision or maintained their vision at baseline, and 26% gained ≥ 15 letters. The patients who have a vision of ≥20/40 at month 18 were 45% compared to 15% at baseline. During the PRN phase (month 3–18), the mean number of reinjections was 3.5 ± 2.5 (range 0–12), the mean number of days that elapsed before the first PRN injection was administered was 155 ± 130 (range 21–448), and the mean number of days between the first and the second PRN injection was 99 ± 67 (range 22–350). Overall, 50% of the patients needed ≤3 additional injections after month 3 and 75% needed ≤4 injections after month 3.

Regeneron and Bayer HealthCare have joined forces and initiated a global development program for VEGF Trap-Eye in NV-AMD. In two parallel phase 3 trials, which have completed recruitments, the companies are evaluating VEGF Trap-Eye administered at the following dosages: 0.5 mg every 4 weeks, 2 mg every 4 weeks, or 2 mg every 8 weeks (following three monthly doses) in direct comparison with ranibizumab (Lucentis; Genentech, Inc.) administered 0.5 mg every 4 weeks according to its U.S. label during the first year of the studies. In the studies, PRN dosing will be evaluated during the second year of each study. The VIEW1 study enrolled patients in the United States and Canada and the VIEW2 study encompassed patients in Europe, Asia Pacific, Japan, and Latin America (Box 11.1).

Tyrosine Kinase Inhibitors

Pazopanib (GlaxoSmithKline, Inc.)

Pazopanib (also known as GW786034) is a tyrosine kinase inhibitor that blocks VEGFR receptor (VEGFR)-1, 2, 3, platelet-derived growth factor receptor (PDGFR), c-kit receptor, fibroblast growth factor receptor 1 (FGFR1),

FGFR3, and c-fms (Fig. 11.1). By blocking the post-receptor cascade, pazopanib theoretically provides a widespread inhibition of angiogenesis. It has varying affinities for different receptors:

VEGFR1≈VEGFR2≈VEGFR3>PDGFRβ≈PDGFRα≈cKit>FGFR1≈FGFR3≈cfms>>other kinases.[22]

Pazopanib was initially developed as an anticancer drug but has been found to inhibit ocular angiogenesis as well. Takashi and colleagues demonstrated that in mouse models, orally administered pazopanib resulted in 93% decrease in the size of CNV lesion compared with vehicle treatment. Periocular injection in similar models resulted in 40% regression in size of CNV, showing that the drug is effective in both locally and systemically administered forms. Another interesting point to note is that pazopanib not only suppresses further growth but also causes regression of the existing CNV lesion.

Pazopanib is being evaluated in several clinical trials as a potential therapeutic agent in patients with NV-AMD. A phase 1 trial designed to establish the safety and tolerability of pazopanib eye drops in humans has been completed on 38 healthy volunteers and elderly subjects with NV-AMD.[23] The trial was a two-part study that assessed the tolerability of single and repeat eye drop dosing. A phase 2 study to evaluate the pharmacodynamics, safety, and pharmacokinetics of pazopanib eye drops in patients with NV-AMD will begin in 2010.[24,25]

Vatalanib (Novartis, Inc.)

Vatalanib (also known as CGP 79787, CGP-797870, PTK/ZK, PTK787, UNII-5DX9U76296, ZK-232934) is an orally administered tyrosine kinase inhibitor. It causes widespread inhibition of multiple VEGFR tyrosine kinases—VEGFR1 (sFlt-1), VEGFR2 (KDR), and VEGFR3 (Flt-4).[26]

Vatalanib has been studied in a number of preclinical studies and has shown promising results. Daily subcutaneous injections of vatalanib in murine models of retinal NV showed significant inhibition of growth of the lesion.[27] Another model showed reduction in angiogenic changes when a single intravitreal injection was administered.[28] Oral administration also worked well to inhibit CNV[29] and NV in the subretinal space.[27] The drug has been used orally in patients with hematologic and solid malignancies; adverse events including fatigue, diarrhea, hypertension, nausea/vomiting have been reported. However, no serious adverse events have been noted with the use of vatalanib thus far.[30]

Clinical safety and efficacy of oral Vatalanib used in combination with verteporfin (Visudyne; Novartis, Inc) or ranibizumab are being evaluated in patients with subfoveal CNV secondary to AMD in a randomized, double-masked, multicenter, phase 1/2 clinical trial (ADVANCE). The study enrolled 50 patients and initially started with three cohorts: Visudyne + PTK787, 500 mg/day; Visudyne + PTK787, 1,000 mg/day; Visudyne + placebo. The protocol was then modified to use ranibizumab with PTK787 for participants in the second cohort so as to reflect the current standard of care for AMD patients. The primary ouwtcome measure was to assess safety of vatalanib in patients with AMD. Assessment of change in visual acuity, macular edema, and fluorescein leakage from baseline were secondary outcome measures.[31]

TG100801 (TargeGen Inc.)

TG100801 is an inactive prodrug, which generates the active molecule TG100572 by deesterification. TG100572 inhibits Src kinases and VEGF and PDGFR kinases. Topical formulation is available and is believed to reach the site of action by penetration through the sclera.[32] Systemic delivery of TG100572 in a murine model of laser-induced CNV caused significant suppression of CNV but with an associated weight loss suggestive of systemic toxicity. To minimize systemic exposure, topical delivery of TG100572 to the eye was explored, and while substantial levels of TG100572 were achieved in the retina and choroid, higher levels were achieved using TG100801. TG100801 is sufficiently small to cross the sclera enabling an effective topical formulation to be developed. Topical TG100801 significantly suppressed laser-induced CNV in mice, reduced fluorescein leakage from the vasculature and retinal thickening measured by optical coherence tomography in a rat model of retinal vein occlusion. The data suggested that TG100801 may provide a new topically applied treatment approach for ocular NV and retinal edema.[32]

A phase 1 trial using TG10081 on 42 healthy volunteers has been completed. Preliminary results suggest that the drug is safe for topical administration in human eyes when used twice a day for 14 days.[33]

Unfortunately, the phase 2 multicenter clinical trial of TG100801 in patients with NV-AMD was discontinued because of keratopathy.[33,34]

Integrin Inhibitors

JSM6427 (Jerini Ophthalmic, Inc.)

Integrins are an important family of cell surface receptors composed of α-β heterodimers. They play important roles in intercellular adhesion, adhesion to the extracellular matrix, and transmitting signals between cells and from the extracellular matrix.[35,36] Different combinations of α-β heterodimers have specific functions in different tissues.[36]

Integrins are believed to be involved in angiogenesis via transmitting signals from the extracellular matrix, and as downstream effectors of growth factors like VEGF, FGF, and others.[36,37] Angiogenic growth factors like FGF and TGF are associated with upregulation of integrin α5β1.[38,39]

Campochiaro and colleagues showed that integrin α5β1 is upregulated in mouse models of CNV and plays an important role in its development and maintenance.[36] Furthermore, they demonstrated that systemic administration of JSM6427, a highly selective competitive antagonist of integrin α5β1, successfully inhibited development of new and promoted regression of established CNV. However, in this study, they were unable to show significant inhibition of CNV following intravitreal administration of JSM6427. The authors suggested that sustained intravitreal drug levels are probably required to provide sufficient inhibition. Endothelial cells in normal vessels are not dependent on α5β1; hence, JSM6427 can provide specific inhibition of pathological CNV.[36] The specificity of the drug for pathological vessels suggests a good safety profile.

A phase 1, open-label study using single and repeated intravitreal dosing of JSM6427 was recruiting patients with subfoveal NV due to AMD. The trial was using the drug in four different concentrations: 1.5, 3, 7.5, or 15 mg/mL. The primary outcome measure was to determine the maximum tolerated dose. Other outcome measures included the pharmacokinetics of JSM6427 following single and multiple intravitreal injections and preliminary data on efficacy.[13] Due to various reasons, the sponsor, Jerini Ophthalmic, Inc., had to discontinue the study. Hopefully, JSM6427 will be evaluated in other studies in the future.

Volociximab (Ophthotech, Inc.)

Volociximab is a chimeric monoclonal IgG4 antibody that binds $\alpha_5\beta_1$ integrin. It was developed for the treatment of solid tumors and is being tested for the treatment of CNV by Ophthotech Corporation. The molecule has been demonstrated to inhibit endothelial cell proliferation and angiogenesis in in vitro assays. When administered by intravitreal injection concurrently with laser-induced Bruch membrane rupture and then weekly, it inhibits the development of laser-induced CNV in cynomolgus monkeys.[40]

A phase 1 dose-escalating trial of intravitreal volociximab in combination with ranibizumab is currently recruiting subjects. The trial has aimed to enroll 50 subjects to establish the safety, tolerability, and pharmacokinetics profile of intravitreal injection of volociximab in subjects with NV-AMD. The primary safety end point aims at determining the presence of any dose-limiting toxicity within a 2-year time frame.

PIGMENT EPITHELIAL–DERIVED FACTOR

Pigment epithelial–derived factor (PEDF) is a protein normally synthesized by the retinal pigment epithelium. It has been identified as an important inhibitor of angiogenesis[41]—ischemic cultured cells are associated with lower levels of PEDF; PEDF levels also have been reported to be lower than normal in ocular diseases like proliferative diabetic retinopathy and CNV.[42,43] PEDF inhibits angiogenesis via various mechanisms, which include inducing apoptosis of endothelial cells[44,45] and downregulating VEGF expression.[46] Furthermore, PEDF is a neuroprotective agent and part of its clinical efficacy may be due to its protective effect on the neurosensory retina.

An E1-, partial E3-, and E4-deleted adenovirus vector was developed to carry the PEDF and formulate the drug—ADGVPEDF.11 (GenVec, Inc.). Intravitreal and subretinal injections of the recombinant adenoviral vector in three different animal models were able to achieve concentrations of PEDF that were sufficiently high to inhibit CNV.[47] Further preclinical studies showed that injections were able to cause regression of established CNV.[48] Although recognized as an antiangiogenic agent at physiological levels, PEDF has been reported to have proangiogenic effects when used at high doses in laser-induced CNV models in mice. The authors suggested that caution should be exercised when using this agent in dose-escalation clinical trials and also mentioned that drug delivery via an adenoviral vector may not produce the same effect.[49]

The safety of AdPEDF in 28 patients with NV-AMD was tested in a phase 1, dose-escalation, multicenter clinical trial as the first study employing gene therapy in NV-AMD. The drug was administered via intravitreal injection. Eight dose levels ranging from 10(6) to 10(9.5) particle units were tested. Safety of the injection was closely monitored in thirteen visits conducted over a year. The injection was well tolerated by most patients, with only minimal transient inflammation noted in a few.[50] Three to six months after injection 50% of the patients treated with 10(6) to 10(7.5) PU and 94% and 71% of those treated with 10(8) to 10(9.5) PU had either stabilization or decrease in size of lesion. In the high-dose group, the effect of the drug on the lesion was sustained at 12 months after injection, when the authors reported a median increase in lesion size of zero disc areas.[50] No serious drug-related adverse effects[51–53] have been reported thus far among the patients in this phase 1 study.

BIOACTIVE LIPIDS

There is increasing recognition that many classes of lipids, especially metabolites of cell membrane components, have a role in signal transduction and in regulation of multiple cellular processes. Lipids with such roles are known as "bioactive lipids." The sphingolipids, formed from the condensation of serine and palmitate, are of particular interest in the regulation of the vascular endothelium. The sphingolipid, sphingomyelin, is an important component of cellular membranes. It is synthesized from and broken down to ceramide, which in turn is broken down by ceramidase to yield sphingosine, and then phosphorylated by the sphingosine kinases (SK1 and SK2) to yield sphingosine-1-phosphate (S1P). S1P is the ligand for five different cell-surface S1P receptors. S1P receptors and SKs have all been shown to be present in the eye.[54]

S1P is intimately involved in regulation of endothelial function. $S1P_1$ receptors are required for recruitment of vascular smooth muscle cells and pericytes during mouse embryonic vessel formation.[55] S1P induces proliferation and migration of human endothelial cells[56] and regulates basal and angiopoietin-1–mediated endothelial permeability.[57] There is extensive cross talk between S1P and vascular endothelial cell growth factor receptors: S1P can activate VEGFR-2 in the absence of VEGF; VEGF sensitizes endothelium to the action of S1P by upregulating its receptors; activated PDGF receptor activates SK1 on the cell membrane, activating S1PR1. S1P has a role in animal models of retinal disease. In mice, an anti-S1P monoclonal antibody inhibits the development of laser-induced CNV.[54]

S1P2 receptor knock-out mice demonstrate reduced angiogenesis in the oxygen-induced retinopathy model.[58] Systemic treatment with a small molecule inhibitor of SK significantly reduced retinal fluorescein leakage in diabetic rats.[59]

Sonepcizumab (iSONEP; Lpath, Inc.), is a humanized monoclonal antibody that specifically binds S1P. Intraocular injection of sonepcizumab significantly reduced macrophage influx into ischemic retina and strongly suppressed retinal NV in mice with oxygen-induced ischemic retinopathy. In mice with laser-induced rupture sites in Bruch membrane, intraocular injection of sonepcizumab significantly reduced the area of CNV and concomitantly reduced fluorescein leakage from the remaining CNV. Four weeks after intraocular injection of up to 1.8 mg of the sonepcizumab in nonhuman primates, electroretinogram and fluorescein angiograms were normal, and light microscopy of ocular sections showed no evidence of structural damage. Data collected from animal studies show that S1P stimulates both choroidal and retinal NV and suggest that sonepcizumab could be considered for evaluation in patients with choroidal or retinal NV.[60]

A monoclonal antibody against S1P has been humanized and is in phase 1 trials as an antiangiogenic agent in cancer treatment. A phase 1 dose-escalating trial is ongoing to evaluate the safety and the preliminary efficacy of single intravitreal injection of five different doses of iSONEP in 15 subjects with NV-AMD. The tested doses range from 0.2 to 1.8 mg, and the subjects will be followed for 12 months.

NICOTINE RECEPTOR ANTAGONISTS

ATG003 (CoMentis, Inc.) is the ophthalmic formulation of the drug mecamylamine. Mecamylamine is a nonspecific antagonist of the nicotine receptor. Nicotine is an alkaloid present in plants such as tobacco and coca. It is fat soluble and can therefore easily cross cell membranes. It is mainly metabolized in the liver to cotinine and excreted in the kidneys.[61] Nicotine binds to acetylcholine receptors (AChRs) located on the cell membrane. Over the last decade, nicotinic receptors have been found to be located in multiple nonneuronal tissues, including human endothelial cells.[62] Kiuchi and colleagues demonstrated in 2008 that nicotine receptors are expressed on retinal and choroidal endothelial cells.[63]

Nicotine receptors are made up of multiple subunits (α1-α10, β1-β4, γ, δ, and ε). Endothelial cells possess an α7 AChR, which, when stimulated, indirectly leads to activation of the integrin $\alpha v\beta 3$ receptor and an intracellular mitogen-activated protein kinase (ERK) pathway that further leads to angiogenesis.[64] Specific antagonists of this receptor such as α-bungarotoxin and [65] as well as the nonspecific antagonist mecamylamine have been shown to inhibit proliferation of endothelial cells from different tissues.[66]

In addition to direct effects mediated via the AChR, nicotine has also been shown to induce angiogenic factors like FGF, PDGF, and VEGF.[67,68] It was also found that nicotine increases the expression of VEGF-2 receptor.[69] Nicotine increased the size of the laser-induced choroidal neovascular lesions in mice, but the CNV was inhibited by subcutaneous infusion of 50 mg/kg/day of mecamylamine. Moreover, mecamylamine inhibited growth of CNV lesion even in the absence of exogenous administration of nicotine, implying that acetylcholine is responsible for stimulating nicotinic receptors in vivo and promoting growth of CNV. It has been demonstrated that topical drops of 0.1% or 1% mecamylamine can significantly decrease CNV in mice.[63] The success of the topical drops in mice led to testing in humans.

Topical formulation of ATG3 (mecamylamine HCl) was evaluated in a phase 1 randomized, double-masked, placebo-controlled study that enrolled 80 healthy volunteers in single and multiple dose ascending regimens for up to 14 days of therapy. Subjects received the eye drops twice daily. There were no study medication-related systemic side effects. Mecamylamine levels in plasma were found to be very low following eye drop application. Two Phase 2 studies, one comparing the safety and efficacy of two formulations of ATG003 (1.0% and 0.3%) versus placebo in patients with neovascular age-related macular degeneration (NV-AMD), and another comparing 1.0% ATG003 versus placebo in patients on treatment with anti-VEGF therapy for NV-AMD have been conducted; the former study has been terminated, the latter is ongoing.[70,71]

mTOR PATHWAY MODULATORS

Sirolimus (MacuSight Inc.)

Sirolimus (rapamycin) is a macrolide antibiotic that is produced naturally by *Streptomyces hygroscopicus*.[72] The mechanism of action of sirolimus in immunomodulation has been described extensively in medical literature.[73–76] Sirolimus binds to FKBP12 forming a complex that binds to the mammalian target of rapamycin (mTOR), inhibiting its function in the mTORC1 complex.[77] mTOR is a key component in the cell's response to insulin, insulin-like growth factors, nutrient levels, hypoxia, and redox status. mTOR forms the complexes mTORC1 and mTORC2.[78] mTORC1 promotes translation by phosphorylating and activating the p70-S6 Kinase 1 (S6K1) and phosphorylating and inactivating eukaryotic initiation factor 4E (eIF4E)-binding protein 1(4E-BP1), which is a repressor of translation.[78] The inhibition of mTOR blocks IL-2–mediated signal transduction pathways. Such blockage arrests cell cycle progression from G1 to S phase in T cells, endothelial cells, osteosarcoma cells, myogenic cell lines, and smooth muscle cells.[74,79] In addition, sirolimus inhibits the production of antibodies.[74,80]

Sirolimus' inhibition of mTOR activity has been shown to impact a number of the components of the angiogenic process. Sirolimus inhibits the production, signaling, and activity of many growth factors reported to be relevant to the development of dry eye syndrome, diabetic retinopathy, and CNV. Moreover, sirolimus can modulate the contribution of progenitor stem cells to CNV, reduce permeability, blunt complement-mediated effects and down-regulate genes involved in the inflammatory process.[81–87]

It is hypothesized that as mTOR plays a critical role in regulating basic cellular functions including cell proliferation, survival, mobility, and angiogenesis, inhibitors of mTOR are expected to show a therapeutic effect in treating dry eye, posterior uveitis, and the pathological angiogenesis of CNV.

Sirolimus underwent phase 1 testing in a randomized, open-label, dose-escalation clinical study. The study aimed at the assessment of safety, tolerability, and preliminary bioactivity of intravitreal or subconjunctival injection of sirolimus in patients with newly diagnosed NV-AMD. The maximum tested doses in this study were 880 and 176 μg for the subconjunctival and the intravitreal routes, respectively.[88]

A total of 30 patients were enrolled in this study. All patients were followed for 12 months after a single injection of sirolimus. The intravitreal and subconjunctival injections of sirolimus were found to be both safe and tolerable in all tested doses when used either as intravitreal or as subconjunctival injections. In addition, sirolimus showed preliminary bioactivity indicated by improvements in visual acuity that were associated with corresponding reductions in retinal thickness as detected by optical coherence tomography. The preliminary findings demonstrated that sirolimus administered via subconjunctival injections (Fig. 11.3) was as effective as sirolimus administered via intravitreal injections (Fig. 11.4).[88] Intravitreal injections, while currently the standard route of administration for AMD therapies, are uncomfortable for many patients and are accompanied by the risk of serious infection in a small percentage of patients. In contrast, subconjunctival injections are designed to offer physicians and patients a less invasive and more convenient procedure.[88]

Currently, Macusight, Inc. is sponsoring a phase 2 clinical trial that is randomizing patients with newly diagnosed subfoveal CNV secondary to AMD into two treatment arms: 1,320 μg of subconjunctival injections and 352 μg of intravitreal injections. Sirolimus will be injected at days 0, 60, and 120 and the patients will be followed up for 12 months following day 0.[89] Another phase 2 study is a randomized, masked, controlled clinical trial that aims at the assessment of the safety and efficacy of combined subconjunctival sirolimus and intravitreal ranibizumab therapy in patients with NV-AMD. A total of 60 patients will be randomized into one of three treatments arms: 440 μg of subconjunctival sirolimus plus 500 μg of intravitreal ranibizumab; 1,320 μg of subconjunctival sirolimus plus 500 μg of intravitreal ranibizumab; and 500 μg of intravitreal ranibizumab plus placebo. The main outcomes will be visual acuity and central macular thickness.[90]

The National Eye Institute is also conducting a study assessing the role of immunomodulatory agents in combination with routine care using antiangiogenic therapies for the treatment of subfoveal CNV secondary to AMD. Twenty patients are to be randomly assigned to one of four study arms: intravenous daclizumab, intravenous infliximab, oral sirolimus, or no study medication. The study will assess recurrence of NV, as well as changes in visual acuity and retinal thickening as measured by optical coherence tomography over 24-week intervals.[91]

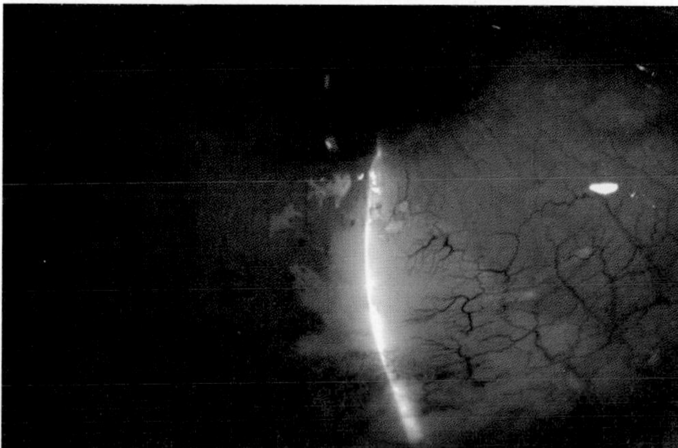

FIGURE 11.3. Slit-lamp image showing white subconjunctival deposits following subconjunctival injection of sirolimus.

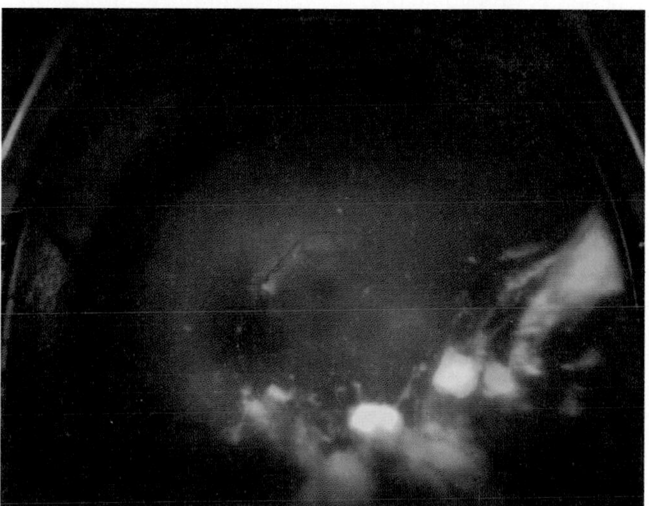

FIGURE 11.4. Wide-angle fundus image showing whitish vitreal deposits of drug materials following intravitreal injection of sirolimus. The image was acquired using Optomap P200MA Camera (OPTOS, Dunfermline, Scotland, UK).

BOX 11.2 Other Trials in Wet Macular Degeneration

ADVANCE Trial: Safety and Efficacy of Oral PTK787 in Patients With Subfoveal CNV Secondary to AMD
Purpose: A phase 1/2 randomized, double-masked, multicenter to compare PK787 (Vatalanib) (tyrosine kinase inhibitor) (Novartis) and ranibizumab in neovascular ARMD.
Status: Completed.
MONET Study: Phase 2 Open-Label Multicenter Study For Age-Related Macular Degeneration Comparing An Investigational Drug PF-04523655 Versus Lucentis In The Treatment Of Subjects With CNV
Purpose: To compare PF-04523655, a synthetic, siRNA that inhibits the expression of the hypoxia-inducible gene, RTP801 gene, and ranibizumab in patients with subfoveal neovascular ARMD.
Method: Please see text for details.
Status: Recruitment phase.
CARE Trial: Safety and Efficacy Study of Small Interfering RNA Molecule (Cand5) to Treat Wet Age-Related Macular Degeneration
Purpose: A phase 2 trial examined the efficacy of bevasiranib (Cand 5) (Acuity Pharmaceuticals), a siRNA that silences production of VEGF, in patients with neovascular ARMD. This siRNA catalytically destroys VEGF mRNA to silence gene expression, thus targeting the production of VEGF. It, however, does not affect the already produced VEGF protein.
Status: Although the phase 2 trials showed the efficacy of the drug, "on March 6, 2009, OPKO decided to terminate the phase 3 clinical trial (COBALT) of bevasiranib based on the recommendation of the Independent Data Monitoring Committee that the bevasiranib clinical trial, as designed, was unlikely to achieve its primary endpoint of reducing vision loss" (OPKO press release).

PF-04523655 (Quark/Pfizer)

PF-4523655 (formerly RTP801i-14) is a synthetic, small interfering RNA (siRNA) that acts via RNA interference to inhibit the expression of RTP801 gene. RTP801 is a hypoxia-inducible gene that was first reported by Quark Pharmaceuticals Inc. in 2002.[92] RTP801 expression acts via the TSC1/TSC2 tumor suppressor complex to inhibit mTOR.[93,94] Expression of the RTP801 gene is dramatically upregulated in response to hypoxia and/or oxidative stress, which leads to the induction of neuronal cell apoptosis. RTP801 is upregulated in the retinas of mice and rats in a model of retinopathy of prematurity, meanwhile, RTP801 knockout mice exhibited attenuated pathology.[95]

As expression of RTP801 is rapidly upregulated in response to ischemia, hypoxia, and/or oxidative stress, it represents a unique gene target that may regulate hypoxia-induced pathogenesis by a mechanism that is independent of growth factors like VEGF. Both geneticin-hibition (RTP801-knockout) and intravitreal injection of PF-04523655 in preclinical animal models of laser-induced CNV led to inhibition of RTP801 expression, induction of expression of antiangiogenic and neurotrophic factors, and subsequent reduction of CNV volume, vessel leakage, and choroid infiltration of inflammatory cells.[96]

In a phase 1 open-label, dose-escalation trial of PF-04523655 delivered by a single intravitreal injection to patients with CNV secondary to AMD is currently ongoing. The study aims to enroll 54 subjects. Subjects are to receive a single intravitreal injection of PF-04523655 in one of nine doses that range between 50 and 3,000 μg. The subjects will be followed for toxic effects for 24 months.[97]

A phase 2 prospective, randomized, dose-ranging study of PF-04523655 in comparison with ranibizumab, for the treatment of subfoveal CNV secondary to AMD (MONET Study), is being planned. The study will determine whether an initial injection of ranibizumab is required before starting PF-04523655. The study will randomize subjects into one of five arms. All subjects will receive an initial dose of 0.5 mg ranibizumab intravitreally. Arm 1 will continue receiving intravitreal ranibizumab alone every 4 weeks until week 12. Arms 2, 3, and 4 will receive different doses of intravitreal PF-04523655 from week 4 to 12 at different time points. Arm 5 will receive a combination of 0.5-mg intravitreal ranibizumab and 1-mg PF-04523655 every 4 weeks from baseline to week 12. The primary outcome measures will be the mean change in the BCVA by week 16. Secondary outcome measures will include the changes in the central retinal thickness as measured by OCT at week 16 compared to baseline, changes in the lesion size as detected by FA at week 16, and the incidence and severity of ocular and systemic adverse events by week 48. The phase 2 study aims at the enrollment of 150 subjects (Box 11.2).[98]

SUMMARY

Throughout the pages of this chapter, we have hoped to give the readers a glimpse of selected future classes of agents that are in clinical testing for NV-AMD, including VEGFR Decoy, Tyrosine Kinase Inhibitors, Integrin Inhibitors, PEDF, Bioactive Lipids, Nicotine Receptor Antagonists, mTOR Pathway Modulators, and siRNA. However,

KEY POINTS

- The VEGF pathway has been inhibited by various means, including blocking antibodies targeted against VEGF or its receptors, soluble decoy receptors that prevent VEGF from binding to its normal receptors, as well as small molecule inhibitors of the tyrosine kinase activity of the VEGFRs.
- VEGF Trap, a fusion protein, is distinguished from ranibizumab by its higher binding affinity for all VEGF-A isoforms and its ability to inhibit other VEGF family members (placental growth factors 1 and 2, VEGF-B, -C, and -D).
- The CLEAR-IT-2 study using VEGF Trap has shown significant visual acuity improvements in patients with neovascular ARMD. The VIEW I and II studies, two phase 3 clinical trials, are going to compare VEGF Trap and ranbizumab in neovascular ARMD.
- Pigment epithelium–derived factor (PEDF) is a potent endogenous angiogenesis inhibitor. A phase 1 clinical trial using intravitreal injection of an adenovirus vector carrying the PEDF gene has been shown to be without any adverse effects.
- Other inhibitors including bioactive lipids, nicotine receptor antagonists, and mTOR pathway modulators are being investigated in clinical trials in neovascular ARMD.

we have not meant to be all-inclusive. In addition, there are several significant areas of therapeutic need not met by the therapies described in this book. Such areas include repair of areas of RPE loss, repair of atrophied choriocapillaris, elimination of the fibrotic component of CNV, and protection against loss of retinal tissue in both neovascular and non-NV-AMD. Hopefully, with the continuing advancements of basic and clinical research, pharmacotherapy for these and other areas will be covered in future editions of *Therapy of Ocular Angiogenesis: Principles and Practices*.

REFERENCES

1. Friedman DS, O'Colmain BJ, Munoz B, et al. Prevalence of age-related macular degeneration in the United States. *Arch Ophthalmol.* 2004;122:564–572.
2. Rein DB, Wittenborn JS, Zhang X, et al. Forecasting age-related macular degeneration through the year 2050: the potential impact of new treatments. *Arch Ophthalmol.* 2009;127:533–540.
3. Holash J, Davis S, Papadopoulos N, et al. VEGF-Trap: a VEGF blocker with potent antitumor effects. *Proc Natl Acad Sci U S A.* 2002;99:11393–11398.
4. Carmeliet P, Moons L, Luttun A, et al. Synergism between vascular endothelial growth factor and placental growth factor contributes to angiogenesis and plasma extravasation in pathological conditions. *Nat Med.* 2001;7:575–583.
5. Asano M, Yukita A, Matsumoto T, et al. An anti-human VEGF monoclonal antibody, MV833, that exhibits potent anti-tumor activity in vivo. *Hybridoma.* 1998;17:185–190.
6. Kamiya K, Konno H, Tanaka T, et al. Antitumor effect on human gastric cancer and induction of apoptosis by vascular endothelial growth factor neutralizing antibody. *Jpn J Cancer Res.* 1999;90:794–800.
7. Kim KJ, Li B, Winer J, et al. Inhibition of vascular endothelial growth factor-induced angiogenesis suppresses tumour growth in vivo. *Nature.* 1993;362:841–844.
8. Prewett M, Huber J, Li Y, et al. Antivascular endothelial growth factor receptor (fetal liver kinase 1) monoclonal antibody inhibits tumor angiogenesis and growth of several mouse and human tumors. *Cancer Res.* 1999;59:5209–5218.
9. Ferrara N, Chen H, Davis-Smyth T, et al. Vascular endothelial growth factor is essential for corpus luteum angiogenesis. *Nat Med.* 1998;4:336–340.
10. Gerber HP, Hillan KJ, Ryan AM, et al. VEGF is required for growth and survival in neonatal mice. *Development.* 1999;126:1149–1159.
11. Gerber HP, Vu TH, Ryan AM, et al. VEGF couples hypertrophic cartilage remodeling, ossification and angiogenesis during endochondral bone formation. *Nat Med.* 1999;5: 623–628.
12. Goldman CK, Kendall RL, Cabrera G, et al. Paracrine expression of a native soluble vascular endothelial growth factor receptor inhibits tumor growth, metastasis, and mortality rate. *Proc Natl Acad Sci U S A.* 1998;95:8795–8800.
13. Millauer B, Longhi MP, Plate KH, et al. Dominant-negative inhibition of Flk-1 suppresses the growth of many tumor types in vivo. *Cancer Res.* 1996;56:1615–1620.
14. Drevs J, Hofmann I, Hugenschmidt H, et al. Effects of PTK787/ZK 222584, a specific inhibitor of vascular endothelial growth factor receptor tyrosine kinases, on primary tumor, metastasis, vessel density, and blood flow in a murine renal cell carcinoma model. *Cancer Res.* 2000;60:4819–4824.
15. Fong TA, Shawver LK, Sun L, et al. SU5416 is a potent and selective inhibitor of the vascular endothelial growth factor receptor (Flk-1/KDR) that inhibits tyrosine kinase catalysis, tumor vascularization, and growth of multiple tumor types. *Cancer Res.* 1999;59:99–106.
16. Wedge SR, Ogilvie DJ, Dukes M, et al. ZD4190: an orally active inhibitor of vascular endothelial growth factor signaling with broad-spectrum antitumor efficacy. *Cancer Res.* 2000;60:970–975.
17. Gerber HP, Kowalski J, Sherman D, et al. Complete inhibition of rhabdomyosarcoma xenograft growth and neovascularization requires blockade of both tumor and host vascular endothelial growth factor. *Cancer Res.* 2000;60:6253–6258.
18. Kuo CJ, Farnebo F, Yu EY, et al. Comparative evaluation of the antitumor activity of antiangiogenic proteins delivered by gene transfer. *Proc Natl Acad Sci U S A.* 2001;98:4605–4610.
19. Nguyen QD, Shah SM, Hafiz G, et al. A phase 1 trial of an IV-administered vascular endothelial growth factor trap for treatment in patients with choroidal neovascularization due to age-related macular degeneration. *Ophthalmology.* 2006;113:1522 e1–1522 e14.
20. Saishin Y, Takahashi K, Lima e Silva R, et al. VEGF-TRAP(R1R2) suppresses choroidal neovascularization and VEGF-induced breakdown of the blood-retinal barrier. *J Cell Physiol.* 2003;195:241–248.

21. Nguyen QD, Shah SM, Browning DJ, et al. A phase 1 study of intravitreal vascular endothelial growth factor trap-eye in patients with neovascular age-related macular degeneration. *Ophthalmology.* 2009;116:2141–2148 e1.
22. Takahashi K, Saishin Y, Saishin Y, et al. Suppression and regression of choroidal neovascularization by the multitargeted kinase inhibitor pazopanib. *Arch Ophthalmol.* 2009;127:494–499.
23. http://www.clinicaltrials.gov/ct2/results?term=NCT00463320., 2007.
24. ClinicalTrials.gov
25. http://www.clinicaltrials.gov/ct2/results?term=NCT00733304., 2008.
26. Emerson MV, Lauer AK. Current and emerging therapies for the treatment of age-related macular degeneration. *Clin Ophthalmol.* 2008;2:377–388.
27. Ozaki H, Seo M-S, Ozaki K, et al. Blockade of vascular endothelial cell growth factor receptor signaling is sufficient to completely prevent retinal neovascularization. *Am J Pathol.* 2000;156:697–707.
28. Maier P, Unsoeld AS, Junker B, et al. Intravitreal injection of specific receptor tyrosine kinase inhibitor PTK787/ZK222 584 improves ischemia-induced retinopathy in mice. *Graefes Arch Clin Exp Ophthalmol.* 2005;243:593–600.
29. Kwak N, Okamoto N, Wood JM, et al. VEGF is major stimulator in model of choroidal neovascularization. *Invest Ophthalmol Vis Sci.* 2000;41:3158–3164.
30. Thomas AL, Morgan B, Horsfield MA, et al. Phase 1 study of the safety, tolerability, pharmacokinetics, and pharmacodynamics of PTK787/ZK 222584 administered twice daily in patients with advanced cancer. *J Clin Oncol.* 2005;23: 4162–4171.
31. Regnery R, Tappero J. Unraveling mysteries associated with cat-scratch disease, bacillary angiomatosis, and related syndromes. *Emerg Infect Dis.* 1995;1:16–21.
32. Doukas J, Mahesh S, Umeda N, et al. Topical administration of a multi-targeted kinase inhibitor suppresses choroidal neovascularization and retinal edema. *J Cell Physiol.* 2008;216:29–37.
33. http://www.targegen.com/news022707.htm. 2007.
34. http://clinicaltrials.gov/ct2/show/NCT00509548?term=TG100801&rank=2., 2007.
35. Hynes RO. Integrins: versatility, modulation, and signaling in cell adhesion. *Cell.* 1992;69:11–25.
36. Umeda N, Kachi S, Akiyama H, et al. Suppression and regression of choroidal neovascularization by systemic administration of an alpha5beta1 integrin antagonist. *Mol Pharmacol.* 2006;69:1820–1828.
37. Maier AK, Kociok N, Zahn G, et al. Modulation of hypoxia-induced neovascularization by JSM6427, an integrin alpha5-beta1 inhibiting molecule. *Curr Eye Res.* 2007;32:801–812.
38. Enenstein J, Waleh NS, Kramer RH. Basic FGF and TGF-beta differentially modulate integrin expression of human microvascular endothelial cells. *Exp Cell Res* 1992;203:499–503.
39. Yeh CH, Peng HC, Huang TF. Cytokines modulate integrin alpha(v)beta(3)-mediated human endothelial cell adhesion and calcium signaling. *Exp Cell Res* 1999;251:57–66.
40. Ramakrishnan V, Bhaskar V, Law DA, et al. Preclinical evaluation of an anti-alpha5beta1 integrin antibody as a novel anti-angiogenic agent. *J Exp Ther Oncol.* 2006;5:273–286.
41. Dawson DW, Volpert OV, Gillis P, et al. Pigment epithelium-derived factor: a potent inhibitor of angiogenesis. *Science.* 1999;285:245–248.
42. Spranger J, Osterhoff M, Reimann M, et al. Loss of the anti-angiogenic pigment epithelium-derived factor in patients with angiogenic eye disease. *Diabetes.* 2001;50:2641–2645.
43. Tong JP, Yao YF. Contribution of VEGF and PEDF to choroidal angiogenesis: a need for balanced expressions. *Clin Biochem.* 2006;39:267–276.
44. Volpert OV, Zaichuk T, Zhou W, et al. Inducer-stimulated Fas targets activated endothelium for destruction by anti-angiogenic thrombospondin-1 and pigment epithelium-derived factor. *Nat Med.* 2002;8:349–357.
45. Elayappan B, Ravinarayannan H, Sardar Pasha SP, et al. PEDF inhibits VEGF- and EPO- induced angiogenesis in retinal endothelial cells through interruption of PI3K/Akt phosphorylation. *Angiogenesis.* 2009;12:313–324.
46. Takenaka K, Yamagishi S, Jinnouchi Y, et al. Pigment epithelium-derived factor (PEDF)-induced apoptosis and inhibition of vascular endothelial growth factor (VEGF) expression in MG63 human osteosarcoma cells. *Life Sci.* 2005;77:3231–3241.
47. Mori K, Duh E, Gehlbach P, et al. Pigment epithelium-derived factor inhibits retinal and choroidal neovascularization. *J Cell Physiol.* 2001;188:253–263.
48. Mori K, Gehlbach P, Ando A, et al. Regression of ocular neovascularization in response to increased expression of pigment epithelium-derived factor. *Invest Ophthalmol Vis Sci.* 2002;43:2428–2434.
49. Apte RS, Barreiro RA, Duh E, et al. Stimulation of neovascularization by the anti-angiogenic factor PEDF. *Invest Ophthalmol Vis Sci.* 2004;45:4491–4497.
50. Campochiaro PA, Nguyen QD, Shah SM, et al. Adenoviral vector-delivered pigment epithelium-derived factor for neovascular age-related macular degeneration: results of a phase 1 clinical trial. *Hum Gene Ther.* 2006;17:167–176.
51. Arand M. RNA interference, anti-integrins and retinol binders. New strategies to control blindness in the elderly. *MMW Fortschr Med.* 2008;150:18.
52. Rasmussen H, Chu KW, Campochiaro P, et al. Clinical protocol. An open-label, phase 1, single administration, dose-escalation study of ADGVPEDF.11D (ADPEDF) in neovascular age-related macular degeneration (AMD). *Hum Gene Ther.* 2001;12:2029–2032.
53. Tomillero A, Moral MA. Gateways to clinical trials. December 2008. *Methods Find Exp Clin Pharmacol.* 2008;30:761–782.
54. Caballero S, Swaney J, Moreno K, et al. Anti-sphingosine-1-phosphate monoclonal antibodies inhibit angiogenesis and sub-retinal fibrosis in a murine model of laser-induced choroidal neovascularization. *Exp Eye Res.* 2009;88:367–377.
55. Liu Y, Wada R, Yamashita T, et al. Edg-1, the G protein-coupled receptor for sphingosine-1-phosphate, is essential for vascular maturation. *J Clin Invest.* 2000;106:951–961.
56. Kimura T, Watanabe T, Sato K, et al. Sphingosine 1-phosphate stimulates proliferation and migration of human endothelial cells possibly through the lipid receptors, Edg-1 and Edg-3. *Biochem J.* 2000;348(pt 1):71–76.
57. Li X, Stankovic M, Bonder CS, et al. Basal and angiopoietin-1-mediated endothelial permeability is regulated by sphingosine kinase-1. *Blood.* 2008;111:3489–3497.

58. Skoura A, Sanchez T, Claffey K, et al. Essential role of sphingosine 1-phosphate receptor 2 in pathological angiogenesis of the mouse retina. *J Clin Invest*. 2007;117: 2506–2516.
59. Maines LW, French KJ, Wolpert EB, et al. Pharmacologic manipulation of sphingosine kinase in retinal endothelial cells: implications for angiogenic ocular diseases. *Invest Ophthalmol Vis Sci*. 2006;47:5022–5031.
60. Xie B, Shen J, Dong A, et al. Blockade of sphingosine-1-phosphate reduces macrophage influx and retinal and choroidal neovascularization. *J Cell Physiol*. 2009;218:192–198.
61. Kilaru S, Frangos SG, Chen AH, et al. Nicotine: a review of its role in atherosclerosis. *J Am Coll Surg*. 2001;193:538–546.
62. Macklin KD, Maus AD, Pereira EF, et al. Human vascular endothelial cells express functional nicotinic acetylcholine receptors. *J Pharmacol Exp Ther*. 1998;287:435–439.
63. Kiuchi K, Matsuoka M, Wu JC, et al. Mecamylamine suppresses basal and nicotine-stimulated choroidal neovascularization. *Invest Ophthalmol Vis Sci*. 2008;49:1705–1711.
64. Heeschen C, Weis M, Aicher A, et al. A novel angiogenic pathway mediated by non-neuronal nicotinic acetylcholine receptors. *J Clin Invest*. 2002;110:527–536.
65. Beckel JM, Kanai A, Lee SJ, et al. Expression of functional nicotinic acetylcholine receptors in rat urinary bladder epithelial cells. *Am J Physiol Renal Physiol*. 2006;290:F103–F110.
66. Ng MK, Wu J, Chang E, et al. A central role for nicotinic cholinergic regulation of growth factor-induced endothelial cell migration. *Arterioscler Thromb Vasc Biol*. 2007;27:106–112.
67. Mousa S, Mousa SA. Cellular and molecular mechanisms of nicotine's pro-angiogenesis activity and its potential impact on cancer. *J Cell Biochem*. 2006;97:1370–1378.
68. Cooke JP. Angiogenesis and the role of the endothelial nicotinic acetylcholine receptor. *Life Sci*. 2007;80:2347–2351.
69. Jacobi J, Jang JJ, Sundram U, et al. Nicotine accelerates angiogenesis and wound healing in genetically diabetic mice. *Am J Pathol*. 2002;161:97–104.
70. http://clinicaltrials.gov/ct2/show/NCT00607750
71. http://clinicaltrials.gov/ct2/show/NCT00414206
72. Tee AR, Blenis J. mTOR, translational control and human disease. *Semin Cell Dev Biol*. 2005;16:29–37.
73. Napoli KL, Taylor PJ. From beach to bedside: history of the development of sirolimus. *Ther Drug Monit*. 2001;23:559–586.
74. Sehgal SN. Rapamune (RAPA, rapamycin, sirolimus): mechanism of action immunosuppressive effect results from blockade of signal transduction and inhibition of cell cycle progression. *Clin Biochem*. 1998;31:335–340.
75. Kahan BD. Sirolimus: a comprehensive review. *Expert Opin Pharmacother*. 2001;2:1903–1917.
76. Sehgal SN. Sirolimus: its discovery, biological properties, and mechanism of action. *Transplant Proc*. 2003;35:7S–14S.
77. Wan X, Helman LJ. The biology behind mTOR inhibition in sarcoma. *Oncologist*. 2007;12:1007–1018.
78. Hay N, Sonenberg N. Upstream and downstream of mTOR. *Genes Dev*. 2004;18:1926–1945.
79. Kwon YS, Hong HS, Kim JC, et al. Inhibitory effect of rapamycin on corneal neovascularization in vitro and in vivo. *Invest Ophthalmol Vis Sci*. 2005;46:454–460.
80. Sehgal SN. Rapamune (Sirolimus, rapamycin): an overview and mechanism of action. *Ther Drug Monit*. 1995;17:660–665.
81. Aronica SM, Gingras AC, Sonenberg N, et al. Macrophage inflammatory protein-1alpha and interferon-inducible protein 10 inhibit synergistically induced growth factor stimulation of MAP kinase activity and suppress phosphorylation of eukaryotic initiation factor 4E and 4E binding protein 1. *Blood*. 1997;89:3582–3595.
82. Castro C, Campistol JM, Sancho D, et al. Rapamycin attenuates atherosclerosis induced by dietary cholesterol in apolipoprotein-deficient mice through a p27 Kip1 -independent pathway. *Atherosclerosis*. 2004;172:31–38.
83. Attur MG, Patel R, Thakker G, et al. Differential anti-inflammatory effects of immunosuppressive drugs: cyclosporin, rapamycin and FK-506 on inducible nitric oxide synthase, nitric oxide, cyclooxygenase-2 and PGE2 production. *Inflamm Res*. 2000;49:20–26.
84. Butzal M, Loges S, Schweizer M, et al. Rapamycin inhibits proliferation and differentiation of human endothelial progenitor cells in vitro. *Exp Cell Res*. 2004;300:65–71.
85. Nuhrenberg TG, Voisard R, Fahlisch F, et al. Rapamycin attenuates vascular wall inflammation and progenitor cell promoters after angioplasty. *FASEB J*. 2005;19:246–248.
86. Humar R, Kiefer FN, Berns H, et al. Hypoxia enhances vascular cell proliferation and angiogenesis in vitro via rapamycin (mTOR)-dependent signaling. *FASEB J*. 2002;16:771–780.
87. Guba M, von Breitenbuch P, Steinbauer M, et al. Rapamycin inhibits primary and metastatic tumor growth by antiangiogenesis: involvement of vascular endothelial growth factor. *Nat Med*. 2002;8:128–135.
88. http://www.macusight.com/investors_media/press_releases/022508.php. 2008.
89. http://www.clinicaltrials.gov/ct2/show/NCT00712491?term=sirolimus+%2BAMD&rank=3. 2008.
90. http://www.clinicaltrials.gov/ct2/show/NCT00766337?term=sirolimus+%2BAMD&rank=4. 2008.
91. http://clinicalstudies.info.nih.gov/detail/A_2006-EI-0111.html. 2006.
92. Shoshani T, Faerman A, Mett I, et al. Identification of a novel hypoxia-inducible factor 1-responsive gene, RTP801, involved in apoptosis. *Mol Cell Biol*. 2002;22:2283–2293.
93. Brugarolas J, Lei K, Hurley RL, et al. Regulation of mTOR function in response to hypoxia by REDD1 and the TSC1/TSC2 tumor suppressor complex. *Genes Dev*. 2004;18:2893–2904.
94. Corradetti MN, Inoki K, Guan KL. The stress-inducted proteins RTP801 and RTP801L are negative regulators of the mammalian target of rapamycin pathway. *J Biol Chem*. 2005;280:9769–9772.
95. Brafman A, Mett I, Shafir M, et al. Inhibition of oxygen-induced retinopathy in RTP801-deficient mice. *Invest Ophthalmol Vis Sci*. 2004;45:3796–3805.
96. http://www.quarkpharma.com/qbi-en/products/pf-4523655/. 2009.
97. http://www.clinicaltrials.gov/ct2/show/NCT00725686?term=redd14np&rank=2. 2009.
98. http://www.clinicaltrials.gov/ct2/show/NCT00713518?term=pf-04523655&rank=1. 2009.

CHAPTER

12

Safety of Anti-VEGF Drugs

David Boyer • Thomas R. Friberg

INTRODUCTION

Vascular endothelial growth factor-A (VEGF-A) is a member of the platelet-derived growth factor family, promotes angiogenesis, and is a powerful inducer of vascular permeability. Other members of the VEGF family include VEGF-B, VEGF-C, VEGF-D, VEGF-E, and placenta growth factor. VEGF-A, arguably the most important, has different isoforms containing 121, 145, 148, 165, 183, 189, or 208 amino acids. VEGF 189 and 208 are strongly heparin bound and are found in the extracellular matrix. VEGF 165 is partially heparin bound and partially diffusible and is the most common isoform expressed in humans. Furthermore, it causes pathologic neovascularization. VEGF 121 is freely diffusible. When plasmin binds to VEGF-A, VEGF-A 110, an active product, is the result. VEGF-A binds to one of the two tyrosine kinase receptors on the endothelial cell membrane, namely, VEGFR1 or VEGFR2. VEGFR2 is assumed to be the receptor that induces neovascularization.[1–3]

In addition to being associated with the formation of pathologic neovascularization in wet related macular degeneration (AMD), diabetic retinopathy, central retinal vein occlusion, and rubeosis iridis, VEGF-A is also a survival factor. It protects hepatocytes and renal cells, and it is necessary for the maintenance of the choriocapillaris, for wound healing, collateral vessel formation in the heart (atherothrombosis), bone growth, endometrial development, and placental vascularization.[1,4,5]

Small amounts of anti-VEGF drugs (pegaptanib, bevacizumab, and ranizumab) are injected intravitreally into the eye for the treatment of choroidal neovascularization (CNV) associated with AMD. Some drugs gain entrance into the systemic circulation at levels that may inhibit normal circulating levels of VEGF-A. In rhesus monkeys following bilateral injections of 0.5mg of pegaptanib, plasma levels of 0.4 μg/mL of the drug were found. Following one intravitreal injection of 3.0-mg pegaptanib in humans, 80 ng/mL was measured in the plasma. After bilateral injection of 0.5 mg in cynomologous monkeys, serum levels up to 150 ng/mL were measured.[6]

The intravenous administration of anti-VEGF (bevacizumab) medications every 2 weeks with other adjuncts for the treatment of cancer patients is associated with an increase in blood pressure, bleeding, proteinuria, and gastrointestinal perforations, and double the risk of thromboembolic events, including stroke and heart attack. Individuals with AMD have an ischemic stroke risk almost twice as high as those without the disease. In the Blue Mountain Eye Study, prior history of stroke predicted a higher incidence of early AMD (RR 2.32, 95% CI: 1.08–5.01). This association remained significant after controlling for conventional cardiovascular risk factors.[7] Because the use of VEGF inhibitors could theoretically be associated with an increased risk of cardiovascular disease, these events need to be studied to determine if the rate of these severe adverse events (SAEs) is increased with the intravitreal administration of anti-VEGF agents. This has further relevance because patients with wet AMD are at a higher risk for cardiovascular disease, hypertension, and peripheral vascular disease.[2,8,9]

The stimulus that causes CNV is not well understood, but blocking VEGF-A by an intravitreal injection is an effective treatment strategy for CNV associated with AMD. Currently, two anti-VEGF therapies are FDA approved for the treatment of CNV due to AMD. The first drug, pegaptanib (Macugen), is an RNA aptamer that binds to VEGF[10] and was approved in 2004, based on the results from the two pivotal phase 3 VISION trials.[11] The second is ranibizumab (Lucentis), a humanized antigen-binding fragment that binds to all bioactive forms of VEGF-A and their degradation products and was approved in 2006 based on data from three phase 3 pivotal trials: MARINA, ANCHOR, and PIER.[12–15] Bevacizumab (Avastin) is a full-length humanized monoclonal antibody that, similar to ranibizumab, binds to VEGF-A. Although bevacizumab is FDA approved for the treatment of breast, colorectal, and lung cancers, it is used frequently off-label by retinal specialists for the treatment of neovascular AMD.

There are theoretical advantages to selective inhibition of VEGF 165, the pathologic isoform associated with CNV, in reducing systemic SAE and maintaining choriocapillaris health. It is important to analyze randomized clinical trials to determine if this is an actual or purely theoretical risk.

SAFETY OF INTRAVITREAL RANIBIZUMAB, PEGAPTANIB, AND BEVACIZUMAB

A total of 3,863 subjects participated in the MARINA, ANCHOR, PIER, FOCUS, and SAILOR trials, out of whom 3,358 received ranibizumab (Regillo, Yue, Shams, AAO 2008; Boyer, "Safety," AAO 2008).[12–17] Ranibizumab injections administered in these trials totaled 30,736 (2-year MARINA, 10,443; 2-year ANCHOR, 5921; 2-year PIER, 1217; 2-year FOCUS, 2189; 1-year SAILOR, 10,966). In the VISION trials, intravitreal pegaptanib injections were administered to 892 of 1,190 patients in the first year and to 374 of 425 patients in the second year. During the first and second years of the VISION trials, patients received 7,545 and 2,663 pegaptanib injections, respectively.[10,11,18] Safety data for year 3 of the VISION trial revealed that 422 subjects received 3,227 injections of either 0.3 or 1 mg of pegaptanib sodium, yet no safety signal for systemic events from the injections was found or suggested from the trial. This will be further discussed in another section.[19]

SAFETY OF INTRAVITREAL BEVACIZUMAB

Intravitreal bevacizumab, while not FDA approved for use in the eye, is used by many retinal specialists in an off-label manner for the treatment of neovascular AMD, diabetic retinopathy, and vascular occlusions. No randomized clinical trials have yet evaluated bevacizumab in neovascular AMD although many small retrospective studies have been published.[19] Two large-scale retrospective analyses have been conducted to evaluate the safety of intravitreal bevacizumab: (a) the Internet-based International Intravitreal Bevacizumab Survey, which collected physician-reported adverse effects (AEs)[20] and (b) the Pan-American Collaborative Retina Study Group (PACORES), an open-label, uncontrolled, multinational, interventional case series involving patients from eight Latin American institutions.[21]

The International Intravitreal Bevacizumab Survey reported safety data from 70 centers involving 7,113 injections in 5,228 patients with various ocular diseases, with a median 3-month follow-up. Indications for treatment were not reported.[20] The most common AEs, reported per injection, potentially related to the procedure were corneal abrasion (0.15%), retinal detachment (0.04%), and mild discomfort (0.14%); the most common ocular AEs potentially related to the drug were inflammation/uveitis (0.14%), acute vision loss (0.07%), subretinal hemorrhage (0.06%), and retinal pigment epithelium (RPE) tears (0.06%). The most frequent systemic AEs potentially related to the drug were increased blood pressure (0.21%) and cerebrovascular accident (0.07%). No long-term follow-up is available, and self-reporting of AEs and SAEs and lack of controlled follow-up of these patients make the information concerning safety in this registry suspectable.

The PACORES reported 12-month pooled safety data from a total of 4,303 intravitreal injections of 1.25- or 2.5-mg bevacizumab in 1,173 consecutive patients (1,310 eyes). Patients in this report had been treated for proliferative diabetic retinopathy, diabetic macular edema, retinal vein occlusion, as well as CNV from any cause, including 345 patients with neovascular AMD.[21] The most common ocular complications, reported per injection, were subconjunctival hemorrhage (19.5%), increased intraocular pressure (IOP) (0.16%), endophthalmitis (0.16%), tractional retinal detachment (0.16%), and uveitis (0.09%). The incidence of AEs in patients with neovascular AMD was not specifically delineated in this study. The combined systemic adverse events were reported in 18 patients (1.5%) and included 7 (0.59%) cases of acute elevation of systemic blood pressure, 6 (0.5%) cerebrovascular accidents, 5 (0.4%) myocardial infarctions (MIs), and 5 (0.4%) deaths. Because this was not a prospective randomized trial and included patients with diseases other than CNV from AMD, it is difficult to draw conclusions on the safety in the AMD population.

The safety of anti-VEGF therapy should be divided into those events related to the injection and those related to the potential risk of the drug locally or by systemic absorption (Box 12.1).

Ocular Adverse Effects

Endophthalmitis

Of the serious ocular AEs reported in the controlled clinical trials reviewed here, endophthalmitis was a rare injection-related AE (Regillo, Yue, Shams, AAO 2008; Boyer,

BOX 12.1 Side Effects of Anti-VEGF Drugs

Ocular side effects
Endophthalmitis
IOP rise
Uveitis
Vitreous hemorrhage
Rhegmatogenous retinal detachment
RPE tear
Cataract
Systemic side effects
Nonocular hemorrhage
ATEs
Death
Contraindication: Pregnancy

"SAILOR," AAO 2008).[11–18] In MARINA, endophthalmitis (including presumed endophthalmitis) was reported in 1.3% of patients using 0.5 mg and 0.8% of patients in the 0.3-mg group cumulative at 2 years in the MARINA trial. In the ANCHOR trial 2-year results, 3 of 277 patients (1.1%) developed presumed endophthalmitis in the study eye (rate per injection = 3/5,921 [0.05%]) and no patient in the 0.3-mg group was reported to have endophthalmitis. In the 1-year SAILOR trial, two (0.2%) subjects in the 0.3-mg dose and five (0.4%) subjects in the 0.5-mg dose group developed endophthalmitis or presumed endophthalmitis. There were no cases reported in the photodynamic therapy (PDT) (ANCHOR) or sham (MARINA) groups. In FOCUS, the rate of endophthalmitis or presumed endophthalmitis (one case the investigator classified as severe uveitis was treated with antibiotics and was included) was 2.1% in patients receiving ranibizumab plus PDT compared with no cases reported among patients receiving PDT alone. The higher rate of endophthalmitis in FOCUS may reflect the use of a lyophilized formulation of ranibizumab during the first year of the study. The rate of endophthalmitis was significantly reduced after the first year of FOCUS[17] when a solution-based formulation of ranibizumab was used in the second year. In PIER, no cases of endophthalmitis were reported in either the sham or ranibizumab-treated groups.

In the first year of VISION, 12 cases (1.3%) of endophthalmitis, including six in the 0.3-mg group, were reported in pegaptanib-treated patients,[18] nine of which were determined to be associated with deviations of the injection preparation protocol, such as failure to use an eyelid speculum. A task force to study the problem of endophthalmitis was convened and the injection protocol was adjusted; in the second year, no cases of endophthalmitis were reported from a total of 2,663 injections.[11] In year 3 of the VISION trial, two cases of endophthalmitis (0.47%) were reported.

Increased Intraocular Pressure

Transient elevations in IOP were commonly seen within the first 30 minutes after intravitreal ranibizumab or pegaptanib sodium injection in the controlled clinical trials due to the volume of drug injected. The pressures seemed to all return to normal during this period. No evidence of persistently elevated IOP was reported with multiple injections of either drug. It should be noted that subjects with preexisting uncontrolled glaucoma in the study eye (defined as IOP ≥ 30 mm Hg despite treatment on antiglaucoma medication) were excluded from participation in the MARINA, ANCHOR, FOCUS, PIER, and SAILOR trials. The VISION trials had no study entry criteria related to presence of glaucoma. Increased incidence of anterior chamber taps was reported after injection of pegaptanib sodium and is probably related to the increased volume (0.09 mL) injected compared to ranibizumab (0.05 mL).

Uveitis

Uveitis was reported among 1.3% of subjects who received 0.3 or 0.5 mg of ranibizumab in the MARINA trial. In the ANCHOR trial, uveitis was reported in 0.7% of subjects receiving 0.5 mg dose and 0% in subjects receiving PDT or 0.3 mg cumulatively at 2 years.[12] In SAILOR, one case of uveitis was reported (0.1%) in the 0.3-mg cohort and 0.2% in the 0.5-mg ranibizumab treatment arm. In FOCUS, 3.8% of patients receiving ranibizumab plus PDT developed uveitis while there was no uveitis in patients receiving PDT alone. Notably, all cases of uveitis in FOCUS were reported during the first year of the study and appeared to be related to the lyophilized formulation of ranibizumab that was used.[17] No cases of uveitis were reported in the PIER trial or even up to 3 years in the VISION trial.

Recently, a cluster of cases of sterile uveitis was reported in Canada following the intravitreal injection of bevacizumab for a variety of ocular conditions. No etiology of this outbreak was found, and the outbreak was self-limited. Since bevacizumab is usually obtained from a compounding pharmacy where intravenous bevacizumab is placed into smaller aliquots, the possibility of contamination is present; however, clinically, this does not appear to have resulted in an increase in endophthalmitis or uveitis. Though uveitis has been reported after bevacizumab, re-treatment using ranibizumab after did not cause an increase or exacerbation of the uveitis. The FC portion of the bevacizumab molecule theoretically may be a reason for an increased incidence of uveitis.[22]

Vitreous Hemorrhage

In ANCHOR, vitreous hemorrhage developed in 1.5% in the 0.3-mg ranibizumab-treated patients compared with 0% in the PDT and 0.5% in 0.5-mg group. In MARINA, 0.8% sham-injected patients and 0.4% in both the 0.3- and 0.5-mg groups had vitreous hemorrhage. In FOCUS, the rate of vitreous hemorrhage was higher among patients receiving PDT (3.6%) compared with patients receiving ranibizumab plus PDT (1.9%). Notably, all cases of vitreous hemorrhage in FOCUS were reported during the first year. No cases of vitreous hemorrhage were reported in PIER. In SAILOR, the rate of vitreous hemorrhage was relatively low in the 0.3-mg (0.3%) and 0.5-mg ranibizumab (0.1%) treatment arms. In VISION, vitreous hemorrhage was reported in 1.8% of patients in the first year, with no cases reported in the second year and 0.24% of patients in the third.

Rhegmatogenous Retinal Detachment

Rhegmatogenous retinal detachment was rarely reported in any of the controlled clinical trials and not commonly seen in private practice as a sequelae of intravitreal injection. Retinal detachments were felt to be related to either the injection or as a natural history event but not to the drug itself. In the MARINA, FOCUS, and PIER trials, no rhegmatogenous retinal detachments were seen among ranibizumab-treated patients. In these trials, one patient receiving sham injection (0.4%; MARINA) developed a rhegmatogenous retinal detachment. In ANCHOR, rhegmatogenous retinal detachment occurred in 1.5% of ranibizumab-treated patients and 0.7% of PDT-treated patients. In SAILOR, one case of rhegmatogenous retinal detachment (0.1%) was noted; this patient was in the 0.3-mg ranibizumab treatment arm. In the first, second, and third years of the VISION trials, 0.4%, 1.2%, and 0.24% of pegaptanib-treated patients, respectively, experienced a rhegmatogenous retinal detachment. In the first year of the VISION trial, 0.2% of patients were reported to have exudative retinal detachments. In PACORES, one case of rhegmatogenous retinal detachment was encountered but was in a mixed treatment group (see section on bevacizumab).

Retinal Pigment Epithelial Tears

In clinical practice, tears of the RPE occur spontaneously and after treatment of CNV with bevacizumab, ranibizumab, or pegaptanib in AMD eyes. These tears usually develop in patients with large fibrovascular pigment epithelial detachments and typically occur within the first 3 months of instituting treatment.[23–31]

RPE tears were relatively rare in all controlled trials of anti-VEGF therapy. In MARINA, ANCHOR, and PIER, a cumulative reading center analysis of RPE tears showed 1.8%, 3.0%, and 1.6% in 0.5, 0.3 mg, and sham groups, respectively. No cases of RPE tears were reported in the VISION trial, though RPE tears have been subsequently reported after pegaptanib treatment for AMD. Similarly, RPE tears have been reported in patients treated with bevacizumab.

The relatively low incidence of RPE tears occurring in clinical trials may be related to the exclusion of eyes in patients with preexisting large serous RPE detachments in the study eye.

Cataract

In MARINA, traumatic cataract was reported in one patient (0.4%) who had received 0.5 mg of ranibizumab. No cases of traumatic cataract were noted in ANCHOR, FOCUS, and PIER. 0.1% of subjects in both doses in SAILOR were reported to have developed a cataract. In the first year of the VISION trials, traumatic cataract was reported in five patients (0.6%) due to contact with and/or penetration of the lens by the injection needle; one of these cases occurred in the 0.3-mg pegaptanib treatment arm. In the second year, no cases of traumatic lens damage were reported. It should be observed that a 27-gauge needle (diameter 0.41 mm) was used in the VISION trials and was an intrinsic part of the injection syringe, whereas a 30-gauge needle (diameter 0.31 mm) was used in ANCHOR, MARINA, FOCUS, PIER, and SAILOR. Many complaints concerning the "sharpness" of the 27-gauge needle were expressed. The increased incidence of lens damage in VISION was possibly related to the difficulty in penetrating the sclera with the larger needle and/or the lack of experience in giving repeated intravitreal injections. In the ranibizumab trials, this may have been reduced by having a sharper, smaller needle and increased experience with giving intraocular injections. At this time, the pegaptanib syringe has been reconfigured and a 30-gauge needle can be chosen for intravitreal injections.

Systemic Adverse Effects

Based on the results of previously reported systemic anti-VEGF treatments, the incidence of MI and Antiplatelet Trialists' Collaboration (APTC) arterial thromboembolic events (ATEs), which include vascular death and death of unknown cause, nonfatal MI, and nonfatal cardiovascular accidents was carefully evaluated.[32]

Entry criteria for MARINA, ANCHOR, PIER, FOCUS, and SAILOR did not exclude patients for any preexisting cardiovascular, cerebrovascular, or peripheral vascular conditions. Exclusion criteria for participants in the VISION trials included MI within 6 months, unstable angina, and cerebrovascular accident within 12 months, New York Heart Association class III (marked limitation even during less than ordinary activity and comfort only at rest) or IV (severe limitations on physical activity and symptoms at rest) heart disease. *It should be noted that investigators in the ranibizumab trials may have selected out patients with New York Heart Association class III or IV and not enrolled them.*

Nonocular Hemorrhage

In MARINA, the rate of nonocular hemorrhage judged serious and nonserious was 5.5% in the sham, 9.2% in the 0.3 mg, and 8.8% in the 0.5 mg. The rate of nonocular hemorrhages reported as serious was 0.8%, 1.3%, and 2.1%, respectively. ANCHOR total hemorrhages serious and nonserious were 4.9%, 8.8%, and 9.3% with serious reported as 0.7%, 2.9%, and 2.1% in the PDT, 0.3 mg, and 0.5 mg groups, respectively. Of the 15 patients who experienced a serious nonocular hemorrhage in MARINA and ANCHOR, epistaxis was the most common (12 of 15 patients; 80%). In SAILOR, the rates of nonocular hemorrhages were 2.9% and 3.1% in the 0.3 and 0.5-mg ranibizumab treatment arms, respectively. In FOCUS, the 2-year incidence of nonocular hemorrhages was similar between the ranibizumab plus PDT (6.7%) and PDT (7.1%) groups; none was reported as serious. In PIER, 3.4% and 6.6% of patients in the 0.3- and 0.5-mg ranibizumab treatment groups, respectively, and 4.8% of patients receiving sham injection experienced a nonocular hemorrhage.

In VISION, the incidence of serious hemorrhagic AEs among patients receiving pegaptanib injection or sham injection was 1% in the first year, and 1% among pegaptanib-treated patients and 2% among sham-injected patients in the second year.

Arterial Thromboembolic Events

ATEs have been noted in colorectal cancer patients receiving intravenous anti-VEGF therapy (bevacizumab).[33] Because intraocular drugs can enter the systemic circulation,[34] ATEs are a potential concern with intravitreal administration of anti-VEGF agents. The identification of ATEs can be challenging due to variable definitions; however, the APTC provides a standard definition of ATEs, including nonfatal MI, nonfatal cerebrovascular accidents (stroke), and vascular deaths.[32]

In MARINA and ANCHOR, the overall APTC ATE rate ranged from 5.1% to 5.7% in the patients treated with 0.5-mg ranibizumab, compared with 4.2% in sham-injected patients and 4.9% in PDT-treated patients (Boyer, "Safety," AAO 2008). In PIER, one APTC ATE (1.7%) was reported in the 0.3-mg ranibizumab treatment arm (Regillo, Yue, Shams, AAO 2008). In FOCUS, the overall rates of APTC ATEs were 4.8% in the ranibizumab-plus-PDT group and 7.1% in the PDT group (Boyer, "Safety," AAO 2008). In SAILOR, the overall APTC ATE rates were 2.6% and 2.8% among patients receiving 0.3 and 0.5 mg of ranibizumab, respectively (Boyer, "Safety," AAO 2008).[35] A meta-analysis of the systemic safety of intravitreal ranibizumab, based on a pooling of first-year data from MARINA, ANCHOR, PIER, FOCUS, and SAILOR and second-year data from MARINA, ANCHOR, PIER, and FOCUS, has shown that overall APTC ATE rates for the total patient population are similar across treatment groups (Boyer "Meta-Analysis" AAO 2008). In the SAILOR trial, there was no control group. Subjects with angiographically-determined CNV received either 0.3 or 0.5mg. The average total number of ranibizumab injections was 4.9 for Cohort 1. The incidence of vascular deaths in the 0.3 mg and the 0.5 mg was 0.8% and 0.7% and 0.7% and 1.5% in nonvascular deaths, respectively. The incidence of death due to unknown cause was 0.1% in both. Stroke rates were 0.7% and 1.2% in the 0.3- and 0.5-mg groups, respectively.

Recently, the results of the HORIZON trial demonstrating the use of ranibizumab in a third and fourth year (Michael Singer ARVO 2009) demonstrated that continued use of ranibizumab, albeit, intermittent injections given at the investigators' discretion, appeared safe. There were three groups: a group of patients who had received constant injections through the 24 months of ANCHOR, and MARINA (n = 600) or a group that crossed over and received ranibizumab treatment (n = 184) or a no-treatment group (n = 69). The mean/median for injections was 3.6/2 in the continued use group and 4.2/3 in the crossover group. The incidence of ocular AEs in the continued-use group was low: 0.2% endophthalmitis and 0.2% uveitis with no cases of retinal tear or vitreous hemorrhage. SAEs, similarly, were low and well balanced. Nonocular hemorrhages were 5.5%, 4.9%, and 4.3%; death 4.7%, 4.3%, and 7.2% and MI 1.5%, 1.6%, and 1.4% in the constant treatment, crossover group and no-treatment group, respectively.

Similarly, in the VISION trial, the incidence of serious ATEs appeared to be equal in the pegaptanib and sham treatment arms (3% each) in the first year. In the second year, the incidence of serious ATEs was lower in the pegaptanib treatment arm (2%) compared with the sham treatment arm (6%). The third- and fourth-year safety reports of subjects in the VISION trial showed no increased incidence in the ATEs than would be expected though the actual number of patients is small. That is, there is no apparent stroke safety signal seen with the use of pegaptanib sodium, and stroke risk is not listed in the package insert. It should be noted that the annual stroke rate for new-onset neovascular AMD in a large sample of Medicare subjects has been reported at 3.8%. Though this appears to be in line with what has been reported in clinical trials, patients enrolled in trials tend to be healthier than the general Medicare population, and therefore, the incidence of ATEs in these trials compared to the natural history is difficult to determine.

Deaths

The rate of vascular death (meeting APTC criteria, including death of an unknown cause) in MARINA was 1.3% in both doses of ranibizumab, ANCHOR, 1.5% or the 0.3-mg dose and 1.4% in the 0.5-mg dose group compared to 1.7% of sham-injected (MARINA) and 2.1% of PDT-treated (ANCHOR) patients. In PIER, one case of vascular death (1.7%) was reported (a patient in the 0.3-mg ranibizumab treatment arm). In FOCUS, one case of vascular death (1.8%) was reported (in PDT-treated patient). In SAILOR, the 1-year incidence was 1.0% and 0.9% in the 0.3- and 0.5-mg dose, respectively.

The nonvascular death rates in MARINA were 0.8% in the 3-mg group and 1.3% in the 0.5-mg group; ANCHOR, 2.2% (0.3 mg) and 0.7% (0.5 mg), compared with 0.8% of sham-injected patients (MARINA) and 1.4% of PDT-treated patients (ANCHOR). In PIER, one case of nonvascular death (1.7%) was reported (sham-injected patient). In FOCUS, one case of nonvascular death (1.0%) occurred (ranibizumab plus PDT–treated patient). In SAILOR, 0.7% and 1.5% in the 0.3 and 0.5 mg, respectively, was noted.

In the first year of the VISION trials, deaths (vascular or nonvascular) occurred in 2% of patients in each of the pegaptanib and sham treatment arms. In the second year of VISION, two deaths (0.2%) were reported; both patients had received pegaptanib.

Systemic Immunoreactivity

Serum samples were taken prior to administration of ranibizumab in the FOCUS, MARINA, and ANCHOR. A number of patients tested positive before injection of the study drug. Though a small percentage of patients converted as the study continued, in all studies, no visual outcome changes or increase in intraocular inflammation was noted in the FOCUS or MARINA trials. However, in the ANCHOR trial, patients who were immunoreactive or became immunoreactive during the course of the study had a higher incidence of uveitis.

Pregnancy

The anti-VEGF drugs pegaptanib, ranibizumab, and bevacizumab are not intended to be used during pregnancy, and most patients with AMD are beyond childbearing age. However, both ranibizumab and bevacizumab are listed on their product label as class C drugs when used during pregnancy, while pegaptanib is a class B drug. That is, pegaptanib, in contrast to the others, has been tested in animals regarding teratogenic effects when given during pregnancy. None were found. With ranibizumab and bevacizumab, these tests were not conducted. As VEGF is needed in angiogenesis, and angiogenesis is a key process during development of the fetus, using these drugs when a patient is pregnant should be avoided. Obviously, appropriate questions should be asked of the patients when using antiangiogenic therapies.

DISCUSSION

The randomized clinical trials for ranibizumab and pegaptanib show that safety profiles appear comparable and serious ocular or non-ocular AEs were similar and rare with both treatments. Retrospective noncontrolled studies of bevacizumab also showed low perinjection rates of serious ocular and nonocular AEs; however, these are all nonrandomized retrospective studies.

Although in the randomized trials, treatment is delivered as monthly intravitreal injections, the risk of serious ocular adverse events, including retinal detachments, vitreous hemorrhage, or endophthalmitis, was uncommon in these trials, and endophthalmitis rates were similar to what has been reported in other large series.

In the FOCUS trial, the higher rate of ocular AEs, mainly uveitis, compared with other ranibizumab trials may reflect the use of a lyophilized formulation of the drug during the first year. Indeed, ocular AEs decreased in the second year, when a solution-based formulation of ranibizumab was used. In PIER, a relatively lower rate of ocular and nonocular AEs was reported with ranibizumab treatment and may reflect the fewer injections administered over the 2 years of this study compared with the 2-year MARINA, ANCHOR, and FOCUS trials.

The detection of systemic AEs is important in trials evaluating any anti-VEGF therapy as systemic administration of anti-VEGF agents (such as bevacizumab) has been associated with an increased risk of ATEs[36] and intravitreal anti-VEGF agents can enter the systemic circulation and therefore pose a theoretical risk of inducing ATEs. The analysis of the MARINA, ANCHOR, FOCUS, PIER, SAILOR, and VISION trials have not shown such a risk. An independent meta-analysis of the ranibizumab trials has shown similar rates of overall APTC ATEs across treatment groups; however, when a regression analysis of confounding factors that may increase the risk of stroke (previous stroke, transient ischemic attack, congestive heart failure, cardiac arrhythmia, age, sex,) was analyzed and the group of stroke patients was arbitrarily divided into three separate groups reflecting high, medium, or low risk and analyzed, there was significant increase in the odds ratio for the 0.5-mg dose (7×) versus control and (4×) in the 0.3-mg group.[37] It is important to realize there were very few patients who had suffered strokes and subset analysis should be interpreted with caution. On the other hand, death rates from stroke increase rapidly over the age of 75. In none of clinical trials or in the meta-analysis were ages of those who suffered a stroke analyzed with respect to possible added risk imported by intravitreal (IVT) injection. Such an analysis, as more events are documented, might have bearing on which anti-VEGF the clinician selects.

With new longer-acting or chronic release anti-VEGF drugs in development, side effects occurring to the choroid or choriocapillaris need to be carefully monitored. The increased pigmentation and choroidal atrophy that are observed in patients receiving chronic therapy monthly treatment need to be monitored carefully. These changes have been attributed to the natural history of AMD, but these changes should be monitored carefully as they may represent a change in the choroid from chronic anti-VEGF treatment. Similarly, it is important to look at future larger meta-analysis to determine small rare systemic changes that will not be seen in smaller randomized clinical trials.

KEY POINTS

- Randomized clinical trials for ranibizumab and pegaptanib show that safety profiles appear comparable, and serious ocular or nonocular AEs were similar and rare with both treatments.
- Retrospective noncontrolled studies of bevacizumab also showed low per-injection rates of serious ocular and nonocular AEs.
- Ocular side effects include endophthalmitis, IOP rise, uveitis, vitreous hemorrhage, rhegmatogenous retinal detachment, RPE tear, and cataract.
- Systemic side effects include nonocular hemorrhage, ATEs, and death.
- Anti-VEGF drugs are contraindicated in pregnancy.
- The analyses of the MARINA, ANCHOR, FOCUS, PIER, SAILOR, and VISION trials have not shown an increased risk of ATEs.

REFERENCES

1. Ferrara N. Vascular endothelial growth factor: basic science and clinical progress. *Endocr Rev.* 2004;25:581–611.
2. Ferrara N. Role of vascular endothelial growth factor in physiologic and pathologic implications. *Semin Oncol.* 2002;29:10–14.
3. Ferrara N, Henzel WJ. Pituitary follicular cells secrete a novel heparin-binding grow endothelial cells. *Biochem Biophys Res Comm.* 1989;161:851–858.
4. Tuñón J, Ruiz-Moreno JM, Mertin-Ventura JL, et al. Cardiovascular risn and antioangiogenic therapy for age-related macular degeneration. *Surv Ophthalmol.* 2009;54(3): 339–348.
5. Zachary I. Signaling mechanisms mediating vascular protective actions of vascular endothelial growth factor. *Am J Physiol Cell Physiol.* 2001;280:C1375–C1386.
6. van Wijngaarden P, Coster DJ, Williams KA. Inhibitors of ocular neovascularization: promises and potential problems. *JAMA.* 2005;293:1509–1513.
7. Dafer RM, Schneck M, Friberg TR, et al. Intravitreal ranibizumab and bevacizumab: a review of risk. *Sem Ophthalmol.* 2007;22:201–204.
8. Duan Y, Mo J, Klein R, et al. Age-related macular degeneration is associated with incident myocardial infarction among elderly Americans. *Ophthalmology.* 2007;114:4.
9. Hurwitz H, Fehrenbacher L, Novotny W Bevacizumab plus irinotecan, flurouracil, and leicovorin for metastatic colorectal cancer. *N Eng J Med.* 2004; 350:2335–2342.
10. Chakravarthy U, Adamis AP, Cunningham ET Jr, et al. Year 2 efficacy results of 2 randomized controlled clinical trials of pegaptanib for neovascular age-related macular degeneration. *Ophthalmology.* 2006;113:1508–1525.
11. D'Amico DJ, Masonson HN, et al. VEGF Inhibition Study in Ocular Neovascularization (VISION) Clinical Trial Group. Pegaptanib sodium for neovascular age-related macular degeneration: two-year safety results of the two prospective, multicenter, controlled clinical trials. *Ophthalmology.* 2006;113:992–1001.
12. Brown DM, Michels M, Kaiser PK, et al. Ranibizumab versus verteporfin photodynamic therapy for neovascular age-related macular degeneration: two-year results of the ANCHOR study. *Ophthalmology.* 2009;116:57–65.
13. Regillo CD, Brown DM, Abraham P, et al. Randomized, double-masked, sham-controlled trial of ranibizumab for neovascular age-related macular degeneration: PIER study year 1. *Am J Ophthalmol.* 2008;145:239–248.
14. Brown DM, Kaiser PK, Michels M, et al. Ranibizumab versus pertepofin for neovascular age-related macular degeneration. *N Engl J Med.* 2006;355:1432–1444.
15. Rosenfeld PJ, Brown DM, Heier JS, et al. Ranibizumab for neovascular age-related macular degeneration. *N Engl J Med.* 2006;355:1419–1431.
16. Antoszyk AN, Tuomi L, Chung CY, *et al.* Ranibizumab combined with verteporfin photosynamic therapy in neovascular age-related macular degeneration (FOCUS): year 2 results. *Am J Ophthalmol.* 2008;145:862–874.e3.
17. Heier JS, Boyer DS, Ciulla TA, et al. Ranibizumab in combination with verteporfin photodynamic therapy in neovascular age-related macular degeneration (FOCUS): year 1 results. *Arch Ophthalmol.* 2006;142:1532–1542.
18. Gragoudas ES, Adamis AP, Cunningham ET Jr, et al. Pegaptanib for neovascular age-related macular degeneration. *N Engl J Med.* 2004;351:2805–2816.
19. Ip MS, Scott IU, Brown GC, et al. Anti-vascular endothelial growth factor pharmacotherapy for age-related macular degeneration: a report by the American Academy of Ophthalmology. *Ophthalmology.* 2008;115(10):1837–1846.
20. Fung AE, Rosenfeld PJ, Reichel E. The International Intravitreal Becacizumab Safety Survey: using the internet to access drug safety worldwide. *Br J Ophthalmol.* 2007;90: 1344–1349.
21. Wu L, Martinez-Castellanos MA, Quiroz-Mercado H, et al. Twelve-month safety of intravitreal injections of bevacizumab (Avastin®): results of the Pan-American Collaborative Retina Study Group (PACORES). *Graefes Arch Clin Exp Ophthalmol.* 2008;246:81–87.
22. Wickremasinghe SS, Michalova K, Gilhotra J, et al. Acute intraocular inflammation after intravitreous injections of bevascizumab for treatment of neovascular age-related macular degeneration. *Ophthalmology.* 2008;115(11):1911–1915; [Epub 2008 Jul 31].
23. Carvounis PE, Kopel AC, Benz MS. Retinal pigment epithelium tears following ranibizumab for exudative age-related macular degeneration. *Am J Ophthalmol.* 2007;143: 504–505.
24. Bakri SJ, Patel SP. Retinal pigment epithelial tear following intravitreal bevacizumab. *Eye* 2007;21:424–425.
25. Dhalla MS, Blinder KJ, Tewari A, et al. Retinal pigment epithelial tear following intravitreal pegaptanib sodium. *Am J Ophthalmol.* 2006;141:752–754.
26. Gelisken F, Ziemssen F, Voelker M, et al. Retinal pigment epithelial tear following intravitreal bevacizumab injection for neovascular age-related macular degeneration. *Acta Ophthalmol Scand.* 2006;84:833–834.
27. Meyer CH, Mennel S, Schmidt JC, et al. Acute retinal pigment epithelial tear following intravitreal bevacizumab (Avastin) injection for occult choroidal neovascularization secondary to age-related macular degeneration. *Am J Ophthalmol.* 2006;142:160–162.
28. Singh RP, Sears JE. Retinal pigment epithelial tears after pegaptanib injection for exudative age-related macular degeneration. *Am J Ophthalmol.* 2006;142:160–2.
29. Chan CK, Meyer CH, Gross JG, et al. Retinal pigment epithelial tears after intravitreal bevacizumab injection for neovascular age-related macular degeneration. *Retina.* 2007;27:541–551.
30. Chang LK, Sarraf D. Tears of the retinal pigment epithelium: an old problem in a new era. *Retina.* 2007;27:523–534.
31. Kook D, Wolf A, Neubauer AS, et al. Retinal pigment epithelial tears after intravitreal injection of bevacizumab for AMD: frequency and progress. *Ophthalmologe.* 2008;105:158–164.
32. Collaborative overview of randomized trials of antiplatelet therapy—I: Prevention of death, myocardial infarction, and stroke by prolonged antiplatelet therapy in various categories of patients. Antiplatelet Trialists' Collaboration. *BMJ.* 1994;308:81–106.
33. Scappaticci FA, Skillings JR, Holden SN, et al. Arterial thromboembolic events in patients with metastatic carcinoma treated with chemotherapy and bevacizumab. *J Natl Cancer Inst.* 2007;99:1232–1239.

34. Cunha-Vaz JG. The blood-ocular battiers: past, present, and future. *Doc Ophthalmol.* 1997;93:149–157.
35. Boyer DS. SAILOR safety outcomes at one year: does ranibizumab increase the risk of thromboembolic events? Presented at: Angiogenesis 2008 Conference; February 23, 2008; Key Biscayne, FL.
36. Chase JL. Clinical use of anti-vascular endothelial growth factor monoclonal antibodies in metastatic colorectal cancer. *Pharmacotherapy*. 2008;28:23S–30S.
37. Boyer DS. Meta-analysis of APTC events in key phase 2 and phase 2 studies with ranibizumab in wet AMD. Presented at: American Academy of Ophthalmology 2008 Annual Meeting; Novermber 8–11, 2008; Atlanta, GA.

CHAPTER

13

Pharmacokinetics of Anti-vascular Endothelium Growth Factor Pharmacological Agents

Leanne T. Labriola • Muge Kesen • Karl G. Csaky

INTRODUCTION

Revascularization is a serious sequela of ocular diseases including age-related macular degeneration, diabetic retinopathy, vascular occlusive disorders, and retinopathy of prematurity. Research has identified vascular endothelium growth factor (VEGF) as one of the main signaling proteins in this process. With this discovery, novel strategies of preventing neovascularization have focused on inhibiting the VEGF molecule. This has led to a new pharmaceutical class of anti-VEGF drugs, including pegaptanib, ranibizumab, and bevacizumab. This chapter discusses the pharmacokinetic and pharmacodynamic properties of these drugs.

CLINICAL PHARMACOLOGY—BACKGROUND

Pharmacokinetics and Pharmacodynamics

Pharmacokinetics interprets how the different tissues and complexes within the body chemically alter the drug. It studies the drug path from its entry to its excretion from the body. Pharmacokinetics includes the mechanisms of drug liberation, absorption, dispersion, metabolism, and elimination from the body. Alternatively, pharmacodynamics is the study of the cascade of reactions from the drug's initial activation as a drug-receptor complex to its final downstream biological effect. Pharmacodynamics identifies how drugs stimulate, depress, destroy, or replace other substances or reactions in the body.

Compartment Models

One goal of pharmacokinetics is to define the drug concentration as a unit of time. Two different rationales are used to accomplish this goal. They include the noncompartmental model and the compartmental model. These models use different equations to estimate the amount of available drug in the body. The validity of the noncompartment model relies on the estimation of the entire dose of the drug. It uses this amount to create an area under the curve (AUC) graph of the concentration verses time. Direct measurements of drug concentration at several time points increase the accuracy of the curve.

The two-compartmental model uses kinetic theory to estimate the concentration of the drug, which is then entered into a linear or exponential equation to plot the concentration verses time graph. Different equations are used to estimate the total amount of drug as it enters and distributes through the central compartment as compared to when it redistributes to the peripheral compartments. Since the distribution of the drug into the various compartments takes place at the same time as the drug is being eliminated from the body, these models are highly complex.

To use these models in research studies, certain assumptions are made. The first is to assume that the magnitude of the effect is proportional to the amount of drug present. The second is to assume that the drug creates a drug-receptor complex that is equal to the total effect of the drug. The third is to assume that the total amount of the receptor is constant. And finally, the fourth is to assume that the concentration of drug in the plasma is equal to the amount of unbound drug in the body. For the study of the pharmacology of the anti-VEGF agents, most of these assumptions have yet to be verified.

OCULAR PHARMACOLOGY

Models for Studying Ocular Pharmacology

Initial studies on the pharmacokinetics of intravitreal drugs have been established using animal models. Animal models can provide basic concepts of drug functioning and identify overall routes of metabolism, distribution and eliminations. In this chapter, we report on pertinent findings from animal studies and explain their contribution to our current understanding of anti-VEGF medications.

However, the use of animal models has several limitations when used as a comparison model for human tissue. These include the differences in anatomical size, tissue properties, and structure. In addition, animal tissue can be damaged or altered from the methods used to harvest and collect the tissue and the need to euthanize the animals to collect data over several time intervals weighs against the overall utility of this method of research.

The size of the eye and its components vary among different species. In current literature, aqueous volume in the rabbit eye is estimated to be 0.25[1] and 0.134 mL in monkeys.[2] These values are similar to human aqueous chamber of 0.25 mL. However, in humans, the vitreous chamber is 4.5 mL. While rats have a vitreous volume of 56 μL, rabbits and monkeys have a vitreous volume ranging from 1.5 to 3 mL, depending on the species (Fig. 13.1).[3]

Another disadvantage is that the components of the vitreous can be different between species, which creates different inherent viscosities and other tissue properties[4] leading to different volumes of distribution in humans, monkey, rabbits, and rats. The structural relationships between tissues are also different between species. For example, the rabbit eye has no fovea.[5] In regard to the vascular system of the retina, the rabbit retina is merangiotic, or partially vascularized, while human retinas are holangiotic, or completely vascularized.[6] Humans have uneven distribution of blood supply to the retina, with higher vascular flow to the macula and lower flow to the peripheral retina. Humans also have higher choroidal blood flow rates than animals. These differences in blood flow would affect the speed and extent of intravascular delivery or elimination of substances and provide a confounding variable when comparing blood flow between species.

An advantage of animal models is that the tissue can be harvested at different time points and analyzed in various preparations. However, this process also has its limitations. For example, with tissue preparation, the

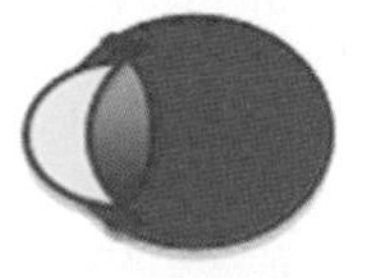

Rabbit:
Aqueous Volume: 0.25 mL
Vitreous Volume: 1.5 – 3 mL

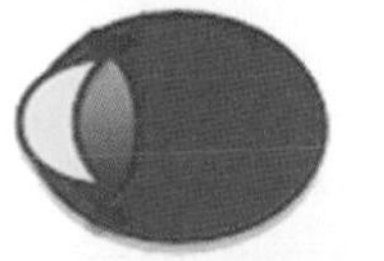

Monkey:
Anterior Volume: 0.134 mL
Vitreous Volume: 1.5 mL – 3 mL

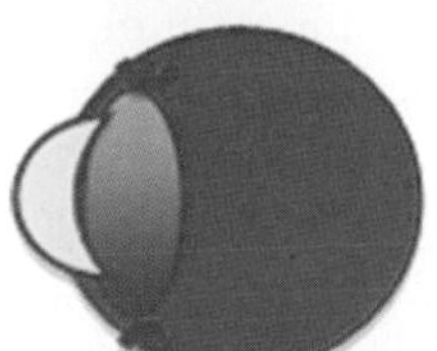

Human:
Anterior Volume: 0.25 mL
Vitreous Volume: 4.5 mL

FIGURE 13.1. Aqueous and vitreous volumes of rabbits, monkeys, and humans.

dynamic relationships between the tissues are lost, the three-dimensional structures are changed, and the tissue becomes a static representation of one segment of time within the study. These changes due to the tissue collection influence the interpretation of the tissue and limit the utility of the final results.

In conclusion, although animal models are advantageous in the fact that they can offer controlled experimental conditions and more invasive strategies can be used for measuring the amount of drug within the tissues, caution has to be used when extrapolating information gained from the studies.

New Technology

New noninvasive modalities are being developed for imaging proteins in the vitreous through radioactive labeling. One example is dynamic contrast-enhanced magnetic resonance imaging (DCE-MRI). This technology uses MRI scans to acquire three-dimensional images in vivo in order to better understand spatial relationships and flow of substances. DCE-MRI is being used in eye research to delineate episcleral outflow pathways, which is just beginning to elucidate the value of this imaging modality in research studies.[7] Similar to DCE-MRI, positron emission tomography uses stereotactic fiduciary markers; specifically,[18] F-fluoromisonidazole and single photon emission computer tomography (SPECT) offer dynamic images of the microenvironment of tumor cells.[8] These images are able to identify the hypoxic centers of tumor cells and may be used in ocular images in the future.

ANTI-VEGF DRUG PHARMACOLOGY

Ocular Barriers to Anti-VEGF Drug Distribution

A major barrier to the flow of substances within the eye is the existence of multiple basement membranes, which include the internal limiting membrane (ILM), the external limiting membrane (ELM), and Bruch membrane. Both the extent of flow impediment and the mechanism in which these membranes can limit flow are still unknown. Contemporary research studies offer opposing theories on these issues. Some authors believe that the membranes can significantly, if not completely, stop molecules from penetrating through the layers of the retina, based on the molecular size. Other groups have shown with their research that even large molecules, such as antibodies, can completely pass through the retina from the inner to outer layers, even going into the choriocapillaris.

The ILM is made from the footplates of Müller cells and attachments to the basal lamina. This structure separates the vitreous from the nerve fiber layer of the retina. Debate exists as to the amount and type of restriction that is created by the ILM. Some research findings suggest that the ILM acts as an impenetrable mechanical filtration barrier as well as a formidable electrostatic barrier,[3,4,9,10] while others studies have show that even large molecules are able to effectively penetrate the ILM.[11] The existence of pores ranging from 10 to 25 μm in size within the ILM[9] supports the argument of a mechanical barrier for this layer. Ranibizuamb, the Fab fragment of bevacizumab, an antibody to VEGF, has been shown to penetrate all layers of the retina, while, a full-sized antibody against the human epidermal growth factor receptor 2 (HER2) could not pass through the layers of the retina.[3] However, critics of the study state that the two groups of comparison were not equal since two different antibodies, the anti-VEGF and anti-HER2, were used. The HER2 is present in many structures within the retina and specific antibody-receptor binding could have occurred at the boundary of the inner retina and limited the overall penetration of the substance. Another study using intravitreal injections showed that the ILM restricted the passage of a 70-kDa molecule of tissue plasminogen activator (tPA), whereas the 20-kDa rhodamine B molecule was able to penetrate this barrier.[10] However, specific binding of one substance and not the other could also have influenced these results since different molecules were compared.

Contrary to the suggestion of the ILM as a mechanical barrier, studies have shown that large molecules, including high molecular weight antibodies, are in fact able to pass through all of the layers of the retina. These molecules include albumin,[12] a tPA analogue called tenecteplase,[13] antibodies against recoverin,[14] melanoma-associated retinopathy antibody,[15] and others.[5,11]

On the outer side of the retina, the *zonular adherents* between the adjacent photoreceptors and Müller cells form the ELM. This is not a true histological membrane and many fenestrations exist within it; however, some authors suggest that this membrane can also offer mechanical or electrostatic resistance to substance flow within the retina.[9]

Deep to the retina, Bruch membrane provides yet another barrier to unwanted substances. It is located between the retinal pigment epithelial cells and the choroid. Bruch membrane specifically has been reported to limit the diffusion of macromolecules, including proteins, oglionucleotides, and genes, from entering the retina.[3,9,16] However, more research needs to be done to delineate the path of flow of molecules that can penetrate the retina and investigate if they disrupt Bruch membrane or use transport mechanisms to cross through it.

Within the eye, the vitreous provides its own type of impediment to the free flow of substances. The vitreous occupies four fifths of the volume of the globe. The vitreal collagen network of fibers and proteoglycan elements creates a barrier to the diffusion of molecules from the anterior hyaloid face to the posterior vitreoretinal surface. The composition of elements include hyaluronan, heparin sulfate, dermatan sulfate, and chondroitin sulfate, which convey an overall negative charge to this matrix, which like the ILM and ELM can create not only a mechanical barrier but also an electrostatic one as well.[9]

Anti-VEGF Ocular Drug Delivery

To date, all of the anti-VEGF agents are delivered by direct intravitreal injection. The absorption of drugs delivered to the eye is influenced by the drug's molecular mass, molecular radius, and solubility. Intravitreal injections essentially have 100% bioavailability to ocular tissues since they are injected at their site of action.

Once the drug is inside the eye, it begins to distribute throughout the vitreous. Fluorescein labeling of molecules and DCE-MRI imaging have shown that molecules exhibit an anterior to posterior concentration gradient within the vitreous humor from a high concentration right behind the lens to a low concentration near the vitreoretinal interface.[7,9] As mentioned earlier, the ocular barriers limit drug dispersion within the eye. The properties of the drug, such as the size, the molecular charge, and the diffusion co-efficient, collectively determine the drug's ability to penetrate the ocular barriers. Recent studies have shown the ability of even larger molecules to pass through the retinal layer, including the blood-ocular barrier. Galbumin, a bovine albumin molecule conjugated with gadolinium, has a molecular weight of 80 kDa and still is capable of penetrating all the layers of the retina. Immunohistochemical tracers and radioactive labeling have been used to confirm the complete transretinal penetration of bevacizumab.[11,17,18] Although the mechanism of retinal penetration has not yet been clearly defined, there is evidence to support an active transport mechanism, similar to that of the nanoparticles, such as endocytosis or transcytosis.[9,17] It is important to understand how larger molecules, such as antibodies, distribute throughout the vitreous since current therapeutic strategies utilize these molecules to deliver target-specific pharmacotherapy.

Drugs that are not metabolized can be eliminated from the eye. Most studies support a first-order elimination model for ocular clearance. However, others have shown that the elimination of different doses of macromolecules, specifically Galbumin, occurred at a constant rate. The terminal vitreous elimination half-lives of the 1 and 0.25 mg/mL of Galbumin were 2 and 0.7 days, respectively.[4] The elimination process showed a steady elimination rate; therefore, this molecule follows a zero-order elimination rate, which is similar to how alcohol is eliminated from systemic circulation.

The major pathways of intraocular drug clearance take place through an anterior route and a posterior route within the eye. The anterior route occurs by the passive diffusion of the drug around the lens into the aqueous chamber and then its excretion via Schlemm canal or the uveoscleral outflow pathway.[19–21] Hydrophilic substances favor this anterior elimination route.[4] The rate of elimination via this route is dependent on the molecular weight and the solubility of the substance. Clearance through the trabecular meshwork and the uveoscleral outflow depends on the permeability of the trabecular meshwork and the episcleral venous pressure. This route can be affected by the factors that alter both the trabecular meshwork or anatomy of the angle of the anterior chamber and the episcleral venous pressure. For example, the rate of clearance can change with inflammation or the disruption of the blood-aqueous barrier in the ciliary epithelium.[22] Overall, this pathway can be slower than the posterior elimination pathway.[22] In spite of this, the anterior elimination route is the major elimination pathway of substances clearance from the vitreous.[19,21]

Medications can also exit the eye through posterior elimination pathways. Posterior pathways include transretinal migration as well as receptor-mediated transcytosis.[7,23] Lipophilic molecules can be more easily excreted through this route since they have to pass through the hydrophobic retinal layers.[4] Drugs that exit through the posterior route do not diffuse directly through the sclera. Instead these substances are eliminated by outflow to through the choroidal circulation.[7] The dynamic properties of the choroid including hydrostatic forces, oncotic pressures, and the fast rate of blood flow combined to eliminate substances through the vascular network of the choriocapillaris. The higher the hydrostatic pressure within the vitreous, the greater the outflow to the episcleral space. In addition, the high extracellular protein levels in the choroid elevate oncotic pressures outside of the vitreous and favor fluid flow across the retina and into the choroid. Lastly, the rapid movement of choroidal blood flow quickly removes the drug from the orbit and expels it through systemic circulation.[7] More research needs to be done to elucidate the exact mechanism of this posterior transport and to delineate the method in which substances can evade the barriers of the posterior blood-ocular barrier.

A specific route for posterior elimination has been shown to be through receptor-mediated transcytosis by the Fc receptor found on tissues that constitute the blood-ocular barrier, such as the surface of the retinal epithelial cells. The Fc Receptor can sequester the drug or help to excrete the drug from the eye. The receptor sequesters the IgG antibody within the endothelium of vessels. This sequestering would extend the half-life of the antibody by preventing its catabolization.[17] In addition, the Fc receptor can aid in transporting the drug through the ocular barriers to eliminate it from the eye. The Fc receptor is able to perform this role in other tissues outside of the eye. In the brain, the Fc receptor can transport IgG molecules by transcytosis across the blood-brain barrier and deliver the entire antibody intact into the bloodstream. In the eye, the Fc receptor was found on lymph vessels and on the epithelial lining of the blood-ocular barrier, a finding that correlates with the presumed role of the receptor of assisting in elimination of drugs through these barriers.[7,23] The discovery of Fc receptors may open a launching platform for new research in ocular pharmacokinetics, which may lead to the identification of other receptor-based transport mechanisms. Research in this field may help to clarify questions on if free drug passage through the blood-retinal barrier is even possible or if all posterior elimination of drugs is receptor-mediated.

PHARMCAOKINETICS OF CURRENT ANTI-VEGF MEDICATIONS

Pegaptanib

Pharmacokinetics

Pegaptanib sodium (Macugen, OIS-Eyetech, NY, USA) is a 28-ribonucleotide molecule with an osmolarity of 280 to 360 mOsm/kg and pH of 6.0 to 7.0 (Drug Insert 2009). Pegaptanib is an aptamer, which is a highly selective derivative of a nucleic acid. Aptamers function by folding into a three-dimensional structure that binds to and directly inhibits the target protein.[24] The target site for pegaptanib is the heparin-binding domain of the proinflammatory $VEGF_{165}$ slice isoform. This region is responsible for intensification of the interaction between the VEGF protein and its receptor that promotes neovascularization. Similar to other aptamers, pegaptanib has a high dissociation constant of 50 pmol/L, making it very effective in binding to $VEGF_{165}$ and inhibiting the amplification of the VEGF receptor signaling cascade.

The high affinity of pegaptanib for its target isoform limits its effects on other splice isoforms of VEGF, such as $VEGF_{120}$, which may create a stable balance of angiogenic precursors and contribute to the overall safety of the drug. In addition, because pegaptanib is an RNA-based molecule, it has little to no toxicity or immunogenicity making it an advantageous therapeutic choice (Fig. 13.2).

Aptamers, however, are limited in their utility by the small molecular sizes, typically 10 to 20 kDa.[24] Their small size allows for rapid elimination from circulation. To address this problem, pegaptanib, has been chemically conjugated to two 20-kDa monomethoxy-polyethylene glycol molecules increasing its overall size and molecular weight to 50-kDa. The addition of these molecules

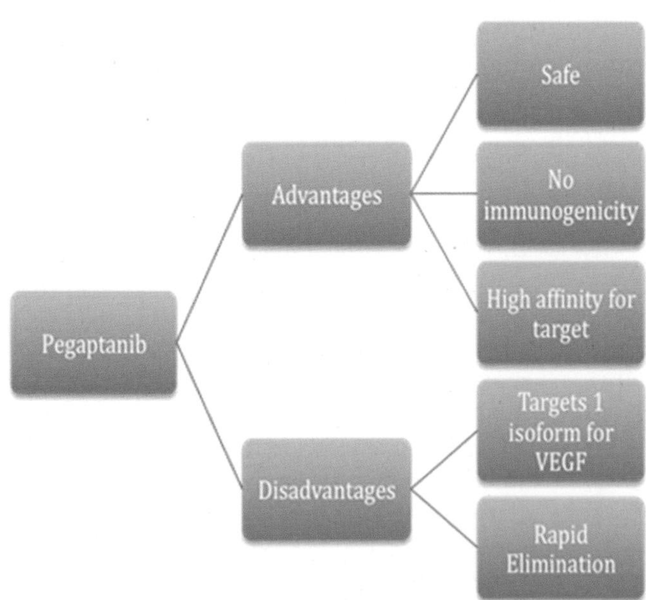

FIGURE 13.2. Advantages and disadvantages of pegaptanib.

to a compound, known as pegylation, limits glomerular excretion and increases the circulatory half-life of the compound.[24] Furthermore, pegylation is thought to increase the stability of pegaptanib and alter its distribution to preferentially target highly vascularized organs.[24]

Absorption

Pegaptanib has a slow systemic absorption, which is the rate-limiting step for this drug.[25]

Distribution

Initial studies in Rhesus Monkeys using radioactive markers provided early information on the pharmacokinetics of the drugs. After injection of 1 and 2 mg of pegaptanib, the vitreous concentrations were 26 and 499 mg/mL, respectively. The vitreous terminal half-life was 94.1 hours for the 1-mg dose and 89.9 hours for the 2-mg dose.[26] This finding reflects a dose-dependant effect of the terminal vitreous half-life of the drug. Twenty-four hours after its administration intravitreously, the drug was detected in the retina, vitreous humor, and aqueous humor within the eye. Twenty-four hours after intravenous administration, the highest concentration outside the eye was found in the kidney.[26] In a rabbit model, an intravitreal injection of 0.5 mg of pegaptanib resulted in initial vitreous of 350 mg/mL, which decreased to 1.7 μg/mL by day 28 of the study.[26] Pegaptanib showed first-order kinetics and was completely eliminated by 84 hours.[26]

After the VISION trial confirmed the safety of the drug, studies were conducted in human patients. A single monocular dose of 3 mg of pegaptanib sodium (ten times the recommended FDA dose) was injected intravitreously. Even at this high dose of pegaptanib, the maximum plasma concentration was only 80 ng/mL, which was reached 1 to 4 days after injection of the drug. Using this information to create an AUC graph and extrapolate the information for other doses of pegaptanib, it was found that an intravitreal injection of 0.5 mg would result in a maximum plasma concentration <10 ng/mL. The plasma half-life of the drug was 10 ± 4 days, and there was no accumulation of the drug in the plasma even after six consecutive weekly doses.[25,26]

Elimination

Because pegaptanib is made from nucleic acids and their site of action is extracellular, it is easily metabolized by the action of endonucleases and exonucleases.[25,26] The accessibility of this drug to degradation processes may explain the reason why pegaptanib does not accumulate in the serum. Pegaptanib is not metabolized by the P450 system.[26] The drug is eliminated primarily in the urine. Rabbit models showed evidence of 2-fluorouridine, a metabolite of pegaptanib, in the urine and plasma after administration.[25] Research suggests that a creatinine clearance of <20 mL/min is associated with a 2.3 times increase in the levels of the drug by AUC calculations.[26] However, pegaptanib has been studied in patients with mild to severe renal impairment, and no dost adjustments are needed with the FDA-recommended 0.3-mg dose.[25]

Ranibizumab

Ranibizumab (Lucentis, Genentech, CA, USA) is a recombinant humanized monoclonal immunoglobulin IgG_1 K-isotype antibody fragment, which binds to the receptor-binding domain of all VEGF isoform, which fully inhibits the protein-receptor complex from being formed, and, therefore, stops all downstream signaling. Ranibizumab was derived by affinity maturation of a humanized Fab fragment of the original monoclonal anti-VEGF antibody and has only one antigen-binding site (Fig. 13.3).[27] Ranibizumab is a 48-kDa antibody. Its pH is 5.5 (drug insert).

Pharmacokinetics

In 2007, Bakri et al. established an experimental rabbit model that was used to study the pharmacokinetics of both bevacizumab and ranibizumab. The same model was used in order to draw comparisons between the two drugs. In the ranibizumab study, 0.5 mg of the drug was injected monocularly into 28 rabbit eyes. Drugs levels were detected using enzyme-linked immunoabsorbant assay of collected samples, namely, aqueous, vitreous, and serum. A noncompartment model was used to create a concentration verses time graph using AUC estimation.[28] The notable quality in this research design is the fact that their drug assay used VEGF molecules to detect the quantity of bound drug in the tissues, instead of simply measuring the free bevacizumab. This imparts greater clinical significance to their result since the bound form of bevacizumab is more representative of the amount of pharmacologically active drug, as we will discuss later in the pharmacodynamic section.

In this model, the maximum vitreous concentration of ranibizumab of 162 μg/mL was reached at day 1. The vitreous terminal half-life for the drug was 2.88 days. A concentration >0.1 μg/mL was measured in the vitreous up to day 29.[28] Their results correlated nicely with the data from Gaudrealut et al.'s study in monkeys, which showed the vitreous terminal half-life of ranibizumab to be 2.9 days. The peak vitreous concentration in Gaudreault et al.'s[29] work was 1,280 μg/mL. The package insert estimates the vitreous terminal half-life to be approximately 9 days (Prod Info LUCENTIS(TM) injection, 2006).

In the aqueous, the maximum concentration was 17.9 μg/mL in rabbits and was reached on day 3. The aqueous terminal half-life was 2.84 days.[28] The maximum aqueous concentration was 57.1 μg/mL in monkeys, with a terminal half-life of 3 days.[29] Both the animal studies show a substantially higher level of ranibizumab in the vitreous humor as compared to the aqueous humor (Fig. 13.4).

Absorption

Studying systemic absorption, Bakri et al.'s[28] experiment with rabbits showed that there was no drug detectable

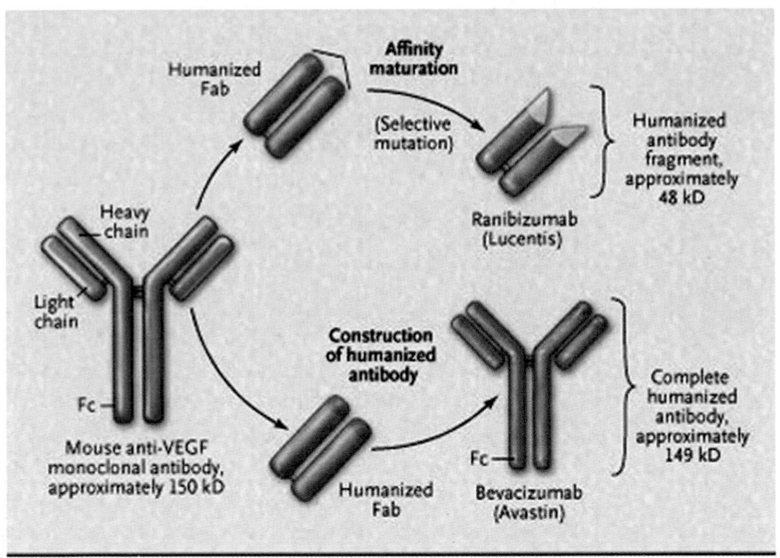

FIGURE 13.3. Relationship between ranibizumab and bevacizumab. Ranibizumab is a recombinant humanized monoclonal IgG1 kappa-isotype antibody fragment (with a molecular weight of about 48 kD). It is produced in an *Escherichia coli* expression system (and thus is not glycosylated) and is designed for intraocular use. Bevacizumab is a recombinant humanized monoclonal IgG1 antibody (with a molecular weight of about 149 kD). It is produced in a Chinese-hamster-ovary mammalian-cell expression system (and thus is glycosylated) and is designed for intravenous infusion. Both the antibody fragment and the full-length antibody bind to and inhibit all the biologically active forms of VEGF A and are derived from the same mouse monoclonal antibody. However, ranibizumab has been genetically engineered through a process of selective mutation to increase its affinity for binding and inhibiting the growth factor. The Fab domain of ranibizumab differs from that of bevacizumab by six amino acids, five on the heavy chain (four of which are in the binding site) and one on the light chain. Not all the intermediate Fabs between the mouse monoclonal antibody and ranibizumab are shown. (Reproduced from Steinbrook R. *N Engl J Med.* 2006;355:1409–1412, with permission.)

both in the contralateral eye and in the serum. This is contradictory to the reports by Gaudreault et al. 2007, which found a maximum serum concentration of 150 ng/mL after a bilateral injection of ranibizumab in a rabbit model. The differences in the detection of serum levels on ranibizumab between these two studies may be reflected in their different use of pharmacokinetic models and their difference in experimental design (Fig. 13.5).

In humans, the product information on ranibizumab states that after monthly intravitreal injection of ranibizumab 0.5 mg, the maximum plasma ranged from 0.3 to 2.36 ng/mL, which is estimated to be 90,000-fold lower than the vitreal concentrations (Prod Info LUCENTIS(TM) injection, 2006) (Table 13.1).

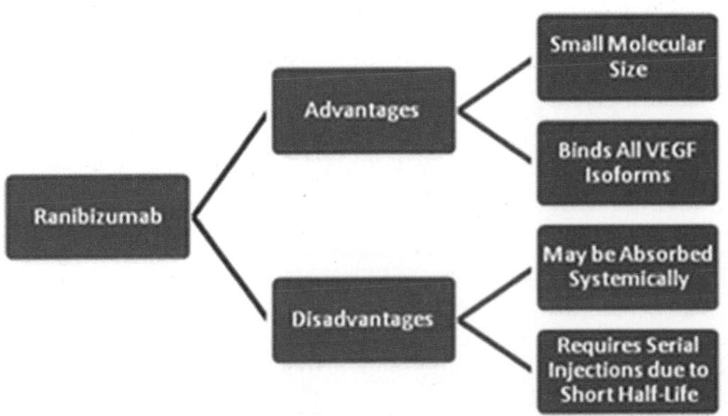

FIGURE 13.4. Advantages and disadvantages of ranibizumab.

Distribution

As the drug distributes through the eye, it is able to penetrate all layers of the retina. Interestingly, the studies proving this result localized the drug both within the intracellular locations between bipolar and photoreceptor cells, as well as, intracellularly internalized by the ganglion and retinal pigment epithelial cells. In addition, the signal was seen below Bruch membrane and throughout the choriocapillaris.[29] This supports the theory that elimination can occur through the outer blood-retinal barrier; however, it is still unclear if this pathway is receptor mediated or if substances can freely diffuse through this tight barrier.

Elimination

Clearance of the drug followed first-order kinetics and was recorded at 0.536 mL/day in rabbits and 0.129 mL/day in monkeys.[28,29] A limited concentration of ranibizumab was found in the serum after injection into a primate model. Reasons include rapid elimination of the drug from the systemic circulation, sequestering of the drug in the vessels walls, or limited transport of the drug into the systemic circulation.

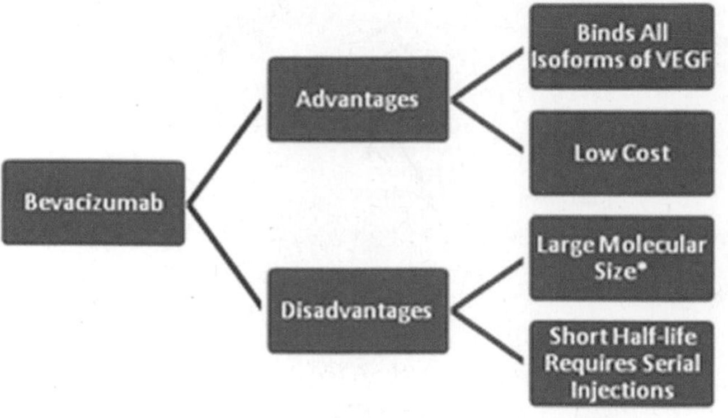

FIGURE 13.5. Advantages and disadvantages of bevacizumab.

Bevacizumab

Bevacizumab (Avastin, Genentech, CA) is a recombinant full-length humanized monoclonal IgG_1 antibody measuring 149 kDa. Bevacizumab is a full-length humanized anti-VEGF monoclonal antibody, which functions similar to ranibizumab by directly inhibiting all of the isoforms of the VEGF molecule from binding to the VEGF receptor, resulting in full inhibition of any downstream proangiogenic receptor signaling (Fig. 13.5).

Pharmacokinetics

Studies of the bevacizumab pharmacokinetics in human revealed a two-compartment model of distribution and elimination for bevacizumab. The work done by Zhu et al. established the following equation for analysis of their model:

$$C(t)=A_0e^{-\alpha t}+B_0e^{-\beta t}$$

In a two-compartment model, the drug penetrates the central compartment, or vitreous first. Then, the drug redistributes to the peripheral compartment and in this model, the retina, choroid, anterior chamber and serum. The first phase when the drug enters the central compartment is so rapid (half-life of 0.5 day) that if early measurements are not taken, it could be missed altogether. This rapid phase may be due to the easy penetration of the drug into the system or to rapid binding of the drug to its target. The second phase, or elimination phase, in this model had a terminal half-life of 6.7 days. In this model, the central compartment was 62 mL and the volume of distribution at stead state was 3.17 mL. The vitreous levels ranged from a maximal concentration of 165 μg/mL at day 2 and decreased over the course of the experiment to a level of 2.63 μg/mL measured at day 101.[6] A significant limitation of this study is the fact that only free bevacizumab could be measured. Ignoring the bound VEGF is ignoring the active form of the drug, which significantly limits the clinical applicability of this information.

Absorption

Results from Bakri et al's study using identical animal models for ranibizumab and bevacizumab, as mentioned above, reported the maximum vitreous concentration of bevacizumab to be 400 μg/mL at day 1, which is higher than that of ranibizumab. The vitreous terminal half-life for the drug was 4.32 days, which is longer than that of ranibizumab. A bevacizumab concentration >0.1 μg/mL was measured in the vitreous until day 30, which is similar to that of ranibizumab. The maximum aqueous concentration was

Table 13.1.

Pharmacokinetic values of ranibizumab based on animal studies

	Rabbit[a]	Monkey[b]	Human[c]
Aqueous maximum concentration	17.9 μg/mL	57.1 μg/mL	
Aqueous terminal ½ life	2.84 days	3 days	
Vitreous maximum concentration	163 μg/mL	1280 μg/mL	
Vitreous terminal ½ life	2.88 days	2.9 days	
Serum maximum concentration	0	150 μg/mL	10 ng/mL
Serum terminal ½ life	N/A	—	10 d

[a]Bakri SJ, et al. Pharmacokinetics of intravitreal bevacizumab (Avastin). *Ophthalmology*. 2007; 114(5):855–859; based on measured amounts in animal models.
[b]Gaudreault J, et al. Pharmacokinetics and retinal distribution of ranibizumab, a humanized antibody fragment directed against VEGF-A, following intravitreal administration in rabbits. *Retina*. 2007;27(9):1260–1266; based on measured amount in animal models.
[c]Chapman JA, Beckey C. Pegaptanib: a novel approach to ocular neovascularization. *Ann Pharmacother*. 2006;40(7–8):1322–1326; based on calculated amounts from a 0.5 mg intravitreal injection.

37.7 μg/mL, reached on day 3. The aqueous terminal half-life was 4.88 days. The maximum serum concentration was 33 μg/mL reached at day 8. The serum terminal half-life was 6.86 days. Serum levels were <1 μg/mL reached by day 29. In this study, bevacizumab was measured in the fellow eye with a maximum aqueous level of 29 ng/mL, which declined over a 4-week period to be undetectable.[28] Research in proliferative diabetic patients also supported the possibility that a monocular injection of bevacizumab could be detected in the contralateral eye.[18] However, more research has to be done to establish if this effect is from a measureable amount of the drug in the contralateral eye or a systemic downregulation of VEGF.

Distribution

Multiple studies have shown bevacizumab's ability to directly penetrate the retina.[5,11,17] Heiduschka et al.'s study used immunohistochemistry and confirmed their findings with radioactive labeling to exquisitely detail the path of bevacizumab after intravitreal injection into monkey eyes. At day 1, bevacizumab was seen in the ILM, ganglion cell layer, and some in the inner plexiform layer. At day 4, the bevacizumab was seen in the inner nuclear layer and outer plexiform layer. At day 7 through 14, the photoreceptors, especially the outer segments, stained positively for bevacizumab. This study reports a time-dependant flow of bevacizumab through the layers of the retina without impediment (Fig. 13.6).

As mentioned previously, studies suggest that the antibody is able to pass through by active transport mechanisms because the intraretinal location of the bevacizumab was seen along side molecules that can assist with active transport. In this study, the drug was colocalized near glial acidic fibrillary protein (GFAP) and vimentin proteins (Fig. 13.7).

The bevacizumab molecules were seen within the outer segments of the photoreceptors inside vesicles believed to be phagosomes. More research needs to be done in this field to confirm these findings, explore their meaning, and outline possible mechanism of transport. In addition, the drug was able to penetrate into the choroid in measurable doses. The serum level of the bevacizumab was measured to be 4% to 5% of the injected intravitreal dose 7 days after its injection.[17]

Elimination

Rabbit models have shown that bevacizumab is eliminated from the vitreous within 4 weeks from its injection. In order to maximize the window of pharmacological activity of the anti-VEGF drugs, researchers have tried to decrease the drugs elimination. The results showed that at 5 weeks, the experimental group, which received topical dorzolamide-timolol (Cosopt, Merk & Co., Inc., New Jersey, USA), had a statistically significant decrease in the central retinal thickness, as measured by optical coherence tomography (OCT) when compared to the control group. However, this effect was not seen at 9 weeks as there was no statistical significance between the groups. Although morphological differences did exist at 5 weeks, this difference was not reflected in the measured visual acuities

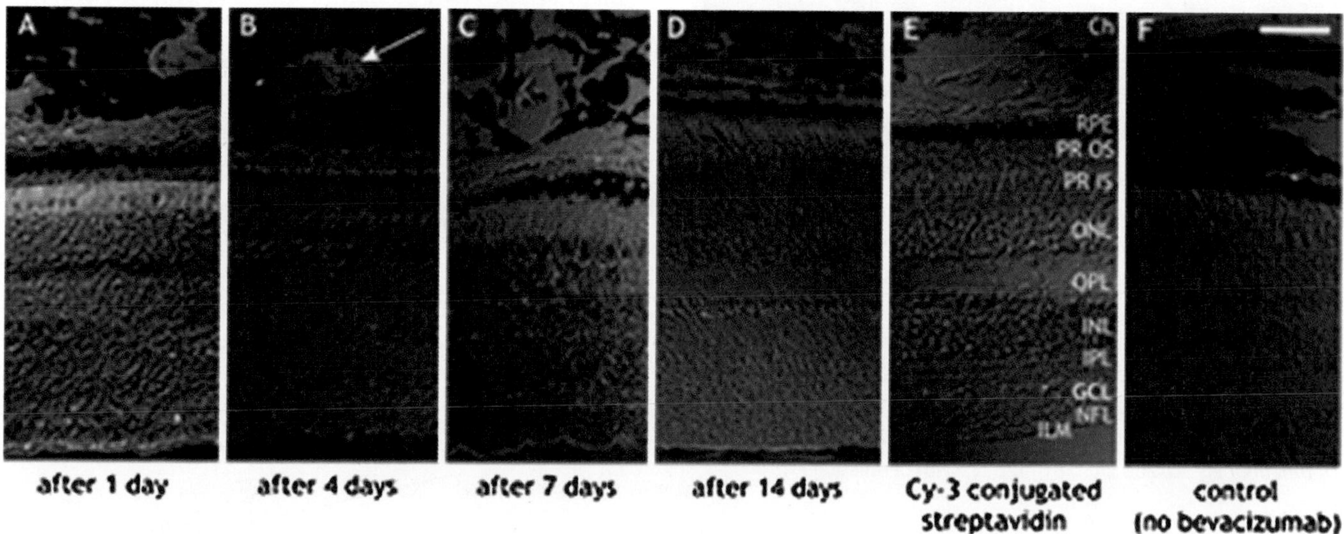

FIGURE 13.6. **A–D:** Time-dependent penetration through the monkey retina of the bevacizumab molecule after its intravitreal injection as detected by a Cy-3-conjugated IgG antibody. For a better orientation, bright-field phase-contrast and fluorescence micrographs have been combined. **E,F:** Images from two control subjects. **E:** Cy-3-conjugated streptavidin was applied to a retinal section obtained 14 days after injection of Avastin. **F:** The Cy-3-conjugated IgG antibody used for bevacizumab detection was applied to a retinal section obtained from the control monkey that did not receive Avastin. The difference between the control and the treated sections **(A)** through **(D)** is clearly visible. NFL, nerve fiber layer. Scale bar, 50 μm. (Reproduced from Heiduschka P. *Invest Ophthalmol Vis Sci.* 2007;48:2814–2823, with permission.)

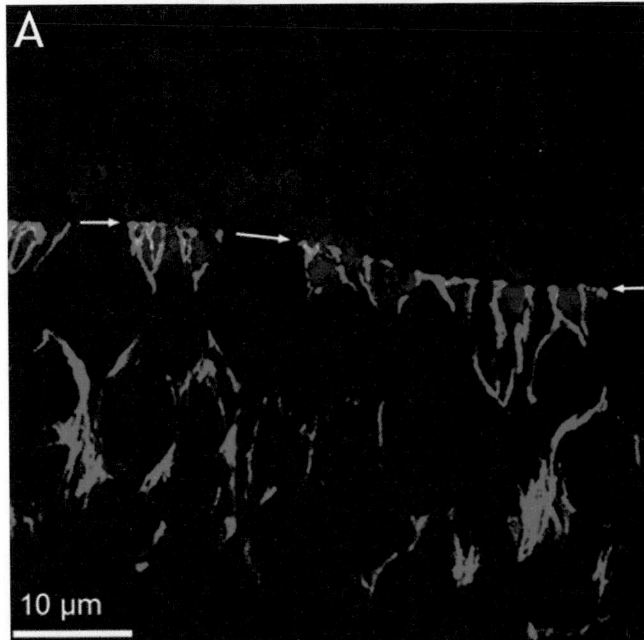

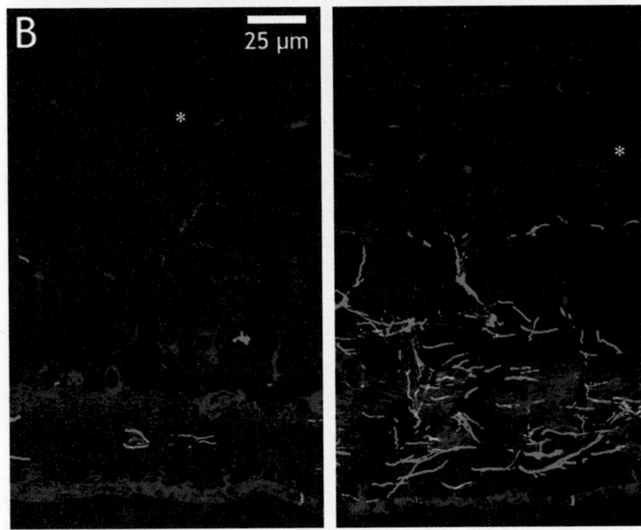

FIGURE 13.7. **A:** Laser scanning micrograph of a retinal section double-stained for bevacizumab (*red*) and vimentin (*green*) 7 days after intravitreal injection of Avastin. **B:** Laser scanning micrograph of a retinal section double-stained for bevacizumab (*red*) and GFAP (*green*) 4 days after intravitreal injection of Avastin. Two different sites of the stained sections are shown that demonstrate local variations in the penetration of bevacizumab and the activation of glial cells (Müller cells and probably astrocytes). (Reproduced from Heiduschka P. *Invest Ophthalmol Vis Sci.* 2007;48:2814–2823, with permission.)

at that time. In conclusion of this study, administration of aqueous suppressants may favorably influence the pharmacokinetics regarding elimination of intravitreal bevacizumab; however, more studies need to be done to ascertain if the difference will lead to a clinical significance such as improvement in visual acuity. However, this study does confirm that a major elimination pathway of intravitreal drugs is via the anterior chamber.

OCULAR PHARMACODYNAMICS

Pharmacodynamics is the study of how a substance interacts with the body in order to produce a specific effect. All pharmacodynamic pathways start with the formation of a drug-receptor complex. The drug-receptor complex creates a permanent chemical change, which activates a membrane receptor that can trigger a downstream signaling cascade. Without the drug-receptor complex, the drug would have no way of influencing the receptor, either by activating it or inhibiting it. Therefore, it will not affect the dynamics of the system.

PHARMACODYNAMICS OF VASCULAR ENDOTHELIAL GROWTH FACTOR

Vascular endothelial growth factor is a proangiogenic cytokine. Under hypoxic conditions, the VEGF molecule binds to the VEGFR-1 and VEGFR-2 receptors, which are the main receptors of VEGF-driven angiogenesis. The activation of the VEGF receptor initiates a dose-dependent tyrosine kinase–dependant pathway that functions to promote endothelial cell proliferation and survival, to induce chemotaxis and gene expression, and to increase vascular permeability and vasodilation.[29,30] To pharmacologically inhibit this neovascularization signal cascade, the drug must inhibit VEGF gene expression, mRNA transcription, protein signaling, or receptor activation. As stated previously in this chapter, ranibizumab and bevacizumab use antibodies that bind to and inhibit the entire VEGF molecule, whereas pegaptanib attaches to the heparin-binding domain of the $VEGF_{165}$ splice isoform to stop the amplification of the VEGF signal (Fig. 13.8). In order for these

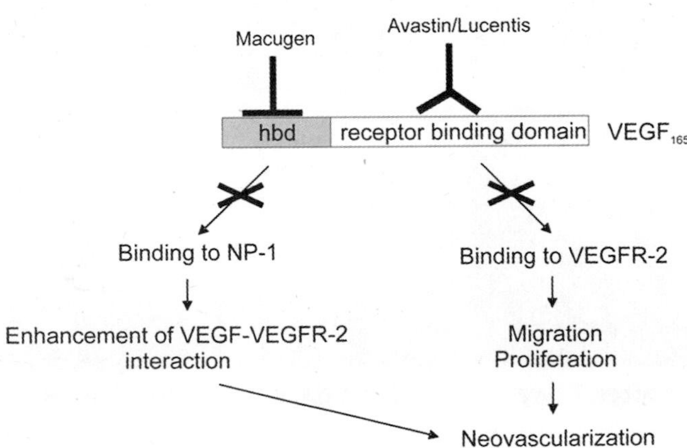

FIGURE 13.8. Schematic model of different pathways inhibited by VEGF antagonists. Bevacizumab and ranibizumab directly inhibit the binding of VEGF to its receptor VEGFR-2 and abrogate VEGF-induced neovascularization. Pegaptanib inhibits the binding to the coreceptor NP-1 and modulates VEGF-induced neovascularization. (Reproduced from Klettner A. *Invest Ophthalmol Vis Sci.* 2008;49:4523–4527, with permission.)

drugs to initiate a pharmacological effect, they must form a drug-receptor complex. Since their target molecule is the VEGF protein or the VEGF splice isoform, this molecule must be present within the eye in order for these drugs to exert an effect. Without the protein present in the system, there would be no binding to the VEGF molecules; therefore, the drugs would have no effect on the signaling cascade. Therefore, it is vital to know when and where VEGF is expressed within the eye.

It is believed that VEGF is expressed at a baseline level, which plays a role in balancing angiogenic factors and possibly influencing neural health. Vascular endothelial growth factor is sensitive to oxidative stress. It is upregulated in hypoxic conditions and downregulated in hyperoxic conditions. Insulin-like growth factor has also been show to increase the production of VEGF.[31] VEGF is produced in retinal pigment epithelial cells, astrocytes, Müller cells, vascular endothelial cell, and ganglion cells.[31] Alternative splice variants of VEGF express different tissue distributions, and $VEGF_{189}$ and $VEGF_{206}$ splice isoforms are membrane bound, while $VEGF_{121}$ and $VEGF_{165}$ splice isoforms are able to diffuse into the vitreous and aqueous compartments.[31] Vascular endothelial growth factor displays a concentration gradient from posterior to anterior within the eye and is excreted via the trabecular meshwork. Simultaneous measurements of VEGF levels in patients with active neovascularization showed that the vitreous humor levels (8.8 ± 9.9 ng/mL) were 60 times more elevated than the aqueous humor levels (5.6 ± 8.6 ng/mL) (p = 0.033).[32] This may be due to the rapid elimination of VEGF through the anterior chamber outflow pathways.

Measuring VEGF in Different Disease States

Vascular endothelial growth factor is consistently elevated in ischemic eyes; however, the degree of elevation shows a wide range of levels that varied over different time points of the disease.[32] Elevated levels of vascular endothelial growth factor were found in patients with proliferative diabetic retinopathy, neovascular glaucoma, retinopathy of prematurity, ischemic central-retinal vein occlusion, vitreous hemorrhage, acute or chronic retinal detachments, and iris neovascularization. Vascular endothelial growth factor was not detected in patients with endophthalmitis, leukemic retinopathy, uveitis, retinitis, and epiretinal membranes. In addition, vascular endothelial growth factor was not detected in patients with choroidal neovascular membranes, possibly because these membranes were inactive at the time of the assay, showing the transient nature of this protein. The highest amounts of VEGF were found in eyes with active proliferative diabetic retinopathy: the VEGF level was 5.6 ± 6.5 ng/mL. Repeat measurements that were performed in the same eyes after photocoagulative laser treatments, which decrease the hypoxic drive of these tissues revealed a decrease in the VEGF level to 1.4 ± 2.0 ng/mL (p = 0.008).[32] Since the rise in VEGF is transient, it is difficult to titrate the appropriate amount of pharmacological therapy that is needed in order to inhibit the full amount of the VEGF protein.

Furthermore, measurements performed on endothelial cells in vitro showed a dose-dependant response to VEGF levels. The maximal effect was produced by 25 ng/mL and half the maximal effect was produced by 1 ng/mL of VEGF.[32] The ability of this small level of VEGF to still show activity would mean that the full amount of VEGF must be inhibited to stop its effect.

High serum and high vitreous VEGF levels were positively correlated with patients who had proliferative diabetic retinopathy and patients with the CC genotype of the VEGF polymorphism. High vitreous levels of VEGF were positively correlated with patient who had proliferative diabetic retinopathy as compared to control eyes without diabetes. Particularly, vitreous VEGF levels were elevated in proliferative diabetic patients with active disease and with macular edema. Vitreous VEGF levels were negatively correlated with the extent of photocoagulation therapy in patients with proliferative diabetic retinopathy, i.e. the greater the extent of the laser treatment, the lower the levels of intravitreal VEGF.[33]

Pharmacodynamic Modeling

With most drugs, the pharmacokinetic model of the drug can be used to predict the amount of drug-receptor complexes that will be formed and, therefore, predict the final pharmacodynamic effect from activation of those receptors. For example, researchers can use pharmacokinetic models to predict the pharmacodynamic effect of alcohol on the body. The amount of alcohol consumed can be used in a pharmacokinetic model to construct a concentration verses time graph in order to estimate the amount of alcohol at any point in time after its consumption. The concentration of alcohol is directly proportional to the amount of effect that it has no the body, or its pharmacodynamic effect. The final effect is based on the assumptions behind basic pharmacological principles. It is important to assume that the amount of alcohol that is measured will all bind to its receptor and be metabolized in the system. Therefore, the total amount of alcohol measured at that time will produce the maximal effect on the subject and the pharmacokinetic model will predict the pharmacodynamic effect on the body. However, this same concept is not true regarding anti-VEGF medications.

Although many research groups have validated the pharmacokinetic models for anti-VEGF drugs, their models cannot accurately predict the final ocular effect of the medication. This is because, unlike alcohol, one of the basic assumptions of pharmacological modeling is not met, which is the fact that the receptor for the drug is not always present within the system. Instead, the receptor for the drug, the VEGF molecule, is transiently produced within the system. Its production depends on the oxygenation level within the ocular tissue. Therefore, under hypoxic conditions, when the VEGF molecule is present, the maximal effect predicted by the pharmacokinetic model may be accurate; however, under high to normal oxygen tension states, when the VEGF molecule is not present in a high concentration, the pharmokinetic model cannot accurately predict the drug's effect on the body. When there is no substrate available to form a drug-receptor complex, the drug exerts no effect on the system no matter how much of the drug is present.

For example, although half of the initial amount of pegaptanib is still present at day 10 after the injection, if there is no VEGF remaining on the tenth day, then the drug will not have a clinical effect. Furthermore, although bevacizumab has been shown to have a longer half-life compared to ranibizumab in animal models, it is not possible to prove that bevacizumab would be a more effective drug unless the VEGF levels and amount of drug-receptor complexes over time are also measured.

Measurement of VEGF Changes with Anti-VEGF Medications

The Heiduschka et al. study provided novel insight into the dynamic interaction of the bevacizumab drug and its VEGF target protein. This research group used immunohistochemical analysis to label the basal amounts of VEGF within a normal monkey eye and the change in VEGF after injection of intravitreal bevacizumab. In the normal monkey eye, VEGF was found mostly in the ganglion cell layer and the inner nuclear layer and, to a lesser extent, in the photoreceptors and the choroidal blood vessel walls. The overall result of injection with bevacizumab was a corresponding decrease of VEGF in that level. Specifically, the first day after injection, the ganglion cell layer had detectable amounts of bevacizumab but no VEGF signal in this level as there was prior to the injection. The VEGF level was also decreased within the choroid at this time, and there was colocalization of VEGF and bevacizumab in the blood vessel walls. Then 14 days after the bevacizumab injection, the drug was detected within the outer segments of the photoreceptors, the choroidal blood vessels and the ILM, while the VEGF protein in these regions was completely diminished except for in some parts of the choriocapillaris. The drug and protein molecules formed a triple-layer appearance in the arteriole walls of the choroid vessels. The inner layer of the blood vessel wall showed pure bevacizumab, while the middle layer had pure VEGF molecule and the outer layer showed both the bevacizumab and VEGF molecules.

The drop in the level of VEGF after the intravitreal injection of bevacizumab is not surprising since the efficacy of bevacizumab has already been outlined. However, the fact that even after 14 days, there was still no detectable levels of VEGF reflects a shut down in the production of the VEGF growth factor since even the basal levels of VEGF were not detected. One explanation for this would be that the formation of the VEGF-bevacizumab complex occupied all the available binding sites of the VEGF molecule; therefore, the antibodies used to label the growth factor in this experiment were unable to bind the molecule, so it might have been present but undetectable by the methods of the assay. Or perhaps, more complex mechanisms exist that affect indirect pathways of VEGF receptor inhibition.

An additional study that provided valuable information was the study by Zhu et al. The major advantage of this study was that they reported on the various isoforms of VEGF in their model. VEGF isoforms were delineated with gel electrophoresis and western blot testing. VEGF levels ranged from 0.2 to 33.9 pg/mL. This dose was dependent on both the amount of bevacizumab and the amount of time elapsed. Furthermore, different isoforms of VEGF were present in different concentrations and showed different dose-correlations with bevacizumab. $VEGF_{165}$ splice isoform was 44% of the total VEGF, making up the largest quantity of isoform present. It showed both a time and bevacizumab dose-response. The $VEGF_{189}$ splice isoform accounted for 37% of the total VEGF and showed a time-related increase to bevacizumab in its amount. The $VEGF_{121}$ splice isoform was 19% of the total VEGF. However, it did not show a time- or dose-dependent response to bevacizumab.[6]

These studies lay the groundwork for understanding the fluctuations of the VEGF protein. Further knowledge of the exact level of VEGF within a diseased eye can lead to improved strategies for targeting and inhibiting this angiogenic signaling cytokine. In future studies, it will be important to continue to quantitate not only the amount of drug present but also the amount of VEGF present within the system.

Therapeutic Dosing Schedules

Identifying the recommended dosing schedule for intravitreal anti-VEGF medications is an important goal for researchers. Although electroretinogram studies have shown that doses as high as 2.5 mg of bevacizumab are nontoxic to the retina,[11] it is not clear if higher dosing of the drug imparts a greater clinical benefit. Large clinical trials have tried to provide clinicians with dosing recommendations. These trials have shown that the amounts of vitreous and serum levels of the anti-VEGF drugs are dose dependent. In the MARINA study, a greater percentage of patients gained 15 letters in the 0.5-mg group (34%) as compared to the reported value of the 0.3-mg group (25%), although this result was not statistically significant. This trend was also seen in the ANCHOR study where 40% of the 0.5-mg group and 36% of the 0.3-mg group gained 15 letters of more of visual acuity. From this data, it seems that a higher vitreous level of ranibizumab may correlate to a larger gain in visual acuity. In comparison, the VISION trial showed that there was no statistical difference between the 0.3-, 1-, or 3-mg dose of pegaptanib in improving visual acuity.[34]

In addition to determining the dose amount, the best schedule for delivering the dose is still unknown. Clinical trials, including VISION, ANCHOR, and MARINA, have all used a standard dosing schedule of every 6 weeks for the VISION study and monthly injections for ANCHOR and MARINA. When dosing schedules were extended to quarterly basis after initial induction, as in the PIER Trial, the overall visual gain was lower that expected. The decrease in visual acuity could correlate with a decrease in vitreal concentrations of ranibizumab to a level below the necessary concentration for the full inhibitory effect on VEGF-induced endothelial cell growth, thereby, allowing VEGF to promote angiogenic factors and potentiate the progression of the sight-threatening choroidal neovascularization in these patients. So the most appropriate dosing schedule would be the one that maintains steady states of the anti-VEGF drug in concentrations adequate enough to inhibit the VEGF receptor when the receptor is present.

Large clinical trials are invaluable to clinical practice. The trials focusing on anti-VEGF medications provide strong results that show an overall positive affect of pharmacotherapy for treating macular degeneration. The results from these studies were revolutionizing and have forever changed the current practice of Ophthalmology in their ability to not only slow vision loss but also improve vision after damage from neovascular macular degeneration. However, to show that the anti-VEGF medication influences the final outcome of visual acuity or OCT thickness, these studies make several assumptions. They assume that there is a constant supply of VEGF within the eye and that as long as the drug is present in the eye, it is exerting an effect on the VEGF level. Some of these trials assume that a gain in vision is directly correlated with the anti-VEGF medication binding to and inhibiting VEGF receptor activation. Although some of these assumptions may be true, the studies do not take the steps to prove these theories within their study. More research is needed to validate the logic behind these clinical trials and explain the assumptions made in their outcome measurements. Overall, the results from these studies should be weighed accordingly when referring to the results from these studies for shaping clinical guidelines.

This disconnect between the conclusions drawn between the pharmacokinetic and pharmacodynamic models makes it difficult to predict the final effect of anti-VEGF medications on the level of VEGF as well as to establish recommendations on dose amounts and schedules that should be used to optimize the effect of the medication. To connect the hypothesis of the study with results that validate the assumptions, some studies measure the amount of VEGF within the tissue and report how it changes with the addition of an anti-VEGF medication. Other studies optimize the conditions using in vitro–controlled experiments to ensure that the VEGF molecule is present within the system.

The in vitro studies of bevacizumab were initially performed by oncologists since bevacizumab is an approved anticancer medication. One of these studies created an endothelial cell culture medium to analyze certain pharmacological aspects of bevacizumab. In this study, bevacizumab showed a dose-dependent response in its ability to inhibit VEGF-induced endothelial growth. The minimal amount of bevacizumab needed to effectively alter the cell growth was 22 ng/mL, while the dose that achieved complete inhibition (which was equal to blocking 50 ng/mL of VEGF) was 500 ng/mL of bevacizumab. Using this information, they reported that a 2.6:1 ratio of bevacizumab to homodimeric VEGF was necessary to reach maximal inhibitory effect of bevacizumab.[30] Since multiple pharmacological models have shown that the clearance of bevacizumab follows first-order kinetics in the plasma as well as in the vitreous and that the rate of systemic drug elimination parallels the rate of vitreous clearance, we can assume that the same ratio will apply within the vitreous. Using this logic and the reported vitreous half-life of bevacizumab as 6.7 days, the complete inhibition of VEGF would be possible for 48 days and a concentration above 22 ng/mL would last 78 days from injection.[6] Clinically, this becomes relevant, since in order to maintain vitreous levels of bevacizumab above 500 ng/mL or the dose necessary for full inhibitory effect on VEGF, intravitreal injections would have to be repeated every 6 to 7 weeks.

Another in vitro study directly compared the effect of clinical doses of bevacizumab and ranibizumab on tissue sheets of retina, retinal pigment epithelium, and choroid. Separate experiments showed that 317 pg/mL of VEGF can be completely neutralized within 6 hours by one dose of 0.25 mg/mL of bevacizumab or 0.125 mg/mL of ranibizumab. The effect of inhibition of VEGF lasted up to 16 hours for both drugs. Each drug was diluted to ascertain the threshold dose for inhibition of VEGF. From this model, bevacizumab and ranibizumab lost their ability to neutralize VEGF at a concentration of 975 and 120 ng/mL, respectively. These results indicate a 17-fold higher binding capacity of ranibizumab as compared to bevacizumab, making even dilute forms of the medication very effective in inhibiting VEGF receptor signaling. Interestingly, in this experiment, pegaptanib did not show any affect on neutralizing the in vitro VEGF levels.[35]

These in vitro experiments call into question the proper dose that should be administered within each injection of the anti-VEGF medications. They suggest that our current clinical doses are exponentially higher than the doses needed to create the same clinical effect. Currently, the idea of using microdoses of bevacizumab is being studied for its use intravenously as a chemotherapeutic agent. Future research needs to be done and supported by clinical trials to determine the appropriate doses for intravitreal use of these medications.

KEY POINTS

- Pharmacokinetics is how the body affects the drug. It includes the study of drug liberation, absorption, dispersion, metabolism, and elimination.
- Pharmacodynamics is how the drug affects the body. It includes analysis of how the drug stimulates, depresses, destroys, or replaces substances within the body.
- Intravitreal drugs are limited in their dispersion by ocular barriers. These barriers include the vitreous, ILM, ELM, and Bruch membrane. Studies have shown that these membranes reduce flow by mechanical and electrostatic barriers.
- Elimination pathways for intravitreal drugs include both anterior and posterior pathways. The anterior pathway eliminates drug through the trabecular meshwork and uveoscleral outflow. The posterior pathway eliminates drug through transretinal migration of substances and receptor-mediated transcytosis.
- Pegaptanib is a highly selective nucleic acid derivative that acts on the heparin-binding domain of VEGF-165 slice isoform. It has a high affinity for its substrate and it has been proven to be safe after intravitreal administration; however, it only works on one isoform of VEGF and it is quickly eliminated from the body. Extrapolation of data from human pharmacokinetic studies of pegaptanib shows that after an intravitreal injection of 0.5 mg, the maximum serum concentration will be approximately 10 ng/mL within the plasma with a plasma half-life of 10 days.
- Ranibizumab and bevacizumab are recombinant humanized monoclonal immunoglobulin IgG1 antibodies. Ranibizumab is a fragment of this antibody, while bevacizumab is the full-length antibody. They bind to the receptor-binding domain of all VEGF isoforms.
- Animal models have shown opposing results if either ranibizumab or bevacizumab is able to penetrate into the serum after intravitreal injection; however, human studies have shown that both of these drugs can be measured in the serum after intravitreal injection; this significance of this observation is still being studied.
- In order for an anti-VEGF medication to be effective, its substrate (the VEGF protein) must be present. The VEGF protein is transiently expressed, and its amount varies in different disease states.
- New research should focus on analyzing VEGF protein in relation to disease state and the change in VEGF protein after the introduction of anti-VEGF medication.

CONCLUSION

Understanding the pharmokinetics and pharmacodynamics of a drug is vital to the safe and effective implementation of the drug in clinical practice. Studies that focus on elucidating the mechanism behind these pharmacological principles offer important treatment guidelines for physicians.

REFERENCES

1. Kim H, Csaky KG, Gravlin L, et al. Safety and pharmacokinetics of a preservative-free triamcinolone acetonide formulation for intravitreal administration. *Retina.* 2006;26(5):523–530.
2. Pederson JE, Gaasterland DE, MacLellan HM. Anterior chamber volume determination in the rhesus monkey. *Invest Ophthalmol Vis Sci.* 1978;17(8):784–787.
3. Mordenti J, Cuthbertson RA, Ferrara N, et al. Comparisons of the intraocular tissue distribution, pharmacokinetics, and safety of 125I-labeled full-length and Fab antibodies in rhesus monkeys following intravitreal administration. *Toxicol Pathol.* 1999;27(5):536–544.
4. Molokhia SA, Jeong EK, Higuchi WI, et al. Transscleral iontophoretic and intravitreal delivery of a macromolecule: study of ocular distribution in vivo and postmortem with MRI. *Exp Eye Res.* 2009;88:418–425.
5. Dib E, Maia M, Longo-Maugeri IM, et al. Subretinal bevacizumab detection after intravitreous injection in rabbits. *Invest Ophthalmol Vis Sci.* 2008;49(3):1097–1100.
6. Zhu Q, Ziemssen F, Henke-Fahle S, et al. Vitreous levels of bevacizumab and vascular endothelial growth factor-A in patients with choroidal neovascularization. *Ophthalmology.* 2008;115(10):1750–1755, 1755 e1.
7. Kim H, Robinson MR, Lizak MJ, et al. Controlled drug release from an ocular implant: an evaluation using dynamic three-dimensional magnetic resonance imaging. *Invest Ophthalmol Vis Sci.* 2004;45(8):2722–2731.
8. Foo SS, Abbott DF, Lawrentschuk N, et al. Functional imaging of intratumoral hypoxia. *Mol Imaging Biol.* 2004;6(5): 291–305.
9. Kim H, Robinson SB, Csaky KG. Investigating the movement of intravitreal human serum albumin nanoparticles in the vitreous and retina. *Pharm Res.* 2009;26(2):329–337.
10. Kamei M, Misono K, Lewis H. A study of the ability of tissue plasminogen activator to diffuse into the subretinal space after intravitreal injection in rabbits. *Am J Ophthalmol.* 1999;128(6):739–746.
11. Shahar J, Avery RL, Heilweil G, et al. Electrophysiologic and retinal penetration studies following intravitreal injection of bevacizumab (Avastin). *Retina.* 2006;26(3):262–269.
12. Takeuchi A, Kricorian G, Yao XY, et al. The rate and source of albumin entry into saline-filled experimental retinal detachments. *Invest Ophthalmol Vis Sci.* 1994;35(11):3792–3798.
13. Kwan AS, Vijayasekaran S, McAllister IL, et al. A study of retinal penetration of intravitreal tenecteplase in pigs. *Invest Ophthalmol Vis Sci.* 2006;47(6):2662–2667.
14. Adamus G, Machnicki M, Elerding H, et al. Antibodies to recoverin induce apoptosis of photoreceptor and bipolar cells in vivo. *J Autoimmun.* 1998;11(5):523–533.
15. Lei B, Bush RA, Milam AH, et al. Human melanoma-associated retinopathy (MAR) antibodies alter the retinal ON-response of the monkey ERG in vivo. *Invest Ophthalmol Vis Sci.* 2000;41(1):262–266.
16. Duvvuri S, Majumdar S, Mitra AK. Drug delivery to the retina: challenges and opportunities. *Expert Opin Biol Ther.* 2003;3(1):45–56.

17. Heiduschka P, Fietz H, Hofmeister S, et al. Penetration of bevacizumab through the retina after intravitreal injection in the monkey. *Invest Ophthalmol Vis Sci*. 2007;48(6):2814–2823.
18. Avery RL, Pearlman J, Pieramici DJ, et al. Intravitreal bevacizumab (Avastin) in the treatment of proliferative diabetic retinopathy. *Ophthalmology*. 2006;113(10):1695 e1–1695 e15.
19. Del Amo EM, Urtti A. Current and future ophthalmic drug delivery systems. A shift to the posterior segment. *Drug Discov Today*. 2008;13(3–4):135–143.
20. Kim H, Csaky KG, Chan CC, et al. The pharmacokinetics of rituximab following an intravitreal injection. *Exp Eye Res*. 2006;82(5):760–766.
21. Byeon SH, Kwon OW, Song JH, et al. Prolongation of activity of single intravitreal bevacizumab by adjuvant topical aqueous depressant (Timolol-Dorzolamide). *Graefes Arch Clin Exp Ophthalmol*. 2009;247(1):35–42.
22. Oishi M, Maeda S, Hashida N, et al. Pharmacokinetic behavior of intravitreal triamcinolone acetonide prepared by a hospital pharmacy. *Jpn J Ophthalmol*. 2008;52(6):489–492.
23. Kim H, Fariss RN, Zhang C, et al. Mapping of the neonatal Fc receptor in the rodent eye. *Invest Ophthalmol Vis Sci*. 2008;49(5):2025–2029.
24. Healy JM, Lewis SD, Kurz M, et al. Pharmacokinetics and biodistribution of novel aptamer compositions. *Pharm Res*. 2004;21(12):2234–2246.
25. Chapman JA, Beckey C. Pegaptanib: a novel approach to ocular neovascularization. *Ann Pharmacother*. 2006;40(7–8): 1322–1326.
26. Kourlas H, Schiller DS. Pegaptanib sodium for the treatment of neovascular age-related macular degeneration: a review. *Clin Ther*. 2006;28(1):36–44.
27. Dadgostar H, Waheed N. The evolving role of vascular endothelial growth factor inhibitors in the treatment of neovascular age-related macular degeneration. *Eye*. 2008; 22(6):761–767.
28. Bakri SJ, Snyder MR, Reid JM, et al. Pharmacokinetics of intravitreal bevacizumab (Avastin). *Ophthalmology*. 2007;114(5):855–859.
29. Gaudreault J, Fei D, Beyer JC, et al. Pharmacokinetics and retinal distribution of ranibizumab, a humanized antibody fragment directed against VEGF-A, following intravitreal administration in rabbits. *Retina*. 2007;27(9):1260–1266.
30. Wang Y, Fei D, Vanderlaan M, et al. Biological activity of bevacizumab, a humanized anti-VEGF antibody in vitro. *Angiogenesis*. 2004;7(4):335–345.
31. Penn JS, Madan A, Caldwell RB, et al. Vascular endothelial growth factor in eye disease. *Prog Retin Eye Res*. 2008; 27(4):331–371.
32. Aiello LP, Avery RL, Arrigg PG, et al. Vascular endothelial growth factor in ocular fluid of patients with diabetic retinopathy and other retinal disorders. *N Engl J Med*. 1994;331(22):1480–1487.
33. Petrovic MG, Korosec P, Kosnik M, et al. Local and genetic determinants of vascular endothelial growth factor expression in advanced proliferative diabetic retinopathy. *Mol Vis*. 2008;14:1382–1387.
34. Gragoudas ES, Adamis AP, Cunningham ET, et al. Pegaptanib for neovascular age-related macular degeneration. *N Engl J Med*. 2004;351(27):2805–2816.
35. Klettner A, Roider J. Comparison of bevacizumab, ranibizumab, and pegaptanib in vitro: efficiency and possible additional pathways. *Invest Ophthalmol Vis Sci*. 2008;49(10): 4523–4527.

CHAPTER

14

Anti-VEGF Therapies for Retinal Neovascularization

Jason Hsu • Allen C. Ho

INTRODUCTION

Until recently, laser panretinal photocoagulation (PRP) has been the standard for treatment of patients with proliferative diabetic retinopathy (PDR) in order to reduce the risk of vision loss. The Diabetic Retinopathy Study (DRS) confirmed that PRP was associated with a 50% reduction in the risk of severe visual loss (visual acuity < 5/200) compared to no treatment.[1,2,3] The Early Treatment of Diabetic Retinopathy Study (ETDRS) further defined the appropriate timing for initiation of PRP.[4] However, laser PRP can be uncomfortable for patients and is not without its potential risks, including visual field constriction, night blindness, macular edema, development or progression of tractional retinal detachment (TRD), and choroidal detachment with possible acute angle closure glaucoma. In addition, only about 60% of patients with PDR seem to respond to PRP laser treatment with regression of neovascularization within 3 months.[5] As a result, many patients require additional laser treatment and about 4.5% ultimately need pars plana vitrectomy despite PRP.[6]

The role of growth factors in the development of retinovascular diseases was first proposed by Michaelson[7] in 1948. It was not until the discovery and cloning of vascular endothelial growth factor (VEGF) in 1989 and the ensuing development of anti-VEGF antibodies that the key role of this factor in retinal neovascularization was realized.[8,9] VEGF levels have been shown to correlate with the severity of PDR and decrease following PRP.[10,11] Injection of VEGF in a primate model produced a retinopathy similar to diabetic retinopathy and even resulted in iris neovascularization.[12,13] Blockage of VEGF was associated with inhibition of iris neovascularization and suppression of retinal neovascularization in primates.[14,15] Given these findings, anti-VEGF treatments have been hypothesized as an alternative treatment for retinal neovascularization.

ANTI-VEGF THERAPIES FOR NEOVASCULARIZATION IN PROLIFERATIVE DIABETIC RETINOPATHY

Pegaptanib

Pegaptanib sodium (Macugen; Eyetech Pharmaceuticals, Inc.; New York, NY and Pfizer Inc.; New York, NY) is an anti-VEGF aptamer that specifically blocks the 165 isoform of VEGF, which is believed to be the predominant isoform responsible for pathological neovascularization. It was the first treatment of its kind approved for intraocular injection by the Food and Drug Administration in the treatment of neovascular age-related macular degeneration. A phase 2 study with pegaptanib was also performed in 172 patients with diabetic macular edema and found that intravitreal injections every 6 weeks for 12 to 30 weeks resulted in better visual acuity outcomes, decreased central retinal thickness, and a reduced need for focal/grid laser at 36 weeks compared to sham injections.[16] At baseline, 19 of these subjects were also noted to have retinal neovascularization. This provided an opportunity to explore the effects of pegaptanib sodium on these patients in a retrospective fashion. Three of the nineteen patients were excluded from this review since one had PRP performed 13 days before randomization and two did not have follow-up photographs. Of the remaining 16 subjects, 8 had prior PRP at least 26 weeks before study entry, 1 had PRP 14 weeks before enrollment, and 1 was treated with PRP 89 days after study enrollment.

Thirteen of the sixteen patients were randomized to the pegaptanib group. Of these, eight (including the one patient who received PRP after study enrollment) showed regression or absence of neovascularization by week 36. None of the three patients in the sham group showed regression. Following cessation of pegaptanib, three of the eight patients who originally showed regression of neovascularization had progression by week 52.

This study was the first report documenting regression of neovascularization in patients with PDR who were given intravitreal anti-VEGF therapy. Although the number of cases was small, they provided the initial evidence for a definitive role of VEGF in retinal neovascularization and confirmed experimental observations in laboratory studies.[17] While spontaneous regression of retinal neovascularization has been reported, such cases are extremely rare.[18] The fact that 62% of the patients with baseline retinal neovascularization who received pegaptanib showed regression in addition to the observation that recurrence of the new vessels occurred in three of the eight cases after discontinuation of the injections seems to suggest a causal relationship.

Bevacizumab

Bevacizumab (Avastin; Genentech, Inc., South San Francisco, California) is a full-length recombinant humanized monoclonal antibody directed against all isoforms of VEGF and approved by the Food and Drug Administration for the treatment of metastatic colorectal cancer.[19,20,21] Shortly after intravitreal bevacizumab was reported to have beneficial effects in patients with neovascular age-related macular degeneration,[22,23] several small case series emerged describing the effects of this treatment on patients with neovascularization due to PDR.

Avery demonstrated the rapidity of regression of iris and retinal neovascularization in a 60-year-old woman who had prior partial PRP 18 months before.[24] One week after intravitreal bevacizumab, both the iris rubeosis and retinal neovascularization were clinically regressed with resolution of neovascular leakage on fluorescein angiography. iedlander and Welch[25] described a 36-year-old patient with advanced PDR and macular edema who received an intravitreal injection of 1.25-mg bevacizumab. Initial visual acuity was 20/100. Eight days later, his visual acuity had improved to 20/40 and the neovascular vessels were no longer apparent. Isaacs and Barry reported a similar result in an asymptomatic 70-year-old patient with neovascularization of the disc (NVD) whose visual acuity was 20/30. Following a single 1.25-mg injection of intravitreal bevacizumab, complete resolution of the NVD was noted at the 1 month follow-up visit and the visual acuity remained stable.[26] Fluorescein angiography showed no evidence of neovascular leakage. No clinical evidence of recurrence of the NVD was seen at the 2 month follow-up. Figure 14.1 shows one of our patients who presented with NVD due to PDR. He received 1.25 mg of intravitreal bevacizumab and returned 2 weeks later with no clinical evidence of NVD (Fig. 14.2).

Mason et al.[27] described three patients who demonstrated rapid regression of neovascularization following a single 1-mg intravitreal bevacizumab injection. One case with prior PRP but active NVD and neovascularization elsewhere (NVE) showed complete regression by 3 weeks postinjection with no recurrence by last follow-up

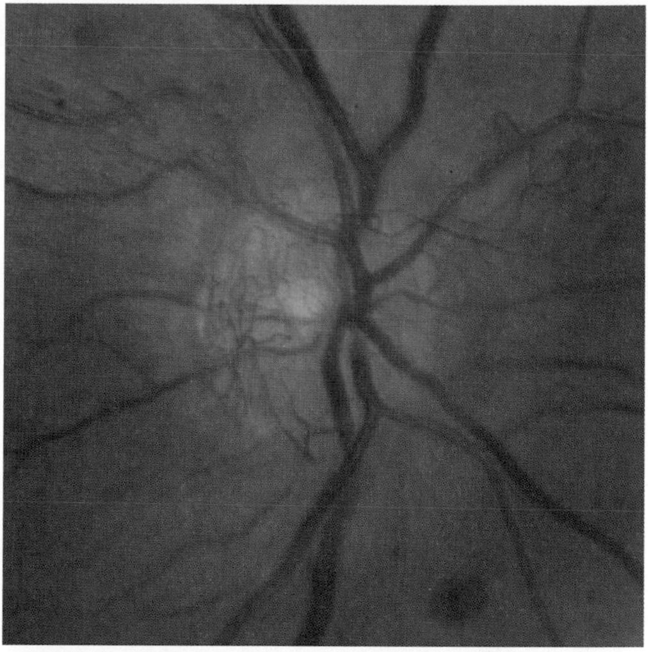

FIGURE 14.1. Color photograph demonstrating disc neovascularization in a diabetic patient prior to intravitreal bevacizumab.

at 10 weeks. A second case with partial PRP presented with severe NVD and NVE. The neovascularization regressed within 2 weeks of an intravitreal bevacizumab injection. Additional PRP was delivered and the patient remained stable until last follow-up at 5 months. The final case presented with severe PDR with a subhyaloid hemorrhage involving the macula. Following intravitreal bevacizumab, regression of the NVD and NVE was noted within

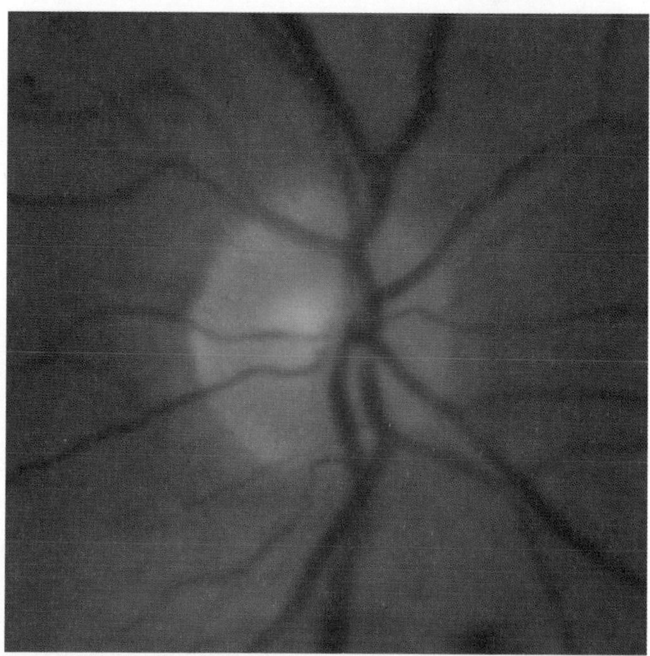

FIGURE 14.2. Color photograph 2 weeks after intravitreal bevacizumab showing marked clinical regression of the disc neovascularization.

3 weeks. One potential benefit of such rapid regression of neovascularization might be prevention of vitreous hemorrhage (VH).

Avery et al.[28] confirmed a biologic effect of intravitreal bevacizumab on regression of retinal and iris neovascularization due to diabetes mellitus. In this retrospective case series, 45 eyes of 32 patients with retinal and/or iris neovascularization received a single dose of intravitreal bevacizumab. Follow-up was short-term, ranging from 1 to 14 weeks with a mean of 5 weeks. The majority of eyes (38 of 45) had received prior PRP. Various doses of intravitreal bevacizumab were tested with two eyes receiving 6.2 μg, five eyes receiving 12.5 μg, one eye receiving 62 μg, two eyes receiving 125 μg, two eyes receiving 625 μg, and 33 eyes receiving 1.25 mg.

All eyes demonstrated partial to complete reduction in leakage of the neovascularization on fluorescein angiography, even with the lowest dose tested. Of 26 eyes with NVD, complete resolution of angiographic leakage was seen in 19 eyes (73%). A fast clinical response was noted with leakage decreasing in as little as 24 hours after the injection. In several cases, the neovascularization seemed to regress with a reduction in the caliber and presence of neovascular vessel perfusion. Following the single injection, time to recurrence of angiographic leakage varied from 2 weeks to beyond 11 weeks. Interestingly, two cases had a mild decrease in leakage from retinal or iris neovascularization in the uninjected fellow eye, suggesting that the intravitreal dose may cross the blood-retinal barrier and reach therapeutic systemic levels. While no adverse events were seen in this short-term study, these findings suggest that systemic side effects may occur even with intravitreal injections and that lower doses may help mitigate the potential risk.

Jorge et al.[29] performed a prospective nonrandomized study of 15 eyes of 15 consecutive patients treated with 1.5 mg of intravitreal bevacizumab for active neovascularization from diabetic retinopathy that was refractory to laser treatment. Complete PRP had to be performed at least 4 months prior to enrollment in the study. Patients were followed for 12 weeks. Mean logMAR visual acuity improved significantly from a baseline of 0.90 (20/160) to 0.76 (20/125) at 1 week, 0.77 (20/125) at 6 weeks, and 0.77 (20/125) at 12 weeks ($p < 0.05$). The mean area of active neovascularization was quantified with fluorescein angiography and was found to decrease significantly from 27.79 mm^2 at baseline to 5.43 mm^2 1 week after intravitreal bevacizumab ($p < 0.05$). Eleven of the fifteen eyes (74%) had decreased leakage while four eyes had no leakage at 1 week (Fig. 14.3). By week 6, no fluorescein leakage was seen in any eye (see Fig. 14.3). However, 12 weeks after the injection, some fluorescein leakage was noted with a mean area of 5.50 mm^2 (see Fig. 14.3), which was still significantly smaller compared to baseline ($p < 0.05$). Some amount of fluorescein leakage was seen in 14 of the 15 eyes (93%). However, no new or enlarged areas of active neovascularization were seen in any patient. No major adverse events were noted. This study was limited due to its small size and short follow-up but confirmed a transient effect of intravitreal bevacizumab on regression of neovascularization, which seems to begin to wear off between 6 and 12 weeks postinjection.

Another retrospective study of 44 eyes of 33 consecutive patients with retinal neovascularization from PDR who were treated with bevacizumab was performed by Arevalo et al.[30] Patients were followed for a mean of 28.4 weeks. Thirty-five eyes received 2.5 mg of intravitreal bevacizumab while the remaining nine eyes received 1.25 mg. Thirty-three eyes had prior PRP. Mean baseline visual acuity was logMAR 1.21 (20/300), and the final visual acuity was logMAR 0.70 (approximately 20/100). Twelve eyes (27.3%) had remained stable, 29 eyes (65.9%) had improved by two or more ETDRS lines, and 3 eyes (6.8%) had decreased by two or more ETDRS lines.

Twenty-seven eyes (61.4%) had total regression of the neovascularization by fundus exam and absence of leakage on fluorescein angiography. An additional 15 eyes (34.1%) had partial regression whereas only 2 eyes (4.5%) demonstrated no regression. Of the eyes with no regression, both had been previously treated with PRP. One eye had received 1.25 mg of intravitreal bevacizumab and progressed to TRD. The second eye developed VH after 2.5 mg of intravitreal bevacizumab. Regression of neovascularization was seen in some eyes as soon as 7 to 15 days after intravitreal bevacizumab. The authors found that the 2.5-mg dose appeared to be more effective than the 1.25-mg dose in inducing complete regression of neovascularization ($p = 0.01$).

Recurrence of neovascularization was seen in 21 eyes (47.7%) at a mean of 12.4 weeks (range = 4–34 weeks) necessitating a second injection. Seven eyes recurred after the second injection at a mean of 17.3 weeks (range = 11–22 weeks) and required a third injection. No local or systemic adverse events were reported over 6 months of follow-up.

As in prior studies, the authors felt that bevacizumab induces faster regression of neovascularization compared to PRP. Due to the longer time to regression with PRP, which is usually on the order of weeks, VH can occur and induce visual loss or prevent completion of the laser treatment. Therefore, bevacizumab may offer multiple benefits including prevention of VH, longer intervals between PRP sessions to lower the risk of complications, and allowing more selective use of PRP.

Minella et al.[31] reported their results of an interventional case series of 15 eyes from 10 patients with bilateral PDR who received intravitreal injections of 1.25-mg bevacizumab. Thirteen eyes had severe PDR with active neovascularization, and two eyes had recurrent VH. They chose to include only patients who had a hemoglobin A1c < 8.5%. Some patients included had prior PRP or

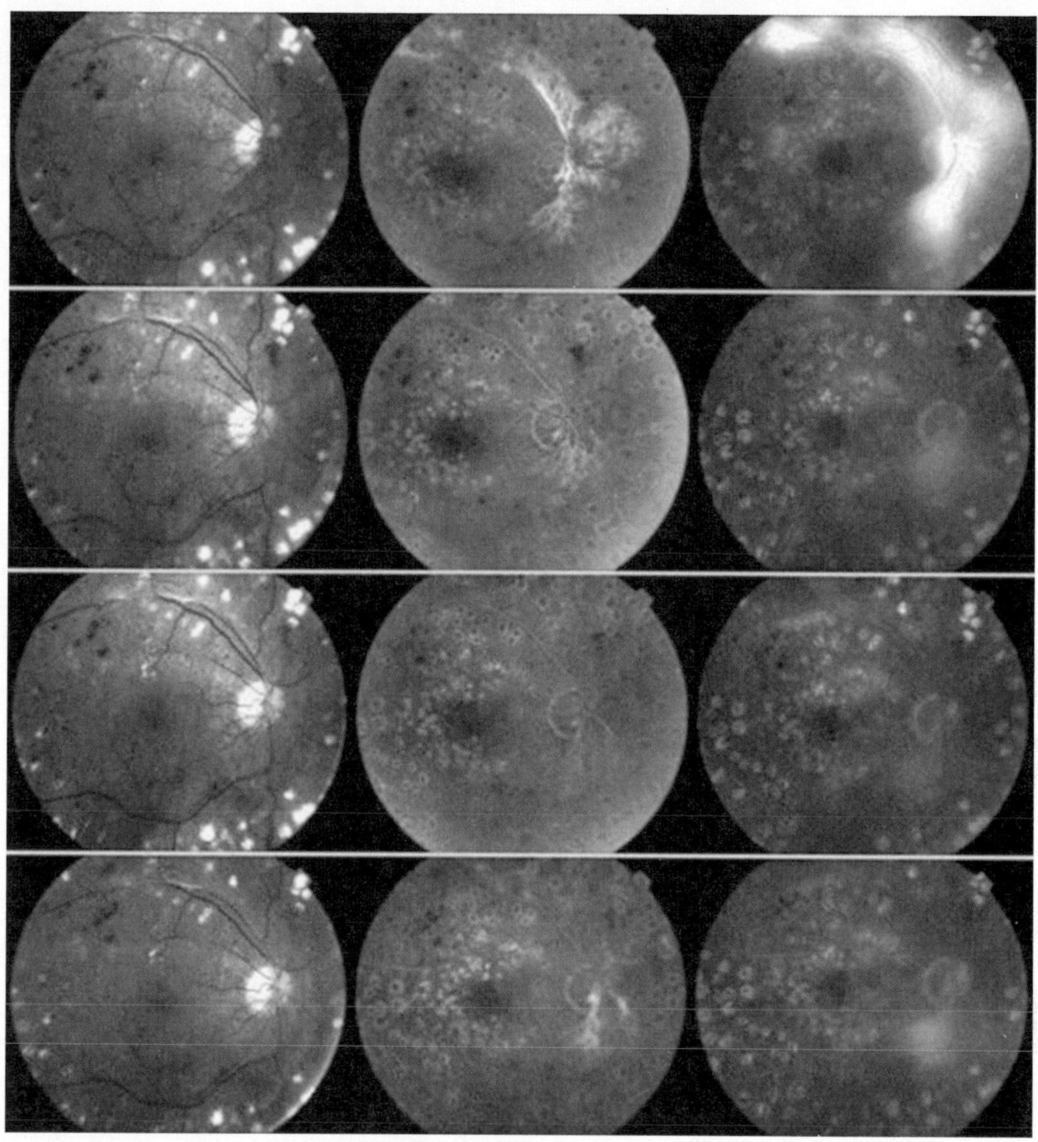

FIGURE 14.3. Red free, early- and late-phase fluorescein angiography from a diabetic patient with persistent active new vessels 5.5 months after panretinal laser photocoagulation (Case 1). **(Top)** Actively leaking new vessels at baseline; some fluorescein leakage also within the macula. **(Top center)** Marked decrease in fluorescein leakage from new vessels noted at baseline could be seen as early as 1 week after an intravitreal injection of 1.5 mg of bevacizumab. **(Bottom center)** At 6 weeks, some staining but no fluorescein leakage from new vessels and within the macula. **(Bottom)** Twelve weeks after injection, minimal fluorescein leakage is observed from new vessels noted at baseline. (Reproduced from Jorge, et al. *Retina.* 2006;26:1009, with permission.)

focal laser therapy. The authors performed quantitative planimetric analysis (QPA) of neovascular area based on the fluorescein angiogram and confirmed a significant reduction from 10.15 mm^2 at baseline to 1.15 mm^2 at month 1 postinjection (p = 0.01). PRP was performed at least 30 days after the initial injection. At 3 months follow-up, the QPA of neovascular area remained stable at 1.07 mm^2. Of eight eyes with 9 months follow-up, the QPA was maintained at 1.28 mm^2. The two eyes with recurrent VH showed both rapid resolution as well as regression of the neovascularization following intravitreal bevacizumab. No systemic or local adverse events were noted.

Bevacizumab Versus PRP Laser

A randomized, prospective fellow-eye controlled clinical trial comparing standard PRP and PRP with concomitant intravitreal bevacizumab was performed by Mirshahi et al.[32]

Eighty eyes of 40 patients with bilateral PDR exhibited high-risk characteristics as defined by the Diabetic Retinopathy Study (i.e., NVD greater than or equal to one-fourth to one-third disc area, any amount of NVD with vitreous or preretinal hemorrhage, or NVE greater than or equal to one-half disc area with preretinal or VH).[33] One eye of each patient was randomly assigned to receive a single 1.25 mg of intravitreal bevacizumab at the time of their first PRP session. All eyes received standard PRP (1,200–1,500 spots, 0.2 seconds duration, 1/2 spot size apart) in three sessions, 1 week apart. Patients were followed for at least 16 weeks. Exclusion criteria included uncontrolled hypertension, myocardial infarction, or cerebrovascular accident within the past 6 months, uncontrolled glaucoma, previous retinal photocoagulation of any kind, and presence of TRD.

At week 6, 35 of the 40 bevacizumab-treated eyes (87.5%) compared to only 10 of the 40 eyes (25%) in the sham group showed complete regression of neovascularization on fluorescein angiography ($p < 0.005$). All patients in the bevacizumab group had at least partial regression though 36 of the 40 patients in the sham group also had at least partial regression (with 26 having partial regression in addition to the 10 with complete regression). However, by week 16, complete regression was only seen in 25% of eyes for each group. Partial regression was noted in 28 eyes in the bevacizumab group and 26 eyes in the sham group. In the bevacizumab group, the strongest determinant of recurrence of neovascularization was the hemoglobin A1c, which was 1.5% higher in those that recurred compared to those that did not ($p = 0.033$). No adverse events were seen in the bevacizumab-treated eyes.

One problem with this fellow-eye controlled study is the report that intravitreal bevacizumab injections may have an effect on the fellow eye.[28] This may explain the relatively high number of patients in the PRP only group that had at least partial regression of neovascularization by week 6. Therefore, it is possible that the difference in regression of neovascularization between the two groups may have been even greater than reported. Nevertheless, this study helps confirm a rapid but transient biological effect of bevacizumab on regression of neovascularization. Despite concomitant PRP, 75% of patients who received bevacizumab still had recurrence of neovascularization at week 16. This suggests that PRP may take longer to induce a permanent downregulation in VEGF and as a result, patients may need repeat intravitreal injections. Alternatively, the initial PRP treatment may have been insufficient.

PRP alone Versus PRP + Bevacizumab

A prospective, randomized study comparing PRP plus 1.5 mg of intravitreal bevacizumab with PRP alone was conducted by Tonello et al.[34] on 30 eyes of 22 patients with high-risk PDR and no prior laser treatments. Patients were followed for 16 weeks. Eight patients with bilateral PDR were included with the eye having the worse best-corrected visual acuity (BCVA) being assigned to PRP plus bevacizumab. In the 15 eyes that received bevacizumab with PRP, the injection was given an hour after completion of the second PRP session at week 3 after initial presentation.

The area of active neovascularization was measured based on fluorescein angiography and was found to decrease significantly in the PRP plus bevacizumab group from 11.15 mm^2 at baseline to 0.62 mm^2 at week 4, 0.67 mm^2 at week 9 and 4.46 mm^2 at week 16. No significant change was seen in the PRP only group with a baseline area of 15.31 mm^2, 14.73 mm^2 at week 4, 14.26 mm^2 at week 9, and 13.58 mm^2 at week 16. Best-corrected visual acuity remained stable in both groups throughout the study at around 20/40. The authors admit that they were hoping to see a protective effect of bevacizumab on preventing macular edema after PRP. However, no patients in the PRP only group developed macular edema, which may have been related to the PRP protocol (not >800 shots at one treatment and spread over two treatments that were 2 weeks apart).

A transient effect of bevacizumab is again suggested by the results of this study with a mild increase in the area of neovascularization from the week 9 to 16 follow-up despite concomitant PRP. It is possible that this trend may have continued if further follow-up were available. In this particular study, no visual acuity benefit was seen and no complications such as VH or TRD occurred even in the PRP only group despite maintaining active neovascular vessels throughout the 4-month duration of the study. Larger studies with longer duration of follow-up will be necessary to determine if bevacizumab provides any additional clinical benefit to PRP alone other than rapid neovascular regression.

Cho et al.[35] conducted a similar prospective, randomized study on 41 eyes of 25 patients with high-risk PDR (Box 14.1). Patients were divided into groups based on presence of clinically significant macular edema (CSME) and the enrolled eye was then randomized to receive either PRP with 1.25 mg of intravitreal bevacizumab or PRP alone. All eyes with CSME received focal/grid laser treatment at the time of PRP. Patients with prior PRP or focal/grid laser as well as hemoglobin A1c exceeding 9.5% were excluded. Nineteen eyes had CSME while 22 eyes did not. Nineteen eyes were randomized to the PRP group and 22 eyes to the PRP plus bevacizumab group. Sixteen patients had bilateral high-risk PDR and had one eye randomized to receive PRP with the fellow eye receiving the PRP plus bevacizumab. For the eyes in the PRP plus bevacizumab group, the injection was delivered 1 week before starting PRP. PRP was delivered in three sessions separated by 1 week with each session involving 300 to 500 shots.

In the PRP only group, BCVA decreased significantly from a baseline of logMAR 0.23 (~20/34) to 0.29 (~20/39) at 3 months ($p = 0.041$). In the PRP plus bevacizumab group, no significant change in visual acuity was noted. Central macular thickness by optical coherence tomography (OCT) also decreased from a baseline of 295 to 240 μm at 1 month ($p = 0.012$) and 237 μm at 3 months ($p = 0.008$).

Looking at eyes that presented with CSME, there was no significant change in visual acuity during the 3-month study in either treatment group. However,

BOX 14.1 Panretinal Photocoagulation Combined with Intravitreal Bevacizumab in High-risk Proliferative Diabetic Retinopathy

Objective: To evaluate the efficacy of intravitreal bevacizumab as an adjunctive treatment to PRP for high-risk PDR with or without CSME.

Methods: A prospective, randomized study was conducted on eyes with high-risk PDR with or without concomitant CSME. Eyes in each group were then randomly assigned to receive PRP or 1.25-mg intravitreal bevacizumab 1 week before starting PRP. Eyes with CSME also received focal/grid laser at the time of initial PRP.

Results: Forty-one eyes of 25 patients were enrolled. Nineteen eyes had CSME. Nineteen eyes were randomized to the PRP group and 22 eyes to the PRP with bevacizumab group (Plus group). BCVA was significantly worse at 3 months ($p = 0.041$) in the PRP group but was unchanged in the Plus group. Central macular thickness decreased significantly at 1 month and 3 months in the Plus group but was unchanged in the PRP group. In eyes with CSME initially, there was no significant change in BCVA in both groups. In eyes without CSME initially, BCVA was significantly worse at 1 month and 3 months ($p = 0.004, 0.016$) in the PRP group but unchanged in the Plus group. The proportion of eyes that developed vitreous hemorrhage was significantly lower in the Plus group ($p = 0.023$).

Conclusions: Intravitreal bevacizumab before PRP may lower the risk of vision loss especially in patients without CSME initially and development of vitreous hemorrhage in patients with high-risk PDR.

Source: Cho WB, Oh SB, Moon JW, et al. Panretinal photocoagulation combined with intravitreal bevacizumab in high-risk proliferative diabetic retinopathy. *Retina.* 2009;29:516–522.

a decrease in central macular thickness was noted on OCT from 359 μm at baseline to 268 μm at 1 month ($p = 0.003$) and 252 μm at 3 months ($p = 0.001$) in the PRP plus bevacizumab group.

In eyes without CSME at presentation, BCVA worsened in the PRP only group from a baseline logMAR 0.18 (about 20/30) to 0.26 (about 20/36) at 1 month ($p = 0.047$) and 0.30 (about 20/40) at 3 months ($p = 0.011$). This was correlated with increasing central macular thickness on OCT. No changes were seen in visual acuity or OCT thickness in the PRP plus bevacizumab group. Four patients developed increased proliferation and VH in the PRP only group. None of these complications were seen in the PRP plus bevacizumab group. No progression to TRD was seen in either group, and no major local or systemic adverse events were noted.

This study supports combination treatment with PRP and bevacizumab for eyes with high-risk PDR, especially in cases with no CSME at baseline, to prevent subsequent macular edema, which has been well described following PRP alone.[36,37] In addition, bevacizumab seemed to lower the risk of subsequent VH developing after PRP. However, the study size is small and the differences in mean visual acuity are also small. The authors admit that Snellen acuities were used rather than ETDRS protocol refractions to measure BCVA. Finally, the follow-up period was relatively short and it is possible that given more time the difference between the PRP only and the PRP plus bevacizumab groups may have disappeared with longer follow-up. Nevertheless, a short-term clinical benefit of bevacizumab may make this a useful adjunct.

While few reports have been published using pegaptanib for retinal neovascularization, they have not shown as dramatic a response compared to bevacizumab. This difference in clinical response may be due to bevacizumab's activity against all isoforms of VEGF while pegaptanib only inactivates the $VEGF_{165}$ isoform.[38] No reports have been published to date involving ranibizumab (Lucentis; Genentech, Inc., South San Francisco, CA) for retinal neovascularization related to PDR. One of the primary goals in designing ranibizumab as a Fab fragment rather than a full-length antibody like bevacizumab is the theoretical improved retinal penetration due to the smaller size. Although this feature may be an important consideration for subretinal neovascularization such as in neovascular age-related macular degeneration, it does not have any advantages in PDR where the pathological neovascularization is preretinal in location. Given the longer predicted half-life of bevacizumab, it may have the overall advantage for treatment in these cases.[39]

ANTI-VEGF THERAPIES FOR VITREOUS HEMORRHAGE IN PROLIFERATIVE DIABETIC RETINOPATHY

Due to the rapid regression of retinal neovascularization with intravitreal bevacizumab, one of the major potential benefits has been purported to be prevention of VH. The next logical topic to explore is the effects of intravitreal bevacizumab in patients with PDR who present with VH already present. Spontaneous resolution of VH usually takes time in part due to continuous bleeding from active neovascularization. Prior to the availability of anti-VEGF therapies, the main options were observation with the hope that PRP can be performed as the hemorrhage begins to clear or surgical intervention to remove the blood with simultaneous PRP.

Anti-VEGF therapies cause regression of neovascular vessels and may decrease any further bleeding, thereby accelerating the rate of VH resolution. This may help decrease the need for vitrectomy. With improved media clarity, PRP laser can then be completed to ensure that the neovascular regression becomes more permanent.

Spaide and Fischer[40] initially reported two patients with VH from PDR who were treated with 1.25 mg of intravitreal bevacizumab. Both patients presented with dense VH that precluded PRP. The first patient was a 68-year-old woman with prior incomplete PRP due to nonclearing VH of several years. Her initial visual acuity was 20/60. A localized extramacular TRD was noted on B-scan ultrasound. One week postinjection, she had improved to 20/40 and showed regression of both the retinal neovascularization and VH. By 3 months postinjection, early signs of reperfusion of retinal neovascularization were noted on clinical exam and fluorescein angiography. An additional injection was given. No progression of the TRD was seen. The second patient was a 38-year-old man with VH and an extramacular TRD. His initial visual acuity was 20/70. One week postinjection, his visual acuity had improved to 20/50 with a reduction in VH. One month postinjection, he was 20/30 with little remaining VH. The fibrovascular proliferation appeared nearly regressed though some leakage was noted on fluorescein angiography. An additional injection was given, and by 1 week later, he had improved to 20/25. At this point, PRP was performed. No progression of the TRD was noted.

An interventional prospective case series of 38 eyes of 38 patients with active PDR who received one to three intravitreal injections of 1.25-mg bevacizumab was performed by Moradian et al.[41] (Box 14.2). Eligible eyes had active neovascularization refractory to prior PRP and/or severe new VH precluding completion of PRP. The first group was given intravitreal bevacizumab at least 3 months after the last session of PRP. The second group was given intravitreal bevacizumab at least 1 month after the onset of VH. Reinjection could occur at intervals of 6 or 12 weeks based on surgeon discretion, if there was incomplete VH resolution and/or inadequate regression of neovascularization.

VH was present in 32 eyes and the severity was found to decrease significantly compared to baseline at the weeks 1-, 12-, and 20-week follow-ups from the first intravitreal bevacizumab injection ($p = 0.014, 0.0001$, and 0.002, respectively). Younger patients tended to show a greater amount of VH resolution. Mean BCVA also improved from approximately 20/270 at baseline to approximately 20/68 at week 20. The study did not show any significant changes in the extent of the fibrovascular tissue during follow-ups through 20 weeks compared to baseline, despite regression of the vascular component. In two cases, progression to TRD occurred 1.5 to 2 months after a second injection of bevacizumab, necessitating vitrectomy. No other local or systemic adverse events were observed. These results should be interpreted with care due to the lack of a control group. The majority of patients had only mild VH at baseline. It is possible that the improvement in visual acuity and resolution of VH may have been no better compared to the natural course without bevacizumab.

BOX 14.2 Intravitreal Bevacizumab in Patients with Vitreous Hemorrhage due to PDR

Objective: To evaluate the effect of intravitreal bevacizumab in eyes with active proliferative diabetic retinopathy (PDR).
Methods: An interventional prospective case series was performed on eyes with active PDR that were given one to three injections of 1.25-mg intravitreal bevacizumab.
Results: Thirty-eight eyes of 38 patients were included and followed for 20 weeks. Thirty-two eyes had vitreous hemorrhage (VH) at baseline. VH resolved significantly after 1 week ($p = 0.014$), 12 weeks ($p = 0.0001$), and 20 weeks ($p = 0.002$).
Conclusions: Intravitreal bevacizumab may induce VH resolution in patients with active PDR..

Source: Moradian S, Ahmadieh H, Malihi M, et al. Intravitreal bevacizumab in active progressive proliferative diabetic retinopathy. *Graefes Arch Clin Exp Ophthalmol.* 2008;246:1699–1705.

A small case series involving four eyes of four patients by Ruiz-Moreno et al.[42] addressed the use of intravitreal bevacizumab in patients with recurrent VH after vitrectomy. All eyes had undergone pars plana vitrectomy with detachment of the posterior hyaloid and PRP. An additional two repeat vitrectomies had been performed for recurrent VH. Patients were hand motions at baseline and had B-scans that confirmed the retina was attached. Monthly injections of 1.25 mg of intravitreal bevacizumab were given until the VH cleared. Two eyes had complete resolution of the VH after two injections while the other two eyes required three. Two eyes had rubeosis iridis at baseline, which resolved after the injection. Patients were followed for 4 months. No adverse reactions were noted.

Instead of injecting bevacizumab postoperatively, Yang et al.[43] performed a prospective, nonrandomized, comparative case study looking at preoperative intravitreal injection of 1.25 mg of bevacizumab 1 week prior to planned vitrectomy surgery for PDR with active fibrovascular proliferation and associated new preretinal or VH. All 16 eyes of 15 patients were left with 10% perfluoropropane (C3F8) tamponade at the end of surgery. Patients with more severe retinopathy possibly requiring silicone oil tamponade were excluded. The authors compared these results with 24 eyes of 24 historical controls that were matched for severity of active fibrovascular proliferation and underwent similar surgery with 10% C3F8 tamponade but did not receive preoperative bevacizumab.

In the study group that received the bevacizumab, all cases showed a decrease in visible neovascularization without an increase in retinal traction 1 week after the injection. Less intraoperative bleeding was noted in the study eyes compared to historical controls with moderate bleeding requiring endodiathermy occurring in only 2 of the 16 (12.5%) in the former group and 13 of the 24 (54.2%) in the control group ($p < 0.01$). The average time to vitreous clearing, defined as the interval between the end of surgery and the time when retinal vessels could be visualized below the gas bubble, was lower in the bevacizumab group (7.2 ± 5.6 days) compared to the control group (15.2 ± 11.4 days, $p = 0.04$). Early recurrent VH was seen in none of the bevacizumab eyes and only one of the control eyes. Late recurrent VH occurred in one eye of each group 3.5 to 4 months after surgery.

Based on this study, pretreatment with intravitreal bevacizumab seems to decrease the risk of intraoperative hemorrhaging and, as a result, postoperative time to vitreous clearing. This may allow for faster visual rehabilitation for patients. No significant difference was found in the incidence of recurrent VH between the two groups. The authors had previously reported a lower likelihood of early recurrent VH in patients who received long-acting gas tamponade prior to the conclusion of surgery, which was done in both the study and control groups.[44]

One further idea is to inject intravitreal bevacizumab at the conclusion of surgery to decrease the risk of postoperative VH, which may result from residual fibrovascular tissue bleeding.[45] The potential benefit would be inhibiting early neovascularization which may be one of the causes of early recurrent VH. However, since VEGF plays an important role in maintaining normal platelet function, the use of bevacizumab could in fact delay the reparative process of injured blood vessels and therefore increase the risk of recurrent VH.[46] In addition, anti-VEGF therapies are unlikely to prevent early bleeding from vessels that have been mechanically injured from surgical manipulation. The effect of anti-VEGF therapies at the conclusion of surgery in order to prevent recurrent VH requires further investigation.

ANTI-VEGF THERAPIES AS AN ADJUNCT PRIOR TO TRACTIONAL RETINAL DETACHMENT REPAIR

Chen and Park[47] first described the use of 1.25 mg of intravitreal bevacizumab prior to surgery in a patient with TRD. At 2 weeks postinjection, significant regression of the neovascularization was noted but the TRD and fibrous scaffolding remained (Figs. 14.4 and 14.5). The patient underwent pars plana vitrectomy, membrane peeling, endolaser, and sulfur hexafluoride (SF6) tamponade. During surgery, minimal bleeding occurred during the segmentation and delamination of the preretinal membranes with many of the epicenters of neovascularization peeling with only blunt dissection. Preoperatively, the visual

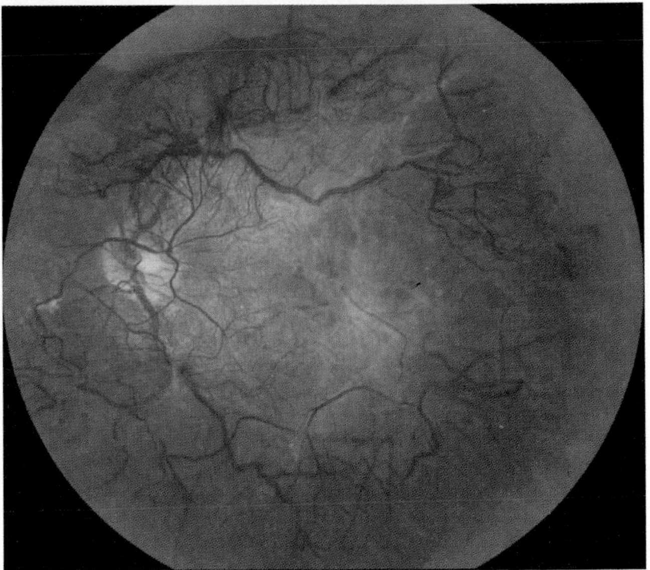

FIGURE 14.4. Color fundus photograph of the left eye demonstrating significant fibrovascular proliferation with TRD prior to intravitreal bevacizumab. (Reproduced from Chen E, Park CH. *Retina.* 2006;26:699, with permission.)

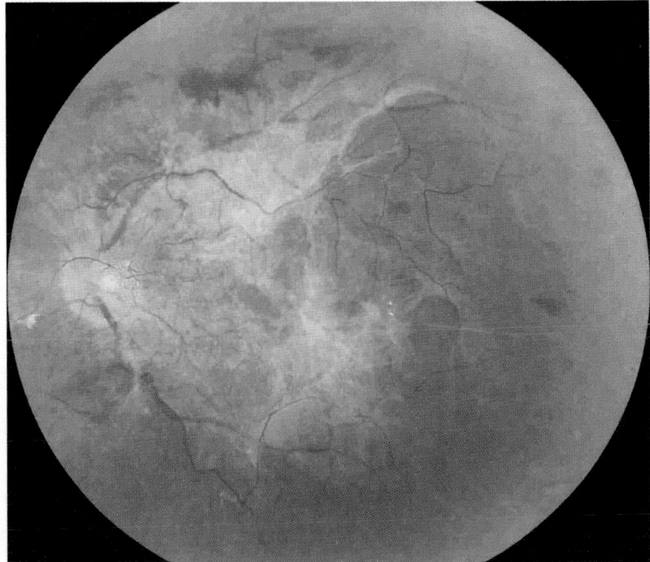

FIGURE 14.5. Color fundus photograph 2 weeks after intravitreal bevacizumab showing significant regression of the neovascularization but persistence of the fibrovascular scaffolding. (Reproduced from Chen E, Park CH. *Retina.* 2006;26:700, with permission.)

acuity was 20/400. One month after surgery, the vision had improved to 20/70 (Fig. 14.6). In conclusion, the authors felt that preoperative use of bevacizumab had made the surgical repair of TRD technically easier.

Yeoh et al.[48] examined the effects of 1.25 mg of intravitreal bevacizumab prior to vitrectomy surgery for TRD or VH in 18 eyes of 16 patients. Inclusion criteria included TRD involving the macula with active neovascularization, rubeosis with VH precluding PRP, severe ischemia on FA, or fellow eye developing rubeosis after vitrectomy. Fifteen eyes had macula-involving TRD and three eyes had non-clearing VH (two had rubeosis and one had severe ischemia on FA). Vitrectomy was performed within 2 weeks of the intravitreal bevacizumab injection, with a mean interval of 9 days (range = 6–14 days). Minimum follow-up was 6 months postoperatively. Five eyes were filled with silicone oil, three with SF6, one with air, and the remaining nine eyes had no tamponade. No adverse events were noted, and no documented progression of the TRD was seen after the injection.

Baseline Snellen visual acuities ranged from 20/120 to hand motions. By 6 months postoperative, 14 eyes had improved, 1 was unchanged, and 3 were worse. Of the worse eyes, two had macular ischemia on fluorescein angiography and one still had silicone oil tamponade. Seven eyes (38.8%) had rebleeding within the 6-month follow-up period, with a mean time to rebleeding of 43.6 days (range = 7–81 days). Six of the seven rebleeds required surgical washout. Based on tamponade, none of the silicone oil eyes rebled, two of the three SF6 eyes rebled, and five of the nine eyes without tamponade rebled. None of the patients with rebleeds were on anticoagulants. Five of the seven rebleeds did not have additional endolaser at the time of surgery. During the surgical washout, a source of the bleeding could only be ascertained in one eye where the patient was seen to have fibrovascular ingrowth at one of the sclerotomies.

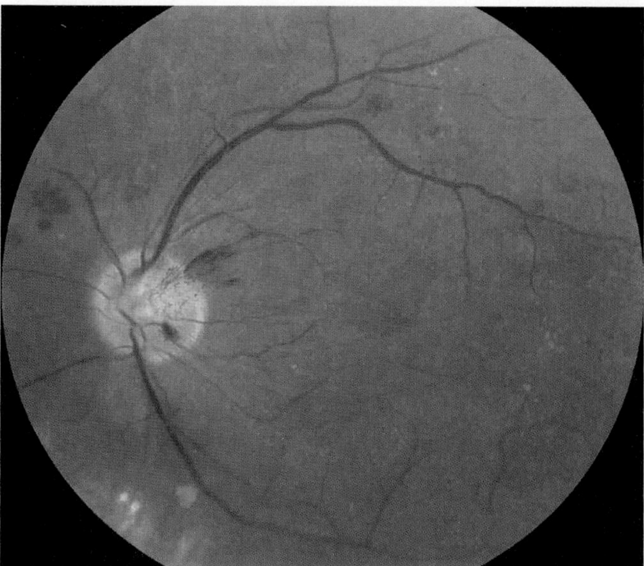

FIGURE 14.6. Postoperative color fundus photograph demonstrating successful removal of the preretinal fibrosis and absence of neovascularization. (Reproduced from Chen E, Park CH. *Retina.* 2006;26:700, with permission.)

This high rate of rebleeding appears to be in the upper range of what has been reported without bevacizumab.[49,50,51] One possible explanation is the severity of the cases selected for preoperative bevacizumab, which placed these eyes at a higher risk for recurrent hemorrhage regardless. Another possibility is that the bevacizumab temporarily causes the vascular component to regress. As a result, the stalks that are opened during delamination, which normally would be treated with intraoperative diathermy, are not apparent at the time of surgery and are only in a temporary state of hemostasis. The authors suggest that additional PRP should be added in all cases in order to reduce the potential of rebleeding as the bevacizumab wears off. Since the preoperative bevacizumab is removed at the time of surgery, they also suggest that an additional injection at the end of the procedure may be helpful in lowering the rebleed rate.

Similar to prior reports, the authors observed that following intravitreal bevacizumab there was significant regression of the active neovascularization, making surgery technically easier since the fibrovascular complex could be readily separated from the retina with less intraoperative hemorrhaging, which in turn provided better visualization. The surgeons involved felt that the fibrovascular membranes subjectively seemed less adherent to the retina compared to cases without preoperative bevacizumab. As a result, intravitreal bevacizumab seems to be most appropriate for cases where there is a significant active vascular component to the fibrovascular proliferation. Eyes in the fibrotic stage may be less likely to benefit to the same extent.

The timing of preoperative bevacizumab may also be critical due to the potential for progression of the TRD. When anti-VEGF therapies are used, the equilibrium between different growth factors affecting active vessel proliferation and fibrosis may shift toward the fibrosis-inducing factors, leading to contraction of the fibrovascular tissue. Ideally, surgery should be performed at the time of greatest regression of the active vascular component but before further fibrous proliferation or contraction occurs in order to minimize progression of TRD. In this series, the earliest interval between bevacizumab injection and surgery was 6 days, which the authors felt was sufficient time. Due to the small sample size and lack of controls, it is difficult to draw any strong conclusions from this article. However, the study provides more evidence in the body of literature to the value of bevacizumab as an adjunct prior to TRD repair.

Ishikawa et al. also reported their experience with 1.25 mg of intravitreal bevacizumab prior to surgery for repair of TRD in eight eyes of six patients with severe

PDR.[52] Patients received the injection 3 to 30 days prior to vitrectomy. All patients showed marked regression of the vascular component of the fibrovascular proliferation. Two of the five eyes that received bevacizumab 7 days or more prior to vitrectomy were found to have strong adhesions of the fibrotic membranes to the retina resulting in some surgical complications. Three eyes that had a shorter interval between the injection and vitrectomy (3 days for 2 eyes and 5 days for 1 eye) showed no firm adhesions. Even in the cases that underwent vitrectomy only 3 days after bevacizumab injection, the authors noted minimal bleeding during surgery. Based on these findings, the authors believe that a shorter interval between injection and surgery may suffice and minimize the risk of complications from increased adherence of the preretinal fibrosis. As before, the small number of patients and retrospective nature of this study without a control group make it difficult to interpret these results.

To date, only Rizzo et al.[53] have performed a small, randomized, prospective study involving 22 eyes of 22 patients with TRD from PDR (Box 14.3). Eleven patients were randomized to preoperative intravitreal injection of 1.25 mg of bevacizumab 5 to 7 days prior to vitrectomy (group 1). The remaining 11 patients underwent surgery without bevacizumab (group 2). All surgeries were carried out using 20-gauge pars plana vitrectomy. The authors created a system of determining the complexity of each case in order to ensure that the two groups were matched. No adverse events were recorded. In addition, no progression of the TRD was seen in the bevacizumab-treated eyes, which may be due to the relatively short interval of 5 to 7 days between injection and surgery.

In the group 1 eyes, remarkable regression of the active neovascular vessels was noted clinically and on fluorescein angiography within 24 to 48 hours postinjection. In order to determine whether there was any difference in ease of surgery, the study explored several different surgical parameters. In group 1, intraoperative hemorrhaging occurred a mean of only five times and required endodiathermy twice. In group 2, it occurred 16 times and required endodiathermy 9 times. In group 1, the surgeon was able to peel a mean of 21 epicenters of neovascularization with blunt dissection and 35 were removed with sharp dissection. However, no blunt dissection was possible in the control group and sharp dissection had to be applied to a mean of 57 epicenters. The average number of instrument exchanges during surgery was 27 in group 1 and 53 in group 2. Mean surgical time was 57 minutes in group 1 and 83 minutes in group 2.

Clinically, mean BCVA improved from logMAR 1.87 (~20/1500) preoperatively to logMAR 0.88 (~20/150) in group 1 at 6 months postoperative. In group 2, no difference was seen with preoperative mean BCVA of logMAR 2.04 (~2/200) and postoperative mean BCVA of logMAR 2.01. Anatomic attachment was confirmed in 11 eyes that had received bevacizumab and only 9 eyes in the control group at the 6-month follow-up.

This study more objectively measured an improvement in the ease of surgery in eyes randomized to receive preoperative intravitreal bevacizumab. The cases were shorter with fewer required instrument exchanges as well as less hemorrhaging and need for intraocular diathermy. Many of these findings were likely due to the relative ease with which the preretinal fibrosis could be dissected from the retina as evidenced by the ability to use blunt dissection much more frequently in the bevacizumab-treated eyes. Less iatrogenic breaks were also seen with none occurring in the bevacizumab eyes and four in the control eyes. Two possible explanations include decreased hemorrhaging leading to better retinal visualization and decreased strength of adhesion between the fibrovascular tissue and the retina.

BOX 14.3 Intravitreal Bevacizumab as a Preoperative Adjunct Before Vitrectomy Surgery in the Treatment of Proliferative Diabetic Retinopathy

Objective: To evaluate the use of preoperative intravitreal bevacizumab in eyes undergoing pars plana vitrectomy for TRD.

Methods: A prospective, randomized study was performed on eyes with TRD due to proliferative diabetic retinopathy. Patients were randomized to no injection or 1.25-mg intravitreal bevacizumab 5–7 days prior to surgery.

Results: Twenty-two eyes of 22 patients were included and followed for 6 months. Eleven eyes received intravitreal bevacizumab preoperatively (group 1), while 11 eyes underwent direct surgery (group 2). Mean surgical time was 57 minutes in group 1 and 83 minutes in group 2. Mean tool exchanges was 27 vs. 53, intraoperative bleeding 5 vs. 15, endodiathermy 2 vs. 9. Mean preoperative BCVA was 1.87 logMAR in group 1 and 2.04 logMAR in group 2. Mean postoperative BCVA at 6 months was 0.88 logMAR in group 1 and 2.01 logMAR in group 2 ($p = 0.01$). Anatomical attachment was achieved in all 11 patients in group 1 and 9 of 11 patients in group 2.

Conclusions: Intravitreal bevacizumab prior to vitrectomy was well tolerated, facilitated surgical repair of TRD, and led to better visual outcomes.

Source: Rizzo S, Genovesi-Ebert F, Di Bartolo E, et al. Injection of intravitreal bevacizumab (Avastin) as a preoperative adjunct before vitrectomy surgery in the treatment of severe proliferative diabetic retinopathy (PDR). *Graefes Arch Clin Exp Ophthalmol.* 2008;246:837–842.

COMPLICATIONS OF ANTI-VEGF THERAPIES IN PROLIFERATIVE DIABETIC RETINOPATHY

A single case report of multiple retinal hemorrhages occurring after intravitreal bevacizumab was reported by Lee and Koh.[54] They described a 65-year-old woman who underwent pars plana vitrectomy, endolaser PRP, phacoemulsification with intraocular lens implantation, and intravitreal injection of 1.25-mg bevacizumab. Her baseline visual acuity was 20/400. One week later, she was noted to have developed multiple, extensive blot retinal hemorrhages throughout the entire fundus. Her visual acuity remained 20/400 and other systemic factors including blood glucose, blood pressure, and serum lipid levels were reported as stable. Nine months later, the hemorrhages were significantly less but the visual acuity remained at 20/200. The authors attribute this reaction to the intravitreal bevacizumab, postulating that the hemorrhages may have resulted from blockade of all VEGF isoforms including the physiological ones leading to ischemia and the retinal hemorrhages.

The same authors also reported a case of worsening macular ischemia following vitrectomy with 2.5 mg of intravitreal bevacizumab for diabetic VH.[55] In this case, the 40-year-old man underwent uncomplicated surgery, but postoperatively, the visual acuity remained unchanged at 20/400. Comparing preoperative and postoperative fluorescein angiograms, the authors noted that the area of the foveal avascular zone had increased from 1.48 to 1.96 mm^2. As before, the authors are concerned that blockade of all VEGF isoforms with bevacizumab, some of which are needed for normal endothelial function, may lead to vasoconstriction, leukocyte adherence, platelet activation, thrombosis, impaired coagulation, vascular inflammation, and atherosclerosis.[56] The end result may be increased ischemia.

Several case reports and series have noted a risk of progression of TRD following intravitreal bevacizumab injection.[57] Tranos et al. reported a 55-year-old woman with VH and a macula-threatening TRD who presented with a visual acuity of 20/40. The patient declined surgery and was treated with PRP plus 1.25 mg of intravitreal bevacizumab. One week later, her visual acuity had worsened to 20/120 and the TRD was now involving the fovea. She underwent surgical repair and improved to 20/40. While the authors observed regression of the vascular component, there seemed to be increased contraction of the fibrovascular membrane leading to progression of the TRD. An alternative explanation might be increased vitreoretinal traction from the actual injection itself due to vitreous incarceration at the injection site. Patients with fibrovascular proliferation adjacent to the macula may be at highest risk for this complication.

The largest retrospective case series to date involved 211 patients who were given 1.25 mg of intravitreal bevacizumab prior to vitrectomy for severe PDR refractory to PRP. Of 211 eyes that were injected prior to vitrectomy, 11 eyes (5.2%) were identified that either developed or had progression of a TRD. All patients had received PRP at least 2 months prior to the intravitreal bevacizumab. The mean time from injection to TRD was 13 days (range = 3–31 days). Mean baseline visual acuity was approximately 20/125. Following TRD development or progression, mean visual acuity dropped to hand motions. One patient developed a retinal break from increased traction and had a combined total tractional-rhegmatogenous retinal detachment 3 weeks after injection. Eight of the eleven eyes subsequently underwent surgery and had a final mean BCVA of 20/160. Compared with baseline BCVA, four eyes had improved, two remained the same, and two lost two or more ETDRS lines.

Since all patients had received PRP at least 2 months prior to intravitreal bevacizumab, the authors suggest a causal relationship between the injection and TRD development or progression, especially given the short mean time interval of only 13 days.[58] They suggest that patients undergoing intravitreal bevacizumab prior to vitrectomy should be scheduled for surgery in a timely fashion since 9 of the 11 eyes (81.8%) developed TRD or progressed by 5 days or more after the injection. All 11 patients were also noted to be insulin dependent and nine had poor glycemic control with hemoglobin A1c of at least 9.5% (mean 10.6%).

While larger doses of intravitreal bevacizumab may theoretically have a longer duration of effect, Avery et al.[28] have previously shown a biological effect with neovascular regression even at lower doses. It is possible that lower doses may provide similar adjunctive benefits prior to vitrectomy without causing as much increased traction. Since these patients are scheduled for surgery soon after the injection anyhow at which time the bevacizumab will be cleared from the vitreous, this may be an alternative way to potentially decrease the risk of TRD development and progression especially in eyes with significant preexisting traction. Further studies will be necessary to confirm this theory.

In addition to progression of TRD after intravitreal bevacizumab, Mitamura et al.[59] reported the development of a macular hole–related retinal detachment (MH-RD). In this case, the 40-year-old man was given 1.25 mg of intravitreal bevacizumab for iris, angle, and retinal neovascularization associated with VH despite PRP 2 months before. He had neovascular glaucoma with an intraocular pressure of 48 mm Hg on maximum medical therapy. The patient did not have a posterior vitreous detachment, and no TRD or macular hole was present on examination prior to the injection. Two weeks later, the vision had dropped from 6/100 to 1/100, and he was noted to have a MH-RD with pseudo-operculum and incomplete PVD confirmed by OCT. The iris, angle, and retinal neovascularization were markedly regressed. Despite surgical repair, the patient's final visual acuity was 1/100. The authors suggest that the bevacizumab induced rapid involution of the

BOX 14.4 Potential Complications of Intravitreal Bevacizumab for Proliferative Diabetic Retinopathy

- Retinal hemorrhages
- Macular ischemia
- Development or progression of TRD
- Development of combined tractional-rhegmatogenous retinal detachment
- Development of macular hole–related retinal detachment
- Increased risk of postoperative vitreous hemorrhage after TRD repair

neovascularization but resulted in accelerated fibrosis and contraction of the posterior hyaloid causing the MH-RD. A summary of these potential complications is presented in Box 14.4.

CLINICAL APPLICATION

Treatment of PDR Without Significant Vitreous Hemorrhage

Based on the findings of the Diabetic Retinopathy Study and the Early Treatment of Diabetic Retinopathy Study, we generally do not initiate treatment for PDR unless high-risk characteristics are present (Fig. 14.7). This is defined as NVD ≥1/3 to 1/2 disc area, any NVD associated with preretinal or VH, or NVE ≥ 1/2 disc area associated with preretinal or VH.

Patients presenting with high-risk PDR, noCSME (defined as retinal thickening at or within 500 μm of the center of the macula, hard exudates at or within 500 μm of the center of the macula associated with adjacent retinal thickening, or a zone or zones of retinal thickening one disc area in size at least part of which is within one disc diameter of the center of the macula), and no significant associated preretinal fibrosis are given an intravitreal injection of 1.25-mg bevacizumab either immediately following PRP or 1 to 2 weeks prior to initiation of PRP. The rationale is to lower the likelihood of VH and potential development of macular edema with PRP. We perform PRP in at least two sessions separated by about 2 weeks with 600 to 800 spots during each session. Our laser parameters include a spot size of 500 μm separated by one burn width and titrated to a moderately intense white burn as described in the DRS.

Patients with high-risk PDR and CSME but no significant associated preretinal fibrosis are typically treated with an intravitreal injection of 1.25-mg bevacizumab initially. One to two weeks later, focal or modified grid laser photocoagulation is performed at the same time as the first session of PRP. The same PRP protocol is used as before, although the first session of PRP is generally performed nasally in order to further reduce the risk of exacerbation of macular edema. One reason behind starting with bevacizumab is to reduce the macular edema, which often allows improved laser uptake with lower energy. A second reason is to potentially lower the risk for VH and worsening of the macular edema with PRP.

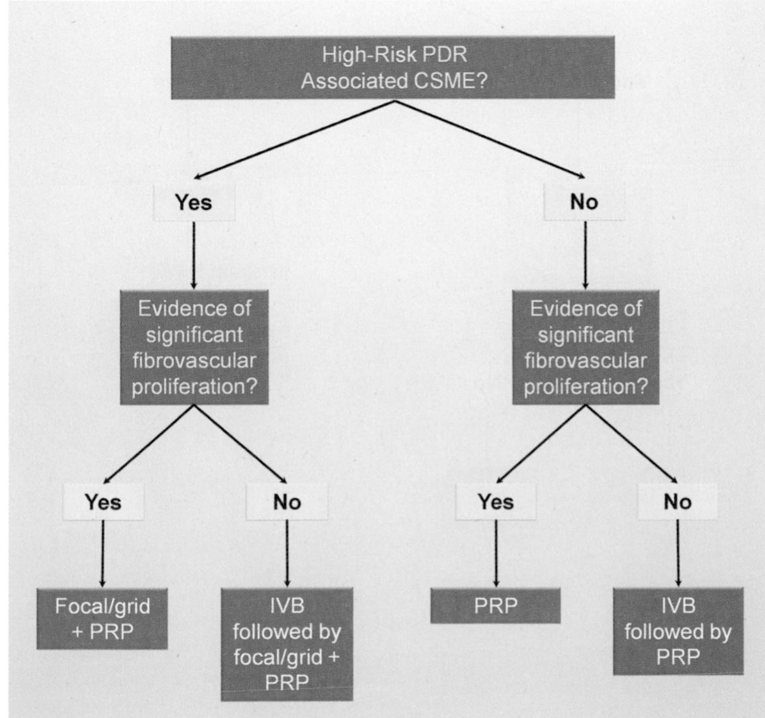

FIGURE 14.7. Approach to a patient with high-risk PDR without vitreous hemorrhage. PRP, panretinal photocoagulation; IVB, intravitreal bevacizumab.

If there is recurrence of retinal neovascularization, we recommend reinjecting 1.25 mg of intravitreal bevacizumab either immediately following or 1 to 2 weeks prior to additional fill-in PRP. Again, the rationale is to minimize the risk of VH and macular edema.

In patients with high-risk PDR and more prominent associated fibrovascular proliferation, we generally will avoid intravitreal bevacizumab due to the risk of TRD development. Instead, we proceed with PRP or PRP with focal/grid, if CSME is present.

Treatment of Vitreous Hemorrhage due to PDR

Our management of patients presenting with VH related to PDR is dependent on the amount of hemorrhage and media opacity (Fig. 14.8). If a clear view of at least some of the periphery can be obtained and we can ascertain by ophthalmoscopy that there is no significant existing fibrovascular proliferation under traction, we generally recommend starting PRP followed by immediate intravitreal injection of 1.25-mg bevacizumab. The concern in these patients is that if there is existing traction under the hemorrhage, the bevacizumab could exacerbate the traction and cause or worsen a TRD. In addition, we like to proceed with PRP while there is a view available since further dispersion of the existing VH or further hemorrhaging itself could preclude PRP at a future date. Patients are instructed to stay upright to allow settling of the hemorrhage inferiorly and are followed every 2 to 4 weeks with further fill-in PRP performed as the hemorrhage continues to clear. If there is worsening or no significant clearing of the hemorrhage within 2 to 3 months, we generally consider proceeding with pars plana vitrectomy and simultaneous PRP endolaser.

If there is no clear view of the fundus in any quadrant, we recommend obtaining a B-scan ultrasound. Should the B-scan show significant TRD involving or threatening the macula, we usually proceed with preoperative intravitreal bevacizumab within 5 days of scheduled pars plana vitrectomy, membrane peeling, and PRP endolaser with gas or oil tamponade as indicated. If the B-scan does not show any areas of TRD, we would consider starting with an intravitreal bevacizumab injection. In these cases, patients need to be followed closely (usually every 2 weeks) with serial B-scan ultrasounds if the view is not clearing since there is a risk that they could develop TRD. Once the view begins to clear, PRP laser should be initiated and filled-in until a full scatter can be completed. In the cases where there is further worsening of hemorrhage, subsequent development of TRD, or no significant clearing of the hemorrhage after 1 to 2 months, we will often recommend proceeding with pars plana vitrectomy.

Treatment of Tractional Retinal Detachment due to PDR

In patients presenting with TRD which is either involving or threatening the macula, we prefer scheduling the patient for surgical repair and proceeding with an intravitreal injection of 1.25-mg bevacizumab no >5 days before the surgery (Fig. 14.9). Our concern with a longer interval

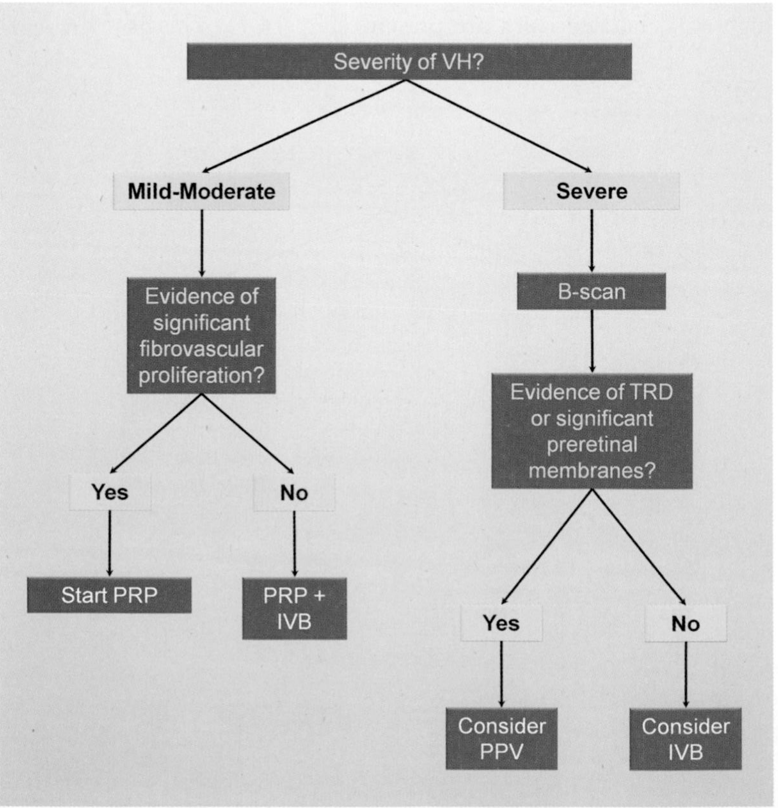

FIGURE 14.8. Approach to a patient with vitreous hemorrhage due to PDR. PRP, panretinal photocoagulation; IVB, intravitreal bevacizumab; TRD, tractional retinal detachment; PPV, pars plana vitrectomy.

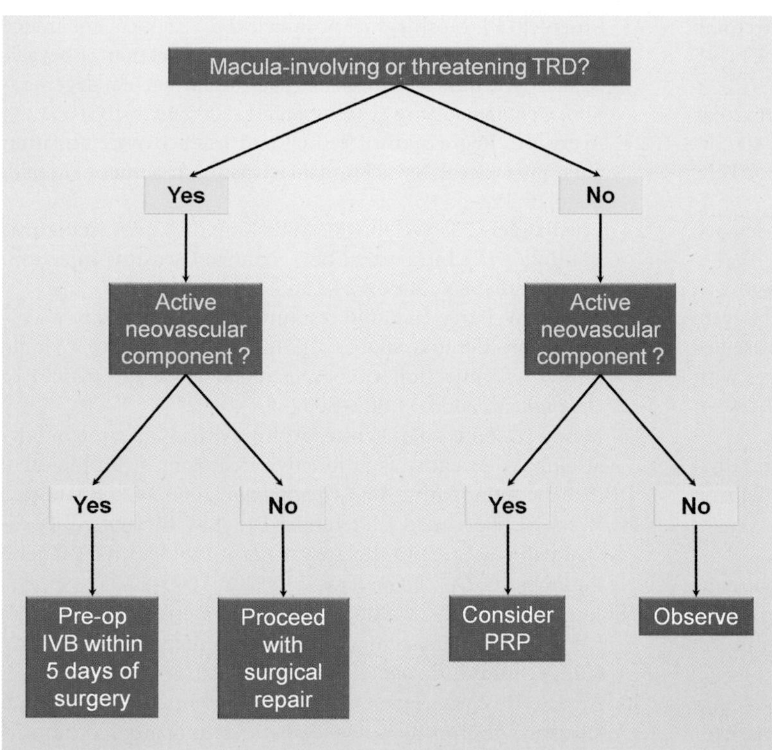

FIGURE 14.9. Approach to a patient with tractional retinal detachment due to PDR. PRP, panretinal photocoagulation; IVB, intravitreal bevacizumab; TRD, tractional retinal detachment.

between injection and surgery is the potential for increased fibrosis and subsequent traction leading to worsening of the TRD.

If the TRD is extramacular and no surgical intervention is planned, we prefer to avoid intravitreal bevacizumab due to the potential for the fibrovascular proliferation to contract and affect the macula. PRP should still be performed if active neovascularization is present but should be kept at least approximately 1 disc diameter from the edge of the fibrovascular proliferation.

KEY POINTS

- VEGF levels are elevated in the aqueous and vitreous of patients with PDR and have been shown to decrease following PRP.
- Anti-VEGF therapies, especially intravitreal bevacizumab, have been shown to induce rapid regression of retinal neovascularization in patients with PDR.
- The effects of intravitreal bevacizumab are transient and therefore PRP is still necessary to allow for a more permanent regression of neovascularization.
- Intravitreal bevacizumab prior to or at the time of initial PRP for PDR may lower the risk of development or worsening of VH and macular edema.
- In patients with VH due to PDR, intravitreal bevacizumab may decrease the risk of further hemorrhage and prevent further fibrovascular proliferation until PRP can be performed.
- In patients with TRD involving or threatening the macula, intravitreal bevacizumab improves the ease of surgical membrane dissection and decreases intraoperative hemorrhage, potentially improving the chance of successful surgical outcomes.
- In patients with significant fibrovascular proliferation, intravitreal bevacizumab may lead to worsening of TRD and should be used with caution in these cases.

REFERENCES

1. The Diabetic Retinopathy Study Research Group. Preliminary report on effects of photocoagulation therapy. *Am J Ophthalmol*. 1976;81:383–397.
2. The Diabetic Retinopathy Study Research Group. Photocoagulation treatment of proliferative diabetic retinopathy: the second report of Diabetic Retinopathy Study findings. *Ophthalmology*. 1978;85:82–106.
3. The Diabetic Retinopathy Study Research Group. Four risk factors for severe visual loss in diabetic retinopathy: the third report from the Diabetic Retinopathy Study. *Arch Ophthalmol*. 1979;97:654–655.
4. Early Treatment of Diabetic Retinopathy Study. Early photocoagulation for diabetic retinopathy. ETDRS Report Number 9. *Ophthalmology*. 1991;98:766–785.
5. Vander JF, Duker JS, Benson WE, et al. Long-term stability and visual outcome after favorable initial response of proliferative diabetic retinopathy to panretinal photocoagulation. *Ophthalmology*. 1991;98:1575–1579.

6. Flynn HW Jr, Chew EY, Simons BD, et al. Pars plana vitrectomy in the Early Treatment Diabetic Retinopathy Study. ETDRS report number 17. *Ophthalmology.* 1992;99:1351–1357.
7. Michaelson IC. The mode of development of the vascular system of the retina, with some observations on its significance for certain retinal diseases. *Trans Ophthalmol Soc U K.* 1948;68:137–180.
8. Ferrara N. Vascular endothelial growth factor: basic science and clinical progress. *Endocr Rev.* 2004;25:581–611.
9. Adamis AP, Shima DT. The role of vascular endothelial growth factor in ocular health and disease. *Retina.* 2005;25:111–118.
10. Adamis AP, Miller JW, Bernal M-T, et al. Increased vascular endothelial growth factor levels in the vitreous of eyes with proliferative diabetic retinopathy. *Am J Ophthalmol.* 1994; 118:445–450.
11. Aiello LP, Avery RL, Arrigg PG, et al. Vascular endothelial growth factor in ocular fluid of patients with diabetic retinopathy and other retinal disorders. *N Engl J Med.* 1994; 331:1480–1487.
12. Tolentino MJ, Miller JW, Gragoudas ES, et al. Intravitreous injections of vascular endothelial growth factor produce retinal ischemia and microangiopathy in an adult primate. *Ophthalmology.* 1996;103:1820–1828.
13. Tolentino MJ, Miller JW, Gragoudas ES, et al. Vascular endothelial growth factor is sufficient to product iris neovascularization and neovascular glaucoma in a nonhuman primate. *Arch Ophthalmol.* 1996;114:964–970.
14. Adamis AP, Shima DT, Tolentino MJ, et al. Inhibition of vascular endothelial growth factor prevents retinal ischemia associated iris neovascularization in a nonhuman primate. *Arch Ophthalmol.* 1996;114:66–71.
15. Aiello LP, Pierce EA, Foley ED, et al. Suppression of retinal neovascularization in vivo by inhibition of vascular endothelial growth factor (VEGF) using soluble VEGF-receptor chimeric proteins. *Proc Natl Acad Sci USA.* 1995;92:10457–10461.
16. Macugen Diabetic Retinopathy Study Group. A Phase 2 randomized double-masked trial of pegaptanib, an anti-vascular endothelial growth factor aptamer, for diabetic macular edema. *Ophthalmology.* 2005;112:1747–1757.
17. Ishida S, Usui T, Yamashiro K, et al. $VEGF_{165}$-mediated inflammation is required for pathological, but not physiological, ischemia-induced retinal neovascularization. *J Exp Med.* 2003;198:483–489.
18. Bandello F, Gass JD, Lattanzio R, et al. Spontaneous regression of neovascularization at the disk and elsewhere in diabetic retinopathy. *Am J Ophthalmol.* 1996;122:494–501.
19. Yang JC, Hawarth L, Sherry RM, et al. A randomized trial of bevacizumab, an anti-vascular endothelial growth factor antibody, for metastatic renal cancer. *N Engl J Med.* 2003; 349:427–434.
20. Kabbinavar F, Hurwitz HI, Fehrenbacher L, et al. Phase 2, randomized trial comparing bevacizumab plus fluorouracil (FU)/leucovorin (LV) with FU/LV alone in patients with metastatic colorectal cancer. *J Clin Oncol.* 2003;21:60–65.
21. Hurwitz H, Fehrenbacher L, Novotny W, et al. Bevacizumab plus irinotecan, fluorouracil, and leucovorin for metastatic colorectal cancer. *N Engl J Med.* 2004;350:2335–2342.
22. Michels S, Rosenfeld PJ, Puliafito CA, et al. Systemic bevacizumab (Avastin) therapy for neovascular age-related macular degeneration: twelve-week results of an uncontrolled open-label clinical study. *Ophthalmology.* 2005;112:1035–1047.
23. Rosenfeld PJ, Moshfeghi AA, Puliafito CA. Optical coherence tomography findings after an intravitreal injection of bevacizumab (Avastin) for neovascular age-related macular degeneration. *Ophthalmic Surg Lasers Imaging.* 2005;36:33133–33135.
24. Avery RL. Regression of retinal and iris neovascularization after intravitreal bevacizumab (Avastin) treatment. *Retina.* 2006;26:352–354.
25. Friedlander SM, Welch RM. Vanishing disc neovascularization following intravitreal bevacizumab (Avastin) injection. *Arch Ophthalmol.* 2006;124:1365.
26. Isaacs TW, Barry C. Rapid resolution of severe disc new vessels in proliferative diabetic retinopathy following a single intravitreal injection of bevacizumab (Avastin). *Clin Exp Ophthalmol.* 2006;34:802–805.
27. Mason JO, Nixon PA, White MF. Intravitreal injection of bevacizumab (Avastin) as adjunctive treatment of proliferative diabetic retinopathy. *Am J Ophthalmol.* 2006;142:685–688.
28. Avery RL, Pearlman J, Pieramici DJ, et al. Intravitreal Bevacizumab (Avastin) in the Treatment of Proliferative Diabetic Retinopathy. *Ophthalmology.* 2006;113:1695–1705.
29. Jorge R, Costa RA, Calucci D, et al. Intravitreal bevacizumab (Avastin) for persistent new vessels in diabetic retinopathy (IBEPE Study). *Retina.* 2006;26:1006–1013.
30. Arevalo JF, Wu L, Sanchez JG, et al. Intravitreal bevacizumab (Avastin) for proliferative diabetic retinopathy: 6-months follow-up. *Eye.* 2009;23:117–123.
31. Minnella AM, Savastano CM, Ziccardi L, et al. Intravitreal bevacizumab (Avastin) in proliferative diabetic retinopathy. *Acta Ophthalmol.* 2008;86:683–687.
32. Mirshahi A, Roohipoor R, Lashay A, et al. Bevacizumab-augmented retinal laser photocoagulation in proliferative diabetic retinopathy: a randomized double-masked clinical trial. *Eur J Ophthalmol.* 2008;18:263–269.
33. Diabetic Retinopathy Study Research Group. Photocoagulation treatment of proliferative diabetic retinopathy. Clinical application of Diabetic Retinopathy Study (DRS) findings. DRS Report Number 8. *Ophthalmology.* 2006;113:1706–1712.
34. Tonello M, Costa RA, Almeida FPP, et al. Panretinal photocoagulation versus PRP plus intravitreal bevacizumab for high-risk proliferative diabetic retinopathy (IBeHi study). *Acta Ophthalmol.* 2008;86:385–389.
35. Cho WB, Oh SB, Moon JW, et al. Panretinal photocoagulation combined with intravitreal bevacizumab in high-risk proliferative diabetic retinopathy. *Retina.* 2009;29:516–522.
36. McDonald HR, Schatz H. Macular edema following panretinal photocoagulation. *Retina.* 1985;5:5–10.
37. McDonald HR, Schatz H. Visual loss following panretinal photocoagulation for proliferative diabetic retinopathy. *Ophthalmology.* 1985;92:388–393.
38. Ferrara N. Vascular endothelial growth factor: basic science in clinical progress. *Endocrinol Rev.* 2004;25:581–611.
39. Mordenti J, Cuthbertson RA, Ferrara N, et al. Comparisons of the intraocular tissue distribution pharmacokinetics and safety of 125 I-labeled Fab antibodies in rhesus monkeys following intravitreal administration. *Toxicol Pathol.* 1999;27:536–544.
40. Spaide RF, Fisher YL. Intravitreal bevacizumab (Avastin) treatment of proliferative diabetic retinopathy complicated by vitreous hemorrhage. *Retina.* 2006;26:275–278.
41. Moradian S, Ahmadich H, Malihi M, et al. Intravitreal bevacizumab in active progressive proliferative diabetic retinopathy. *Graefes Arch Clin Exp Ophthalmol.* 2008;246:1699–1705.

42. Ruiz-Moreno JM, Montero JA, Lugo F, et al. Intravitreal bevacizumab in recurrent diabetic vitreous hemorrhage after vitrectomy. *Acta Ophthalmol*. 2008;86:231–232.
43. Yang CM, Yeh PT, Yang CH, et al. Bevacizumab pretreatment and long-acting gas infusion on vitreous clear-up after diabetic vitrectomy. *Am J Ophthalmol*. 2008;146:211–217.
44. Yang CM, Yeh PT, Yang CH. Intravitreal long-acting gas in the prevention of early postoperative vitreous hemorrhage in diabetic vitrectomy. *Ophthalmology*. 2007;114:710–715.
45. Charles S, Rosenfeld PJ, Gayer S. Medical consequences of stopping anticoagulant therapy before intraocular surgery or intravitreal injections. *Retina*. 2007;27:813–815.
46. Mosesson MW. Fibrinogen and fibrin structure and functions. *J Thromb Haemost*. 2005;3:1894–1904.
47. Chen E, Park CH. Use of intravitreal bevacizumab as a preoperative adjunct for tractional retinal detachment repair in severe proliferative diabetic retinopathy. *Retina*. 2006;26:699–700.
48. Yeoh J, Williams C, Allen P, et al. Avastin as an adjunct to vitrectomy in the management of severe proliferative diabetic retinopathy: a prospective case series. *Clin Exp Ophthalmol*. 2008;36:449–454.
49. Yeh PT, Yang CM, Yang CH, et al. Cryotherapy of the anterior retina and sclerotomy sites in diabetic vitrectomy to prevent recurrent vitreous hemorrhage. *Ophthalmology*. 2005;112:2095–2102.
50. West J, Gregor Z. Fibrovascular ingrowth and recurrent haemorrhage following diabetic vitrectomy. *Br J Ophthalmol*. 2000;84:822–825.
51. Schiff WM, Banle GR, Hwang JC, et al. Diabetic vitrectomy. Influence on lens status upon anatomic and visual outcomes. *Ophthalmology*. 2007;114:544–550.
52. Ishikawa K, Honda S, Tsukahara Y, et al. Preferable use of intravitreal bevacizumab as a pretreatment of vitrectomy for severe proliferative diabetic retinopathy. *Eye*. 2009;23: 108–111.
53. Rizzo S, Genovesi-Ebert F, Di Bartolo E, et al. Injection of intravitreal bevacizumab (Avastin) as a preoperative adjunct before vitrectomy surgery in the treatment of severe proliferative diabetic retinopathy (PDR). *Graefes Arch Clin Exp Ophthalmol*. 2008;246:837–842.
54. Lee CS, Koh HJ. Multiple retinal haemorrhages in diabetic retinopathy after adjunctive intravitreal bevacizumab (Avastin) with pars plana vitrectomy. *Acta Ophthalmol*. 2008;86:812–813.
55. Lee SJ, Koh HJ. Enlargement of the foveal avascular zone in diabetic retinopathy after adjunctive intravitreal bevacizumab (Avastin) with pars plana vitrectomy. *J Ocul Pharmacol Ther*. 2009;25:173–174.
56. Mourad JJ, des Guetz G, Debbabi H, et al. Blood pressure rise following angiogenesis inhibition by bevacizumab. A crucial role for microcirculation. *Ann Oncol*. 2008;19: 927–934.
57. Tranos P, Gemenetzi M, Papandroudis A, et al. Progression of diabetic tractional retinal detachment following single injection of intravitreal Avastin. *Eye*. 2008;22:862.
58. Arevalo JF, Maia M, Flynn HW, et al. Tractional retinal detachment following intravitreal bevacizumab (Avastin) in patients with severe proliferative diabetic retinopathy. *Br J Ophthalmol*. 2008;92:213–216.
59. Mitamura Y, Ogata K, Oshitari T, et al. Retinal detachment with macular hole following intravitreal bevacizumab in patient with severe proliferative diabetic retinopathy. *Br J Ophthalmol*. 2008;92:717–718.

CHAPTER

15

Anti-VEGF Therapies in Diabetic Macular Edema

P.S. Silva • Z.A. Haddad • J.K. Sun • J.D. Cavallerano • L.P. Aiello

INTRODUCTION

For the past 20 years, diabetic retinopathy (DR) has remained the most common cause of blindness in the working age adult population in the United States and other developed countries.[1–3] DR is the most frequently occurring microvascular complication of diabetes, affecting nearly all persons with 15 or more years of diabetes.[4,5] Diabetic macular edema (DME) is a manifestation of DR that may occur in any stage of the retinopathy and often leads to loss of central vision.[6–8] The natural course of DME is characterized by chronic continued retinal vascular leakage and retinal thickening, often with intraretinal lipid deposition.[6] The Wisconsin Epidemiologic Study of Diabetic Retinopathy reported that over a 10-year period, DME was present in 24% of patients and visually threatening clinically significant macular edema (CSME) was present in 10% of patients.[7,8] DME is more common in type 2 diabetes patients on insulin than in type 1 diabetes patients, and prevalence increases in both types as the duration of diabetes increases.[8] The involvement of the center of the macula has been shown to be an important predictor in determining visual outcome among patients with CSME.[9–11] If left untreated, 24% of eyes with CSME and 33% with center involving CSME will have moderate visual loss (MVL; i.e., a doubling of the visual angle) within 3 years.[12] The Early Treatment Diabetic Retinopathy Study (ETDRS) established focal/grid laser photocoagulation as the standard of care in the treatment of CSME.[12] Focal/grid laser was shown to be effective at reducing the risk of MVL by 50%, but 15% of laser treated patients in the ETDRS continued to develop MVL after 3 years.[12] This continued development of visual loss following focal/grid laser has encouraged investigators to search for novel treatment modalities in the management of eyes with DME.

Rationale

Focal/grid laser is currently the only treatment modality for CSME that has been validated for long-term safety and efficacy by multiple large clinical trials.[12–14] Despite its proven benefit, focal/grid laser does not directly address the underlying pathophysiologic mechanisms of DME, and this may explain suboptimal response and continued visual loss in spite of adequate laser treatment in some patients.[15] Furthermore, the pathogenesis of DME is multifactorial and likely involves multiple mechanisms including inflammation,[16] angiogenesis,[17,18] endothelial junctional dysfunction,[19,20] and contribution from different growth factors[21,22] all of which contribute to significant variability in the response to specific treatment modalities.

Vascular endothelial growth factor (VEGF) has been shown to play a central role in the pathophysiologic process underlying neovascular eye diseases.[17,18] As such, anti-VEGF-based agents have emerged as a novel, highly specific treatment modality for retinal vascular pathology. Diabetic retinal neovascularization has been shown to be exquisitely sensitive to treatment with VEGF inhibitors, with regression of the neovascularization beginning as early as one day after treatment with complete regression commonly observed[23] (Fig. 15.1). Studies of limited size and duration suggest that the anti-VEGF treatment response may be more variable for DME, suggesting that DME is a multifactorial process involving pathways in addition to VEGF (Fig. 15.2). Determining the optimal treatment for DME has remained elusive and has prompted significant research and development of anti-VEGF and similarly based DME treatment modalities.

Presently, there are many agents that target different points of the pathophysiologic cascade theorized to underlie the development of DME (Table 15.1). There are drugs that directly inhibit the VEGF molecule such as the anti-VEGF aptamer pegaptanib (Macugen; OSI Pharmaceuticals, Melville, NY), the monoclonal antibody fragment ranibizumab (Lucentis; Genentech Inc., San Francisco, CA), and the full-length monoclonal antibody bevacizumab (Avastin; Genentech Inc., San Francisco, CA). Modified soluble VEGF receptor analog VEGF-Trap (Regeneron Pharmaceuticals, Tarrytown, NY) is also being studied. It is a fusion protein of portions of VEGF-R1 and VEGF-R2 and the Fc region of human IgG that binds all VEGF isoforms with higher affinity than anti-VEGF

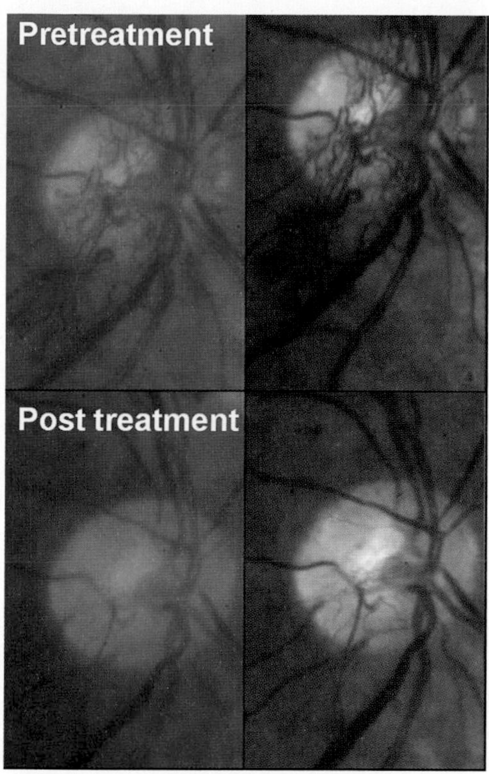

FIGURE 15.1. Anti-VEGF agents have been shown to be effective in inducing temporary regression of retinal neovascularization. Retinal neovascularization on the optic nerve shows marked regression following a single intravitreal injection of bevacizumab. (Images courtesy of Robert Avery MD, Santa Barbara, CA.)

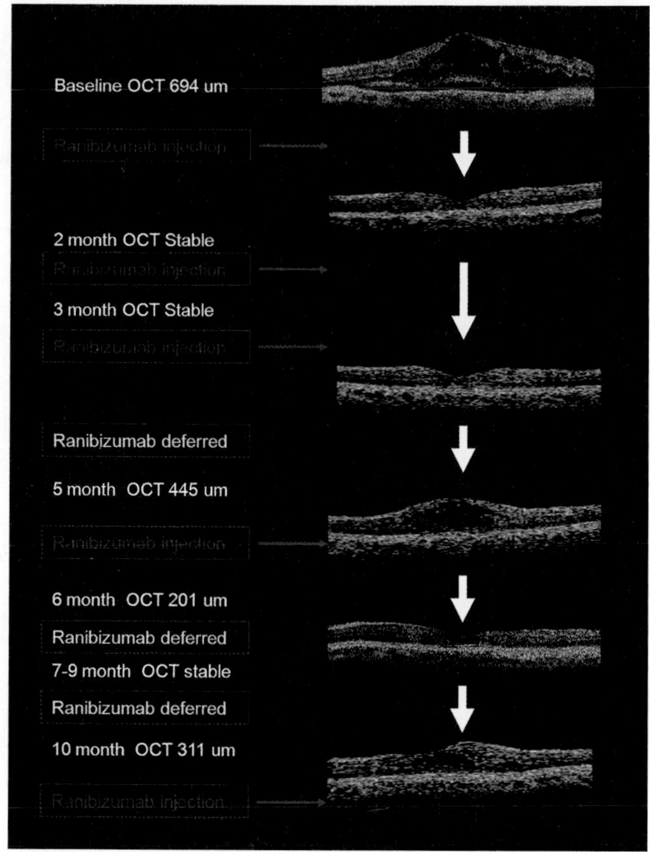

FIGURE 15.2. The responses of diabetic macular edema to intravitreal anti-VEGF agents have significant variability and require repeated injections to prevent the recurrence. Following injections of ranibizumab, there is a substantial reduction in retinal thickness but the edema recurs when injections are withheld. (Images from the Beetham Eye Institute Image Library.)

antibodies. Other treatment modalities include small interfering RNAs (siRNAs) bevasiranib (Opko Health Inc., Miami, FL), Rapamycin (Sirolimus, MacuSight Inc, Union City, CA), and Sirna-027 (Sirna Therapeutics, San Francisco, CA). They inactivate mRNA ultimately by inhibiting mRNA translation, which suppresses VEGF production and VEGF receptor production. Oral agents with ocular bioavailability such as Vatalanib (PTK-787; Novartis International, Basel, Switzerland), which is an inhibitor of VEGF receptor tyrosine kinases, Ruboxistaurin (Eli Lilly, Indianapolis, IN), an oral protein kinase C β (PKC β) inhibitor, and oral and topically active multitarget kinase inhibitors (such as Src kinase inhibitors) have received significant interest. The future may lie in the development of treatment regimens that act on different points along multiple pathways responsible for the development of DME. The targeting of multiple points along more than one pathway may increase the clinical effectiveness and robustness of the therapeutic effect. Additionally, having a wide selection of highly specific agents may promote the development of an optimal treatment strategy tailored to the needs of a specific patient.

As of June 2009, there are 145 registered clinical trials assessing the efficacy or safety of response of various regimens in the treatment of DME. Twenty-two trials specifically target VEGF or VEGF-related pathways. A summary of the important highlights and results of published trials is presented in Table 15.2.

Pegaptanib

Pegaptanib (Macugen, OSI Pharmaceuticals, Melville, NY) is a ribonucleic acid aptamer that selectively binds to the VEGF165 isoform. Trials utilizing pegaptanib provided the proof of principle evidence regarding the effectiveness of anti-VEGF agents in the treatment of neovascular and exudative retinal disease. In December 2004, it was the first anti-VEGF agent to be approved by the United States Food and Drug Administration (U.S. FDA) for the treatment of neovascular wet age-related macular degeneration (AMD). Clinical trials assessing its efficacy and safety in the treatment of DME are currently ongoing.

In a prospective, randomized, double-masked, controlled multicenter phase 2 trial, pegaptanib (0.3, 1.0, or 3 mg) versus sham injection was administered at 6-week intervals via intravitreal injection in 172 subjects with

Table 15.1.

Agents currently being investigated in clinical trials for the treatment of DME[a]

Agent	Route of Administration	Class	Mechanism	Manufacturer	Stage of Development
Pegatanib (Macugen)	Intravitreal injection	Anti-VEGF aptamer	Blocks VEGF165 isoform	OSI/Eyetech	FDA approved, Off-label use
Ranibizumab (Lucentis)	Intravitreal injection	Monoclonal antibody fragment	Blocks all VEGF-A isoforms	Genentech	FDA approved, Off-label use
Bevacizumab (Avastin)	Intravitreal injection	Monoclonal antibody	Blocks all VEGF-A isoforms	Genentech	FDA approved, Off-label use
VEGF-trap	Intravitreal injection	Decoy receptor	Block all VEGF isoforms and PGF	Regeneron	Clinical trial use
Ruboxistaurin (Arxxant)	Oral	PKC β inhibitor	Selective inhibitor of PKC β isoform	Eli Lilly	Clinical trial use
PF-04523655	Intravitreal injection	siRNA	Blocks RTP801 pathway	Pfizer	Clinical trial use
Rapamycin (Sirolimus)	Subconjunctival injection	Macrolide	mTOR inhibitor	MacuSight Inc	FDA approved, Off-label use
Bevasiranib (Cand5)	Intravitreal injection	siRNA	silences the mRNA encoding for VEGF	Opko Health	Clinical trial use
Efalizumab (Raptiva)	Subcutaneous injection	Monoclonal antibody	Immunosuppressant binds to CD11a	Genentech	Withdrawn from the market
Triamcinolone Acetonide (Trivaris, Triessense, Kenalog)	Intravitreal injection, periocular injection	Corticosteroid	Multiple physiologic effects, Anti-inflammatory, Inhibits VEGF and VEGF gene expression	Allergan, Alcon, Bristol-Myers Squibb	FDA approved, Off-label use
Dexam-ethasone (Posudex, SK-0503)	Intravitreal implant	Corticosteroid	Multiple physiologic effects, Anti-inflammatory, Inhibits VEGF and VEGF gene expression	Allergan, Sanwa Kagaku Kenyusho	Clinical trial use
Fluocinolone Acetonide (Retisert, Ilivien)	Intravitreal implant	Corticosteroid	Multiple physiologic effects, Anti-inflammatory, Inhibits VEGF and VEGF gene expression	Bausch & Lomb, Alimera Sciences	Clinical trial use
Methotrexate	Intravitreal injection	Antimetabolite	Inhibits dihydrofolate reductase	Multiple, generic formulation	FDA approved, off-label

[a] http://clinicaltrials.gov/ accessed 5/27/2009.
VEGF, vascular endothelial growth factor; PDF, placental growth factor; PKC β, protein kinase C β isoform; siRNA, small interfering RNA; mTOR, mammalian target of rapamycin.

center-involving DME (Fig. 15.3).[24] Intravitreous pegaptanib (0.3, 1, 3 mg) or sham injections were performed at study entry, week 6, and week 12 with additional injections and/or focal photocoagulation as needed for another 18 weeks. Final assessments were conducted at week 36. Median VA was better at week 36 with 0.3 mg (20/50), as compared with sham (20/63) ($p = 0.04$). A larger proportion of those receiving 0.3 mg as compared with sham gained 10 or more letters in VA (approximately two lines) (34% vs. 10%; $p = 0.003$) or 15 or more letters (18% vs. 7%; $p = 0.12$). Mean central retinal thickness decreased by 68 µm with 0.3 mg versus an increase of 4 µm with sham ($p = 0.02$). Larger proportions of those receiving 0.3 mg had an absolute decrease of both ≥100 µm (42% vs. 16%; $p = 0.02$) and

Table 15.2.

Randomized controlled trials evaluating pharmacological therapies in DME

Agent	Clinical Trial	Study design (n)	Inclusion Criteria	Intervention	Follow-up	Results	Safety/Comments
Pegatanib (Macugen)	Cunningham et al.[24]	Randomized, double-masked, placebo-controlled, dose-ranging, multicenter trial (172 patients)	-Center-involved DME -Photocoagulation could be safely withheld for 16 wk -BCVA between 20/50 and 20/320	-Intravitreous pegaptanib (0.3 mg, 1 mg, 3 mg) or sham injections at study entry, week 6, and week 12 -Additional injections and/or focal laser as needed for another 18 wk	36 wk	- Median BCVA was better at week 36 with 0.3 mg (20/50) compared to sham (20/63) (p = 0.04). -34% of those receiving 0.3 mg gained >10 letters compared to 10% sham (p = 0.003) -18% of those receiving 0.3 mg gained >15 letters compared to 7% sham (p = 0.7) -Mean CST decreased by 68 µm with 0.3 mg compared to an increase of 4 µm with sham (p = 0.02) -49% of those receiving 0.3 mg absolute decrease of 100 µm compared to 42% of sham (p = 0.02). -Photocoagulation was deemed necessary in 25% of each pegaptanib arm compared to 48% of sham (p = 0.04)	-All pegaptanib doses were well tolerated. -Endophthalmitis occurred in 1 of 652 injections (0.15%/injection) -Not powered sufficiently to detect a difference between the different dosages -Focal laser treatment deferred at baseline, laser treatment control arm was not utilized in the trial
Ranibizumab (Lucentis)	Chun et al.[42]	Dose-escalating pilot study (0.3 mg: 5 patients; 0.5 mg: 5 patients)	-Center-involved DME -BCVA between 20/63 and 20/400	-Intravitreal ranibizumab (two doses used) at study entry, month 1 and 2	24 months	-At 3 mo, the low-dose group (0.3 mg) gained a mean of 12.0 letters and the high-dose group (0.5 mg) gained 7.8 letters from baseline -Decrease in central retinal thickness in the low-dose group (45.3 µm) and the high-dose group (197.8 µm) at 3 mo	-No systemic adverse events were reported -Mild-to-moderate ocular inflammation in five patients

(Continued)

Table 15.2.

Randomized controlled trials evaluating pharmacological therapies in DME (*Continued*)

Agent	Clinical Trial	Study design (n)	Inclusion Criteria	Intervention	Follow-up	Results	Safety/Comments
	Nguyen et al.[43]	Nonrandomized Clinical trial (10 patients)	-Center-involved DME -BCVA between 20/40 and 20/320	-Intravitreal 0.5 mg of ranibizumab at study entry, month 1, 2, 4, and 6	9 mo	-At 7 months, improvement in mean BCVA was 12.3 letters and median 11 letters -BCVA at baseline was 20/80, improved to 20/40 at month 7 ($p = 0.05$). -Mean foveal thickness decreased by 85% (from mean 503 µm to 257 µm at month 7).	-No adverse or systemic side effects—Plateau in degree of reduction of foveal thickening during the month 1 to 3 -Additional benefit achieved during every other month dosing.
Ruboxistaurin (Arxxant)	PKC-DRS2 Group[50]	Randomized, double-masked, placebo-controlled, parallel, multicenter trial (685 patients)	-ETDRS retinopathy levels of ≥47A and ≤53E, -BCVA ≥ 45 letters	-Placebo or ruboxistaurin (32 mg) administered orally once daily	36 mo	-Treatment was associated with less progression of DME to within 100 µm of the macular center (68% vs. 50%, $p = 0.003$) - 26% less frequent application initial focal laser in eyes without prior history of focal treatment ($p = 0.008$)	
	Davis et al.[51]	Randomized, double-masked, placebo-controlled, parallel, multicenter trial (686 patients)	-DME not within 300 µm of the center of the macula; -ETDRS retinopathy level between 20 and 47A -BCVA 75 or more letters, no history of PRP or focal/grid laser	- Placebo or ruboxistaurin (32 mg) administered orally once daily	36 mo	-Treatment was associated with a delay in progression of DME to a sight-threatening stage ($p = 0.054$ [unadjusted]; Cox proportional hazards model, hazards ratio = 0.66; 95% confidence interval, 0.47–0.93; $p = 0.02$) -In patients with moderately severe to very severe nonproliferative DR with long-standing severe DME, ruboxistaurin-treated patients showed a 30% reduction in rate of visual loss over 36 months in treatment group compared to placebo (0.47 vs. 0.67 letters per month $p = 0.022$).	

Agent	Clinical Trial	Study design (*n*)	Inclusion Criteria	Intervention	Follow-up	Results	Safety/Comments
Bevacizumab (Avastin)	Bonini-Filho et al.[31]	-Multicenter, nonrandomized clinical trial (10 consecutive patients)	-DME with CMT >250 μm, and "severe" capillary loss within 1,500 μm of the center of the macula (as assessed by FA according to ETDRS criteria) -BCVA 20/40 or worse -No history of prior focal laser or vitrectomy -No history of panretinal photocoagulation in the last 6 months	-1.5 mg (0.06 mL) of intravitreal bevacizumab at baseline with reinjections at 8-wk interval if subretinal or intraretinal fluid were persistent or recurrent on OCT	1 y	-Mean logMAR ETDRS BCVA was 0.786 ($20/125^{-1}$) at baseline and 0.558 ($20/80^{-2}$) at week 54 ($p < 0.008$) -The mean CMT (μm)/TMV (mm^3) values were, respectively, 472.6/10.9 at baseline and 274.6/8.7 at week 54 ($p < 0.007$) -Bevacizumab reduced dye leakage on FA -No worsening of macular ischemia	-No control arm
	Scott et al.[32]	-Randomized phase 2 trial on 121 eyes	-Center involved DME -CST ≥250 μm -BCVA 20/32–20/320 -No history of treatment for DME in the past 3 mo -No history of vitrectomy -No history of panretinal photocoagulation in the last 4 mo	A-Focal laser at baseline ($n = 19$) B-1.25 mg of intravitreal bevacizumab at baseline and 6 wk ($n = 22$) C-2.5 mg of intravitreal bevacizumab at baseline and 6 wk ($n = 24$) D-1.25 mg of intravitreal bevacizumab at baseline and sham injection at 6 wk ($n = 22$) E-1.25 mg of intravitreal bevacizumab at baseline and 6 wk with laser photocoagulation at 3 wk ($n = 22$)	70 wk (only results at 24 wk are included in report)	-Groups B and C had greater reduction in CST at 3 wk and one line increase in median VA over 12 wk compared to A -No difference between B and C -CST reduction >11% present in 43% in bevacizumab-treated eyes and 28% in laser-treated eyes at 3 wk and 37% and 50%, respectively at 6 wk -No benefit or adverse effect from combining laser with bevacizumab injection	-Endophthalmitis in 1 eye -Adverse events not attributed to bevacizumab: Myocardial infarction ($n = 2$), congestive heart failure ($n = 1$), hypertension ($n = 3$), worsened renal function ($n = 3$) -A beneficial effect of laser could be observed if follow-up was longer -Modest sample size and short follow-up -Phase 3 trial needed to determine if bevacizumab is beneficial

(Continued)

Table 15.2.

Randomized controlled trials evaluating pharmacological therapies in DME (*Continued*)

Agent	Clinical Trial	Study design (*n*)	Inclusion Criteria	Intervention	Follow-up	Results	Safety/Comments
	Ahmadieh et al.[35]	-Prospective, placebo-controlled, randomized clinical trial on 115 eyes	-CSME unresponsive to previous laser treatment (last session being more than 3 mo prior to enrollment) - VA better than 20/40	A-Three injections of bevacizumab (1.25 mg/0.05 mL) at 6-wk intervals (n = 41) B-Combined 1.25 mg/0.05 mL bevacizumab and 2 mg/0.05 mL triamcinolone followed by two injections of bevacizumab at 6-wk intervals (n = 37) C-Sham injection (n = 37)	24 wk	-At week 24, change in CMT compared to baseline was −95.7 µm in group A, −92.1 µm in group B, and +34.9 µm in group C -Improvement of BCVA was initiated at weeks 6 and 12 in groups B and A respectively -No significant differences in anatomical and visual outcomes in groups A and B	- Anterior chamber inflammation in one fifth of the patients in groups A and B for 1 wk with no sequelae -IOP rise in 8.1% of patients in group B -Addition of triamcinolone in the first injection induced earlier visual improvement but no significant additive effect later during follow-up -Longer follow-up needed
	Soheilian et al.[37]	-Randomized three-arm clinical trial on 150 eyes	-CSME with no prior treatment -VA 20/240–20/300	A-1.25 mg of intravitreal bevacizumab (n = 50) B-1.25 mg of bevacizumab and 2 mg of triamcinolone (n = 50) C-Focal or modified grid laser (n = 50) -Retreatment was performed at 12-wk intervals whenever indicated (persistent CSME with VA worse than 20/40)	36 wk	-VA improvement >2 Snellen lines at 36 wk was detected in 37%, 25%, and 14.8% of patients in groups A, B, and C, respectively (improving effect persisted longer in group A (up to 36 wk) than in group B (up to 12 weeks) -VA changes at 36 wk were −0.28 logMAR, -0.04 logMAR, and +0.01 logMAR in groups A, B and C, respectively (p = 0.053) - Intravitreal bevacizumab injection in patients with DME yielded a better visual outcome at 24 wk compared with macular laser	- IOP rise in 16% of patients in group B controlled by drops -Mild anterior chamber reaction in 20% and 18% of eyes in groups A and B, respectively lasting 1 wk -VA improvement in group B had a shorter duration than in group A (12 vs. 36 wk) probably secondary to cataract progression, ocular hypertension, and adverse effects of triamcinolone preservatives

Agent	Clinical Trial	Study design (n)	Inclusion Criteria	Intervention	Follow-up	Results	Safety/Comments
						-CMT changes were not significant among the three groups except at 6 wk and the reduction of CMT was greater in group A -72% of patients required only one injection of bevacizumab, 22% and 6% of eyes required a second and third injection, respectively -No adjunctive effect of triamcinolone	-A more beneficial effect of laser could be seen with longer follow-up -The laser arm had a better baseline visual acuity that could bias the results -This study is currently being extended for up to 2 y
	Faghihi et al.[38]	-Prospective, randomized clinical trial on 130 eyes	DME	A-1.25 mg intravitreal bevacizumab ($n = 42$) B-1.25 mg bevacizumab and 2 mg triamcinolone acetonide ($n = 41$) C- Macular laser photocoagulation ($n = 47$)	16 weeks	-At week 6, CMT reductions were greater in groups A and B compared to C ($p < 0.001$) -At week 16, the response was not stable for group A ($p < 0.001$), but group B maintained its superior status to group C ($p < 0.001$) -At week 16, visual acuities were unchanged for groups A and C and improvement in group B was marginal and at most was 0.1 log MAR	

(Continued)

Table 15.2.

Randomized controlled trials evaluating pharmacological therapies in DME (*Continued*)

Agent	Clinical Trial	Study design (n)	Inclusion Criteria	Intervention	Follow-up	Results	Safety/Comments
VEGF-trap	Do et al.[46]	-Phase 1 exploratory study of five eyes	DME	-Single intravitreal injection of VEGF trap	6 wk	-At 6 wk, 4/5 patients had a 31% reduction in OCT-measured foveal thickness ($p = 0.06$) -At 6 wk, 4/5 patients had a median improvement of three letters	- No serious side effects - A larger phase 2 study is underway
Bevasiranib (Cand5)	Singerman[56]	-RNAi assessment of C and 5 in patients with DME (RACE trial) Phase 2, randomized, controlled trial on 48 patients	DME	-Three injections of either 0.2, 1.5 or 3 mg of intravitreal bevasiranib every 4 wk	52 wk	-At 4 wk, VA decreased and retinal thickness increased, this reverted on the second month -91% of patients had stabilization of vision throughout 6–12 wk	- Four patients had iritis/uveitis -Phase 3 trial is underway with initiation of therapy by ranibizumab followed by bevasiranib every 8–12 wk thereafter

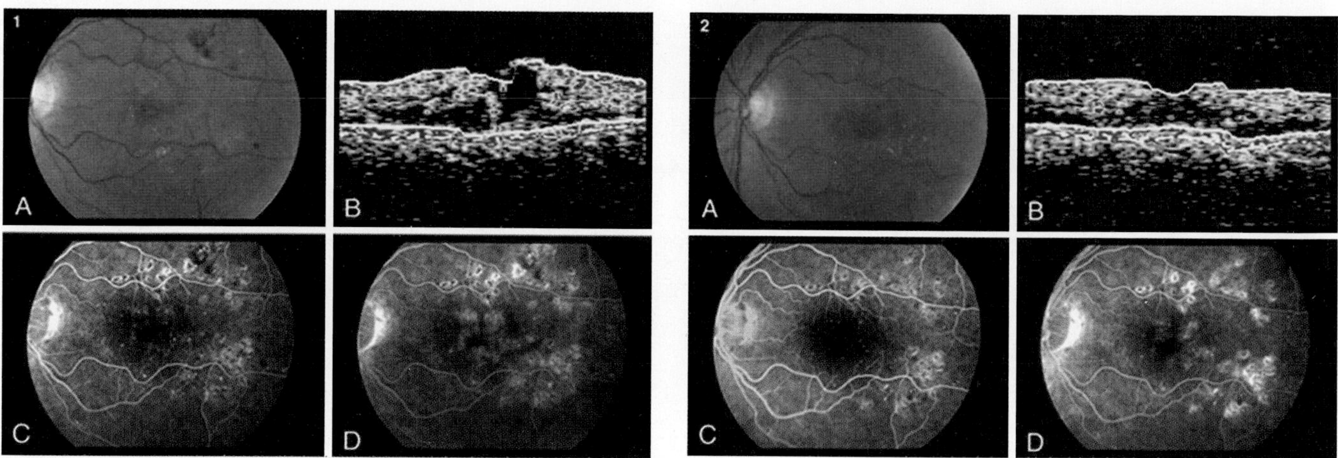

FIGURE 15.3. 1: From a representative subject, a baseline color fundus photograph (A), OCT image (B), and serial fluorescein angiographic images (C, D) before treatment with intravitreous pegaptanib, 0.3 mg, show intraretinal hemorrhage, microaneurysm formation, and exudates; a retinal thickness of 422 μm with cystic spaces evident at the center of the macula; and progressive development of diabetic macular edema (D). Previous focal laser photocoagulation scars are apparently superior and temporal to the fovea (C, D). Visual acuity at time of study entry was 68 Early Treatment Diabetic Retinopathy Study chart letters (Snellen acuity, 20/50). Laser photocoagulation was given 6 months before enrollment. **2:** From the same subject as in Figure 5.3A, a week-36 color fundus photograph (A), OCT image (B), and serial fluorescein angiographic images (C, D) after 4 intravitreous injections (at day 0, week 6, week 12, and week 24) of pegaptanib, 0.3 mg, show partial resolution of retinal microaneurysms, hemorrhages, and exudates; a marked decrease in retinal thickness to 267 μm; complete resolution of the intraretinal cystic spaces; and decreased perifoveal leakage corresponding to the anatomic changes observed on OCT, version 2. Visual acuity at week 36 was 79 Early Treatment Diabetic Retinopathy Study chart letters (Snellen acuity, 20/25). No focal laser photocoagulation treatments were given after enrollment. (Reproduced with permission from Cunningham et al. *Ophthalmology.* 2005;112:1747–175.)

≥75 μm (49% vs. 19%; p = 0.008). Photocoagulation was deemed necessary in fewer subjects in each pegaptanib arm (0.3 mg vs. sham, 25% vs. 48%; p = 0.04). All pegaptanib doses were well tolerated. Despite the observed differences in the efficacy of the three dosages, the study was not powered sufficiently to detect a difference between the different dosages. Furthermore, the eyes enrolled had focal laser treatment deferred at baseline and a laser treatment control arm was not utilized in the trial. It is unknown if these results are better than if focal photocoagulation had been given at study entry and it is unknown if these beneficial outcomes would provide lasting benefit that would persist for at least 3 years as is seen with focal/grid laser.[25] All pegaptanib doses were well tolerated. Endophthalmitis occurred in 1 of 652 injections (0.15%) and was not associated with severe visual loss.

Currently, a phase 2/3 randomized, controlled, double-masked, multicenter, comparative trial, in parallel groups is ongoing to further investigate the observed benefit seen in the initial phase 2 trial. Intravitreal injections of 0.3 mg pegaptanib will be given as often as every 6 weeks for 2 years in patients with center-involving DME with an open-label 3-year extension (ClinicalTrials.gov identifier: NCT00605280). The primary outcome measure is the proportion of patients after 1 year who experience an improvement in vision from baseline in the treatment group compared to the sham injection group. The trial has been completed with 260 subjects enrolled and preliminary unpublished results suggesting significant benefit with intravitreal pegaptanib treatment. The mean visual acuity gain in ETDRS letters with pegaptanib treatment compared to sham at one and two years were 5.2 vs 1.2 (p = 0.05) and 6.1 vs 1.3 (p = 0.01) respectively. The percentage of patients gaining ≥ 10 ETDRS letters at 2 years was significantly large in patients receiving pegaptanib treatment compared to sham (37% vs 20%, p=0.0005). Adverse events were reported to be consistent with those observed in clinical trials of pegaptanib in patients with neovascular AMD (Box 15.1).

Bevacizumab

Bevacizumab (Avastin, Genentech Inc., San Francisco, CA) is a full-length humanized monoclonal antibody that inhibits all isoforms of VEGF-A. It has two binding sites compared to ranibizumab. It has a molecular weight of 149 kDa whereas ranibizumab has a molecular weight of 48 kDa. Ranibizumab has a threefold to sixfold higher affinity to VEGF compared to bevacizumab.[26] Being larger, bevacizumab has a longer half-life. Bevacizumab was approved by the FDA in February 2004 for the treatment of metastatic colorectal cancer, metastatic breast cancer, and non–small cell lung cancer.[27] It has been used as an off label treatment for AMD, proliferative diabetic retinopathy (PDR), radiation retinopathy, uveitic macular edema,

BOX 15.1 Clinical Trials in DME

DRCR.net Trial with Bevacizumab in DME

Purpose: A randomized Phase 2 trial to provide data on the short-term effect of intravitreal bevacizumab for DME. Five groups: (a) focal photocoagulation, (b) intravitreal injection of 1.25 mg of bevacizumab at baseline and 6 weeks, (c) intravitreal injection of 2.5 mg of bevacizumab at baseline and 6 weeks, (d) intravitreal injection of 1.25 mg of bevacizumab at baseline and sham injection at 6 weeks, or (e) intravitreal injection of 1.25 mg of bevacizumab at baseline and 6 weeks with photocoagulation at 3 weeks.

Results: Compared with group A, groups B and C had a greater reduction in CST at 3 weeks and about 1 line better median VA over 12 weeks. There were no meaningful differences between groups B and C in CST reduction or VA improvement. A CST reduction >11% (reliability limit) was present at 3 weeks in 36 of 84 (43%) bevacizumab-treated eyes and 5 of 18 (28%) eyes treated with laser alone, and at 6 weeks in 31 of 84 (37%) and 9 of 18 (50%) eyes, respectively. Combining focal photocoagulation with bevacizumab resulted in no apparent short-term benefit or adverse outcomes.

Conclusions: Intravitreal bevacizumab can reduce DME in some eyes "but the study was not designed to determine whether treatment is beneficial. A phase 3 trial would be needed for that purpose." (DRCR Network. *Ophthalmology.* 2007;114:1860–1867.)

READ-2 Trial: Ranibizumab for Edema of the mAcula in Diabetes

Purpose: A Phase 2 randomized, open-label, parallel assignment, safety/efficacy study to compare intravitreal ranibizumab and focal/grid laser treatment in DME. *Group 1:* Intravitreal ranibizumab (0.5 mg), *Group 2:* Focal/grid laser, *Group 3:* A combination of ranibizumab 0.5 mg and focal/grid laser.

Results: At month 6, the mean gain in BCVA was significantly greater in group 1 (+7.24 letters) compared with group 2 (-0.43 letters) and group 3 (+3.80 letters). Excess foveal thickness was reduced by 50%, 33%, and 45% in groups 1, 2, and 3, respectively. During a span of 6 months, ranibizumab injections by the study protocol had a significantly better visual outcome than focal/grid laser treatment in patients with DME. (Nguyen et al. *Ophthalmology.* 2009;116:2175–2181.) At year 1, the mean gain in BCVA was +6.46 letters, +4.48 letters and + 2.08 letters in Groups 1, 2, and 3, respectively. (Do et al. Presented at the AAO Meeting, 2009.)

Status: Active, not recruiting.

RESOLVE Trial: Safety and Efficacy of Ranibizumab in DME With Center Involvement (Novartis)

Purpose: A randomized, double-masked, multicenter, Phase 2 study assessing the safety and efficacy of two concentrations (3 and 5 mg) of intravitreal Ranibizumab compared with nontreatment control for the treatment of DME with center involvement. (Clinicaltrials.gov Identifier: NCT00284050.)

Status: Completed.

REVEAL Trial: Efficacy and Safety of Ranibizumab (Intravitreal Injections) in Patients With Visual Impairment Due to Diabetic Macular Edema

Purpose: A randomized, double-masked, multicenter Phase 3 study to confirm the efficacy and safety of ranibizumab (0.5 mg) as adjunctive therapy when added to laser photocoagulation and/or mono-therapy in patients with visual impairment due to DME. *Arm 1:* Raninibizumab + sham laser, *Arm 2:* sham injection + laser, *Arm 3:* Ranibizumab + laser. (Clinicaltrials.gov Identifier: NCT00989989.)

Status: Ongoing.

RIDE/RISE Trial: A Study of Ranibizumab Injection in Subjects with CSME With Center Involvement Secondary to Diabetes Mellitus (Genentech)

Purpose: A phase 3, double-masked, multicenter, randomized, sham injection-controlled study of the efficacy and safety of ranibizumab injection in patients with center involving CSME secondary to diabetes mellitus. Monthly intravitreal injections of ranibizumab for 24 months. The primary efficacy outcome measure is the proportion of subjects who gain at least 15 letters in BCVA compared with baseline. (RIDE Clinicaltrials.gov Identifier: NCT00473382 and RISE Clinicaltrials.gov identifier: NCT00473330.)

Status: Active, not recruiting patients.

vein occlusions, and DME.[28] It has attracted interest partly because of its significantly lower cost and presumably (but unproved) similar efficacy to ranibizumab, given the similarities in molecular structure.

In a large interventional retrospective multicenter study from six different countries, 101 eyes of 82 patients with diffuse DME were randomized to either 1.25 or 2.5 mg of primary intravitreal bevacizumab injection. All patients were followed for 12 months (mean 57.6 ± 8.4 weeks). The mean number of intravitreal bevacizumab injections per eye was three (range: 1–2 injections) at a mean interval of 14.1 ± 10.5 weeks. Best corrected visual acuity (BCVA) in the 1.25 mg group at 1 month improved from 20/190 (logMAR = 0.97) to 20/85 (logMAR 0.62)(p = 0.0001). This improvement was maintained throughout the follow-up period. The mean final BCVA at 12 months was 20/76 (logMAR = 0.58) ($p < 0.001$). In the 1.25 mg group, the mean central macular thickness (CMT) decreased from 419.1 ± 201.1 μm at baseline to 268.2 ± 95.5 μm at 12 months ($p < 0.0001$). Similar visual and anatomic improvement was seen in the 2.5 mg group with no difference in the results. Adverse events included transient high blood pressure in one patient (1.2%), transient increased intraocular pressure in one eye (1%), and tractional retinal detachment in one eye (1%). Therefore, over a 12-month period, intravitreal bevacizumab at a dose of either 1.25 or 2.5 mg resulted in equal anatomic and visual improvement in 49.5% of patients with minimal, if any, serious side effects. The maximum benefit was seen during the first month and was maintained over 12 months and 82.2% of eyes had reduced risk of VA loss. Comparing eyes that had one or two injections to those that had three or more injections, a significant drop in BCVA at 6 months was seen in the former group, suggesting that repetitive injections are needed with at least three injections per year.[29]

A prospective, noncomparative case series on 126 patients evaluated the effect of 1.25 mg bevacizumab on chronic (>12 months) diffuse macular edema not responsive to previous treatments; 62% had received focal laser treatment, 38% panretinal laser treatment, 11% vitrectomy, and 41% intravitreal injection of triamcinolone. Patients were followed every 4 weeks for up to 12 months. Only 59 patients completed the 12 months follow-up. Thirty-eight percent of patients did not receive focal laser treatment prior to enrollment because of extensive macular ischemia, close proximity of the source of leakage to the fovea as assessed by fluorescein angiography (FA), and anatomic alterations of the retina such as cystoid spaces reflecting the chronicity of the macular edema; however, the investigators did not withhold photocoagulation from any patient, if indicated. Patients had additional injections at 4-week intervals if they responded to the previous injection by retinal thickness reduction or visual acuity improvement. Injections were postponed if either no further reduction of retinal thickness was noted on optical coherence tomography (OCT) scans or no further improvement of VA was measured. The decision to perform a reinjection was based on the recurrence of macular edema (change in OCT > 100 μm centrally) and associated deterioration of VA (>5 ETDRS letters) during follow-up. Patients were classified as nonresponders if there was no change in retinal thickness detected after three injections and no further reinjections were performed. No other treatments including laser photocoagulation were applied during the study period. Within this period, 48% received at least three intravitreal injections of bevacizumab. Mean diameter of foveal avascular zone (FAZ) was 858 ± 341 μm. Forty-four percent had FAZ > 800 μm indicating marked macular ischemia. Mean VA at baseline was 40.3 ETDRS letters. Mean VA change was −1.6 ETDRS letters at 6 months ($p = 0.3$) and +5.1 ETDRS letters at 12 months ($p = 0.02$). Throughout follow-up, VA changes were not significant except at 12 months. Mean central retinal thickness on OCT was 463 μm at baseline, 374 μm at 6 months ($p < 0.001$), and 357 μm at 12 months ($p < 0.001$). Macular ischemia did not progress as a result of injections, and the FAZ diameter was not found to be related to central retinal thickness or visual acuity. There was no correlation between the visual and anatomic outcomes. Age, prior treatments, and central retinal thickness were not predictive of visual outcome. The authors concluded that patients with advanced stages of macular edema (diffuse and chronic) not responsive to prior treatments had long-term decrease in central retinal thickness after repeated injections of bevacizumab; however, a better functional outcome could be achieved if macular ischemia was not present and if tighter inclusion criteria were applied.[30]

Bonini-Filho et al. noted more favorable changes in BCVA and in CMT and total macular volume (TMV) in patients with DME and "severe capillary loss" after treatment with bevacizumab. This was a multicenter, open-label, nonrandomized study on 10 consecutive patients with DME, CMT > 250 μm, and "severe" capillary loss within 1,500 μm of the center of the macula (as assessed by FA according to ETDRS criteria). Patients received 1.5 mg (0.06 mL) of intravitreal bevacizumab at baseline with reinjections at 8-week intervals if subretinal or intraretinal fluid were persistent or recurrent on OCT. Main outcome measures were changes in BCVA and OCT variables (CMT and TMV) at 1 year. The mean logMAR ETDRS BCVA was 0.786 ($20/125^{-1}$) at baseline, 0.646 ($20/80^{-2}$) at week 8, 0.580 ($20/80^{-1}$) at week 16, 0.574 ($20/80^{-1}$) at week 24, and 0.558 ($20/80^{-2}$) at week 54. A significant change in BCVA was noted at all follow-up visits ($p < 0.008$) compared to baseline. The mean CMT (μm)/TMV (mm^3) values were, respectively, 472.6/10.9 at baseline, 371.4/9.9 at week 8, 359.5/9.8 at week 16, 323.9/9.4 at week 24, and 274.6/8.7 at week 54. Compared with baseline, a significant change in both CMT and TMV was noted only at 24 and 54 weeks ($p < 0.007$). At 54 weeks, bevacizumab reduced dye leakage on FA compared to baseline with no worsening of macular ischemia in all patients. The improvement in BCVA and in OCT variables at week 24 was maintained up to week 54, even after a period of approximately 6 months (30 weeks) with no additional reinjections. This study, however, was limited by its small sample size and by having no control arm.[31]

The Diabetic Retinopathy Clinical Research Network (DRCR.net) conducted a randomized phase 2 clinical trial evaluating the effect of intravitreal bevacizumab on DME over a 70-week period. Efficacy was assessed at 12 weeks and safety at 24 weeks. One-hundred-twenty-one eyes with center involving DME, CST of ≥275 μm on OCT, and BCVA ranging from 20/32 to 20/320 were randomly assigned to one of the five groups: 19 eyes were randomized to focal laser at baseline, 22 eyes to 1.25 mg of intravitreal avastin injection at baseline and 6 weeks, 24 eyes to 2.5 mg of intravitreal avastin injection at baseline and 6 weeks, 22 eyes to 1.25 mg of intravitreal avastin injection at baseline and sham injection at 6 weeks, and 22 eyes to 1.25 mg of intravitreal avastin injection at baseline and 6 weeks with laser photocoagulation at 3 weeks. At baseline, median central subfield thickness (CST) was 411 μm and median Snellen VA equivalent was 20/50. Compared with the laser group, the second and third groups had a greater reduction in CST at 3 weeks and about one line better median visual acuity over 12 weeks. There were no meaningful differences in CST observed with bevacizumab relative to photocoagulation after the 3-week time point. There was no benefit demonstrated by using the larger dose of avastin. A CST reduction >11% (the reliability limit) was present at 3 weeks in 36/84 (43%) bevacizumab-treated eyes and in 5/18 (28%) eyes treated with laser alone, and at 6 weeks in 31/84 (37%) and 9/18 (50%) eyes, respectively. There appeared to be no short-term benefit to combining focal photocoagulation with bevacizumab; however, a beneficial effect of combining focal laser with bevacizumab injection could occur over a time longer than the duration of the study. Systemic safety evaluation of bevacizumab was limited by the modest sample size and the short follow-up; however, few adverse events were reported. Endophthalmitis developed in one eye. During the first 24 weeks, two patients treated with bevacizumab had myocardial infarction without attributing the cause to the drug, one patient had congestive heart failure, three patients had elevated blood pressure, and three patients had worsened renal function.[32] A large phase 3 randomized clinical trial is needed to determine if there is a clinically meaningful benefit of intravitreal avastin injection for DME.

In a retrospective study, 11 previously vitrectomized eyes with internal limiting membrane peel and persistent DME showed no improvement after three intravitreal avastin injections at 6 months. This result could be secondary to the rapid wash out of the drug in vitrectomized eyes. The study was limited by its small sample size and short follow-up.[33]

There have been additional studies comparing bevacizumab to triamcinolone and evaluating triamcinolone as an adjunct to bevacizumab in treating DME. A prospective comparative interventional case series compared the effect of an intravitreal injection of bevacizumab with that of triamcinolone acetonide for DME on 28 eyes of 14 patients with bilateral DME. Each patient received an intravitreal injection of 4 mg triamcinolone acetonide in one eye and 1.25 mg bevacizumab in the other eye. Subjects were followed for 24 weeks after the injection. At week 1, foveal thickness and VA in the triamcinolone group improved from 522.3 ± 91.3 μm and 0.64 ± 0.28 logMAR at baseline to 342.6 ± 85.5 μm and 0.33 ± 0.21 logMAR. The central foveal thickness remained at this level till week 12, whereas in the bevacizumab group, the foveal thickness and VA improved from 527.6 ± 78.8 μm and 0.61 ± 0.18 logMAR at baseline to 397.6 ± 103.0 μm and 0.37 ± 0.17 logMAR. The central foveal thickness remained at this level till week 4; however, DME recurred in both groups at 24 weeks with the triamcinolone group faring better. The foveal thickness and visual acuity were 410.4 ± 82.4 μm (p = 0.002) and 0.47 ± 0.25 logMAR at 24 weeks in the triamcinolone group and 501.6 ± 92.5 μm (p = 0.012) and 0.61 ± 0.17 logMAR in the bevacizumab group. In summary, bevacizumab led to a 24% reduction in foveal thickness at week 1 that persisted till week 4, then decreased gradually to a 5% reduction by week 12. Triamcinolone led to a 35% reduction in foveal thickness at week 1 that persisted until week 12. The modest improvement seen in the bevacizumab group could be explained by the fact that only one injection was given during the follow-up period; triamcinolone is a multipotency drug that targets different pathophysiologic pathways in DME; injecting bevacizumab in one eye could have some effect on the fellow eye, biasing the results with triamcinolone; and lastly, the central retinal thickness in this subgroup of patients was higher at baseline compared to other studies.[34]

A prospective, placebo-controlled, randomized clinical trial compared intravitreal bevacizumab with triamcinolone to intravitreal bevacizumab without triamcinolone for refractory DME. One-hundred-fifteen eyes of 101 patients with refractory DME were randomly assigned to one of the three study arms: (a) three injections of intravitreal bevacizumab (1.25 mg/0.05 mL) at 6-week intervals, (b) combined intravitreal injections of bevacizumab and triamcinolone (1.25 mg/0.05 mL and 2 mg/0.05 mL, respectively) followed by two intravitreal injections of bevacizumab at 6-week intervals, and (c) sham injection (control group). CMT was reduced significantly in both the bevacizumab and combination groups. At week 24, CMT change compared to the baseline was −95.7 μm (95% CI, −172.2 to −19.26) in the bevacizumab group, −92.1 μm (95% CI, −154.4 to −29.7) in the combination group, and +34.9 μm (95% CI, 7.9 to 61.9) in the control group. There was a significant difference between each of the two treatment groups and control groups (p = 0.012 and 0.022, respectively). Improvement of BCVA was measured at weeks 6 and 12 in the bevacizumab/triamcinolone group and the bevacizumab groups, respectively. Compared to baseline, BCVA at 24 weeks in the bevacizumab and bevacizumab/triamcinolone groups was significantly better than the control group (p = 0.01 and 0.006, respectively); however, there was no significant difference in the change of CMT and BCVA between the bevacizumab and bevacizumab/triamcinolone groups (p = 0.99). Elevation of IOP occurred in three eyes (8.1%) in the bevacizumab and triamcinolone groups. The study results suggest that by adding triamcinolone in the first injection, earlier visual improvement can be achieved; however, there was no demonstrated significant additive effect during later follow-up.[35]

Paccola et al.[36] randomly assigned 28 patients to receive a single intravitreal injection of either 4 mg/0.1 mL triamcinolone acetonide or 1.5 mg/0.06 mL bevacizumab. CMT was significantly reduced in the intravitreal triamcinolone group compared with the bevacizumab group at weeks 4, 8, 12, and 24 ($p < 0.05$). LogMAR best-corrected visual acuity was significantly higher at weeks 8 (0.69; ~20/100^{+1}) and 12 (0.74; ~20/100^{-2}) in the intravitreal triamcinolone group compared with the bevacizumab group at weeks 8 (0.83; ~20/125^{-1}) and 12 (0.86; ~20/160^{+2}) ($p < 0.05$), also suggesting that a single intravitreal injection of triamcinolone may offer certain advantages over bevacizumab in the short-term management of refractory DME; however, a significant change from baseline in mean intraocular pressure was seen at week 4 (+2.25 mm Hg) in the intravitreal triamcinolone group ($p < 0.0001$).

Soheilian et al.[37] conducted a randomized three-arm clinical trial comparing intravitreal bevacizumab injection alone or in combination with intravitreal triamcinolone acetonide versus macular laser photocoagulation as a primary treatment of DME. One-hundred-fifty eyes of 129 patients with clinically significant DME and no previous treatment were randomly assigned to one of the three groups: (a) 1.25 mg of intravitreal bevacizumab injection (50 eyes), (b) 1.25 mg of intravitreal bevacizumab and 2 mg of intravitreal triamcinolone (50 eyes), and (c) the laser group (50 eyes). Whenever indicated, retreatment was performed at 12-week intervals. The bevacizumab group had better visual acuity outcomes at 36 weeks compared with the combination and laser groups with a logMAR change of −0.28±0.25 compared with baseline ($p = 0.053$). Significant CMT reduction was observed in all groups only up to 6 weeks; however, CMT changes were not significant among the groups in all visits. Retreatment up to 36 weeks was required for 14 eyes in the bevacizumab group, 10 eyes in the combination group, and 3 eyes in the laser group. Only one intravitreal bevacizumab injection was required in 72% of cases in the first group. Visual acuity improved by two or more Snellen lines at 36 weeks in 37%, 25%, and 14.8% of patients in the bevacizumab, combination, and laser groups, respectively. Intravitreal bevacizumab injection in patients with DME yielded a better visual outcome at 24 weeks compared with macular photocoagulation with no additive effect from triamcinolone; however, this finding did not correlate with a similar anatomic outcome. The better results seen with the bevacizumab group could be secondary to cataract progression or adverse effects from the triamcinolone preservatives. A more beneficial effect of laser could be seen with a longer follow-up. This study is currently being extended for up to 2 years.

Faghihi et al.[38] showed that a single intravitreal bevacizumab injection or triamcinolone plus bevacizumab injection had significantly greater macular thickness reduction at 16 weeks in comparison to standard laser treatment; however, the response for bevacizumab alone was short-lived compared with the combination group (bevacizumab and triamcinolone) maintaining their superiority to the laser group at week 16 ($p < 0.001$). Visual acuity improvement in the combination group was marginal and at most was 0.1 logMAR and did not correlate with the reduction in the retinal thickness.

Currently, there are seven active clinical trials designed to test the effect of bevacizumab on DME. They include head-to-head trials comparing intravitreal bevacizumab injection to intravitreal ranibizumab or triamcinolone acetonide injection. Clinical trials testing the efficacy of combined intravitreal bevacizumab with triamcinolone acetonide injection and intravitreal bevacizumab as an adjunct to pars plana vitrectomy are also underway. Posterior subtenons injection of avastin for DME is being investigated as well.

A phase 4 interventional, randomized, double-masked trial is underway to compare the effect of intraocular bevacizumab with intraocular triamcinolone in patients with CSME (TRIASTIN) (ClinicalTrials.gov identifier: NCT00682539). This study is currently recruiting patients. Patients with center involved CSME will be randomized to either intravitreal injection of 2.5 mg avastin or 8 mg triamcinolone. In order to be eligible, patients should have a CMT of at least 300 µm in the central subfield as measured by OCT with no history of systemic corticosteroids intake within the past 3 months prior to enrollment or concurrent corticosteroid use. In the avastin arm, intravitreal injection is given monthly for the first 3 months after which a sham injection will be performed if the CMT is <300 µm. Patients in the triamcinolone arm will be injected with triamcinolone monthly for the first 2 months. At month 3, they will receive a sham injection. After 3 months, reinjection of triamcinolone is performed if the CMT stays more than 300 µm or else they will receive a sham injection. Primary outcome measure is to evaluate the efficacy of avastin as assessed by ETDRS visual acuity and CMT on OCT over a 12-month period.

A phase 2 randomized, double-blind, uncontrolled study compared over 6 months a single intravitreal injection of 4 mg triamcinolone acetonide to 1.25 mg of bevacizumab in 13 patients with DME and CST greater than 300 µm (Tribeva-DME). This study has recently been completed (ClinicalTrials.gov identifier: NCT00874744). The results are not yet available. Primary outcome measure included treatment efficacy, and secondary outcome measures included visual acuity and intraocular pressure differences at baseline and follow-up visits (4, 12, and 24 weeks) in the same treatment group and between both treatment arms.

In addition, a phase 4 interventional, double-blind, randomized clinical trial is currently recruiting patients to compare the efficacy of intravitreal injections of triamcinolone and bevacizumab individually or simultaneously for the treatment of DME with a central thickness >275 µm on OCT (ATEMD) (ClinicalTrials.gov identifier: NCT00737971). It is currently recruiting patients for a total sample size of 300 patients randomized to intravitreal bevacizumab injection (0.05 mL/1.25 mg), triamcinolone (0.1 mL/4 mg), or a combination of intravitreal triamcinolone + bevacizumab administered on day 0, week 4, and week 8. The primary outcome measure is ETDRS Snellen visual acuity measured monthly, and secondary outcome measures are intraocular pressure and retinal thickness by OCT. The study is still currently recruiting participants with an enrollment target of 300 subjects.

A single posterior subtenon's capsule injection of bevacizumab (2.5 mg /0.1 mL) is being investigated in a phase 4 trial for DME with no prior treatment and a retinal thickness of ≥250 µm (ClinicalTrials.gov identifier: NCT00567372). Macular volume, macular thickness, and BCVA will be assessed at baseline, weeks 3, 6, and 12.

The study has not been completed, and is still recruiting participants.

A head-to-head phase 3 trial comparing intravitreal bevacizumab to ranibizumab for persistent DME and persistent PDR after laser treatment is currently recruiting patients. The primary outcome measures will be the effect on macular edema and neovascularization, and the absolute change in visual acuity (ClinicalTrials.gov identifier: NCT00545870).

The 12 month results from a prospective single center randomized trial of intravitreal bevacizumab or laser therapy in the management of diabetic macular edema (BOLT study) is presented in Box 15.2.

BOX 15.2 BOLT Study: Intravitreal Bevacizumab or Laser Therapy for DME

Objectives: To determine if repeated treatment with intravitreal bevacizumab results in superior outcomes compared to modified ETDRS laser treatment in patients with persistent CSME.

Methods: Prospective, randomized, masked, single-center, 2-year, 2-arm clinical trial in which 80 eyes of 80 patients with center-involving CSME, no evidence of substantial macular ischemia (foveal avascular zone <1000 μm in greatest linear dimension and no severe perifoveal intercapillary loss on fluorescein angiography), and at least 1 prior macular laser treatment were randomized to either bevacizumab (6 weekly; minimum of 3 injections and maximum of 9 injections in the first 12 months) or laser (4 monthly; minimum of 1 treatment and maximum of 4 treatments in the first 12 months). The primary end point was the difference in ETDRS best-corrected visual acuity (BCVA) at 12 months between the bevacizumab and laser arms.

Results: The baseline mean ETDRS BCVA was 55.7+/-9.7 in the bevacizumab arm and 54.6+/-8.6 in the laser arm. The mean ETDRS BCVA at 12 months was 61.3+/-10.4 in the bevacizumab arm and 50.0+/-16.6 in the laser arm (P = 0.0006). At 12 months, the bevacizumab arm gained a median of 8 ETDRS letters, whereas the laser arm lost a median of 0.5 ETDRS letters (P = 0.0002). The odds of gaining at least 10 ETDRS letters over 12 months were 5.1 times greater in the bevacizumab group than in the laser group (adjusted odds ratio, 5.1; 95% confidence interval, 1.3-19.7; P = 0.019). The median number of injections was 9 in the bevacizumab arm, and the median number of treatments was 3 in the laser arm.

Conclusions: The study provides evidence to support the use of bevacizumab in patients with center-involving CSME without advanced macular ischemia.

Source: Michaelides M, Kaines A, Hamilton RD, et al. A prospective randomized trial of intravitreal bevacizumab or laser therapy in the management of diabetic macular edema (BOLT study) 12-month data: report 2. Ophthalmol. 2010;117:1078-1086.

Ranibizumab

Ranibizumab (Lucentis, Genentech Inc., San Francisco, CA) is a monoclonal antibody fragment derived from the same parent antibody as bevacizumab that is directed toward human VEGF. Unlike pegaptanib that targets only the VEGF165 isoform, both bevacizumab and ranibizumab block all isoforms of VEGF-A. Ranibizumab is much smaller than the parent antibody and has been "affinity enhanced" to provide for a stronger binding to VEGF-A.[39] The smaller molecular size of Ranibizumab allows for a faster penetration into the retina and a more rapid elimination from systemic circulation compared to bevacizumab.[40,41] Ranibizumab was granted U.S. FDA approval in June 2006 for the treatment of neovascular AMD. Currently, it is the approved anti-VEGF agent proven to provide the most gain in vision in patients with choroidal neovascularization secondary to AMD; as such, its application in the treatment of DME and PDR is the subject of rigorous investigation.

Initial pilot clinical trials reported a series of 10 consecutive patients who received intravitreal injections of ranibizumab (0.3 mg in five patients or 0.5 mg in the next five patients) at baseline, month 1, and month 2.[42] At 3 months, the low-dose group (0.3 mg) gained a mean of 12.0 letters and the high-dose group (0.5 mg) gained 7.8 letters from baseline (Fig. 15.4). There was a significant decrease in central retinal thickness in the low-dose group (45.3 μm) and the high-dose group (197.8 μm) at 3 months as well.

In the phase 1, ranibizumab for edema of the macula in diabetes (READ-1), a second series of 10 patients with chronic DME received intravitreal injections of ranibizumab (0.5 mg) at baseline and months 1, 2, 4, and 6.[43] The mean and median improvement in visual acuity at 7 months were 12.3 and 11 letters, respectively, an improvement of approximately more than two lines. The visual acuity at baseline was 20/80, which improved to 20/40 at month 7 (p = 0.05). The mean foveal thickness decreased by 85% (from mean 503–257 μm at month 7). No adverse or systemic side effects were reported. On the basis of the encouraging results from these pilot studies, there are 16 larger phase 2 and 3 trials with ranibizumab that are currently ongoing with eight trials still recruiting patients.

The READ-2 Study: **R**anibizumab for **E**dema of the m**A**cula in **D**iabetes (ClinicalTrials.gov identifier: NCT00407381) will compare intravitreal injections of 0.5 mg of ranibizumab to focal/grid laser photocoagulation and a combination of ranibizumab plus laser for the treatment DME. The primary outcome measure will be improvement in vision of 15 or more letters or achieving a final vision of 50 letters or better if baseline vision was 40 letters. Outcomes will be assessed at 6, 12, 24, and 36 months. The study is still ongoing and the preliminary 6 month results are presented in Box 15.1.

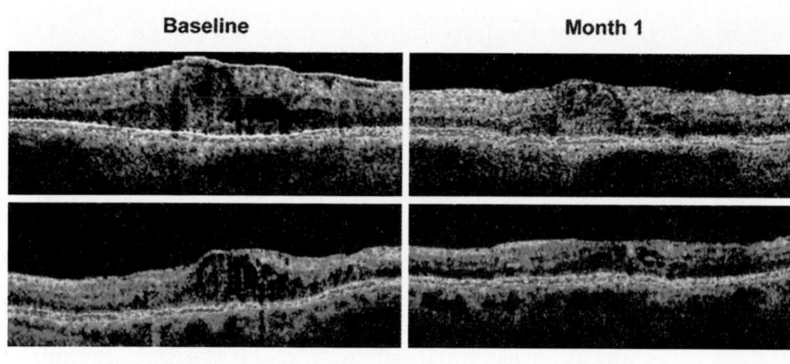

FIGURE 15.4. OCT images of the study eye retina of case 1 at baseline and months 1, 3, and 6. Case 1 had received 0.3 mg of ranibizumab. (Reproduced with permission from Chun et al. *Opthalmology.* 2006;113:1706–1712.)

The RESOLVE (ClinicalTrials.gov identifier: NCT00-284050): Randomized, Double-Masked, Multicenter, Phase 2 Study Assessing the Safety and Efficacy of Two Concentrations of Ranibizumab (Intravitreal Injections) Compared with Nontreatment Control for the Treatment of DME with Center Involvement, and the RESTORE (ClinicalTrials.gov identifier: NCT00687804): Efficacy and Safety of Ranibizumab (Intravitreal Injections) in Patients With Visual Impairment Due to Diabetic Macular Edema, and RESTORE Ext (ClinicalTrials.gov identifier: NCT00906464) will provide information on the efficacy and safety of the ranibizumab in the treatment of DME. The RESTORE trial is expected to be completed by December 2009 with open-label extension. RESTORE Ext will continue to evaluate patients for an additional 24 months with completion expected by January 2012.

There are several ongoing multicenter, randomized, controlled phase 3 trials involving intravitreal ranibizumab or in combination with focal/grid laser for the treatment of DME, compared to focal/grid laser alone, or a head-to-head comparison with bevacizumab are being conducted which will aid in determining the role of ranibizumab in the management of DME.

The RISE (ClinicalTrials.gov identifier: NCT00-473330): A Phase 3, Double-Masked, Multicenter, Randomized, Sham Injection-Controlled Study of the Efficacy and Safety of Ranibizumab Injection in Subjects with Clinically Significant Macular Edema With Center Involvement Secondary to Diabetes Mellitus and the RIDE (ClinicalTrials.gov identifier: NCT00473382): A Phase 3, Double-Masked, Multicenter, Randomized, Sham Injection-Controlled Study of the Efficacy and Safety of Ranibizumab Injection in Subjects with Clinically Significant Macular Edema With Center Involvement Secondary to Diabetes Mellitus, will assess the proportion of subjects who gain at least 15 letters compared with baseline at 24 months comparing two concentrations of intravitreal ranibizumab and sham injections. Both trials are expected to end by October 2012.

The DRCR.net trial, LRT for DME (ClinicalTrials.gov identifier: NCT00444600): Intravitreal Ranibizumab or Triamcinolone Acetonide in Combination With Laser Photocoagulation for Diabetic Macular Edema, will evaluate intravitreal injections of triamcinolone or ranibizumab compared to focal/grid laser in the treatment of center-involved DME. The study is still ongoing and the 12 month results are presented in Box 15.3. A second DRCR.net trial LRT for DME + PRP (ClinicalTrials.gov identifier: NCT00445003): Intravitreal Ranibizumab or Triamcinolone Acetonide as Adjunctive Treatment to Panretinal Photocoagulation (PRP) for PDR will evaluate the efficacy of adjunct injection of triamcinolone or an intravitreal injection of ranibizumab with PRP compared to PRP and focal laser in preventing loss of vision and exacerbation of DME after PRP treatment. The primary outcome measure will be vision at 14 weeks adjusted for baseline acuity. A target of 381 patients will be enrolled with an estimated completion date in 2010.

VEGF Trap

VEGF Trap (Regeneron Pharmaceuticals, Tarrytown, NY) is a 110-kDa soluble protein that contains extracellular VEGF receptor sequences fused to an IgG backbone.[44] It is similar to bevacizumab and ranibizumab in that it blocks all isoforms of VEGF and placental growth factor.[45] The predicted biological activity of intravitreal administered VEGF Trap at 10 weeks after injection has been shown in animal models to be comparable to the activity of ranibizumab at 30 days.[39] This prolonged biological activity can be explained by the higher VEGF-binding affinity of VEGF Trap but the exact duration of intravitreal action remains unknown.[39] An exploratory study to assess the safety and bioactivity of a single 4.0 mg intravitreal injection of VEGF-trap in patients with DME was performed in five patients with encouraging results.[46] At 6 weeks following the injection, four of the five patients showed reduction in OCT-measured foveal thickness (median 74 μm; 31% reduction from baseline, $p = 0.0625$) and four of the five showed improvement in BCVA (median improvement of three letters). No significant ocular adverse events were reported following the injection. Currently, a Phase 2, doubled-masked, randomized study of the efficacy and safety of VEGF-Trap in subjects with DME is currently recruiting participants (ClinicalTrials.gov Identifier NCT00789477). Approximately 200 subjects will be

BOX 15.3 DRCR Trial with Ranibizumab in Diabetic Macular Edema. Protocol I

Objective: To determine if ranibizumab therapy alone or in combination with laser, or if triamcinolone in combination with laser, might result in improved outcomes compared with laser alone for treatment of DME.

Methods: A multicenter, randomized clinical trial in which eyes (854) with visual acuity 20/32 to 20/320 and DME involving the fovea were randomized to sham injection + prompt laser, 0.5 mg ranibizumab + prompt laser, 0.5 mg ranibizumab + deferred (> or =24 weeks) laser, or 4 mg triamcinolone + prompt laser. Retreatment followed an algorithm facilitated by a web-based, real-time data-entry system.

Results: The 1-year mean change in the visual acuity letter score from baseline was significantly greater in the ranibizumab + prompt laser group (+9+/-11, P<0.001) and ranibizumab + deferred laser group (+9+/-12, P<0.001) but not in the triamcinolone + prompt laser group (+4+/-13, P=0.31) compared with the sham + prompt laser group (+3+/-13). Reduction in mean central subfield thickness in the triamcinolone + prompt laser group was similar to both ranibizumab groups and greater than in the sham + prompt laser group. In the subset of pseudophakic eyes at baseline (n=273), visual acuity improvement in the triamcinolone + prompt laser group appeared comparable to that in the ranibizumab groups. No systemic events attributable to study treatment were apparent. Three eyes (0.8%) had injection-related endophthalmitis in the ranibizumab groups, whereas elevated intraocular pressure and cataract surgery were much more frequent in the triamcinolone + prompt laser group. Two-year visual acuity outcomes were similar to 1-year outcomes.

Conclusions: Intravitreal ranibizumab with prompt or deferred laser is more effective through at least 1 year compared with prompt laser alone for the treatment of DME involving the central macula. Ranibizumab as applied in this study, although uncommonly associated with endophthalmitis, should be considered for patients with DME and characteristics similar to those in this clinical trial. In pseudophakic eyes, intravitreal triamcinolone + prompt laser seems more effective than laser alone but frequently increases the risk of intraocular pressure elevation.

Source: Elman MJ, Aiello LP, Beck RW, et al. Randomized trial evaluating ranibizumab plus prompt or deferred laser or triamcinolone plus prompt laser for diabetic macular edema. Ophthalmology 2010;117(6):1064-77.

randomized in the United States, Canada, Australia, and EU. It is estimated to be completed by February 2011.

Ruboxistaurin

Ruboxistaurin (Arxxant, Eli Lily Co, Indianapolis, IN) is an orally active selective inhibitor of PKC β, which has effectively modest ability to modulate VEGF.[47] PKC β inhibition has been shown to ameliorate renal and retinal blood flow abnormalities, increased retinal vascular permeability, and retinal neovascularization associated with diabetes and diabetes-like processes in animals.[48] In the PKC β Inhibitor-Diabetic Retinopathy Study 2 (PKC-DRS2), oral administration of 32 mg/day ruboxistaurin reduced sustained MVL (≥15-letter loss on the ETDRS BCVA chart sustained ≥6 months) in patients with moderately severe to very severe nonproliferative DR from 9.1% in placebo-treated patients to 5.5% (40% risk reduction, $p = 0.034$).[49] When CSME was >100 μm from the center of the macula at baseline, ruboxistaurin treatment was associated with less progression of DME to within 100 μm of the macular center (68% vs. 50%; $p = 0.003$) and application of initial focal laser treatment in eyes without prior history of such treatment at baseline was less frequent by 26% ($p = 0.008$).[49] Currently, a phase 3 clinical trial is ongoing to further evaluate if ruboxistaurin can slow development of center-involved DME (ClinicalTrials.gov identifier: NCT00090519). The primary outcome measure is the mean duration of definite center-involved DME at 36 months, 731 patients are enrolled and the results are expected by late 2010.

The PKC-Diabetic Macular Edema Study (PKC-DMES), which was designed to evaluate the safety and efficacy of ruboxistaurin on non–center-involved DME (>300 μm from the macular center), showed that daily oral administration of ruboxistaurin compared to placebo may delay progression of DME to a sight-threatening stage ($p = 0.054$ [unadjusted]; Cox proportional hazards model, hazards ratio = 0.66; 95% confidence interval, 0.47–0.93; $p = 0.02$).[50] An analysis of patients in the PKC-DRS2 with moderately severe to very severe nonproliferative DR with long-standing severe DME showed a 30% reduction in rate of visual loss over 36 months in ruboxistaurin-treated patient compared to placebo (0.47 vs. 0.67 letters per month; $p=0.022$).[51] Currently, a phase 3 clinical trial is ongoing and recruiting patients to test the hypothesis that oral administration of ruboxistaurin for approximately 24 months will reduce the baseline to endpoint changes in macular thickness, as measured by OCT, in patients with CSME. A target enrollment of 300 patients is expected with the study completion date set for December 2010.

Rapamycin

Rapamycin (Sirolimus, MacuSight Inc, Union City, CA) is a macrolide that is a specific inhibitor of mTOR (mammalian target of rapamycin), a regulatory protein kinase, which regulates cell growth, proliferation, motility, and survival. Inhibition of mTOR downregulates hypoxia-inducible factor-1, which moderates production of VEGF. It specifically inhibits VEGF through two separate pathways: the inhibition of mTOR causes a decrease in production of VEGF; further downstream, it also decreases the response of endothelial cells to VEGF activation through downregulation of intracellular signaling.[52,53]

The initial multicenter, open-label phase 1 dose escalation study was conducted in 50 patients with DME (ClinicalTrials.gov identifier: NCT00401115). Patients were randomly assigned to receive either a single intravitreal (IVT) (44, 110, 176, 264, or 352 μg) or a single subconjunctival (220, 440, 880, 1,320, or 1,760 μg) rapamycin injection.[54] BCVA was assessed by ETDRS protocol, and CST as determined by OCT was interpreted by an independent reading center at 14, 45, 90, and 180 days. No dose-limiting toxicities were observed and no serious ocular adverse events probably or possibly related to the study drug were reported. A statistically significant treatment effect ($p < 0.05$) was observed at 14, 45, and 90 days. Mean BCVA improvements were 8.8 ± 4.4, 11.4 ± 7.6, and 7.4 ± 8.6 letters at 14, 45, and 90 days, respectively, following a single 440 μg subconjunctival injection. Anatomical changes were also observed, with mean OCT reductions of 33 ± 60, 78 ± 50, and 54 ± 93 μm at 14, 45, and 90 days, respectively. Similar changes were observed following a single 352 μg IVT injection, with mean BCVA improvements of 11.6 ± 7.7, 6.4 ± 7.1, and 7.8 ± 2.2 letters, and mean OCT reductions 72 ± 53, 42 ± 39, and 61 ± 47 μm at 14, 45, and 90 days, respectively. These functional and anatomical improvements persisted through 180 days following a single injection.

A phase 2, randomized, double-masked, placebo-controlled, dose-ranging clinical study to assess the safety and efficacy of subconjunctival injections of rapamycin in patients with DME is ongoing (ClinicalTrials.gov identifier: NCT00656643). Three dosages of two subconjunctival injections of rapamycin will be evaluated (220, 440, and 880 μg) and compared to placebo. The primary outcome measure is ETDRS best-corrected visual acuity at 180 days. Secondary outcome measures will include foveal OCT CST and safety, both at 180 days. An estimated 120 patients will be enrolled, and the anticipated study completion date is March 2012.

A concurrent National Eye Institute–sponsored pilot study will independently evaluate the efficacy of rapamycin in the treatment of DME (ClinicalTrials.gov identifier: NCT00711490). An initial five participants will be enrolled into this open-label pilot study. After receiving two 20 μL (440 μg) subconjunctival injections in the study eye at baseline and month 2, the participants will be reevaluated every 2 months for at least 1 year for possible additional injections. During follow-up, participants will not undergo reinjection if they show significant clinical improvement, defined as no intraretinal fluid or cysts present on OCT or 100% reduction in excess retinal thickness over 225 μm on OCT or no leakage on FA. Beginning at month 4, participants will be assessed for treatment failure, defined as loss of 15 or more letters of vision compared to baseline at two consecutive visits or a 50% or greater increase in total retinal thickness as measured by OCT at two consecutive visits. Individual participants will be required to suspend treatment and withdraw from study therapy at any visit in which they are deemed a treatment failure. The primary outcome is the change in BCVA in the study eye at 6 months compared to baseline. The study is currently still recruiting patients.

Bevasiranib

Bevasiranib (Cand5, Opko Health Inc, Miami, FL) is a synthetic double-stranded siRNA oligonucleotide. Its mechanism of action relies on RNA interference, which allows a single siRNA to guide the cleavage of thousands of mRNAs, resulting in highly specific and effective gene silencing. Preclinical studies have shown that bevasiranib selectively silences the mRNA encoding for VEGF.[56] A phase 2 randomized, double-masked dose comparison, safety and efficacy study of the bevasiranib for the treatment of DME has been completed (ClinicalTrials.gov identifier: NCT00306904). Three dosage of bevasiranib (3.0, 1.5, and 0.2 mg) given 4 weeks apart were evaluated. They were monitored for safety for 52 weeks. Initially, retinal thickness increased and visual acuity decreased at week 4. However, the effect on both retinal thickness and visual acuity reverted by the second month. Ninety-one percent of patients had stabilization of vision through 6 to 12 weeks, and four patients developed uveitis/iritis.[57] A phase 3 trial is currently in the planning stages, with ranibizumab used for initiation of therapy followed by intravitreal injections of bevasiranib every 8 to 12 weeks (Box 15.4).

PF-04523655

PF-04523655 (Pfizer, New York, NY) is a novel siRNA that uses RNA interference technology to silence the expression of the RTP-801 gene. The RTP-801 gene has been shown to cause the upregulation of VEGF in hypoxic conditions, implying its role in proliferative retinopathies.[57] The Pfizer DEGAS trial is a phase 2, prospective, randomized, multicenter, comparative study evaluating the efficacy and safety of PF-04523655 compared to laser in the treatment of DME (ClinicalTrials.gov identifier: NCT00701181). The primary outcome measure is the mean change from baseline in the BCVA at 24 months. The study is currently recruiting patients, and approximately 160 patients will be enrolled from the United States, EU, and India. It is estimated to be completed by July 2012.

Methotrexate

Methotrexate (MTX) is an antimetabolite, which competitively inhibits the enzyme dihydrofolate reductase. It has been systemically used as a cancer chemotherapeutic agent and as a steroid-sparing agent in noninfectious uveitis.[58] Intravitreal MTX has been widely used to treat refractory ocular lymphoma and a dose of 400 μg has been shown to be clinically well tolerated.[59] Currently, a nonrandomized, uncontrolled, pilot study is underway to evaluate intra-

BOX 15.4 Clinical Trials in DME

RACE Trial: Safety and Efficacy Study of siRNA Molecule (Cand5) to Treat DME

Purpose: A Phase 2 trial to evaluate the pharmacokinetics, safety, and preliminary efficacy of three doses of Cand5 (Opko Health) in DME patients. Cand5 is a siRNA molecule that selectively silences the mRNA encoding for VEGF.

Conclusions: Initially, retinal thickness increased and visual acuity decreased at week 4. However, the effect on both retinal thickness and visual acuity reverted by the second month. Ninety-one percent of patients had stabilization of vision through 6 to 12 weeks. (Clinicaltrials.gov Identifier: NCT00306904.)

Status: Completed.

DA VINCI Trial: DME and VEGF Trap-Eye: Investigation of Clinical Impact

Purpose: A Phase 2 double-masked, randomized, controlled study of the safety, tolerability, and biological effect of repeated intravitreal administration of VEGF Trap-Eye (Regeneron) in patients With DME (four different doses of VEGF Trap Eye vs. non-drug injection). (Clinicaltrials.goc Identifier: NCT00789477.)

Status: Active, not recruiting.

DEGAS Trial: Prospective, Randomized, Multi-Center, Comparator Study Evaluating Efficacy and Safety of PF-04523655 Versus Laser in Subjects With DME

Purpose: A phase 2 prospective, randomized study to compare the effectiveness of the drug, PF-04523655 (Pfizer), with the standard laser therapy in DME. The PF-04523655 is a novel siRNA that silences the expression of the RTP-801 gene that has been shown to cause the upregulation of VEGF in hypoxia. (Clinicaltrials.gov Identifier: NCT00701181.)

Status: Recruiting.

vitreal methotrexate in patients with recalcitrant DME (ClinicalTrials.gov identifier: NCT00779142). Intravitreal methotrexate 200 μg will be administered once or twice depending on the therapeutic response over a 6-month period. The primary outcome measure is the occurrence of a 40% decrease in CST on OCT at the end of 3 months after the last intraocular injection. The study is currently recruiting patients with a target of five patients with the estimated completion date of September 2010.

Multi-targeted kinase inhibitors

Early preclinical animal studies have shown promising orally and topically active kinase inhibitors that may be effective in the treatment of DME. Topically active Src kinase inhibitors have been shown to be particularly promising in that Src kinase activity appears critical only for VEGF-induced permeability and may be dispensable for mitogenic, neurotrophic, antiapoptotic, and other effects of VEGF.[60,61] Thus, inhibiting Src kinase may prevent VEGF-associated vascular permeability while preserving its angiogenic and cell-survival activities.[61,63] The compound TG100572, a multitargeted kinase inhibitor, which potentially inhibits VEGF, PDGF, and FGF receptor kinases as well as the Src family of kinase blocked proliferation and induced apoptosis of cycling vascular endothelial cells in vitro and, when administered systemically, suppressed choroidal neovascularization[63]; however, significant toxicity was encountered. This toxicity was avoided with the topical administration of the prodrug, TG100801, which resulted in local penetration and subsequent significant levels of TG100901 and TG100572 in the posterior segment of the eye.[63] Scheppke et al.[62] and Doukas et al.[63] have shown in a murine model that topically applied Src kinase inhibitor, TG100801, may have clinical utility based on its ability to suppress retinal vascular leakage by inhibiting the Src and VEGFR families of tyrosine kinases.

Adverse Effects

Systemic Side Effects

VEGF is required for normal wound healing and endochondral bone formation. It plays an important role in the female reproductive cycle through endometrial development and placental vascularization. VEGF also controls vascular tone, glomerulogenesis, and renal glomerular capillary function. Its systemic inhibition therefore could theoretically result in impairment of wound healing, bleeding, inhibition of bone growth, infertility, hypertension, and proteinuria.[64]

Following ischemic events, VEGF has a pivotal role in promoting collateral vessels formation, which is particularly important in diabetic persons who are at increased risk of having cardiovascular and peripheral vascular events. Therefore, long-term systemic VEGF inhibition can have increased risk of ischemic and thromboembolic events. These events were noticed in colon cancer patients receiving intravenous anti-VEGF as chemotherapy. The risk of such events was found to be 5%.[64,65]

Although commonly administered intravitreal doses of anti-VEGF therapy are approximately 1/400 or less of the usual systemic dose, the possibility of systemic adverse side effects nevertheless exists. A meta-analysis of all randomized clinical trials on ranibizumab for AMD, which included the MARINA, ANCHOR, and FOCUS studies, evaluated the 2-year incidence of cerebrovascular accidents and myocardial infarction in the ranibizumab-treated subjects (n = 859) compared to sham-treated subjects (n = 434).[66] There was an increased incidence of cerebrovascular accidents in the ranibizumab-treated subjects (n = 19, 2.2%) compared to sham-treated subjects (n = 3, 0.7%) (p = 0.045; OR 3.24; CI 0.96–10.95).[66] There was no apparent association between ranibizumab treatment and myocardial infarction. It should be noted that this was a meta-analysis of three different studies and does not conclusively demonstrate the substantial presence or extent of risk of these treatments.

Ocular Side Effects

Ocular adverse events resulting from the intravitreal injection itself include endophthalmitis, ocular inflammation, retinal detachment, vitreous hemorrhage, and traumatic cataract. Data from over 2,009 injections administered in clinical trials employing the same standardized procedure for the preparation and intravitreal injection using preservative-free triamcinolone in prefilled syringes have reported only one case of endophthalmitis (0.05%).[67] In all cases, the risk for serious adverse event is <1.5% per patient per year.[68]

Apart from the procedure itself, VEGF blockade has potential intraocular side effects. VEGF is secreted by retinal cells. The basal expression of VEGF by the neural retina approaches 15 to 20 pg/mg of protein. It has a role in retinal vascular homeostasis, neuroprotection, photoreceptor differentiation, and survival.[65] Inhibiting VEGF secretion from retinal pigment epithelial cells can cause regression of the choriocapillaris.[69] The development of a VEGF inhibitor that blocks the pathological effects of VEGF while sparing its physiological effects may be optimal. Further safety data on the long-term intraocular effects of anti-VEGF therapy are also needed.

CONCLUSION

There are numerous anti-VEGF agents currently under evaluation as novel therapeutic interventions for DME. Multiple studies suggest that there may be at least short-term benefits from anti-VEGF treatment for DME in terms of visual acuity improvement and decrease in retinal edema. However, the long-term safety and efficacy of anti-VEGF therapies for DME have not yet been clearly established although extensive data will become available in the coming year. Systemic glycemic control and control of coexisting systemic risk factors remain the standard of care for patients with DME with, pending new data from the trials described, the appropriate application of focal/grid laser treatment in patients with CSME.[14,70] Results obtained with focal/grid laser are currently the benchmark by which novel treatments are assessed in clinical trials for the treatment of DME.

A potential algorithm in the management of patients with DME is presented in Figure 15.5. Current ongoing trials, including studies that evaluate anti-VEGF therapy in combination with laser and/or intravitreal steroid, will help to further elucidate the long-term safety and efficacy of anti-VEGF agents for DME. The results from these trials may expand or alter current treatment algorithms by increasing the array of available therapies for DME and identifying relative efficacies of individual treatments.

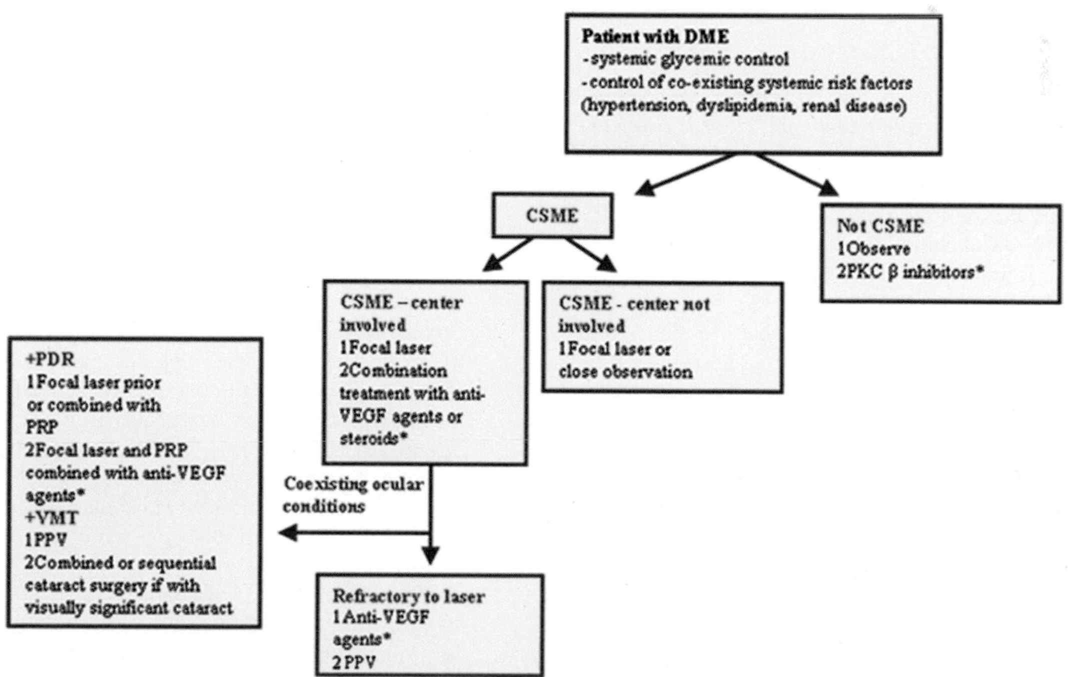

FIGURE 15.5. Potential approach in the management of diabetic macular edema. *Limited to clinical trials or off-label use. DME, diabetic macular edema; CSME, clinically significant macular edema; VEGF, vascular endothelial growth factor; PKC β, protein kinase C β; PDR, proliferative diabetic retinopathy; PRP, panretinal photocoagulation; PPV, par plana vitrectomy.

KEY POINTS

- Macular edema is a common cause of visual loss in patients with diabetes, untreated 33% of patients with center-involved CSME will experience MVL.
- The extent of VEGF involvement in the multifactorial pathogenesis of DME is not yet fully determined.
- Intravitreal ranibizumab with prompt or deferred (≥24 weeks) focal/grid laser have superior functional (visual acuity) and anatomic (OCT measured retinal thickness) outcomes compared with focal/grid laser treatment alone.
- Intravitreal anti-VEGF treatment with prompt or deferred laser should be considered for patients with center-involved DME and VA 20/32 or worse, but careful monitoring is required, as retreatment often needed, even after full resolution of edema.
- In patient groups with macular edema presentations that have not been evaluated (such as edema not involving the center or those with excellent vision) focal/grid laser remains a primary treatment modality pending further clinical trial data.
- Additional clinical trials evaluating anti-VEGF therapies are underway and will provide additional data in this and coming years.

REFERENCES

1. Centers for Disease Control and Prevention. *National diabetes fact sheet: General information and national estimates on diabetes in the United States, 2007*. Atlanta, GA: U.S. Department of Health and Human Services, Centers for Disease Control and Prevention, 2008.
2. Kempen JH, O'Colmain BJ, Leske MC, et al. The prevalence of diabetic retinopathy among adults in the United States. *Arch Ophthalmol*. 2004;122:552–563.
3. Wild S, Roglic G, Green A, et al. Global prevalence of diabetes: estimates for the year 2000 and projections for 2030. *Diabetes Care*. 2004;27:1047–1053.
4. Klein R, Klein BE, Moss SE, et al. The Wisconsin epidemiologic study of diabetic retinopathy. II. Prevalence and risk of diabetic retinopathy when age at diagnosis is less than 30 years. *Arch Ophthalmol*. 1984;102:520–526.
5. Klein R, Klein BE, Moss SE, et al. The Wisconsin epidemiologic study of diabetic retinopathy. III. Prevalence and risk of diabetic retinopathy when age at diagnosis is 30 or more years. *Arch Ophthalmol*. 1984;102:527–532.
6. Ferris FL III, Patz A. Macular edema. A complication of diabetic retinopathy. *Surv Ophthalmol*. 1984;28 Suppl: 452–461.
7. Klein R, Klein BE, Moss SE, et al. The Wisconsin Epidemiologic Study of Diabetic Retinopathy. XV. The long-term incidence of macular edema. *Ophthalmology*. 1995;102:7–16.
8. Klein R, Klein BE, Moss SE, et al. The Wisconsin epidemiologic study of diabetic retinopathy. IV. Diabetic macular edema. *Ophthalmology*. 1984;91:1464–1474.
9. Browning DJ, Glassman AR, Aiello LP, et al. Relationship between optical coherence tomography-measured central retinal thickness and visual acuity in diabetic macular edema. *Ophthalmology*. 2007;114:525–536.
10. Browning DJ, Altaweel MM, Bressler NM, et al. Diabetic macular edema: what is focal and what is diffuse? *Am J Ophthalmol*. 2008;146:649–655.
11. Danis RP, Glassman AR, Aiello LP, et al. Diurnal variation in retinal thickening measurement by optical coherence tomography in center-involved diabetic macular edema. *Arch Ophthalmol*. 2006;124:1701–1707.
12. Early Treatment Diabetic Retinopathy Study research group. Photocoagulation for diabetic macular edema. Early Treatment Diabetic Retinopathy Study report number 1. *Arch Ophthalmol*. 1985;103:1796–1806.
13. Diabetic Retinopathy Clinical Research Network. A randomized trial comparing intravitreal triamcinolone acetonide and focal/grid photocoagulation for diabetic macular edema. *Ophthalmology*. 2008;115:1447–1449.
14. Aiello LM, Ferris FL III. Photocoagulation for diabetic macular edema. *Arch Ophthalmol*. 1987;105:1163.
15. Joussen AM. Therapeutic approached to (diabetic) macular edema. In Joussen AM, Gardner TW, Kirchhof B, et al., eds. *Retinal Vascular Disease*. Heidelberg, Germany: Springer-Verlag, 2007:353–376.
16. Kern TS. Contributions of inflammatory processes to the development of the early stages of diabetic retinopathy. *Exp Diabetes Res*. 2007;2007:95–103.
17. Aiello LP, Avery RL, Arrigg PG, et al. Vascular endothelial growth factor in ocular fluid of patients with diabetic retinopathy and other retinal disorders. *N Engl J Med*. 1994;331:1480–1487.
18. Miller JW, Adamis AP, Shima DT, et al. Vascular endothelial growth factor/vascular permeability factor is temporally and spatially correlated with ocular angiogenesis in a primate model. *Am J Pathol*. 1994;145:574–584.
19. Antonetti DA, Barber AJ, Hollinger LA, et al. Vascular endothelial growth factor induces rapid phosphorylation of tight junction proteins occludin and zonula occluden 1. A potential mechanism for vascular permeability in diabetic retinopathy and tumors. *J Biol Chem*. 1999;274:23463–23467.
20. Miyamoto K, Khosrof S, Bursell SE, et al. Prevention of leukostasis and vascular leakage in streptozotocin-induced diabetic retinopathy via intercellular adhesion molecule-1 inhibition. *Proc Natl Acad Sci USA*. 1999;96: 10836–10841.
21. Schroder S, Palinski W, Schmid-Schonbein GW. Activated monocytes and granulocytes, capillary nonperfusion, and neovascularization in diabetic retinopathy. *Am J Pathol*. 1991;139:81–100.
22. Aiello LP, Bursell SE, Clermont A, et al. Vascular endothelial growth factor-induced retinal permeability is mediated by protein kinase C in vivo and suppressed by an orally effective beta-isoform-selective inhibitor. *Diabetes*. 1997;46: 1473–1480.
23. Avery RL. Regression of retinal and iris neovascularization after intravitreal bevacizumab (Avastin) treatment. *Retina*. 2006;26:352–354.

24. Cunningham ET Jr, Adamis AP, Altaweel M, et al. A phase 2 randomized double-masked trial of pegaptanib, an anti-vascular endothelial growth factor aptamer, for diabetic macular edema. *Ophthalmology*. 2005;112:1747–1757.
25. Beck RW, Edwards AR, Aiello LP, et al. Three-year follow-up of a randomized trial comparing focal/grid photocoagulation and intravitreal triamcinolone for diabetic macular edema. *Arch Ophthalmol*. 2009;127:245–251.
26. Chen Y, Wiesmann C, Fuh G, et al. Selection and analysis of an optimized anti-VEGF antibody: crystal structure of an affinity-matured Fab in complex with antigen. *J Mol Biol*. 1999;293:865–881.
27. Mulcahy MF, Benson AB III. Bevacizumab in the treatment of colorectal cancer. *Expert Opin Biol Ther*. 2005;5:997–1005.
28. Bhagat N, Grigorian RA, Tutela A, et al. Diabetic macular edema: pathogenesis and treatment. *Surv Ophthalmol*. 2009;54:1–32.
29. Arevalo JF, Sanchez JG, Fromow-Guerra J, et al. Comparison of two doses of primary intravitreal bevacizumab (Avastin) for diffuse diabetic macular edema: results from the Pan-American Collaborative Retina Study Group (PACORES) at 12-month follow-up. *Graefes Arch Clin Exp Ophthalmol*. 2009;247:735–743.
30. Kook D, Wolf A, Kreutzer T, et al. Long-term effect of intravitreal bevacizumab (avastin) in patients with chronic diffuse diabetic macular edema. *Retina*. 2008;28:1053–1060.
31. Bonini-Filho M, Costa RA, Calucci D, et al. Intravitreal bevacizumab for diabetic macular edema associated with severe capillary loss: one-year results of a pilot study. *Am J Ophthalmol*. 2009;147:1022–1030.
32. Scott IU, Edwards AR, Beck RW, et al. A phase 2 randomized clinical trial of intravitreal bevacizumab for diabetic macular edema. *Ophthalmology*. 2007;114:1860–1867.
33. Yanyali A, Aytug B, Horozoglu F, et al. Bevacizumab (Avastin) for diabetic macular edema in previously vitrectomized eyes. *Am J Ophthalmol*. 2007;144:124–126.
34. Shimura M, Nakazawa T, Yasuda K, et al. Comparative therapy evaluation of intravitreal bevacizumab and triamcinolone acetonide on persistent diffuse diabetic macular edema. *Am J Ophthalmol*. 2008;145:854–861.
35. Ahmadieh H, Ramezani A, Shoeibi N, et al. Intravitreal bevacizumab with or without triamcinolone for refractory diabetic macular edema; a placebo-controlled, randomized clinical trial. *Graefes Arch Clin Exp Ophthalmol*. 2008; 246:483–489.
36. Paccola L, Costa RA, Folgosa MS, et al. Intravitreal triamcinolone versus bevacizumab for treatment of refractory diabetic macular oedema (IBEME study). *Br J Ophthalmol*. 2008;92:76–80.
37. Soheilian M, Ramezani A, Obudi A, et al. Randomized trial of intravitreal bevacizumab alone or combined with triamcinolone versus macular photocoagulation in diabetic macular edema report 2. *Ophthalmology*. 2009;116:1142–1150.
38. Faghihi H, Roohipoor R, Mohammadi SF, et al. Intravitreal bevacizumab versus combined bevacizumab-triamcinolone versus macular laser photocoagulation in diabetic macular edema. *Eur J Ophthalmol*. 2008;18:941–948.
39. Stewart MW, Rosenfeld PJ. Predicted biological activity of intravitreal VEGF Trap. *Br J Ophthalmol*. 2008;92:667–668.
40. Bakri SJ, Snyder MR, Reid JM, et al. Pharmacokinetics of intravitreal ranibizumab (Lucentis). *Ophthalmology*. 2007;114:2179–2182.
41. Bakri SJ, Snyder MR, Reid JM, et al. Pharmacokinetics of intravitreal bevacizumab (Avastin). *Ophthalmology*. 2007; 114:855–859.
42. Chun DW, Heier JS, Topping TM, et al. A pilot study of multiple intravitreal injections of ranibizumab in patients with center-involving clinically significant diabetic macular edema. *Ophthalmology*. 2006;113:1706–1712.
43. Nguyen QD, Tatlipinar S, Shah SM, et al. Vascular endothelial growth factor is a critical stimulus for diabetic macular edema. *Am J Ophthalmol*. 2006;142:961–969.
44. Holash J, Davis S, Papadopoulos N, et al. VEGF-Trap: a VEGF blocker with potent antitumor effects. *Proc Natl Acad Sci USA*. 2002;99:11393–11398.
45. Saishin Y, Saishin Y, Takahashi K, et al. VEGF-TRAP(R1R2) suppresses choroidal neovascularization and VEGF-induced breakdown of the blood-retinal barrier. *J Cell Physiol*. 2003; 195:241–248.
46. Do DV, Nguyen QD, Shah SM, et al. An exploratory study of the safety, tolerability and bioactivity of a single intravitreal injection of vascular endothelial growth factor Trap-Eye in patients with diabetic macular oedema. *Br J Ophthalmol*. 2009;93:144–149.
47. Xia P, Aiello LP, Ishii H, et al. Characterization of vascular endothelial growth factor's effect on the activation of protein kinase C, its isoforms, and endothelial cell growth. *J Clin Invest*. 1996;98:2018–2026.
48. Ishii H, Jirousek MR, Koya D, et al. Amelioration of vascular dysfunctions in diabetic rats by an oral PKC beta inhibitor. *Science*. 1996;272:728–731.
49. Aiello LP, Davis MD, Girach A, et al. Effect of ruboxistaurin on visual loss in patients with diabetic retinopathy. *Ophthalmology*. 2006;113:2221–2230.
50. PKC-DMES Study Group. Effect of ruboxistaurin in patients with diabetic macular edema: thirty-month results of the randomized PKC-DMES clinical trial. *Arch Ophthalmol*. 2007;125:318–324.
51. Davis MD, Sheetz MJ, Aiello LP, et al. Effect of ruboxistaurin on the visual acuity decline associated with long-standing diabetic macular edema. *Invest Ophthalmol Vis Sci*. 2009;50:1–4.
52. Guba M, von Breitenbuch P, Steinbauer M, et al. Rapamycin inhibits primary and metastatic tumor growth by antiangiogenesis: involvement of vascular endothelial growth factor. *Nat Med*. 2002;8:128–135.
53. Luan FL, Ding R, Sharma VK, et al. Rapamycin is an effective inhibitor of human renal cancer metastasis. *Kidney Int*. 2003;63:917–926.
54. Blumenkranz MS, Dugel PU, Solley DM, et al. A randomized dose-escalation trial of locally-administered sirolimus to treat diabetic macular edema. Annual Meeting of the Association for Research in Vision and Ophthalmology 2009 Fort Lauderdale, Florida 2008.
55. Dykxhoorn DM, Palliser D, Lieberman J. The silent treatment: siRNAs as small molecule drugs. *Gene Ther*. 2006;13:541–552.
56. Singerman LJ. A Phase 2, pharmacokinetic, randomized, double-masked, controlled, dose comparison study of Cand5 for intravitreal injection for the treatment of diabetic macular edema. 25th Annual Meeting of the American Society of Retina Specialists 2007;Indian Wells, CA.

57. Brafman A, Mett I, Shafir M, et al. Inhibition of oxygen-induced retinopathy in RTP801-deficient mice. *Invest Ophthalmol Vis Sci*. 2004;45:3796–3805.
58. Samson CM, Waheed N, Baltatzis S, et al. Methotrexate therapy for chronic noninfectious uveitis: analysis of a case series of 160 patients. *Ophthalmology.* 2001;108:1134–1139.
59. Velez G, Yuan P, Sung C, et al. Pharmacokinetics and toxicity of intravitreal chemotherapy for primary intraocular lymphoma. *Arch Ophthalmol*. 2001;119:1518–1524.
60. Ferrara N, Gerber HP, LeCouter J. The biology of VEGF and its receptors. *Nat Med*. 2003;9:669–676.
61. Alon T, Hemo I, Itin A, et al. Vascular endothelial growth factor acts as a survival factor for newly formed retinal vessels and has implications for retinopathy of prematurity. *Nat Med*. 1995;1:1024–1028.
62. Scheppke L, Aguilar E, Gariano RF, et al. Retinal vascular permeability suppression by topical application of a novel VEGFR2/Src kinase inhibitor in mice and rabbits. *J Clin Invest*. 2008;118:2337–2346.
63. Doukas J, Mahesh S, Umeda N, et al. Topical administration of a multi-targeted kinase inhibitor suppresses choroidal neovascularization and retinal edema. *J Cell Physiol*. 2008;216:29–37.
64. van Wijngaarden P, Coster DJ, Williams KA. Inhibitors of ocular neovascularization: promises and potential problems. *JAMA*. 2005;293:1509–1513.
65. Simo R, Hernandez C. Intravitreous anti-VEGF for diabetic retinopathy: hopes and fears for a new therapeutic strategy. *Diabetologia*. 2008;51:1574–1580.
66. Ueta T, Yanagi Y, Tamaki Y, et al. Cerebrovascular accidents in ranibizumab. *Ophthalmology*. 2009;116:362.
67. Bhavsar AR, Ip MS, Glassman AR. The risk of endophthalmitis following intravitreal triamcinolone injection in the DRCRnet and SCORE clinical trials. *Am J Ophthalmol*. 2007;144:454–456.
68. Jager RD, Aiello LP, Patel SC, et al. Risks of intravitreous injection: a comprehensive review. *Retina*. 2004;24:676–698.
69. Blaauwgeers HG, Holtkamp GM, Rutten H, et al. Polarized vascular endothelial growth factor secretion by human retinal pigment epithelium and localization of vascular endothelial growth factor receptors on the inner choriocapillaris. Evidence for a trophic paracrine relation. *Am J Pathol*. 1999;155:421–428.
70. Aiello LP, Cahill MT, Wong JS. Systemic considerations in the management of diabetic retinopathy. *Am J Ophthalmol*. 2001;132:760–766.

CHAPTER

16

Steroids for Diabetic Macular Edema and Neovascular Age Related Macular Degeneration

Felix Y. Chau • Daniel F. Kiernan • Jennifer I. Lim

INTRODUCTION

Ocular steroids for the treatment of diabetic macular edema (DME) and neovascular age-related macular degeneration (NVAMD) have been utilized in an evolving treatment strategy over the course of many years. The unifying principle behind using steroids for treating these conditions is that steroids are capable of reducing the vascular permeability of capillary endothelial cells, suppressing vascular endothelial growth factor (VEGF) production, and reducing the inflammatory response that contributes to both DME and NVAMD. Over the last few years, studies have compared ocular steroid treatment for DME (sub Tenon's or intravitreal) with focal laser and anti-VEGF agents for treating DME. Steroid therapy has also been compared with PDT and anti-VEGF agents for treating NVAMD. This chapter will review the underlying principles behind using steroids for DME and NVAMD, review current studies evaluating steroid use for treating DME and NVAMD, and offer expert opinion Jennifer Lim (JL) regarding the role of steroids for DME and NVAMD for the future (Box 16.1).

MOLECULAR MECHANISMS

Since Machemer and Peyman first suggested the use of the vitreous as a depot for drug delivery to the retina and conducted the first experiments using intravitreal steroids,[1–3] intravitreal and other means of delivering steroids to the retina have been employed with various scientific rationales. Inflammation, especially leukostasis within capillaries, is known to result in increased vascular permeability and subsequent fluid accumulation in the retina in both DME[4] and NVAMD.[5] Steroids can reduce retinal edema in both these conditions by reducing inflammation.

The exact anti-inflammatory mechanism of corticosteroids is still not fully understood. Corticosteroids may induce lipocortin synthesis, which subsequently inhibits phospholipase A2 in its production of arachadonic acid.[6] The decreased production of arachadonic acid in turn results in reduced synthesis of its inflammatory cascade derivatives such as prostaglandins and leukotrienes.[6] Steroids may thus reduce the chemical signals for inflammation.[6]

Steroids may also reduce leukocyte adhesion and extravasation that occur during inflammation by reducing the expression of immunoglobulin superfamily molecules during endothelial cell activation. Immunoglobulin superfamily molecules such as intercellular adhesion molecule (ICAM)-1, vascular cell adhesion molecule (VCAM)-1, and major histocompatibility complex (MHC)-I and -II are expressed during vascular endothelial cell activation during the process of inflammation. These adhesion molecules help leukocytes adhere to the endothelial cell surface from the circulating blood stream and assist in their extravasation from the blood stream into the surrounding tissue. Triamcinolone acetonide has been found to reduce the cytokine-induced expression of ICAM1, MHC-I, and MHC-II antigen by choroidal endothelial cells as well as to reduce the permeability of choroidal endothelial cell monolayers in vitro.[7–9] By reducing choroidal endothelial cell adhesion molecule expression and permeability, triamcinolone acetonide may have a therapeutic role in treating these inflammation-related contributors to NVAMD.[5] Similarly, by reducing retinal vascular endothelial cell expression of molecules such as ICAM-1 and CD-18 and by reducing leukocyte adhesion to retinal vascular endothelial cell walls, steroids may reduce the inflammation-related contributors to DME.[4,10–13]

In addition to reducing inflammation and its associated increase in vascular permeability in DME and NVAMD, steroids may also reduce vascular permeability and retinal edema mediated in part by VEGF. VEGF has been found to increase vascular permeability through breakdown of the blood-retina barrier and is considered one of the mediators

BOX 16.1 How do I Approach DME and Neovascular ARMD?

At present, the evidence-based approach to management of DME points to the use of primary laser photocoagulation as the best choice of available treatments. The DRCR showed us definitively that although there may be an early improvement in visual acuity with IVTA, the long-term visual results are indeed better with laser alone. In addition, the high rate of complications associated with IVTA deters me from using these drugs as a first-line treatment.

However, when an eye has had a "full" focal grid treatment and still has macular edema with leakage on the fluorescein angiogram, I would consider adjunctive drug therapy. At present, our choices include intravitreal anti-VEGF drugs or steroids. I would consider using these prescriptions in an attempt to thin the retina and perhaps improve visual acuity. In addition, the use of a drug that has a different mechanism of action, aside from laser, may be beneficial. Of course, this is not proven and experimental.

I am eagerly awaiting the results of the dexamethasone implant study for DME (Allergan study). The dexamethasone implant has a longer duration of action and has a lower rate of intraocular pressure elevation than available steroids. It may be a reasonable treatment for eyes with refractory macular edema. Perhaps, this drug could be combined with laser treatment.

For neovascular AMD, anti-VEGF treatment has clearly become the standard of care. I rarely use steroids or PDT for neovascular AMD currently, but these may have a future role as adjuncts to anti-VEGF treatment as current trials are investigating combination therapy with different steroids and doses of PDT along with anti-VEGF treatment.

—Jennifer Lim,MD

of edema in DME[14–16] and a major mediator of choroidal neovascularization (CNV) and edema in NVAMD.[17] VEGF is thought to increase retinal vascular permeability in DME via several theories including (a) phosphorylation of the tight junctional protein occludin, which causes disruption of the tight junctional complex and (b) FAS-mediated endothelial cell apoptosis.[14–16,18] VEGF's major role in the formation of CNV and its resulting fluid accumulation in the retina in NVAMD has resulted in anti-VEGF therapies becoming the current standard of care in treatment of NVAMD.[19] As steroids have been found to inhibit the expression of VEGF and the VEGF gene,[20,21] steroids in principle should reduce the VEGF-mediated components of DME and NVAMD.

STEROID FORMULATIONS FOR DME AND NVAMD

Triamcinolone acetonide has been used clinically for the inhibition of neovascularization and reduction of retinal edema. Triamcinolone is a conventional steroid, with typical glucocorticoid and mineralocorticoid anti-inflammatory activity.[6] In ophthalmic practice, it is available as an injectable suspension, usually either 4 or 20 mg. Although many commercial preparations exist, the most commonly used preparation is Kenalog-40 (triamcinolone acetonide, Bristol-Myers-Squibb, Peapack, NJ). Triamcinolone does not achieve significant systemic serum levels when injected intravitreally;[22] however, differences in particle size (<1 to >20 mm) may contribute to variability in clearance times and durations of action following vitreous injection.[23] Although they are effective angiostatic agents, glucocorticoids are associated with significant ocular side effects, including the development of posterior subcapsular cataracts and ocular hypertension and iatrogenic glaucoma in sensitive patients.

Various rationales have led to the use of triamcinolone acetonide as an intravitreal injection for steroid treatment of the retina. Steroids given topically, systemically, or injected into the subconjunctival or sub-Tenon's space often do not reach sufficiently high intraocular concentrations to achieve therapeutic levels or have serious systemic side effects when given long term.[6] In contrast to soluble substances injected into the eye that leave the globe within hours to days, triamcinolone acetonide is normally in crystalline form of variable particle sizes that can be injected as a suspension. As solid crystals, triamcinolone is a more ideal steroid than soluble forms of steroid for achieving long-lasting concentrations of drug over time within the eye. Additionally, systemic concentrations of triamcinolone in the venous blood after intravitreal injection have been measured as insignificant compared to physiologic serum cortisol levels, suggesting intravitreal triamcinolone (IVTA) is ideally suited for treating the retina at high concentration with minimal systemic side effects.[24]

Like triamcinolone, anecortave acetate has also been used for reducing retinal neovascularization and edema. Anecortave acetate (Retaane, Alcon Laboratories, Fort Worth, TX) is an artificially modified steroid that was specifically designed to eliminate the undesired side effects of glucocorticoids while enhancing angiostatic activity. It is synthesized by removing the 11b-hydroxyl group on the B ring of the steroid nucleus and by replacing it with a C9-11 double bond to form a unique pregnan cortisene compound. The altered structural configuration confers distinct angiostatic capabilities, inhibiting multiple steps in the neovascularization process, including initiation of the angiogenic cascade and elaboration of the angiogenic growth factors VEGF and insulin-like growth factor (IGF)-1 and their receptors.[25–28] Initial studies in chick embryos and mouse intraocular tumors demonstrated that anecortave effectively inhibited newly forming small vessels, whereas existing normal vessels were unaffected.[29–33]

Dexamethasone has the highest relative strength of any other steroid used in ophthalmic practice.[6,34] A single dose of 0.18 mg/mL dexamethasone is equivalent to 1 mg/mL triamcinolone in terms of equal corticosteroid efficacy and is short acting, with faster clearance from the vitreous.[35] Intravitreal dexamethasone has been shown to suppress streptozotocin-induced leukostasis in diabetic rats[36] and VEGF-induced blood-retinal barrier breakdown in rabbits[37] via VEGF and ICAM-1 inhibition within the retinal vasculature. When administered as treatment pulses, it may be less likely to result in glaucoma or cataract progression than other sustained-delivery steroids.[38,39] Triple therapy using photodynamic therapy (PDT), intravitreal dexamethasone, and anti-VEGF agents is currently being assessed in patients with NVAMD for maintenance of visual acuity and reduction in the frequency of treatment of AMD patients.[38–41] Dexamethasone in a sustained release implant has also previously been used to treat macular edema secondary to diabetes, uveitis, and vein occlusions[42] and recently gained FDA approval for treating macular edema from vein occlusions. It is currently being studied more carefully in treating DME.

Fluocinolone is another potent corticosteroid with high glucocorticoid receptor affinity. As an intravitreal implant that provides sustained release fluocinolone over about 2.5 years, the Retisert device has been U.S. FDA approved for the treatment of noninfectious posterior uveitis.[43] Cataracts and increased intraocular pressure are common side effects requiring surgical or medical management. In vitro studies using human retinal pigment epithelial (ARPE-19) cells have suggested fluocinolone inhibits VEGF expression via glucocorticoid receptors and inhibits tumor necrosis factor-alpha (TNF-alpha)–induced angiogenesis in chick chorioallantoic membrane.[44] These suggest a potential role along with anti-VEGF therapy for fluocinolone in treating NVAMD. Furthermore, the fluocinolone intravitreal implant was also found to help reduce DME and improve visual acuity in a 3-year study, although glaucoma-related complications and cataracts were again significant side effects.[45]

STEROIDS AND DME: PRIOR STUDIES AND FUTURE DIRECTIONS

Triamcinolone Acetonide for DME

Potential benefits of steroids over focal and grid laser for DME include absence of damage to retinal tissue that would be caused by laser and broader treatment of the retina for more diffuse DME not easily treated by focal or grid laser. With these theoretical advantages, steroid treatment for DME has progressed from case reports in 2001 to randomized, controlled clinical trials comparing intravitreal steroids with placebo, focal/grid laser, and other controls as of 2009.[46–52]

As shown in Table 16.1, many permutations of comparing IVTA at different doses against various control groups (placebo injection, observation, and later focal/grid laser) have suggested a trend of transient improvement of DME and visual acuity that gradually declines over a dose-dependent time. Early case studies of eyes with DME refractory to laser suggested the role of IVTA as alternative treatment. In 2001, Jonas et al.[46] performed one of the first intravitreal injections of triamcinolone acetonide (20 mg) in an eye with declining vision from DME refractory to grid laser treatment and found improvement in acuity from 0.10 to about 0.40 in 2 months. In 2002, Martidis et al.[47] treated 16 eyes with DME that failed to respond to at least two laser sessions with 4 mg of triamcinolone acetonide (Figs. 16.1 to 16.3).[47] Vision improved by 2.4, 2.4, and 1.3 Snellen lines at the 1-, 3-, and 6-month follow-up intervals, respectively, with corresponding decreases in optical coherence tomography (OCT) central macular thicknesses of 55%, 57.5%, and 38%, respectively. Some cases did result in intraocular pressure increases above 21 mm Hg requiring topical treatment.[47]

Further studies, many with control groups for comparison, clarified the potential role of triamcinolone for DME. In an inter-eye comparison in 2004, Jonas et al.[53] also found that steroid-treated eyes (20–25 mg triamcinolone) compared to observed eyes more often had two or more lines of Snellen visual acuity improvement (55% vs. 25%) or three or more lines of Snellen visual acuity improvement (35% vs. 10%). In the same year in a case series study, Jonas et al.[54] also estimated that 20 to 25 mg of triamcinolone produces a maximum visual improvement within 1 to 7 months with return to baseline vision in 8 to 9 months. In 2004, Sutter et al. performed in a randomized controlled trial comparing 4 mg IVTA in 34 eyes with placebo injection in 35 eyes. The steroid-treated eyes more often showed a gain of five letters or more (55% vs. 16%).[55] Also in 2004, Ciardella et al.[56] in a case series of 30 eyes found that 4 mg triamcinolone resulted in improved logMAR visual acuities; vision improved from a baseline of 0.17 ± 0.12 to 0.34 ± 0.18, 0.36 ± 0.16, and 0.31 ± 0.17 at 1, 3, and 6 months respectively with a reduction in hard exudates (Fig. 16.4).[56] The mean interval between first and second injections was 5.7 ± 2.7 months. The mean interval between second and third injections was 5.7 ± 3.3 months. Intraocular pressure rises above 21 mm Hg occurred in 40% of eyes. Correlating with other studies showed improved visual acuity, Ozkiris et al.[57] found in 2004 that 8 mg triamcinolone given to 40 eyes with DME resulted in significant improvements in pattern electroretinogram: with a mean follow-up of 6 months, both the mean visual acuity and mean p50 amplitude pERG improved. In 2005, Jonas et al.[58] determined that lower degrees of macular ischemia, higher preoperative visual acuity, and higher degrees of macular edema in diffuse DME correlated with improvement in

Table 16.1.

IVTA at Different Doses Compared with Control Groups

Author	Year	Dosage (mg)	Eyes	Design	Results (experimental % vs. control %)
Jonas and Sofker	2001	20–25	1	Case report	Vision increase
Martidis et al.	2002	4	16	Case series	Increased vision, IOP
Jonas et al.	2003	20–25	36	Comparative NR	Increased VA, IOP
Massin et al.	2004	4	30	Inter-eye	Reduced macular thickness
Jonas et al.	2004	20–25	40	Inter-eye	Two line Snellen improvement (55% vs. 25%) Three line Snellen improvement (35% vs. 10%)
Jonas et al.	2004	20–25	38	Case series	Maximum visual improvement 1–7 mo Return to baseline 8–9 mo
Sutter	2004	4	69	Double masked	5+ letter gain (55% vs. 16%) Placebo controlled RCT
Bakri et al.	2004	4	19	Case series	
Ciardella et al.	2004	4	30	Case series	Baseline 0.17–0.34, 0.36, 0.31 at 1, 3, 6 mo Reduction in hard exudates Interval between repeat injections 5.7 mo IOP > 21 mm Hg in 40%
Ozkiris	2004	8	40	Case series	Improved pattern ERG
Bandello	2004	4	1	Case report	IVTA with PRP
Karacorlu	2004	4	1	Case report	Regression of NV in PDR
Avitable	2005	4	63	Randomized	IVTA better than laser DME and vein occlusion
Zacks and Johnson	2005	4	4	Case series	IVTA with PRP
Jonas et al.	2005	20-25	53	Case series	Degree of macular edema, VA, ischemia Relates to visual increase after IVTA
Jonas	2005	20-25	4	Case series	Reincrease in vision after reinjection
Spandau	2005	2-13	27	Randomized	Dosage dependence on duration of effect
Lam et al.	2007	4	111	RCT	IVTA + grid not better than IVTA Grid laser worst outcome
Grover et al.	2008	Variable, F, D	632	Meta-analysis	IVTA or implants may improve vision in Persistent, refractory DME
DRCR	2008	4,1	840		At 2 y, focal/grid laser more effective And with fewer side effects than IVTA
DRCR	2009	4,1	306		At 3 y, focal/grid laser more effective Most eyes with 4 mg IVTA need CE/IOL

visual acuity after treatment with IVTA. In 2005, Spandau et al.[50] in a prospective, randomized, double-masked interventional study of 27 eyes comparing doses of 2 mg (8 eyes), 5 mg (10 eyes), and 13 mg (9 eyes) of triamcinolone found more pronounced treatment effect and longer duration in the 13 mg group than the 5 and 2 mg groups. In 2007, Lam et al.[59] discovered in a randomized study of 111 eyes with DME comparing 4 mg triamcinolone (IVTA) combined with grid laser versus IVTA alone or grid laser alone that IVTA combined with grid laser was not better than IVTA alone, and that grid laser alone had the worst visual outcomes.

In 2008, with many published independent studies looking at steroid treatment for macular edema, Grover et al.[51] performed a meta-analysis of 632 eyes with DME from seven studies—four using IVTA and three using a fluocinolone acetonide implant (FAI) or dexamethasone drug delivery system (DDS).[51] The study found visual improvement (improved mean difference in LogMAR visual acuity) with IVTA compared with controls at 3 months (−0.15 LogMAR, 7.5 letters), 6 months (−0.23 LogMAR, 11.5 letters), 9 months (−0.29 LogMAR, 14.5 letters), and 24 months (−0.11 LogMAR, 5.7 letters). The relative risk

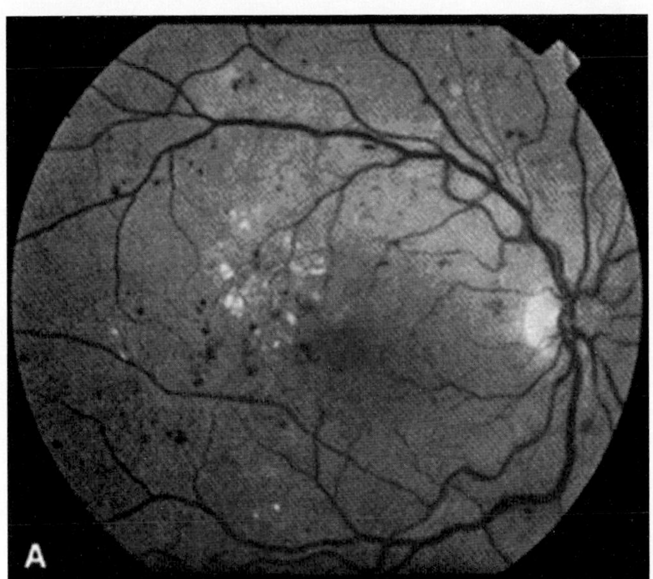

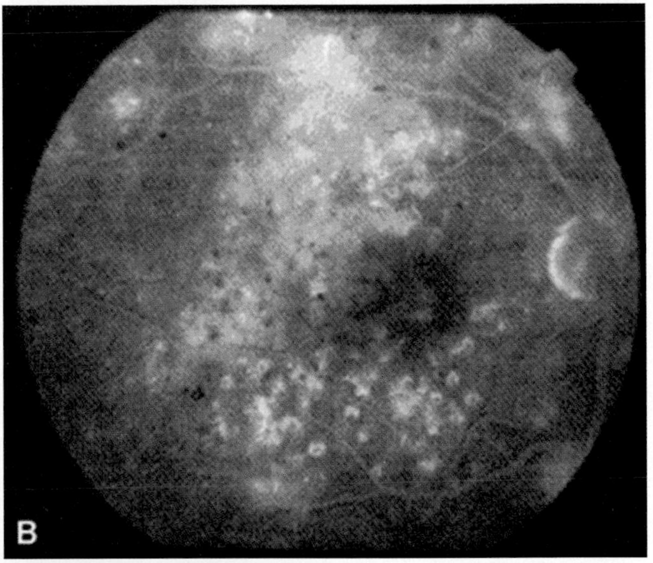

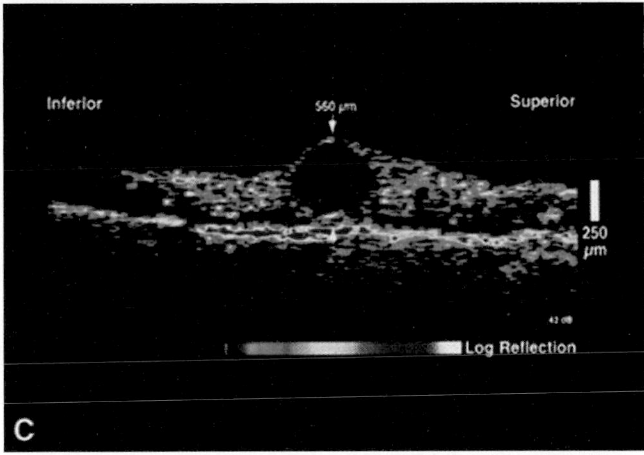

FIGURE 16.1. Nonproliferative diabetic retinopathy with chronic clinically significant macular edema. **A:** A color photograph after three laser sessions (6/30/98) showing multiple microaneurysms with hard exudate. Clinically, there was persistent thickening under the fovea with cystoid spaces. **B:** Fluorescein angiography corresponding to color photograph confirms diffuse macular leakage. Note the multiple laser scars surrounding the fovea. **C:** An OCT cross section corresponding to the color photograph shows persistent macular edema with development of large cystoid spaces. Visual acuity measures 20/50. Additional laser photocoagulation was performed.

for improving one or more lines in visual acuity was 2.85 at 3 months, 1.25 at 6 months, and 2.17 at 24 months, all in favor of IVTA. Mean improvements in OCT retinal thickness were −131.97 μm at 3 months, −135 μm at 6 months, −133 μm at 9 months, and −59 μm at 24 months, all in favor of IVTA. Improved clinical outcomes of FAI and DDS trials were also reported. Elevated IOP and cataract progression occurred with IVTA but seemed manageable.[51]

In 2008, as a potentially definitive study comparing IVTA with focal/grid laser for DME, the Diabetic Retinopathy Clinical Research Network (DRCR.net) completed the 2-year follow-up for a multicenter, randomized, controlled clinical trial comparing 1 mg IVTA, 4 mg IVTA, and focal/grid laser.[52] In this trial, 840 eyes with DME involving the fovea with visual acuities 20/40 to 20/320 were randomized to focal/grid laser ($n = 330$), 1 mg ($n = 256$), or 4 mg ($n = 254$) triamcinolone (IVTA). Retreatment was allowed for persistent or new edema at 4 months intervals. At 4 months, there was a greater positive treatment response on visual acuity in the 4 mg IVTA group compared with laser or 1 mg IVTA. However, at 1 year, little difference was found in visual acuity among the groups, and from 16 months to the 2 year primary outcome assessment, the laser group had superior visual acuities and better safety profiles (fewer eyes with intraocular pressure increases and cataracts) than either the 1 or 4 mg triamcinolone groups. OCT central subfield retinal thicknesses similarly showed greater initial treatment effect in the 4 mg group at 4 months, with later superior improvements for the laser treatment group at 2 years compared to both the 1 and 4 mg IVTA groups. The improvements in visual

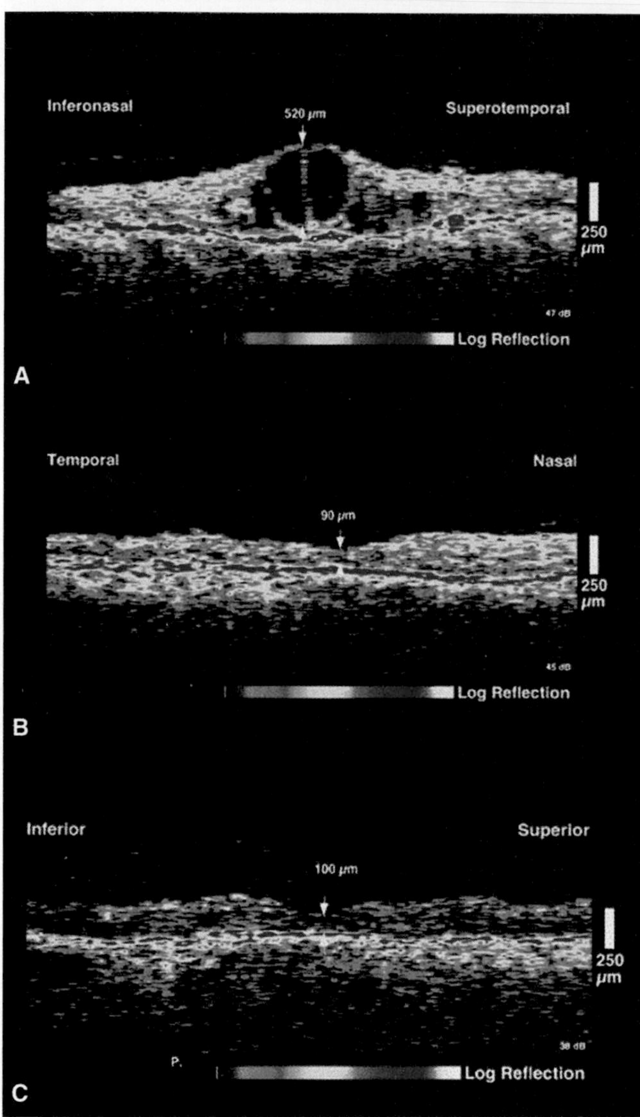

FIGURE 16.2. Nonproliferative diabetic retinopathy with chronic clinically significant macular edema. **A:** An OCT cross section and macular map before IVTA. A total of five laser sessions had been performed previously. Note prominent cystoid spaces involving the fovea with diffuse macular edema. Visual acuity had declined progressively to 20/200. **B:** An OCT cross section 1 month after IVTA. Chronic macular thickening and cystoid spaces have resolved completely, and vision has returned to 20/60. **C:** An OCT cross section 3 months after IVTA. The macular edema remains controlled, and vision remains stable. (Reproduced from Martidis, et al. *Ophthalmology.* 2002;109:920, with permission.)

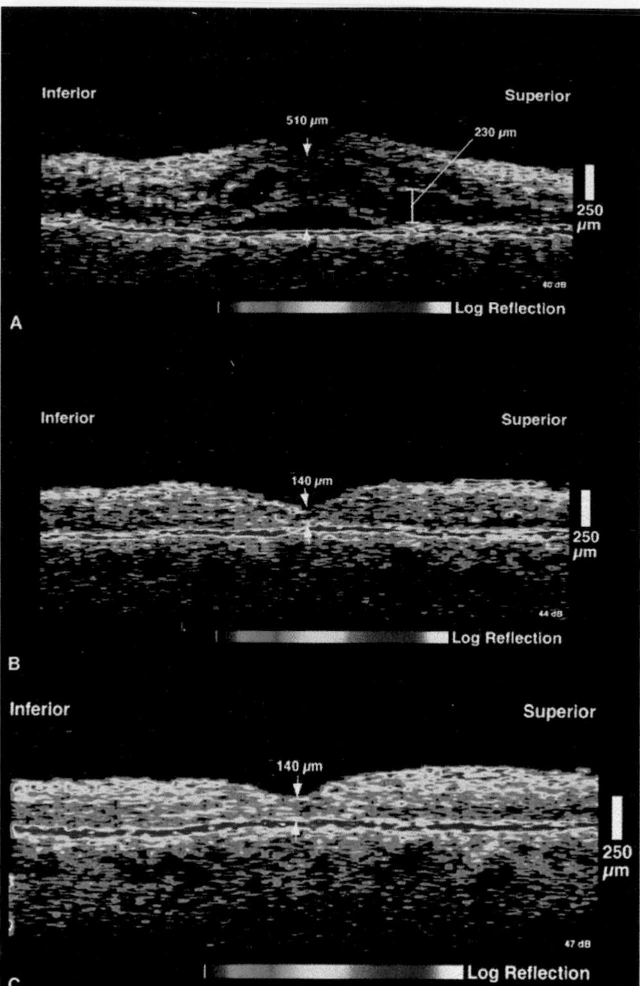

FIGURE 16.3. Proliferative diabetic retinopathy with chronic clinically significant macular edema. **A:** An OCT cross section before IVTA. Note the persistent macular thickening and cystoid macular edema despite two prior laser sessions. Visual acuity measures 20/80. **B:** An OCT cross section 1 month after IVTA shows resolution of macular edema with improvement of visual acuity to 20/50. **C:** An OCT cross section 3 months after IVTA shows sustained control of macular edema; visual acuity measures 20/60. (Reproduced from Martidis, et al. *Ophthalmology.* 2002;109:920, with permission.)

acuity by laser in this study were consistent with prior findings in the ETDRS in eyes with CSDME treated with focal/grid laser with similar entry criteria to the eyes enrolled in this study. In conclusion, the study stated that while IVTA likely is superior to the natural, untreated course of CSME over 2 years, the results suggest that focal/grid laser is more effective than IVTA in improving visual acuity and reducing OCT-measured retinal thickening in the long term.[52]

Furthermore, the study also found that laser had fewer side effects than IVTA, especially regarding ocular hypertension, glaucoma, and the need for cataract surgery.[52] In terms of ocular hypertension and glaucoma, more eyes in the 4 mg IVTA group (40%) than in the 1 mg IVTA group (20%) or laser group (10%) had one of the following at one or multiple visits from baseline: (a) increased intraocular pressure of 10 mm Hg or more above baseline, (b) intraocular pressure of 30 mm Hg or more, and (c) initiation of intraocular pressure-lowering medications (if not being treated at the study entry) or a diagnosis of glaucoma ($p < 0.001$ for all three pair-wise comparisons). Glaucoma surgery was only required in the 4 mg IVTA group (4 eyes: 2 filtering surgeries, 1 laser trabeculoplasty, 1 ciliary body destruction). For phakic eyes at baseline, cataract surgery was required before the 2-year

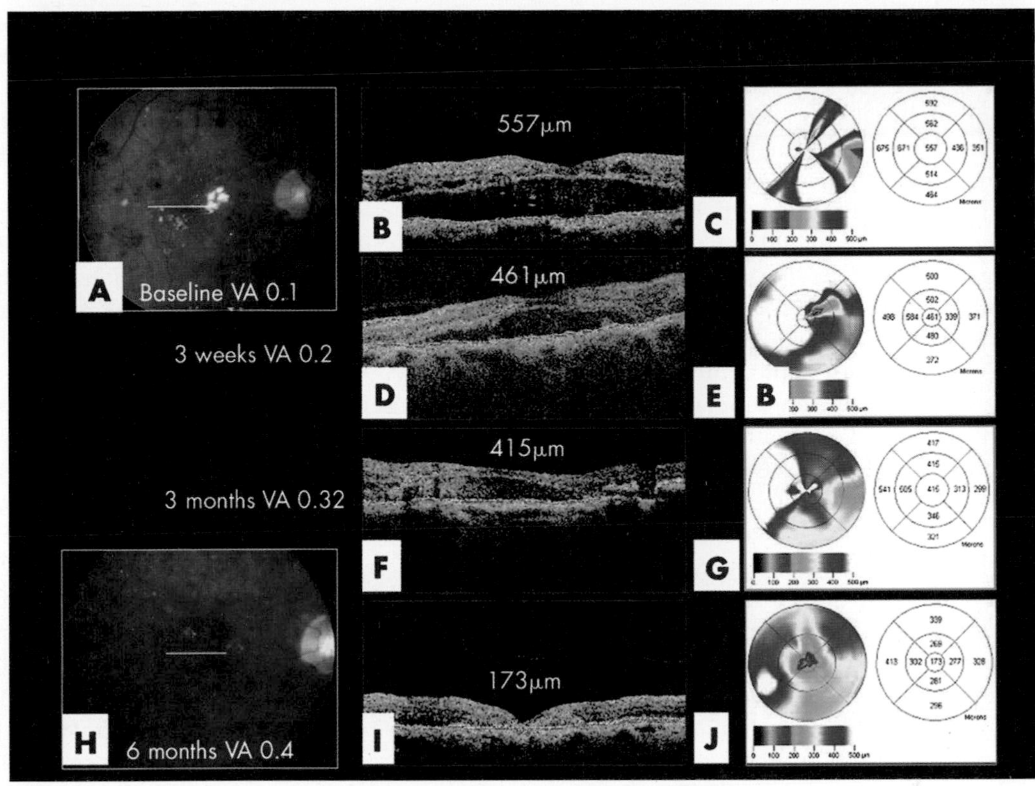

FIGURE 16.4. A 69-year-old diabetic man with reduced visual acuity in the right eye to the level of 0.1 secondary to diffuse diabetic macular edema. He had two previous laser treatments in the right eye. IVTA acetonide 4 mg in 0.1 mL was injected one time in the right eye. **A:** Clinical fundus photograph of the right eye at baseline demonstrated the presence of background diabetic retinopathy. There was diffuse macular edema, hard exudates, and intraretinal hemorrhages at the posterior pole. The white line represents the area scanned with the OCT. **B:** OCT cross section scan through the macula confirmed the presence of macular edema. There were intraretinal fluid-filled cystoid spaces and serous elevation of the neurosensory retina. The macular thickness in the fovea measured by OCT was 557 μm. **C:** False color topographic map of the macula demonstrated diffuse macular thickening. In the false color map, white corresponds to the area of maximal thickening and blue corresponds to the less thick areas. **D:** One month after IVTA, the visual acuity had improved to 0.2. The central macular thickness was decreased to 461 μm. OCT scan through the macula demonstrated slight resolution in the macular edema. **E:** False color topographic map of the macula demonstrated some reduction in retinal thickness especially in the inferonasal macula. **F:** Three months after IVTA, visual acuity had improved to 0.32. There was partial resolution of the serous neurosensory detachment in the macula by OCT. **G:** False color topographic map of the macula confirmed the partial resolution of the macular edema. There was still thickening temporally (*white*). **H:** Clinical photograph of the same eye 6 months after IVTA revealed resolution of the macular edema and reduction in the number of hard exudates at the posterior pole. Visual acuity had improved to 0.4. The white line represents the area scanned with the OCT. **I:** OCT scan through the fovea demonstrated almost total resolution of the serous neurosensory macular elevation. There was also disappearance of the intraretinal cystoid spaces. Central macular thickness was 173 μm. **J:** False color topographic map confirmed the presence of diffuse flattening of the macula. (Reproduced from Ciardella, et al. *Br J Ophthalmol.* 2004;88:1131, with permission)

outcome visit more often in eyes in the 4 mg IVTA group (51%) than in the 1 mg IVTA group (23%) or laser group (13%; $p < 0.001$ for all three pair-wise comparisons).[52]

For the 3-year follow-up of this DRCR study, 306 eyes were available for further analysis (Fig. 16.5).[60] From 2 to 3 years, more eyes improved than worsened in all three treatment groups. The change in visual acuity letter score from baseline to 3 years was a gain of five letters in the laser group and no letters in each triamcinolone group. For the duration of the 3-year study, the probability of requiring cataract surgery was 31%, 46%, and 83% in the laser, 1 mg, and 4 mg triamcinolone groups, respectively. IOP rose by more than 10 mm Hg at any visit in 4%, 18%, and 33% of eyes in the laser, 1mg, and 4 mg triamcinolone groups, respectively. These findings were consistent with the 2-year results suggesting continued superior benefit in focal/grid laser–treated eyes compared to IVTA-treated eyes with less risk of visually significant cataract or elevated intraocular pressure. Indeed, most eyes in the 4 mg IVTA group required cataract surgery.[60]

While establishing focal/grid laser as the gold standard of care in treating DME, the DRCR studies above are most applicable to eyes still amenable to additional focal/grid laser, an explicit part of the DRCR's entry criteria for these studies.[52] Eyes with prior laser treatment were enrolled in the study only if judged by the investigator to have potential benefit from additional laser treatment —enrolled eyes were not considered refractory to additional laser.[52] Eyes with DME that are refractory to focal/grid laser, pseudophakic, and nonglaucomatous with no history of steroid response may still be viable candidates for intravitreal steroid as suggested by prior case series, inter-eye studies, and earlier randomized trials of eyes with laser-refractory DME. In addition, combination treatments using focal laser treatment and triamcinolone have yet to be evaluated and compared. This is currently being assessed in the DRCR Protocol I study.

While not replacing laser treatment, steroids may have a role as adjunctive treatment for DME along with laser photocoagulation. In the DRCR Protocol I study, intravitreal ranibizumab or triamcinolone acetonide is being used in combination with laser photocoagulation for DME.[61] As shown in Figures 16.1 and 16.1a, some patients may have superior improvement in vision and edema without significant intraocular pressure increases with triamcinolone combined with laser compared to laser alone. The patient in Figures 16.1 and 16.1a was a participant in the DRCR Protocol I, with the left eye randomized to IVTA along with laser while the right eye was randomized to laser alone. Sham injections were also given to both eyes. After 48 weeks, there was marked improvement in vision and edema in the steroid- and laser-treated left eye compared to the laser-alone-treated right eye. Final conclusions from this DRCR study—to determine if anti-VEGF treatment or triamcinolone may provide significant benefit along with laser for DME—are pending.

Sustained Release Fluocinolone, Dexamethasone, and Triamcinolone for DME

New devices providing sustained release of triamcinolone at lower doses and alternative steroid formulations may provide other treatment options for eyes with laser-refractory DME. In 2006, a 3-year randomized controlled clinical trial comparing a fluocinolone acetonide intravitreal implant (0.59 mg) versus laser or observation was completed in 197 patients with DME.[45] In this study, by 36 months, more fluocinolone-treated eyes had three or more lines of improvement in visual acuity (28% vs. 15%, $p < 0.05$), but 95% of phakic eyes required cataract extraction, 35% had intraocular pressure rise, 28% required filtering surgery, and 5% required device explantation because of IOP elevations.[45]

In 2007, a sustained release dexamethasone intravitreous DDS was superior to observation in treating 315 eyes with persistent macular edema (>90 days) from diabetes, vein occlusions, uveitis, and other causes.[42] At 90 days, an improvement in BCVA of 10 or more letters was reached by a greater proportion of patients in the dexamethasone DDS 700 μg group (35%) or 350 μg group (24%) compared to observed patients (13%, $p < 0.05$).[42] Increased intraocular pressure of 10 mm Hg or higher occurred in 11% of DDS-treated patients over 3 months.[42] This dexamethasone DDS was recently FDA approved for macular edema from vein occlusions as the Ozurdex implant (Allergan). The role of this dexamethasone implant in treating DME is still under investigation; at present, the Ozurdex data for DME are not yet available.

In 2009, a phase 1 study using a new device (Verisome, ICON Bioscience, Sunnyvale, CA) to release triamcinolone acetonide at low dose (1.1 μg/mL) over a sustained period of 12 months for eyes with chronic cystoid macular edema from venous occlusive disease was reported.[62] For the 13.8 mg cohort of patients, the mean central subfield OCT thickness decreased from a baseline of 518.2 to 225.4 μm at day 120 with one patient requiring Ahmed shunt placement for elevated intraocular pressure.[62] This device has not yet been tested in DME patients.

For patients with DME refractory to further laser treatment, these sustained release steroid devices may serve as potential treatment options as long as cataracts and possible glaucoma are monitored and treated appropriately.

STEROIDS AND NVAMD: PRIOR STUDIES AND FUTURE DIRECTIONS

CNV beneath the retina or retinal pigment epithelium is the most common cause of irreversible retinal damage and visual loss in patients with age-related macular degeneration (AMD). The gold standard treatment for this condition is an intravitreal injection of humanized monoclonal antibodies, antibody fragments or aptamers, target VEGF receptors, blocking a major step in angiogenesis.[63] However, experimental and clinical evidence indicate that the processes of inflammation and neovascularization are intrinsically connected, with multiple factors leading aberrant subretinal blood vessel formation. Numerous inflammatory cytokines, growth factors, and intracellular adhesion molecules[64] are associated with increased vascular permeability, breakdown of the blood-retinal barrier, remodeling of the extracellular matrix and upregulation of proangiogenic factors.[33] Specific cell types, including macrophages, contribute to this phenomenon through expression of inflammatory cytokines[65] and have been found in pathologic samples from donors with AMD.[66]

Pharmacologic strategies using steroids to target the inflammatory-angiogenesis cascade in CNV formation have been widely used for many years. Steroids inhibit proinflammatory cell types including macrophages and leukocytes,[34] prevent extracellular matrix remodeling,[33] suppress VEGF expression in smooth muscle cells,[20] and inhibit other proangiogenic cytokines such as interleukin-6 (IL-6).[67] Additionally, steroids induce lipocortin synthesis,

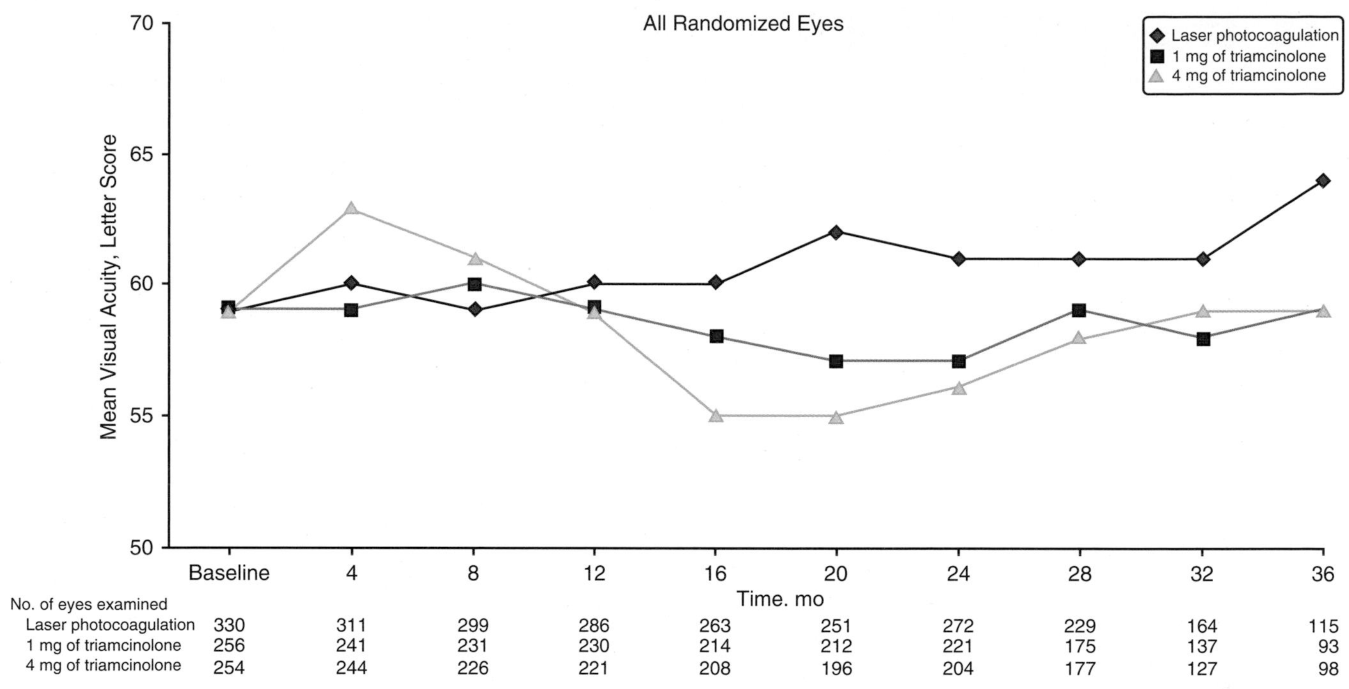

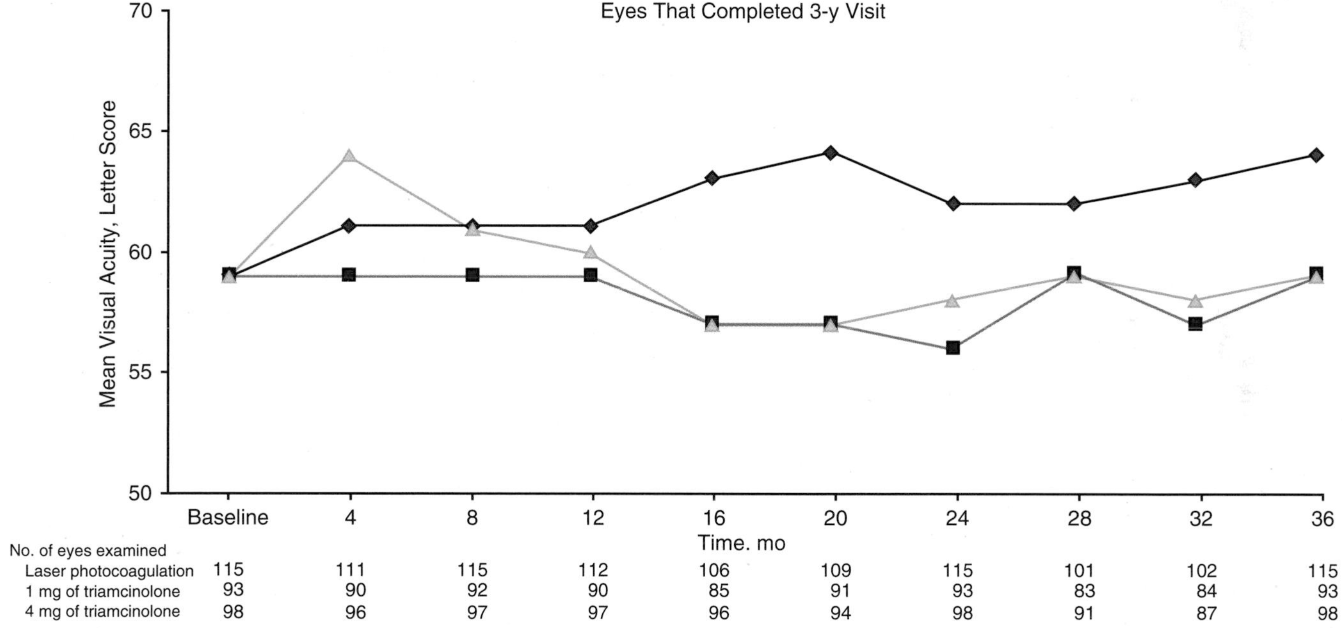

FIGURE 16.5. Mean visual acuity at each visit according to treatment group. Three-year follow-up of a randomized trial comparing focal/grid photocoagulation and IVTA for DME. (Reproduced from DRCR Network. *Arch Ophthalmol.* 2009;127:245, with permission.)

leading to sequential downstream inhibition of inflammatory mediators including phospholipase A2, arachadonic acid, prostaglandins, and leukotrienes.[68] The synergistic mechanisms of steroids including inhibition of angiogenesis and prevention of blood-retinal barrier breakdown led to their use for the treatment of AMD.

Triamcinolone Acetonide for NVAMD

Intravitreal injection of triamcinolone has been used for both the primary treatment of and as an adjunct to PDT for exudative AMD.[69] Early in vitro studies of epithelial cells exposed to stimulators of I-CAM expression such as interferon gamma or tumor necrosis factor suggested that triamcinolone significantly decreased induced vascular permeability through normalization of transepithelial resistance to fluid flow and junctional morphology.[70] Experimental studies in rats that received krypton laser burns to induce CNV demonstrated that eyes that received IVTA had no development of CNV compared to 69% of saline-injected eyes. This implies that triamcinolone caused

BOX 16.2 Trials using Steroids in Neovascular ARMD

VISTA Trial
Study of combined Visudyne therapy with Kenalog in CNV secondary to AMD (see Chapter 23)

VERITAS Trial
Verteporfin IVTA Acetonide Study (see Chapter 23)

LUCEDEX Trial: A Prospective Study Comparing Ranibizumab Plus Dexamethasone Combination Therapy versus Ranibizumab Monotherapy for Wet AMD

Purpose
A Phase 1/2 prospective randomized, safety study comparing intravitreal ranibizumab and dexamethasone combination therapy with intravitreal ranibizumab monotherapy in neovascular ARMD. Arm 1: same day combination therapy with 0.05 mL dose intravitreal dexamethasone injection (10 mg/mL vial) and a single 0.5 mg intravitreal ranibizumab injection, Arm 2: intravitreal injection of 0.5 mg ranibizumab.
Status: Ongoing.

PDEX II Trial: Triple therapy using PDT, intravitreal dexamethasone and intravitreal Ranibizumab injections versus monotherapy with intravitreal Ranibizumab alone

Purpose
A prospective, Phase 2 randomized, masked, efficacy pilot study to compare triple combination therapy of intravitreal ranibizumab, dexamethasone, and PDT with intravitreal ranibizumab monotherapy in neovascular ARMD. *Group 1:* One 500 μg dose (0.05 mL) intravitreal dexamethasone (10 mg/mL vial) in combination with Visudyne PDT and 0.5 mg intravitreal Ranibizumab injection on the same day. *Group 2:* One 0.5 mg intravitreal Ranibizumab injection. Group 1 patients will receive retreatment on a PRN basis, whereas Group 2 patients every 4 weeks for 12 months.
Status: Ongoing.

RADICAL Trial: Reduced Fluence Visudyne Anti-VEGF-Dexamethasone In Combination for AMD Lesions (see Chapter 23)

potent inhibition of fibrovascular proliferation.[71] Based on these and other results demonstrating its antiangiogenic and antiedematous effects,[7–9,39,72–77] triamcinolone has been used in humans for the treatment of exudative AMD. Initial, nonrandomized studies with small numbers of patients demonstrated an apparent benefit in visual acuity with triamcinolone treatment at various doses compared to the natural disease course, including minimally classic and occult lesions for which PDT could not be applied.[5,69,78–86] However, the effect appears to decline after only a few months. Repeated injections often showed decreased efficacy despite IOP elevation and cataract progression that were seen in significant number of treated patients who then required topical treatment or surgery to manage as a result. Subsequent larger, prospective trials found a similar indication of tachyphylaxis.[87–89] For example, Gilles et al.[89] found that a single dose of 4 mg IVTA had no effect on the risk of loss of visual acuity during the first year of the study, despite a significant antiangiogenic effect found 3 months after treatment. Although treatment seems to have a beneficial short-term effect on visual acuity and CNV lesion size, current consensus is that IVTA has a transient effect with a significant side effect risk profile and should not be used as a monotherapy for exudative AMD (Box 16.2).

Triamcinolone Acetonide and PDT with Verteporfin for NVAMD

Despite the disappointing long-term results as a monotherapy, considerable enthusiasm developed for the use of IVTA combined with PDT with verteporfin (Visudyne, Novartis Pharmaceuticals Corporation, East Hanover, NJ) as a treatment for exudative AMD.[39,90] PDT leads to selective cytotoxicity of vascular endothelial cells through production of oxidative radicals but may cause upregulation of VEGF and induce leakage from CNV shortly after treatment.[91,92] Therefore, combining PDT with an antiangiogenic agent such as a steroid may have added benefit compared to PDT alone. Spaide et al. evaluated 26 eyes, which received PDT immediately followed by an intravitreal injection of 4 mg of triamcinolone, with retreatment based on fluorescein angiographic evidence of leakage at 3-month follow-up intervals. Patients were subdivided into those who had or had not received prior PDT. In the treatment-naïve group, significant visual acuity gains were seen at 3 and 6 months, and approximately 30% of patients had an improvement of at least three lines. Conversely, in the previously PDT-treated group, no patients required retreatment but no significant visual acuity gains were seen at 3 or 6 months, and only one patient had an improvement of at least three lines at each time point. This small study concluded that combination triamcinolone and PDT therapy for exudative AMD may have significant benefit especially for treatment-naïve patients, but most patients still required retreatment at 3 months similar to the Treatment of AMD with PDT (TAP) and Verteporfin in Photodynamic Therapy (VIP) trials (Figs. 16.6 and 16.7).[39,93,94]

Longer-term studies of IVTA as an adjunctive treatment to PDT with verteporfin demonstrated safety and visual

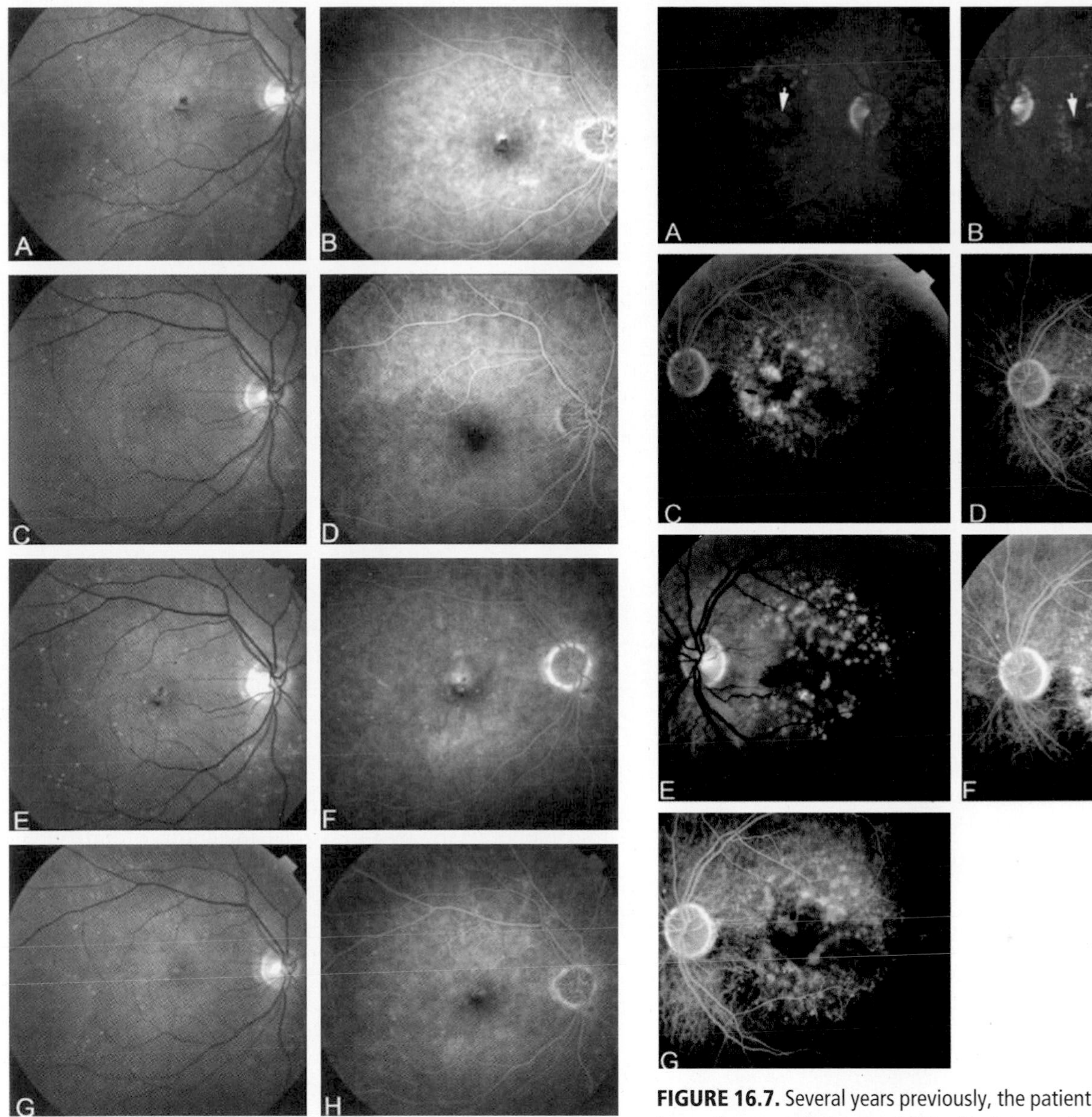

FIGURE 16.6. This patient presented with CNV in the superior fovea of the right eye. Note the pattern of hemorrhages **(A)** and the leakage seen during fluorescein angiography **(B)**. His initial visual acuity was 20/50. When examined 6 months after one treatment, the neovascularization was not visible by either ophthalmoscopy **(C)** or fluorescein angiography **(D)**. His visual acuity was 20/25. Nine months after the first treatment, the patient was asymptomatic, and visual acuity was 20/25. The pattern of hemorrhage **(E)** and leakage seen during fluorescein angiography **(F)** was quite similar to that seen at baseline. The patient was treated with another session of PDT and IVTA. When examined 12 months after initial presentation, he was seen to have nearly complete resorption of hemorrhage **(G)** and no sign of leakage **(H)** during fluorescein angiography. His visual acuity was 20/30. (Reproduced from Spaide, et al. *Retina.* 2005;25:685, with permission.)

FIGURE 16.7. Several years previously, the patient underwent thermal laser photocoagulation for CNV in the right eye (*arrow*) **(A)**. In the left eye **(B)**, he had a hemorrhage located in a symmetrical location (*arrow*). The neovascularization was not well defined **(C)**. Visual acuity was 20/60. The patient was treated with combined PDT and IVTA; 6 months after treatment, visual acuity was 20/40, and there was no evidence of neovascularization **(D)**. Nine months after the first treatment, the patient returned with a hemorrhage **(E)** that was similar in appearance to that seen at presentation with leakage seen during fluorescein angiography **(F)**. He underwent repeated treatment with combined PDT and IVTA; when examined 12 months after presentation, his visual acuity was 20/40 with no evidence of neovascularization **(G)**. (Reproduced from Spaide, et al. *Retina.* 2005;25:685, with permission.)

stabilization in the first 3 to 24 months for lesions with some classic component in >50% of patients[95] and gradual visual improvement in most patients.[35,95] Retreatment rates were lower compared with triamcinolone monotherapy trials, although a significant number of eyes developed cataract (27%–50%) or required glaucoma therapy (21%–25%) or glaucoma surgery (1%) due to increased intraocular pressure. Another group used modified indocyanine green–mediated PDT in combination with IVTA and found similar results in terms of stability or improvement in visual acuity and decrease of subretinal fluid, though over a more limited follow-up period (3–26 months).[96] Specific anatomic changes have also been associated with decreased combination treatment efficacy. One study of patients with chorioretinal anastomosis associated with neovascular AMD showed initial improvement over the first year, but significant visual loss due to CNV recurrence after 2 years.[97]

Anecortave Acetate for NVAMD

Anecortave acetate (Retaane, Alcon, Fort Worth, TX) is a synthetic steroid devoid of glucocorticoid activity with a potent antiangiogenic activity.[25–28,98] It is a slow-release depot suspension, 15 mg delivered via a juxtascleral sub-Tenon retrobulbar injection every 6 months. A trial of 128 eyes of 128 patients found that a single 15 mg injection was safe and resulted in greater stabilization and improvement of visual acuity when compared to the placebo group in AMD patients with subfoveal CNV.[99,100] A phase 3 clinical trial comparing a posterior juxtascleral administration of anecortave acetate for depot suspension 15 mg every 3 months with 15 mg every 6 months versus 30 mg every 6 months during 24 months is ongoing.[101] However, in light of the significant benefits of intravitreal anti-VEGF agents, juxtascleral anecortave may be a second-line, vision-conserving therapeutic option for fibrotic lesions in patients who fail primary intravitreal treatment.[102]

Anecortave Acetate and Photodynamic Therapy with Verteporfin for NVAMD

A prospective, multicenter, randomized study compared 1-year safety and efficacy data regarding posterior juxtascleral depot (PJD) injections of anecortave acetate with PDT in patients with CNV due to AMD. Five hundred thirty-six patients were randomized in a 1:1 ratio to receive either anecortave acetate 15 mg or PDT with verteporfin. Patients who were assigned to PDT were given up to four PDT treatments at 3-month intervals based upon fluorescein angiography. Before the first anecortave acetate injection, patients were given a sham PDT treatment, which was repeated every 3 months if there was evidence of leakage on fluorescein angiogram. Patients in the PDT group were given a sham PJD procedure at the start of the study and at month 6. The main outcome was the percentage of patients losing fewer than three Snellen lines at month 12. At 1 year, the mean change in visual acuity from baseline was not clinically significant between groups, leading the authors to conclude that posterior sub-Tenon's injections of anecortave acetate was comparable to PDT for maintaining vision in patients with subfoveal CNV secondary to AMD.[103]

Squalamine for NVAMD

Squalamine lactate (Evizon, Genaera, New York, NY) is a naturally occurring steroidal compound derived from dogfish shark fin and which inhibits cell membrane Na^+/H^+ exchange and functions as a calmodulin chaperone, suppressing endothelial cell proliferation.[104] It also inhibits iris neovascularization when administered by intravenous injection, although it is ineffective when administered by intravitreal injection.[105,106] Squalamine has been shown to induce regression of experimental retinopathy of prematurity in a mouse model.[107] Although several phase 2 and 2 trials have been initiated to determine the safety and efficacy of intravenous squalamine for the treatment of exudative AMD, all have been terminated prior to completion and without reporting clinical results.[108]

Combination Double and Triple Therapy for NVAMD

Despite the almost complete replacement of intravitreal steroid monotherapy by intravitreal injections of anti-VEGF agents, there is interest in developing combination therapies using PDT with verteporfin, anti-VEGF agents, and IVTA acetonide or dexamethasone (Figs. 16.8 and 16.9) in order to decrease the frequency and cost of treatment while maximizing the visual outcomes and minimizing side effects. Randomized, phase 2 and 3 studies designed to evaluate various combination treatments include the following:

1. intravitreal injection of either a 1 or 4 mg of triamcinolone (TA) or no injection with PDT **(VISTA)**,
2. one of two different doses of TA in combination with PDT plus intravitreal pegaptanib **(VERITAS)**,
3. triple therapy using PDT, intravitreal dexamethasone, and intravitreal ranibizumab (Lucentis, Genentech, South San Francisco, CA) injections versus monotherapy with intravitreal Ranibizumab alone **(PDEX II)**,

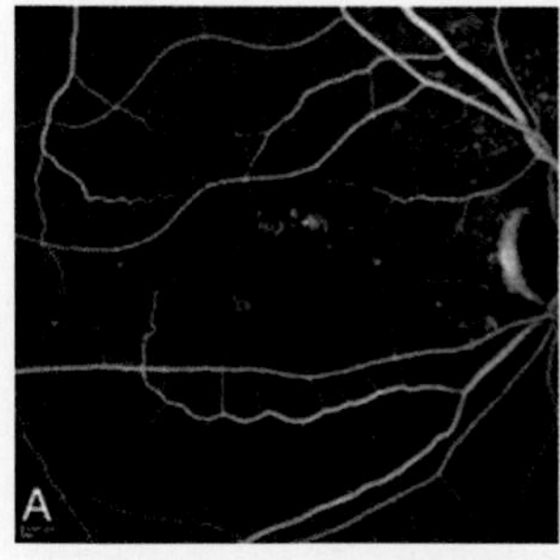

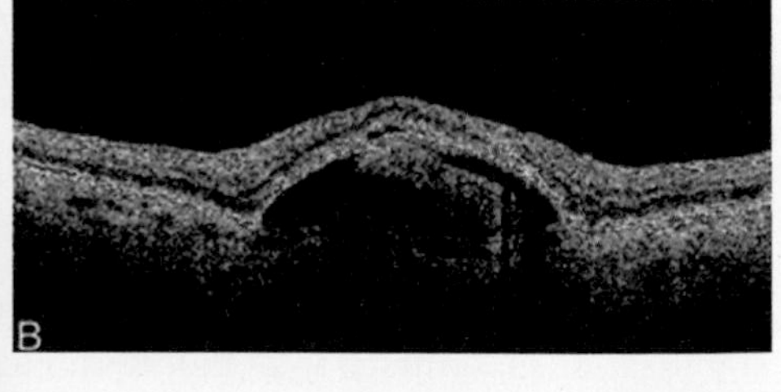

FIGURE 16.8. A: Baseline fluorescein angiogram (FA) of treatment-naïve patient showing CNV with minimally classic vascular leakage and presumed retinal angiomatous proliferation lesion (RAP). **B:** OCT of same patient showing a pigment epithelial detachment (PED) and subretinal fluid. The patient received same-day triple therapy with reduced fluence PDT (25 J/cm²), intravitreal dexamethasone (200 μg), and intravitreal bevacizumab (1.25 mg). (Reproduced from Bakri et al. *Retina.* 2009;29:573, with permission.)

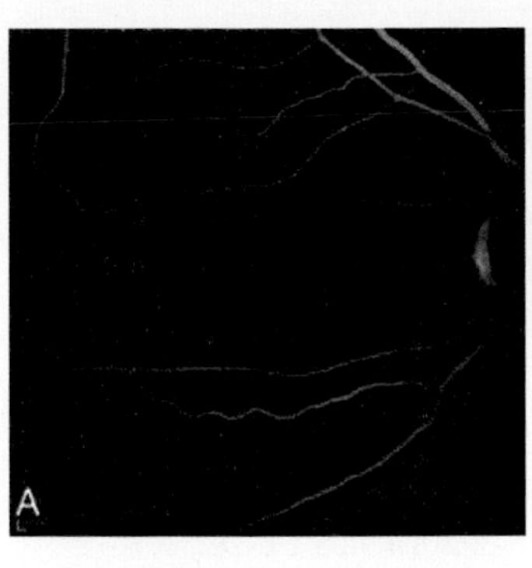

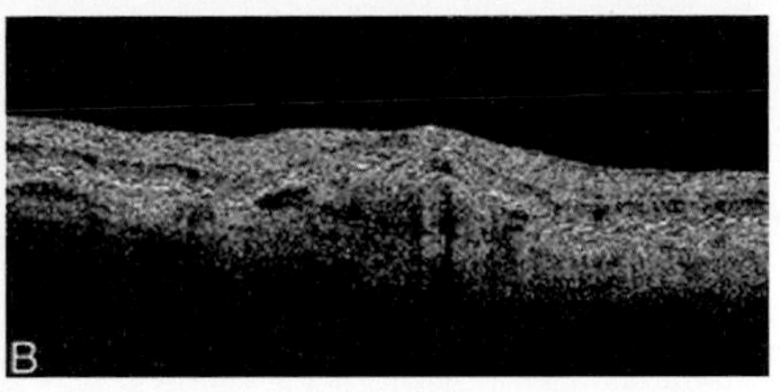

FIGURE 16.9. **A:** Repeat FA at 6 months of the same patient from Figure 16.8 showing resolution of RAP lesion and vascular leakage after triple therapy. The patient received no other treatments in the 6-month interim. **B:** OCT of same patient showing PED still present but subretinal fluid nearly resolved. (Reproduced from Bakri et al. *Retina.* 2009;29:573, with permission.)

4. double- and triple- anti-VEGF-dexamethasone therapy arms with reduced fluence PDT (**RADICAL**), and
5. ranibizumab plus dexamethasone compared to ranibizumab alone without the use of PDT (**LuceDex**).

Another trial investigated whether a triple therapy with bevacizumab (Avastin, Genentech, South San Francisco, CA), half fluence PDT, and preservative free triamcinolone acetonide (**VERTACL**) was terminated due to poor enrollment.[109] Long-term results from these trials may facilitate individualized treatments for AMD patients that include adjunctive steroids along with anti-VEGF therapy.

KEY POINTS

- Intravitreal steroids have been shown to be inferior to laser photocoagulation—the current standard of care—for treatment of DME in eyes still treatable by laser.
- Intravitreal steroids have significant side effects including cataract and glaucoma-related complications.
- Intravitreal steroids may still have a therapeutic role in laser-refractory cases of DME or as an adjunct to laser for DME.
- The role of newer sustained release steroid devices in DME and NVAMD has yet to be defined.
- Intravitreal steroids in various formulations may have an adjunctive role in treating neovascular AMD along with anti-VEGF therapy—the standard of care—and PDT.

Support: National Eye Institute of the National Institute of Health EY001792 Core Grant and Gerhard Cless Retina Research Fund.

REFERENCES

1. Peyman GA, Herbst R. Bacterial endophthalmitis. Treatment with intraocular injection of gentamicin and dexamethasone. *Arch Ophthalmol-Chic.* 1974;91:416–418.
2. Tano Y, Chandler D, Machemer R. Treatment of intraocular proliferation with intravitreal injection of triamcinolone acetonide. *Am J Ophthalmol.* 1980;90:810–816.
3. McCuen BW, Bessler M, Tano Y, et al. The lack of toxicity of intravitreally administered triamcinolone acetonide. *Am J Ophthalmol.* 1981;91:785–788.
4. Joussen AM, Poulaki V, Le ML, et al. A central role for inflammation in the pathogenesis of diabetic retinopathy. *FASEB J.* 2004;18:1450–1452.
5. Penfold PL, Gyory JF, Hunyor AB, et al. Exudative macular degeneration and intravitreal triamcinolone. A pilot study. *Aus N Z J Ophthalmol.* 1995;23:293–298.
6. Jermak CM, Dellacroce JT, Heffez J, et al. Triamcinolone acetonide in ocular therapeutics. *Surv Ophthalmol.* 2007;52:503–522.
7. Penfold PL, Wen L, Madigan MC, et al. Triamcinolone acetonide modulates permeability and intercellular adhesion molecule-1 (ICAM-1) expression of the ECV304 cell line: implications for macular degeneration. *Clin Exp Immunol.* 2000;121:458–465.
8. Penfold PL, Wen L, Madigan MC, et al. Modulation of permeability and adhesion molecule expression by human choroidal endothelial cells. *Invest Ophthalmol Vis Sci.* 2002;43:3125–3130.
9. Penfold PL, Wong JG, Gyory J, et al. Effects of triamcinolone acetonide on microglial morphology and quantitative expression of MHC-II in exudative age-related macular degeneration. *Clin Experiment Ophthalmol.* 2001;29:188–192.
10. Miyamoto K, Khosrof S, Bursell SE, et al. Prevention of leukostasis and vascular leakage in streptozotocin-induced diabetic retinopathy via intercellular adhesion molecule-1 inhibition. *Proc Natl Acad Sci U S A.* 1999;96:10836–10841.
11. Barouch FC, Miyamoto K, Allport JR, et al. Integrin-mediated neutrophil adhesion and retinal leukostasis in diabetes. *Invest Ophthalmol Vis Sci.* 2000;41:1153–1158.
12. Tamura H, Miyamoto K, Kiryu J, et al. Intravitreal injection of corticosteroid attenuates leukostasis and vascular leakage in experimental diabetic retina. *Invest Ophthalmol Vis Sci.* 2005;46:1440–1444.
13. Kern TS. Contributions of inflammatory processes to the development of the early stages of diabetic retinopathy. *Exp Diab Res.* 2007;95–103.
14. Aiello LP, Bursell SE, Clermont A, et al. Vascular endothelial growth factor-induced retinal permeability is mediated by protein kinase C in vivo and suppressed by an orally effective beta-isoform-selective inhibitor. *Diabetes.* 1997;46:1473–1480.
15. Antonetti DA, Barber AJ, Hollinger LA, et al. Vascular endothelial growth factor induces rapid phosphorylation of tight junction proteins occludin and zonula occluden 1. A potential mechanism for vascular permeability in diabetic retinopathy and tumors. *J Biol Chem.* 1999;274:23463–23467.

16. Senger DR, Galli SJ, Dvorak AM, et al. Tumor cells secrete a vascular permeability factor that promotes accumulation of ascites fluid. *Science.* 1983;219:983–985.
17. Rosenfeld PJ, Rich RM, Lalwani GA. Ranibizumab: Phase 3 clinical trial results. *Ophthalmol Clin N Am.* 2006;19:361–372.
18. Joussen AM, Poulaki V, Mitsiades N, et al. Suppression of Fas-FasL-induced endothelial cell apoptosis prevents diabetic blood-retinal barrier breakdown in a model of streptozotocin-induced diabetes. *FASEB J.* 2003;17:76–78.
19. Rosenfeld PJ, Brown DM, Heier JS, et al. Ranibizumab for neovascular age-related macular degeneration. *N Engl J Med.* 2006;355:1419–1431.
20. Nauck M, Karakiulakis G, Perruchoud AP, et al. Corticosteroids inhibit the expression of the vascular endothelial growth factor gene in human vascular smooth muscle cells. *Eur J Pharmacol.* 1998;341:309–315.
21. Nauck M, Roth M, Tamm M, et al. Induction of vascular endothelial growth factor by platelet-activating factor and platelet-derived growth factor is downregulated by corticosteroids. *Am J Respir Cell Mol Biol.* 1997;16:398–406.
22. Andrade RE, Muccioli C, Farah ME, et al. Intravitreal triamcinolone in the treatment of serous retinal detachment in Vogt-Koyanagi-Harada syndrome. *Am J Ophthalmol.* 2004;137:572–574.
23. Francis BA, Chang EL, Haik BG. Particle size and drug interactions of injectable corticosteroids used in ophthalmic practice. *Ophthalmology.* 1996;103:1884–1888.
24. Degenring RF, Jonas JB. Serum levels of triamcinolone acetonide after intravitreal injection. *Am J Ophthalmol.* 2004;137:1142–1143.
25. Yang R, McCollum G, Bingaman D, et al. The effect of anecortave acetate on VEGF message and protein levels in hypoxic muller cells and in RAT OIR. *Invest Ophthalmol Vis Sci.* 2005;46:E-Abstract 4177.
26. Liu C, Gu X, Wang W, et al. Local delivery of anecortave acetate inhibits the expression of retinal IGF-1/IGF-1 receptor in the rat OIR model. *Investig Ophthalmol Vis Sci.* 2005;46:E-Abstract 4135.
27. Folkman J, Ingber DE. Angiostatic steroids. Method of discovery and mechanism of action. *Ann Surg.* 1987;206:374–383.
28. Folkman J, Weisz PB, Joullié MM, et al. Control of angiogenesis with synthetic heparin substitutes. *Science.* 1989;243:1490–1493.
29. Clark AF. Preclinical efficacy of anecortave acetate. *Surv Ophthalmol.* 2007;S2 Suppl 1:S26–S43.
30. Miller JW, Walsh AW, Kramer M, et al. Photodynamic therapy of experimental choroidal neovascularization using lipoprotein-delivered benzoporphyrin. *Arch Ophthalmol.* 1995;113:810–818.
31. Miller JW, Schmidt-Erfurth U, Sickenberg M, et al. Photodynamic therapy with verteporfin for choroidal neovascularization caused by age-related macular degeneration: results of a single treatment in a phase 1 and 2 study. *Arch Ophthalmol.* 1999;117:1161–1173.
32. Schmidt-Erfurth U, Miller JW, Sickenberg M, et al. Photodynamic therapy with verteporfin for choroidal neovascularization caused by age-related macular degeneration: results of retreatments in a phase 1 and 2 study. *Arch Ophthalmol.* 1999;117:1177–1187.
33. Bressler NM, Treatment of Age-Related Macular Degeneration with Photodynamic Therapy (TAP) Study Group. Photodynamic therapy of subfoveal choroidal neovascularization in age-related macular degeneration with verteporfin: two-year results of 2 randomized clinical trials-tap report 2. *Arch Ophthalmol.* 2001;119:198–207.
34. Kreines K, Weinberg IC. The selection of adrenocorticosteroid preparations. *Ohio State Med J.* 1975;71:698:703–706.
35. Augustin AJ, Schmidt-Erfurth U. Verteporfin therapy combined with intravitreal triamcinolone in all types of choroidal neovascularization due to age-related macular degeneration. *Ophthalmology.* 2006;113:14–22.
36. Wang K, Wang Y, Gao L, et al. Dexamethasone inhibits leukocyte accumulation and vascular permeability in retina of streptozotocin-induced diabetic rats via reducing vascular endothelial growth factor and intercellular adhesion molecule-1 expression. *Biol Pharm Bull.* 2008;31:1541–1546.
37. Edelman JL, Lutz D, Castro MR. Corticosteroids inhibit VEGF-induced vascular leakage in a rabbit model of blood-retinal and blood-aqueous barrier breakdown. *Exp Eye Res.* 2005;80:249–258.
38. Heier JS, Boyer DS, Ciulla TA, et al. Ranibizumab combined with verteporfin photodynamic therapy in neovascular age-related macular degeneration: year 1 results of the FOCUS Study. *Arch Ophthalmol.* 2006;124:1532–1542.
39. Spaide RF, Sorenson J, Maranan L. Photodynamic therapy with verteporfin combined with intravitreal injection of triamcinolone acetonide for choroidal neovascularization. *Ophthalmology.* 2005;112:301–304.
40. Bakri SJ, Couch SM, McCannel CA, et al. Same-day triple therapy with photodynamic therapy, intravitreal dexamethasone, and bevacizumab in wet age-related macular degeneration. *Retina.* 2009;29:573–578.
41. Liggett PE, Colina J, Chaudhry NA, et al. Triple therapy of intravitreal triamcinolone, photodynamic therapy, and pegaptanib sodium for choroidal neovascularization. *Am J Ophthalmol.* 2006;142:1072–1074.
42. Kuppermann BD, Blumenkranz MS, Haller JA, et al. Randomized controlled study of an intravitreous dexamethasone drug delivery system in patients with persistent macular edema. *Arch Ophthalmol.* 2007;125:309–317.
43. Jaffe GJ, Martin D, Callanan D, et al. Fluocinolone acetonide implant (Retisert) for noninfectious posterior uveitis: thirty-four-week results of a multicenter randomized clinical study. *Ophthalmology.* 2006;113:1020–1027.
44. Ayalasomayajula SP, Ashton P, Kompella UB. Fluocinolone inhibits VEGF expression via glucocorticoid receptor in human retinal pigment epithelial (ARPE-19) cells and TNF-alpha-induced angiogenesis in chick chorioallantoic membrane (CAM). *J Ocul Pharmacol Ther.* 2009;25:97–103.
45. Pearson P, Levy B, Comstock T, et al. Fluocinolone acetonide intravitreal implant to treat diabetic macular edema: 3-year results of a multi-center clinical trial. Association for Research in Vision and Ophthalmology Annual Meeting, 2006. Poster #5442.
46. Jonas JB, Söfker A. Intraocular injection of crystalline cortisone as adjunctive treatment of diabetic macular edema. *Am J Ophthalmol.* 2001;132:425–427.
47. Martidis A, Duker JS, Greenberg PB, et al. Intravitreal triamcinolone for refractory diabetic macular edema. *Ophthalmology.* 2002;109:920–927.

48. Jonas JB, Kreissig I, Söfker A, et al. Intravitreal injection of triamcinolone for diffuse diabetic macular edema. *Arch Ophthalmol-Chic.* 2003;121:57–61.
49. Massin P, Audren F, Haouchine B, et al. Intravitreal triamcinolone acetonide for diabetic diffuse macular edema: preliminary results of a prospective controlled trial. *Ophthalmology.* 2004;111:218–224; discussion 224–225.
50. Spandau UH, Derse M, Schmitz-Valckenberg P, et al. Dosage dependency of intravitreal triamcinolone acetonide as treatment for diabetic macular oedema. *Br J Ophthalmol.* 2005;89: 999–1003.
51. Grover D, Li TJ, Chong CC. Intravitreal steroids for macular edema in diabetes. *Cochrane Database Syst Rev.* (Online) 2008;CD005656.
52. Diabetic Retinopathy Clinical Research Network. A randomized trial comparing intravitreal triamcinolone acetonide and focal/grid photocoagulation for diabetic macular edema. *Ophthalmology.* 2008;115:1447–1449, 1449.e1–e10.
53. Jonas JB, Harder B, Kamppeter BA. Inter-eye difference in diabetic macular edema after unilateral intravitreal injection of triamcinolone acetonide. *Am J Ophthalmol.* 2004;138:970–977.
54. Jonas JB, Degenring RF, Kamppeter BA, et al. Duration of the effect of intravitreal triamcinolone acetonide as treatment for diffuse diabetic macular edema. *Am J Ophthalmol.* 2004;138: 158–160.
55. Sutter FK, Simpson JM, Gillies MC. Intravitreal triamcinolone for diabetic macular edema that persists after laser treatment: three-month efficacy and safety results of a prospective, randomized, double-masked, placebo-controlled clinical trial. *Ophthalmology.* 2004;111:2044–2049.
56. Ciardella AP, Klancnik J, Schiff W, et al. Intravitreal triamcinolone for the treatment of refractory diabetic macular oedema with hard exudates: an optical coherence tomography study. *Br J Ophthalmol.* 2004;88:1131–1136.
57. Ozkiris A, Evereklioglu C, Oner A, et al. Pattern electroretinogram for monitoring the efficacy of intravitreal triamcinolone injection in diabetic macular edema. *Documenta ophthalmologica. Adv Ophthalmol.* 2004;109:139–145.
58. Jonas JB, Martus P, Degenring RF, et al. Predictive factors for visual acuity after intravitreal triamcinolone treatment for diabetic macular edema. *Arch Ophthalmol-Chic.* 2005; 123:1338–1343.
59. Lam DS, Chan CK, Mohamed S, et al. Intravitreal triamcinolone plus sequential grid laser versus triamcinolone or laser alone for treating diabetic macular edema: six-month outcomes. *Ophthalmology.* 2007;114:2162–2167.
60. Diabetic Retinopathy Clinical Research Network (DRCR.net), Beck RW, Edwards AR, et al. Three-year follow-up of a randomized trial comparing focal/grid photocoagulation and intravitreal triamcinolone for diabetic macular edema. *Arch Ophthalmol-Chic.* 2009;127:245–251.
61. DRCR Protocol I. Available from: http://public.drcr.net/DRCRnetstudies/studies/ProtocolI_lrtdme/ProtIInfo.html. Accessed on Nov 5,2009
62. Lim JI, Wieland MR, Fung A, et al. A phase 1 study evaluating the safety and evidence of efficacy of IBI-20089. A triamcinolone intravitreal injection formulated with the verisome™ drug delivery technology. Patients with cystoid macular edema. Association for Research in Vision and Ophthalmology Annual Meeting, 2009:Program 5395/Poster A346.
63. Nowak JZ. Age-related macular degeneration (AMD): pathogenesis and therapy. *Pharmacol Rep.* 2006;58:353–363.
64. Eyetech Study Group. Anti-vascular endothelial growth factor therapy for subfoveal choroidal neovascularization secondary to age-related macular degeneration: phase 2 study results. *Ophthalmology.* 2003;110:979–986.
65. Grossniklaus HE, Ling JX, Wallace TM, et al. Macrophage and retinal pigment epithelium expression of angiogenic cytokines in choroidal neovascularization. *Mol Vis.* 2002;8: 119–126.
66. Bhutto IA, McLeod DS, Hasegawa T, et al. Pigment epithelium-derived factor (PEDF) and vascular endothelial growth factor (VEGF) in aged human choroid and eyes with age-related macular degeneration. *Exp Eye Res.* 2006;82: 99–110.
67. Crum R, Szabo S, Folkman J. A new class of steroids inhibits angiogenesis in the presence of heparin or a heparin fragment. *Science.* 1985;230:1375–1378.
68. Duguid IG, Boyd AW, Mandel TE. Adhesion molecules are expressed in the human retina and choroid. *Curr Eye Res.* 1992;Suppl 11:153–159.
69. Jonas JB. Intravitreal triamcinolone acetonide: a change in a paradigm. *Ophthalmic Res.* 2006;38:218–245.
70. Spaide RF, Sorenson J, Maranan L. Combined photodynamic therapy and intravitreal triamcinolone for nonsubfoveal choroidal neovascularization. *Retina.* 2005;25:685–690.
71. Ciulla TA, Criswell MH, Danis RP, et al. Intravitreal triamcinolone acetonide inhibits choroidal neovascularization in a laser-treated rat model. *Arch Ophthalmol.* 2001;119:399–404.
72. Jonas JB, Söfker A. Intravitreal triamcinolone acetonide for cataract surgery with iris neovascularization. *J Cataract Refract Surg.* 2002;28:2040–2041.
73. Jonas JB, Kreissig I, Degenring RF. Neovascular glaucoma treated by intravitreal triamcinolone acetonide. *Acta Ophthalmol Scand.* 2003;81:540–541.
74. Bonanomi MT, Susanna R. Intravitreal triamcinolone acetonide as adjunctive treatment for neovascular glaucoma. *Clinics (Sao Paulo).* 2005;60:347–350.
75. Danis RP, Bingaman DP, Yang Y, et al. Inhibition of preretinal and optic nerve head neovascularization in pigs by intravitreal triamcinolone acetonide. *Ophthalmology.* 1996;103: 2099–2104.
76. Penn JS, Rajaratnam VS, Collier RJ, et al. The effect of an angiostatic steroid on neovascularization in a rat model of retinopathy of prematurity. *Invest Ophthalmol Vis Sci.* 2001;42:283–290.
77. Wang YS, Friedrichs U, Eichler W, et al. Inhibitory effects of triamcinolone acetonide on bFGF-induced migration and tube formation in choroidal microvascular endothelial cells. *Graefes Arch Clin Exp Ophthalmol.* 2002;240:42–48.
78. Challa JK, Gillies MC, Penfold PL, et al. Exudative macular degeneration and intravitreal triamcinolone: 18 month follow up. *Aus N Z J Ophthalmol.* 1998;26:277–281.
79. Danis RP, Ciulla TA, Pratt LM, et al. Intravitreal triamcinolone acetonide in exudative age-related macular degeneration. *Retina.* 2000;20:244–250.
80. Jonas JB, Degenring RF, Kreissig I, et al. Exudative age-related macular degeneration treated by intravitreal triamcinolone acetonide. A prospective comparative nonrandomized study. *Eye (London, England).* 2005;19:163–170.

81. Jonas JB, Kreissig I, Degenring R. Repeated intravitreal injections of triamcinolone acetonide as treatment of progressive exudative age-related macular degeneration. *Graefes Arch Clin Exp Ophthalmol.* 2002;240:873–874.
82. Jonas JB, Kreissig I, Hugger P, et al. Intravitreal triamcinolone acetonide for exudative age related macular degeneration. *Br J Ophthalmol.* 2003;87:462–468.
83. Jonas JB, Akkoyun I, Budde WM, et al. Intravitreal reinjection of triamcinolone for exudative age-related macular degeneration. *Arch Ophthalmol.* 2004;122:218–222.
84. Jonas JB, Kreissig I, Degenring RF. Factors influencing visual acuity after intravitreal triamcinolone acetonide as treatment of exudative age related macular degeneration. *Br J Ophthalmol.* 2004;88:1557–1562.
85. Jonas JB, Spandau UH, Harder B, et al. Intereye difference in exudative age-related macular degeneration with minimally classic or occult subfoveal neovascularization after unilateral intravitreal injection of triamcinolone acetonide. *Am J Ophthalmol.* 2005;139:1073–1079.
86. Nicolò M, Ghiglione D, Lai S, et al. Intravitreal triamcinolone in the treatment of serous pigment epithelial detachment and occult choroidal neovascularization secondary to age-related macular degeneration. *Eur J Ophthalmol.* 2005;15: 415–419.
87. Jonas JB, Spandau UH, Kamppeter BA, et al. Follow-up after intravitreal triamcinolone acetonide for exudative age-related macular degeneration. *Eye (London, England).* 2007;21:387–394.
88. Ranson NT, Danis RP, Ciulla TA, et al. Intravitreal triamcinolone in subfoveal recurrence of choroidal neovascularisation after laser treatment in macular degeneration. *Br J Ophthalmol.* 2002;86:527–529.
89. Gillies MC, Simpson JM, Luo W, et al. A randomized clinical trial of a single dose of intravitreal triamcinolone acetonide for neovascular age-related macular degeneration: one-year results. *Arch Ophthalmol.* 2003;121:667–673.
90. Arroyo JG, Michaud N, Jakobiec FA. Choroidal neovascular membranes treated with photodynamic therapy. *Arch Ophthalmol.* 2003;121:898–903.
91. Fingar VH. Vascular effects of photodynamic therapy. *J Clin Laser Med Surg.* 1996;14:323–328.
92. Krammer B. Vascular effects of photodynamic therapy. *Anticancer Res.* 2001;21:4271–4277.
93. Verteporfin Roundtable 2000 and 2001 Participants, Treatment of age-related macular degeneration with photodynamic therapy (TAP) study group principal investigators, Verteporfin in photodynamic therapy (VIP) study group principal investigators. Guidelines for using verteporfin (visudyne) in photodynamic therapy to treat choroidal neovascularization due to age-related macular degeneration and other causes. *Retina.* 2002; 22:6–18.
94. Rechtman E, Danis PR, Pratt LM, et al. Intravitreal triamcinolone with photodynamic therapy for subfoveal choroidal neovascularisation in age related macular degeneration. *Br J Ophthalmol.* 2004;88:344–347.
95. Augustin AJ, Schmidt-Erfurth U. Verteporfin and intravitreal triamcinolone acetonide combination therapy for occult choroidal neovascularization in age-related macular degeneration. *Am J Ophthalmol.* 2006;141:638–645.
96. Arevalo JF, Garcia RA, Mendoza AJ. Indocyanine green-mediated photothrombosis with intravitreal triamcinolone acetonide for subfoveal choroidal neovascularization in age-related macular degeneration. *Graefes Arch Clin Exp Ophthalmol.* 2005;243:1180–1185.
97. Silva RM, Cachulo ML, Figueira J, et al. Chorioretinal anastomosis and photodynamic therapy: a two-year follow-up study. *Graefes Arch Clin Exp Ophthalmol.* 2007;245: 1131–1139.
98. Clinical Trial of Visudyne with Kenalog. Available from: http://www.clinicaltrial.gov/ct2/results?term=VISUDYNE±±With±Kenalog. Accessed on Nov 5, 2009.
99. D'Amico DJ, Goldberg MF, Hudson H, et al. Anecortave acetate as monotherapy for the treatment of subfoveal lesions in patients with exudative age-related macular degeneration (AMD): interim (month 6) analysis of clinical safety and efficacy. *Retina.* 2003;23:14–23.
100. D'Amico DJ, Goldberg MF, Hudson H, et al. Anecortave acetate as monotherapy for treatment of subfoveal neovascularization in age-related macular degeneration: twelve-month clinical outcomes. *Ophthalmology.* 2003;110:2372–2383; discussin 2384–2385.
101. Clinical Trial of RETAANE. cited; Available from: http://www.clinicaltrial.gov/ct2/show/NCT00299507?term=RETAANE&rank=4. Accessed on Nov 5, 2009.
102. Aggermann T, Haas P, Binder S. Anecortave acetate for fibrotic lesions with presence of residual peripheral activity in age-related macular degeneration. *Ann Ophthalmol (Skokie, Ill).* 2008;40:28–30.
103. Slakter JS, Bochow TW, D'Amico DJ, et al. Anecortave acetate (15 milligrams) versus photodynamic therapy for treatment of subfoveal neovascularization in age-related macular degeneration. *Ophthalmology.* 2006;113:3–13.
104. Pietras RJ, Weinberg OK. Antiangiogenic steroids in human cancer therapy. Evidence-based complementary and alternative medicine. *eCAM.* 2005;2:49–57.
105. Genaidy M, Kazi AA, Peyman GA, et al. Effect of squalamine on iris neovascularization in monkeys. *Retina.* 2002;22: 772–778.
106. Jones SR, Kinney WA, Zhang X, et al. The synthesis and characterization of analogs of the antimicrobial compound squalamine: 6 beta-hydroxy-3-aminosterols synthesized from hyodeoxycholic acid. *Steroids.* 1996;61:565–571.
107. Higgins RD, Yan Y, Geng Y, et al. Regression of retinopathy by squalamine in a mouse model. *Pediatr Res.* 2004;56:144–149.
108. Clinical Trial of Squalamine for AMD. Available from: http://www.clinicaltrial.gov/ct2/results?term=Squalamine±AND±AMD. Accessed on Nov 5, 2009.
109. Clinical Trial of Combination Therapy for AMD. Available from: http://www.clinicaltrial.gov/ct2/results? term=combination±therapy±for±AMD. Accessed on Nov 5, 2009.

CHAPTER 17

Anti-VEGF Therapies in Retinopathy of Prematurity

Tushar Ranchod • Antonio Capone, Jr.

INTRODUCTION

Retinopathy of prematurity (ROP) remains a leading cause of blindness worldwide.[1] ROP is characterized by avascular peripheral retina, intraocular dysregulation of vascular endothelial growth factor (VEGF), and pathologic vasculogenesis.

Retinal vascular development begins prior to the fourth month of gestation, with vessels emanating from the optic nerve and growing steadily toward the ora serrata as the fetus approaches term.[2] This process may be interrupted by premature birth, resulting in a spectrum of abnormalities known as ROP. At the mildest end of the spectrum, retinal vascular growth may slow down before resuming a normal growth pattern. At the most severe end of the spectrum, normal vascular growth within the plane of the retina ceases and aberrant vasculature grows in the form of intraretinal shunt vessels as well as neovascular networks extending into the vitreous gel. This neovascularization can mature into fibrovascular preretinal tractional bands, which result in tractional retinal detachment.

VASCULAR ABNORMALITIES IN ROP

Intraretinal shunting in ROP occurs along the border of vascular and avascular retina.[3] If persistent, the changes in vascular flow eventually cause vascular tortuosity upstream and downstream until peripapillary tortuosity and venous dilatation occur and are identified as "plus" disease (Fig. 17.1). The presence of plus disease is therefore a proxy for persistent VEGF dysregulation and aberrant retinal vascularization.

The pathogenesis of extraretinal neovascularization in ROP shares common characteristics with proliferative retinal neovascularization seen in diabetes mellitus, retinal vascular occlusions, and a variety of other retinal diseases. Retinal ischemia from a variety of causes may result in elevated intravitreal VEGF levels, which in turn stimulate retinal neovascularization.[4,5]

CLINICAL STAGES OF ROP

The clinical stages of ROP have been described in the International Classification of Retinopathy of Prematurity (ICROP), which was updated most recently in 2005.[6] Stage 1 is a discrete demarcation line between vascular and avascular retina. Stage 2 is a ridge, which rises above the plane of the retina between vascular and avascular retina (Fig. 17.2). Stage 3 is fibrovascular proliferation extending from the ridge into the preretinal vitreous gel (Fig. 17.3). Fibrovascular traction may progress to a tractional retinal detachment. Stage 4 denotes a partial retinal detachment, with Stage 4a denoting a detachment sparing the fovea and Stage 4b involving the fovea (Fig. 17.4). Stage 5 describes a total retinal detachment.

The stages of ROP are described by the number of clock hours involved as well as the zones in which they occur. The retina is divided into Zone 1 posteriorly, which is centered on the optic disc and extends as a circle with a radius equal to twice the distance from the disc to the fovea. Zone 2 extends from the edge of Zone 1 to the nasal ora serrata. The residual crescent of retina remaining temporally is Zone 3.

"Plus" disease is an additional critical variable in the description of ROP. As mentioned above, intraretinal shunts may form within the ridge between vascular and avascular retina, and the resulting vascular flow abnormalities eventually cause dilatation and tortuosity of the peripapillary retinal vessels.

In the latest update of the ICROP, aggressive posterior ROP (APROP) is classified as a discrete form of ROP. APROP progresses rapidly with vascular tortuosity and dilatation in all four quadrants, usually a Zone 1 or posterior Zone 2 location, and frequent progression to Stage 5 ROP if untreated.[6]

INCIDENCE OF ROP

Not all premature infants develop ROP, and the development of ROP is best predicted by low birthweight and early gestational age. The incidence of ROP is approximately 68% in infants born below 1,250 g, with the incidence

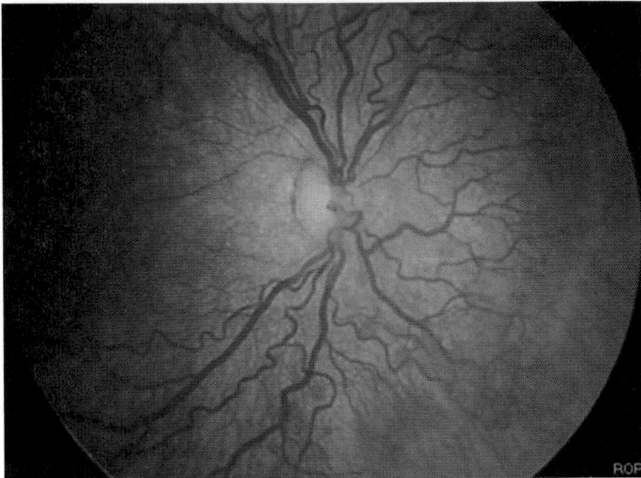

FIGURE 17.1. Plus disease. Intraretinal vascular shunting may progress to peripapillary vascular tortuosity and venous dilatation known as "Plus" disease.

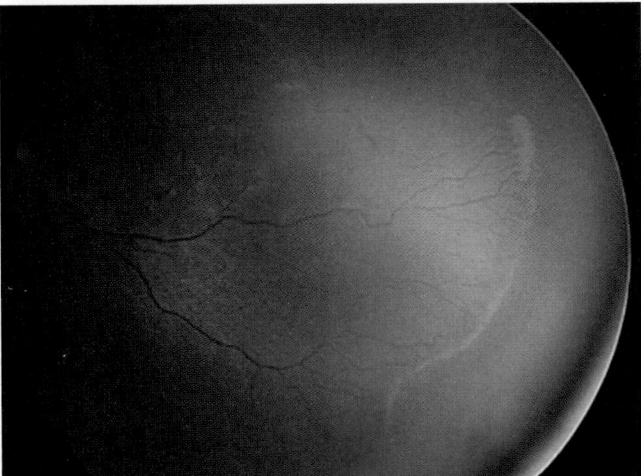

FIGURE 17.2. Stage 2 ROP. In stage 2 disease, a ridge rises above the plane of the retina between vascular and avascular retina. Intraretinal shunt vessels lie within the ridge.

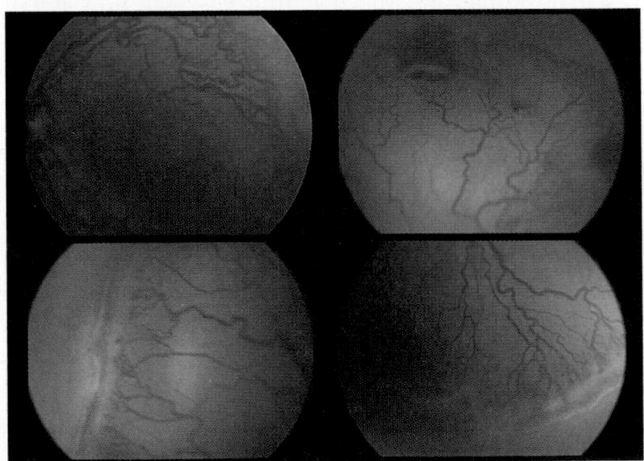

FIGURE 17.3. Stage 3 ROP. Stage 3 is comprised of fibrovascular proliferation extending from the ridge into the vitreous gel.

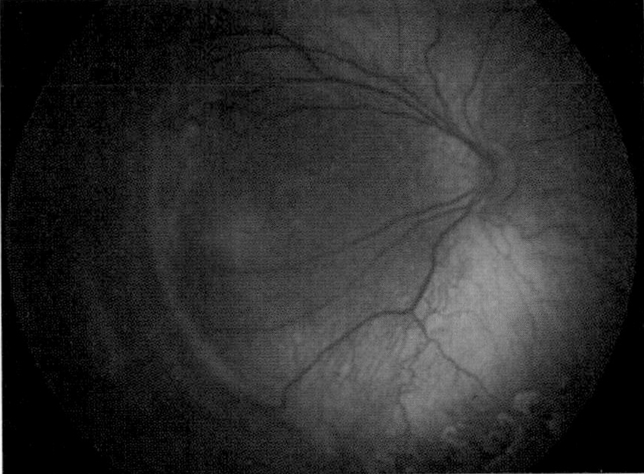

A

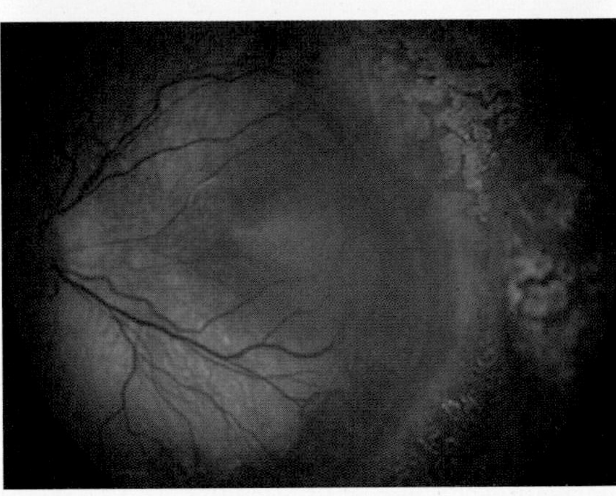

B

FIGURE 17.4. The images (**(A)** right eye top, **(B)** left eye bottom) show bilateral Stage 4b, or macula-involving, detachments, which extend posteriorly from the temporal ridges with neovascularization.

rising to 93% of infants born below 750 g. Similarly, the incidence of ROP is approximately 14% in infants born after 32 weeks gestational age, and the incidence rises to 89% in infants born before 27 weeks.[7]

Most newborns with ROP develop manifestations of disease at fairly predictable intervals, with initial manifestations around 32 weeks postmenstrual age (PMA). Infants who progress to the threshold for ablative treatment usually do so by 37 weeks PMA.[8–11] Approximately 10% of infants with ROP ultimately require treatment, and of the group requiring treatment, approximately 10% progress to retinal detachment despite sufficient laser treatment.[12,13] The exception to this relatively predictable timeline of disease development is a subset of patients with APROP, which progresses early and rapidly to retinal detachment despite timely ablation.[6]

CURRENT MANAGEMENT OF ROP

Infants who reach a treatment threshold of ROP are currently managed with ablation of avascular retina (Box 17.1). Cryotherapy was initially used in the Cryotherapy for

BOX 17.1 Pivotal Trials of Peripheral Retinal Ablation for ROP

CRYO ROP Study: CRYO-ROP

Purpose: To examine the role of cryotherapy in preventing severe vision loss in stage 3 ROP infants.

Method: In this randomized, prospective study, ROP babies with five or more contiguous, or eight cumulative 30 degree sectors (clock hours) of stage 3+ ROP in Zone 1 or 2 were treated with transscleral cryotherapy to the avascular retina (applied in one eye when there was threshold retinopathy in both eyes, or in half the eyes when the threshold severity existed in only one eye). An unfavorable outcome was defined as posterior retinal detachment, posterior retinal fold (usually involving the macula), or retrolental tissue that obscured the view of the posterior pole.

Results: At 12 months, whereas 43% of untreated eyes had an unfavorable outcome, there was significantly less unfavorable outcome in the eyes that received cryotherapy (21.8%).

Conclusions: These data support the efficacy of cryotherapy in reducing the risk of unfavorable ocular outcome from threshold ROP. It is recommended that cryotherapy be considered for both eyes whenever stage 3+ ROP involves the posterior retina (Zone 1) of both eyes. (Palmer, *Doc Ophthalmol.* 1990;74:245.)

ET ROP Study: Early Treatment for ROP

Purpose: To examine the efficacy of ablative treatment in ROP infants with bilateral high-risk prethreshold disease.

Methods: One eye was randomized to early retinal ablative treatment (mostly laser, some cryo) and the fellow eye managed conventionally (control eye). The primary outcome was visual acuity assessed by masked testers using the Teller acuity card procedure. Structural examinations were performed at 6 and 9 months.

Results: Grating acuity results showed a reduction in unfavorable visual acuity outcomes with earlier treatment, from 19.8% to 14.3%. Unfavorable structural outcomes were reduced from 15.6% to 9.0% at 9 months. Further analysis supported retinal ablative therapy for eyes with type I ROP, defined as Zone 1, any stage ROP with plus disease; Zone 1, stage 3 ROP without plus disease; or Zone 2, stage 2 or 3 with plus disease.

Conclusion: Early treatment of high-risk prethreshold ROP significantly reduced unfavorable outcomes in both primary and secondary (structural) measures. (Good, ETROP Group, *Trans Am Ophthalmol Soc.* 2004;102:233.)

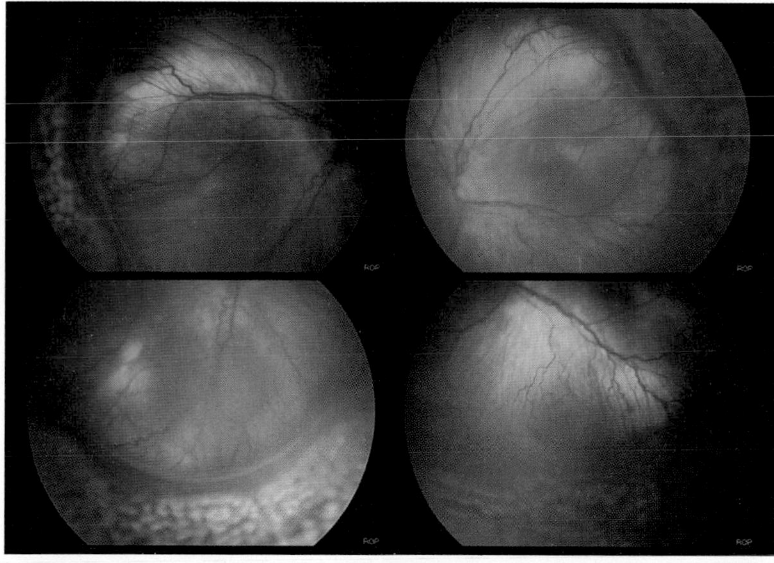

FIGURE 17.5. Laser peripheral laser ablation for threshold ROP. Current standard of care treatment for threshold ROP is thermal laser ablation of the retinal periphery from the ora serrata to the border of vascular and avascular retina.

Retinopathy of Prematurity (CRYO-ROP) trial, but cryotherapy was supplanted by laser photocoagulation in later trials such as the Early Treatment of Retinopathy of Prematurity (ETROP) study. More recent trials have demonstrated superior visual and structural outcomes with laser, which has replaced cryotherapy as the standard-of-care means of peripheral retinal ablation[9,13–15] (Fig. 17.5).

Most cases of disease progression following laser ablation result from inadequate treatment or a delay in treatment after reaching threshold. Even in experienced hands, complete ablation in a single session may be difficult. The border between vascular and avascular retina may be particularly difficult to identify in cases of aggressive posterior disease, due to so-called flat neovascularization characterized by velvety and indistinct edges.[16] Consequently, a second session of laser photocoagulation is often appropriate in eyes with APROP in order to identify and treat any residual skip areas.

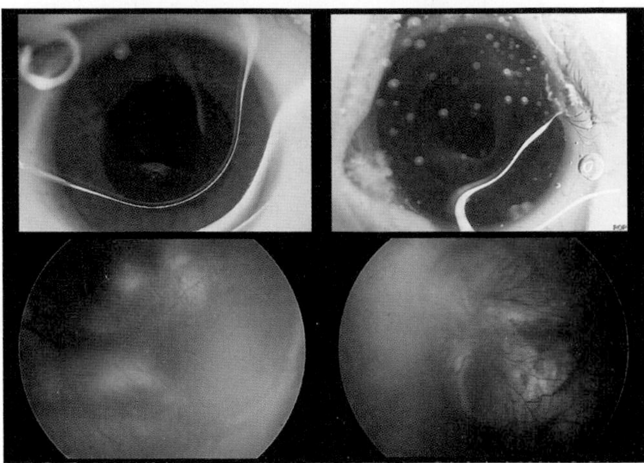

FIGURE 17.6. Poor pupillary dilation or media opacities may prevent the direct visualization needed to deliver peripheral ablation. Diffuse vitreous hemorrhage (**upper left**) may completely obscure the fundus. Persistent tunica vasculosa lentis (**upper right**) may contribute to poor pupillary dilation. Focal or sectoral vitreous hemorrhage (**lower left and right**) may allow incomplete peripheral ablation.

Treatment from the ora serrata to the border of vascularized retina is critical, but complete ablation by laser or cryotherapy is not always possible. In some cases, complete laser ablation may be limited by the surgeon's view (Fig. 17.6). Iris neovascularization and persistent tunica vasculosa occur more commonly in advanced cases of ROP and APROP and may contribute to poor pupillary dilation. The surgeon's view may be limited by hyphema due to iris neovascularization or by vitreous or subhyaloid hemorrhage due to retinal neovascularization, thereby precluding complete laser ablation.

Under ideal circumstances, only about 1% to 2% of newborns with ROP should experience poor structural outcomes, since adequate laser limited poor outcomes to 9% of cases in the ETROP trial, and tertiary care centers have reported good structural and visual outcomes in approximately 90% of cases, which progress to subtotal retinal detachment.[7,17–19] The actual percentage of poor outcomes may remain higher than 2% due to limitations in manpower, an inability to predict which newborns will develop severe disease, and an incomplete arsenal of treatment options to cover all clinical scenarios. The last few years have seen an increased understanding of the pathophysiology of ROP, including the role of VEGF and the potential use of antiangiogenic pharmacologic therapies in the treatment of ROP.

EFFECT OF PERIPHERAL ABLATION ON VEGF LEVELS

The clinical staging of ROP has been used in clinic trials to determine the threshold for peripheral retinal ablative treatment. The CRYO-ROP study demonstrated treatment benefits based on a threshold of five contiguous or eight noncontiguous clock hours of stage 3 disease. The ETROP subsequently redefined the threshold for treatment as Zone 1 disease of any stage with plus disease; stage 3 in Zone 1 regardless of plus disease; or stage 2 or 3 disease in Zone 2 in the presence of plus disease.

Animal models of ROP have demonstrated that the avascular peripheral retina is responsible for producing abnormally high VEGF levels associated with ROP.[20] Presumably, laser photocoagulation of peripheral avascular retina decreases VEGF production by ablating hypoxic tissue and thereby reducing the stimulus for VEGF production.[3] Clinically, regression of ROP is usually seen following peripheral laser ablation, with resolution of plus disease and regression of fibrovascular proliferation.

Peripheral ablation is not universally effective in eliciting regression of ROP. This is particularly true for APROP, which typically afflicts profoundly premature neonates.[6] In this subset of infants, progression of ROP to bilateral retinal detachment and blindness may occur despite timely and complete peripheral retinal ablation.

ROLE OF VEGF IN ROP: A TWO-STAGE PROCESS

Vascularization of the human retina begins early in the second trimester, extending radially from the optic disc and reaching the retinal periphery by approximately 36 to 40 weeks of gestation.[2] VEGF plays a crucial role in this process. As the neurosensory retina matures and metabolic demands increase, a relative hypoxia occurs in the avascular peripheral retina. VEGF is released by the avascular tissue, and the resulting VEGF gradient drives retinal vascularization toward the retinal periphery.[21,22]

VEGF dysregulation in the premature infant occurs in two stages. In the first stage, retinal vascular maturation slows as intravitreal VEGF levels decrease in the presence of the relatively hyperoxic ex utero environment. In the second stage, retinal vasculature grows aberrantly as endogenous and intravitreal VEGF levels increase secondary to prolonged persistence of avascular retina.[3]

Upon delivery, the newborn enters a relatively hyperoxic environment compared to the womb. Because complete retinal vascularization does not occur until full term, premature infants are delivered into a hyperoxic environment while the peripheral retina remains incompletely vascularized.[21] Hyperoxia acts to downregulate VEGF produced by the avascular peripheral retina, and the normal process of retinal vascularization is impeded. In most premature infants, retinal vascularization is delayed but eventually resumes without significant sequelae. However, in some infants, the prolonged tissue hypoxia experienced by avascular retinal periphery causes an abnormal increase in VEGF production.[4,22] Instead of resuming the normal maturation process, pathologic angiogenesis occurs and intraretinal shunting and extraretinal neovascularization may develop.

The two-stage dysregulation hypothesis of VEGF in ROP is based in part based on animal models. The first stage of VEGF dysregulation was clearly demonstrated by Pierce et al.[23] in a mouse model. Mice placed in a hyperoxic environment at 7 days of age displayed decreased retinal VEGF expression and also developed vascular obliteration. Intravitreal injection of VEGF prevented vascular obliteration, thereby confirming VEGF downregulation as the proximal source of vascular dysgenesis.

The progression of retinal neovascularization (the second stage of ROP), mediated by VEGF, has been demonstrated in a rat model. Intravitreal injection of anti-VEGF antibodies significantly reduced retinal neovascularization compared to fellow eyes of rat pups exposed to elevated oxygen levels after birth.[24]

RELATIONSHIP OF OXYGEN AND VEGF LEVELS

When ROP was first described, the disease was attributed to high levels of neonatal oxygen exposure. A hypoxic stimulus for neovascularization was proposed, and oxygen was considered a possible treatment modality for ROP. However, the Cooperative Study of Retrolental Fibroplasia in 1956 demonstrated that administration of 50% oxygen to premature infants for 4 weeks actually increased rates of ROP and vision loss compared to lower oxygen delivery.[25]

Evidence for a hypoxic stimulus gained traction again as research demonstrated a relationship between hypoxia and angiogenic stimuli. The Supplemental Therapeutic Oxygen for Prethreshold ROP (STOP-ROP) study examined whether supplemental oxygen might decrease the rate of prethreshold ROP.[8] Premature infants with oxygen saturations <94% on room air were randomized to a conventional oxygen saturation target (89%–94%) or supplemental oxygen with an increased target (96%–99%). A total of 649 infants were enrolled in the study. The oxygen supplementation group demonstrated a slightly lower rate of progression from prethreshold to threshold ROP (48% vs. 41%), but this difference was not statistically significant. A subgroup analysis of patients without plus disease showed a more pronounced decrease in disease progression (32% vs. 46%), suggesting that oxygen supplementation might reduce disease severity if given early enough. However, the STOP-ROP study also highlighted possible adverse effects of aggressive oxygen supplementation. The oxygen supplementation group demonstrated an increased incidence of pneumonia and exacerbation of chronic lung disease, stayed in the hospital longer, and remained on diuretics for longer compared to the conventional target group.

Studies such as STOP-ROP accounted for the hypoxic drive for retinal neovascularization mediated by VEGF, which is now understood to comprise the second stage of ROP. The first stage of the disease, however, results from the relatively hyperoxic ex utero environment, which impedes retinal vascular growth in the premature neonate. As appreciation grew for the first stage, several studies examined whether lower oxygen saturations might reduce the incidence of ROP in premature infants.

A study by Chow et al.[26] in 2003 examined the incidence of ROP before and after the institution of tighter guidelines for oxygen administration in premature infants with birthweight <1,250 g. The new guidelines aimed to reduce hyperoxic and hypoxic fluctuations with a target oxygen saturation of 85% to 93%. The incidence of stage 3 and 5 ROP dropped from 12.5% to 2.5% after adoption of the new protocol, supporting the role of oxygen fluctuations in stimulating ROP.

Studies by Wright et al. in 2006 and Tokuhiro et al. in 2009 examined the incidence of ROP after adoption of reduced oxygen protocols, and both found reductions in threshold ROP with the newer reduced oxygen saturation targets.[27,28] These studies taken together supported the theory that lower oxygen saturation targets more closely mimic the in utero environment and, thereby, limit the hyperoxic stimulus in the first stage of ROP.

The two-stage theory of ROP implies that lower oxygen targets in the immediate postnatal period might allow retinal vascularization to proceed, while higher oxygen targets might inhibit VEGF-induced neovascularization as premature infants reach term. Sears et al.[29] examined this hypothesis by comparing the incidence of ROP before and after the adoption of a protocol for reduced oxygen (target oxygen saturation of 85%–92%) prior to 34 weeks PMA and elevated targets (92%–97%) after 34 weeks PMA.[29] The incidence of ROP decreased from 35% to 13% and the incidence of threshold disease decreased from 7% to 1% with the new protocol.

FACTORS OTHER THAN VEGF

While the role of VEGF in ROP is supported by a large body of literature, several other factors crucial to disease development have been elucidated recently. Consequently, the two stages of disease progression are increasingly understood in terms of multiple growth factors, both independent and interdependent.

Erythropoietin (Epo), a growth factor secreted by the fetal liver and adult kidney, mediates retinal angiogenesis using a pathway apparently independent from that of VEGF. Like VEGF, Epo is oxygen sensitive, with downregulation in the presence of hyperoxia and upregulation in the presence of hyperoxia.[30] The delivery of Epo to premature infants for the treatment of anemia resulted in increased incidence of treatment-requiring ROP, just as one might expect with the exogenous delivery of VEGF during the second phase of ROP development.[31] Modulation of Epo may prove beneficial in the treatment or prevention of ROP if these initial findings are borne out in further studies.

Insulin-like growth factor-1 (IGF-1), a growth factor transmitted maternally to the developing fetus, appears to be necessary for normal angiogenesis. The presence of VEGF is necessary for angiogenesis as well, but VEGF alone is insufficient based on studies in which IGF-1-knockout mice demonstrated deficient retinal vascular development but were rescued by exogenous IGF-1 delivery.[32,33] Serum levels of IGF-1 increase as the fetus approaches term, and premature infants, therefore, experience a relative deficiency of IGF-1 in the immediate postpartum period. Since IGF-1 acts as a critical cofactor for VEGF activity, vascular development is inhibited during this period. As the neonate matures and begins producing endogenous IGF-1, VEGF activity ensues and may stimulate retinal neovascularization.[34] Modulation of IGF-1 and its related pathways during the immediate postpartum period may play a role in preventing ROP, particularly as the relationship between IGF-1 and VEGF is further clarified.

ANTI-VEGF THERAPY FOR ROP

The advent of anti-VEGF drugs has raised the possibility of treating selected cases of ROP off-label with these medications. The rationale for this approach is drawn from intravitreal VEGF concentration data in human infants with ROP.

In a recently published study, we examined undiluted vitreous samples at the time of surgical repair from the midvitreous of children who developed stage 4 ROP despite standard of care laser.[5] At the time of surgery, the eyes were graded and divided into two groups—vascularly active and vascularly inactive—and compared to a control group consisting of children undergoing cataract surgery for uncomplicated congenital cataract. We measured all isoforms of VEGF by enzyme-linked immunosorbent assay (ELISA). Our findings confirmed that upregulation of VEGF occurs in ROP and that abnormally high levels are present in eyes developing retinal detachments with persistent vascular activity. Such eyes are potential candidate for anti-VEGF medications.

As VEGF is required in the developing retina for normal angiogenesis, the goal of treatment is to quench the excessive levels of VEGF in the vitreous rather than to penetrate retinal tissue. Furthermore, as VEGF activity is endogenously downregulated around the time of the due date, it is likely that premature infants will only require one or perhaps two injections of anti-VEGF medications to prevent progression of disease. For this reason, bevacizumab (Avastin, Genentech, South San Francisco, CA) is a more desirable drug than ranibizumab (Lucentis, Genentech, South San Francisco, CA) for treatment of ROP. While the two medications work through an identical mode of action, bevacizumab is a larger molecule than ranibizumab and may, therefore, penetrate the retina to a lesser degree. Since intraretinal VEGF is desired for continued retinal vascular maturation, less retinal penetration is preferable in this case.

STUDIES OF ANTI-VEGF THERAPY FOR ROP

Several small case series in the literature have documented the use of intravitreal bevacizumab in eyes with APROP refractory to peripheral ablation as well as in eyes with threshold or advanced ROP either as primary or adjunctive therapy[35,36] (Table 17.1).

Nazari et al.[36] injected bevacizumab in 12 eyes of six patients who demonstrated progressive disease after laser treatment, with regression in all treated eyes by a mean of 11 days. Chung et al.[37] combined laser ablation with intravitreal bevacizumab in both eyes of one patient, with prompt and sustained regression in both eyes.

Kusaka et al.[35] treated 23 eyes of 14 patients refractory to laser treatment. Vascular activity decreased in 14 of 15 patients who underwent fluorescein angiography, but three patient developed new or progressive tractional retinal detachment. Twenty eyes underwent vitrectomy after bevacizumab injection.

Mintz-Hittner[38] reported the use of bevacizumab in 22 eyes of 11 patients with stage 3 disease in Zone 1 or posterior Zone 2, of which only one was described as APROP. All eyes showed regression without retinal detachment at 13 to 85 weeks of follow-up. However, other reports have described tractional retinal detachment following bevacizumab injection.[39,40]

The largest experience to date of intravitreal bevacizumab for treatment of ROP is a combined series from Mexico, Portugal, and New York City.[41] Fifty-three eyes of 27 patients were injected with bevacizumab. Eyes were divided into three groups: progression to subtotal retinal detachment despite peripheral ablation (Group 1), threshold ROP with poor visualization preventing peripheral ablation (Group 2), and high-risk threshold or prethreshold ROP without prior treatment (Group 3). The authors reported that all eyes responded favorably with respect to neovascularization, but five eyes with advanced ROP worsened anatomically. No serious systemic adverse events were appreciated. Longer-term follow-up of 18 of these patients demonstrated uncomplicated regression in all eyes by 38 weeks after injection, with the exception of two eyes in Group 1 requiring vitrectomy.[42] The vitrectomized eyes remained stable with attached retinas at 38 weeks of follow-up.

ANTI-VEGF DOSING FOR ROP TREATMENT

Prior studies of intravitreal bevacizumab for ROP have used doses ranging from 0.4 to 1.25 mg. The ideal dose is unclear. Measurements of intravitreal VEGF levels in patients with ROP demonstrated a maximal level of

Table 17.1.

Reported cases of intravitreal bevacizumab for retinopathy of prematurity (ROP)

Author, Year	Patients	Eyes	Stage of Disease	Dose	Injections[a]	Outcomes After Injection
Chung[37]	1	2	APROP	0.75 mg	1	Combined with laser OU Regression OU
Honda[39]	1	1	St3 in Z1, s/p laser	0.4 mg	1	Acute progression of TRD
Kusaka[35]	14	23	All eyes s/p laser 3 eyes St 3 18 eyes St 4a 2 eyes St 4b	0.5 mg	1	Combined with vitrectomy in 8 eyes Subsequent vitrectomy in 12 eyes Decreased vascularity 14/15 eyes on IVFA New/progressive TRD in 3 patients
Lalwani[40]	3	5	Case 1: VH OU, no laser Case 2: Z1, plus s/p laser OU Case 3: ERD OU, no laser	1.25 mg ×1 0.63 mg ×7	1–2	All eyes stable except RRD in one eye Subsequent laser in all eyes
Martinez-Castellanos[41]	27	53	Group 1: St4 s/p laser Group 2: Threshold, poor view Group 3: Threshold, no laser	1.25 mg	1	Regression all eyes Resolution of ERD without surgery in 1 eye
Mintz-Hittner[38]	11	22	St 3 in Z1/ posterior Z2	0.625 mg	1	Regression in all eyes
Nazari[36]	6	12	APROP, St3, s/p laser	0.625 mg	1	Regression in all eyes
Nonobe[58]	6	6	4 eyes St 4b 2 eyes St 5	0.75 mg	1	All St 4b eyes and 1 St 5 eye attached after one subsequent procedure (SB or lens/vit). One St 5 eye attached after three procedures for RRD.

[a] Number of injections per eye.
ERD, exudative retinal detachment; IVFA, intravenous fluorescein angiogram; RRD, rhegmatogenous retinal detachment; SB, scleral buckle; St3, Stage 3 ROP; St4, Stage 4 ROP; St5, Stage 5 ROP; TRD, tractional retinal detachment; lens, lensectomy; VH, vitreous hemorrhage; vit, vitrectomy; Z1, Zone 1; Z2, Zone 2.

3,500 pg/mL of vitreous (Fig. 17.7), which corresponds to approximately 34 ng of bevacizumab assuming a 1:1 binding ratio of bevacizumab to VEGF.[5] The injection of 0.5 mg of bevacizumab in an infant eye may therefore represent more than a 1,000-fold excess of drug delivery. Some excess of drug delivery may be appropriate since hypoxic retina presumably stimulates VEGF production on an ongoing basis, and limited data suggest that the delivery of anti-VEGF antibodies may stimulate further VEGF production.[24,43] At the present, the ideal amount of intravitreal antibody per injection remains undetermined as the exact binding ratio of antibody to VEGF and the rate of continued VEGF production following anti-VEGF injection both remain to be quantified.

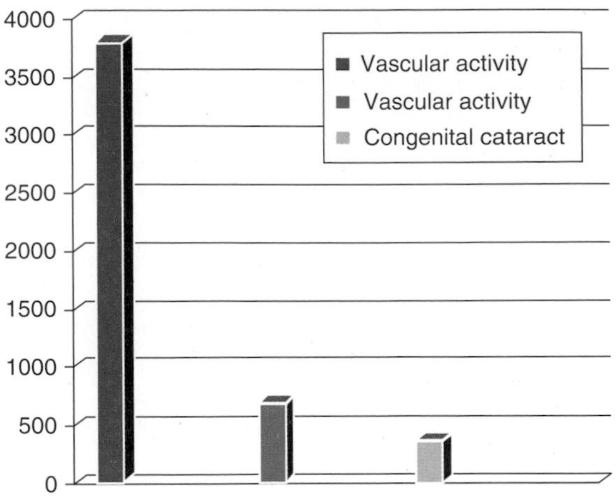

FIGURE 17.7. Intravitreal VEGF levels in ROP. Vitreous samples were taken at the time of vitrectomy for Stage 4a ROP. The sample included 12 patients with significant vascular activity, 10 with minimal vascular activity, and a control group of patients undergoing vitrectomy for congenital cataract.

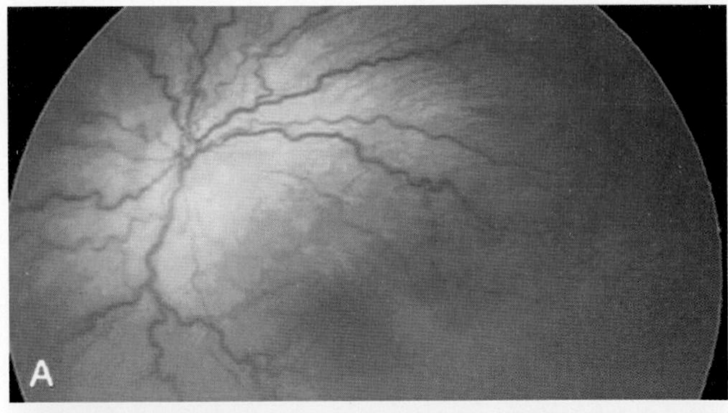

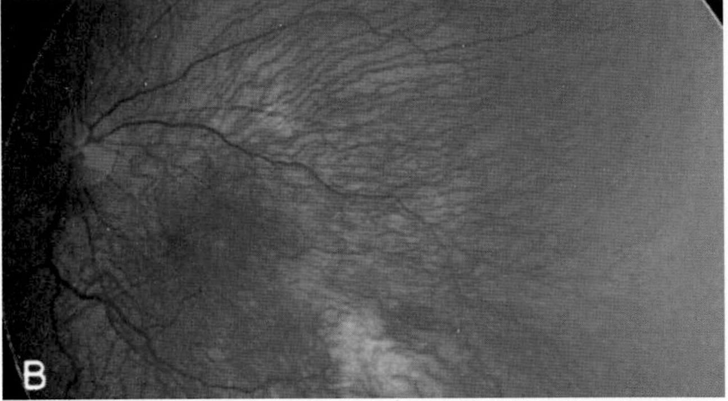

FIGURE 17.8. A: Aggressive posterior ROP in Zone 1 is shown (in the left eye) at 10.3 weeks of life in an infant weighing 515 g at birth (gestational age, 23 weeks). **B:** After intravitreal injection of bevacizumab, the same area at 44.9 weeks of life reveals decreased plus disease and continued anterior vascularization of the retina. (Reproduced from Mintz-Hittner HA, Kuffel RR Jr. *Retina.* 2008;28:831–838, with permission.)

FUTURE OF ANTI-VEGF THERAPY FOR ROP

The next appropriate step would be a prospective clinical trial to evaluate the safety and efficacy of treatment with bevacizumab for improving structural outcomes in ROP. This is the mission of the Pan-VEGF Blockade for the Treatment of Retinopathy of Prematurity (BLOCK-ROP) study, a multicenter prospective longitudinal cohort study including 11 clinical centers in the United States and Canada. The Coordinating Center and Reading Center are located at William Beaumont Hospital in Royal Oak, Michigan (Fig. 17.8).

Phase 2 of the BLOCK-ROP study aims to evaluate the ability of intravitreal bevacizumab to curtail progression from prethreshold to threshold ROP. Secondarily, the study aims to evaluate the efficacy of bevacizumab at improving structural outcomes in ROP with or without subsequent treatment such as peripheral laser ablation or vitrectomy.

Patients with prethreshold disease will be randomized in a 1:1:1 ratio into three groups. Group 1 will receive a single intravitreal bevacizumab injection of 0.75 mg/0.03 mL in one eye and standard-of-care peripheral laser ablation in the fellow eye. Group 2 will receive a single intravitreal bevacizumab injection of 0.625 mg/0.025 mL in one eye and peripheral laser ablation in the fellow eye. Group 3 will receive peripheral laser ablation in both eyes.

Study groups 1 and 2 will use volumes that are reduced compared to the adult treatment volume. This smaller volume should reduce the risk of elevated intraocular pressure and the need for paracentesis. The vitreous levels of VEGF in premature eyes are much higher than those in adult eyes. Therefore, it is anticipated that most, if not all, bevacizumab will be bound to VEGF in the vitreous, markedly reducing the availability of bevacizumab to escape into systemic circulation. One goal of BLOCK-ROP is the determination of an optimal intravitreal bevacizumab dose for use in ROP.

The three-arm study design will also provide valuable data by comparing fellow eyes to treatment eyes. Patients with ROP often develop high myopia. The precise mechanism and relationship between myopia and peripheral retinal ablative treatment remain unclear, but laser appears to limit myopic progression somewhat compared to cryotherapy.[44] If myopia is in fact related to peripheral retinal ablation, the comparison of intravitreal bevacizumab in one eye and laser ablation in the fellow eye may reveal anisometropia related to the different treatments.

The comparison of fellow eyes between treatment groups may also reveal the possible effects of intravitreal bevacizumab on the fellow eye. Studies in adults receiving bevacizumab have indicated a possible fellow eye effect, while other studies have failed to demonstrate a significant decrease in fellow eye intravitreal VEGF levels.[45,46] By comparing laser-treated fellow eyes in groups 1 and 2 to laser-treated eyes in group 3, the BLOCK-ROP study may be able to demonstrate the presence or absence of a clinically meaningful fellow eye effect after intravitreal bevacizumab injection for ROP.

The scientific argument in favor of an anti-VEGF therapeutic approach for ROP is compelling. However, accrual of early phase trial data is appropriate given the vulnerabilities of the target population. In the absence of reliable ocular and systemic safety data, caution is warranted regarding the use of anti-VEGF agents in premature neonates outside the construct of a well-designed clinical trial.

Surgical Implications of Anti-VEGF Therapy Versus Peripheral Retinal Ablation

Peripheral retinal ablation and intravitreal anti-VEGF therapy share a common endpoint of limiting retinal exposure to excess VEGF, thereby stopping the progression of ROP. However, the two treatments may differ significantly with respect to anatomic progression. If intravitreal bevacizumab is proven safe and effective in the treatment of ROP, an evaluation of posttreatment surgical results will be important.

Peripheral laser ablation creates a full-thickness chorioretinal adhesion. In cases of progressive tractional retinal detachment, prior peripheral ablation prevents total retinal detachment (Stage 5 ROP) from occurring. When such cases require vitrectomy, the anatomic differences between eyes with and without prior laser become significant. In eyes with prior laser, a peripheral surgical space exists and the surgeon may be able to safely enter this space and relax peripheral vitreoretinal traction. In eyes without prior laser, the retina may detach to the ora serrata and thereby prevent safe surgical entry through the pars plana or pars plicata.

Intravitreal injection also poses additional relative risks in eyes with impending or existing retinal detachments (Stage 4 or 5). The use of bevacizumab is analogous in this way to its use in patients with proliferative diabetic retinopathy. In patients with diabetic tractional retinal detachment, intravitreal bevacizumab decreases the vascularity of proliferative tissue and thereby decreases the risk of intraoperative hemorrhage. However, bevacizumab may also accelerate fibrovascular contraction and thereby cause or worsen the severity of tractional retinal detachment. Similarly, the literature contains several cases of intravitreal bevacizumab for ROP in which accelerated fibrosis caused or worsened Stage 4 ROP.[39,40]

SYSTEMIC EXPOSURE TO ANTI-VEGF AGENTS

Intravitreal injection of anti-VEGF agents is likely to result in some level of systemic exposure. Intravitreal bevacizumab has been used extensively in adults for a wide variety of conditions, and evidence of systemic sequelae has been minimal. Neonates, however, are likely to be more vulnerable to the effects of systemic anti-VEGF exposure.

During embryogenesis, vascular development occurs through the processes of vasculogenesis and angiogenesis. Vasculogenesis is the de novo growth of vessels resulting from mesodermal differentiation into vascular endothelium, while angiogenesis is the growth of new vessels as branches from existing vessels.[47] VEGF is the primary mediator of angiogenesis, and suppression of VEGF on a systemic level may impede normal vascular development in a variety of organ systems.[48] Consequently, intravitreal injection of anti-VEGF agents must account for the possibility of extraocular side effects in the premature neonate.

GENETIC SUSCEPTIBILITY TO VEGF DYSREGULATION AND ROP

Numerous studies have delineated the role of VEGF in the pathogenesis of ROP, but no clear explanation exists for the vastly different rates of disease progression in patients with similar clinical risk factors. Studies of ROP concordance rates in twins suggest a genetic predisposition to more severe disease.[49] However, studies of individual genes have not yielded consistent correlations with clinical progression of disease.

The signaling pathways potentially involved in VEGF dysregulation are complex. The Wnt pathway is perhaps the best studied of these and plays a role in vasculogenesis (de novo synthesis of vascular channels) of the retina. Frizzled-4 acts as a receptor in the Wnt signaling pathway, and the receptor is activated by a variety of ligands including Wnt-3a, Wnt-8, Wnt-5a, and Norrin (Drenser KA, unpublished data). Furthermore, multiple distinct pathways exist downstream of the activated receptor-ligand complex. The precise relationships between these signaling pathways and retinal levels of VEGF, insulin-like growth factor 1 (IGF-I), tumor necrosis factors alpha and beta, angiopoietin II and other factors are unclear. Consequently, each of the abovementioned pathway components is a candidate for genetic predisposition to advanced ROP, but these components likely represent only a minority of all components involved in relevant signaling pathways.

The study of genetic predisposition to ROP has taken a shotgun approach, focusing on a few specific candidate genes or alleles rather than the entire signal pathway upstream to VEGF. This approach may explain why low serum levels of IGF-I and high vitreous levels of VEGF correlate with ROP severity but no study of any single gene has yielded a consistent causal relationship.[5,32,50–56]

Studies of alleles for VEGF and IGF-1 have occasionally identified alleles correlated with ROP development or severity, but allelic variation has poor predictive value and some studies with positive findings directly contradict each other.[51,52,56,57]

If VEGF is the common downstream dysregulated factor in patients with advanced ROP, many upstream genetic alterations could potentially start the cascade of dysregulation. The pathways involved in VEGF regulation are sufficiently complex that logically identifying candidate genes may be inadequate. Effective genetic evaluation for predisposition to ROP requires the evaluation of large cohorts of newborns for a wide variety of mutations in a prospective manner in order to identify the precise upstream source of VEGF dysregulation in any given infant. Such genetic identification could help predict disease development as well as potentially identify therapies beyond direct anti-VEGF blockade.

KEY POINTS

- ROP occurs in two stages: inhibition of vascularization due to the relative hyperoxia of the ex utero environment, and a subsequent neovascular stimulus from hypoxic avascular peripheral retina.
- Plus disease, comprised of peripapillary vascular tortuosity and venous dilatation, is the consequence of retinal vascular shunting within the ridge between vascular and avascular retina. Plus disease is therefore a proxy for persistent VEGF dysregulation.
- Intravitreal VEGF levels are elevated in patients with ROP, and VEGF levels increase with greater vascular activity.
- The current standard of care treatment for threshold ROP is peripheral retinal laser ablation from the ora serrata to the edge of vascularized retina. Peripheral laser destroys the avascular retina, which produces VEGF and, thereby, drives retinal neovascularization.
- Modifications to oxygen exposure during the two stages of ROP may mitigate disease progression. Further studies are needed to confirm this possibility.
- Intravitreal bevacizumab has been used in numerous case series for treatment of Stage 3 and 4 ROP. Most cases regressed while a few progressed to tractional retinal detachments. Systemic side effects have not been noted, but the number of patients injected to date is insufficient to detect all possible side effects including any possible detrimental effects on normal angiogenesis.
- The BLOCK-ROP study is a randomized prospective study comparing two doses of intravitreal bevacizumab with standard-of-care peripheral laser ablation for threshold ROP.

REFERENCES

1. Repka MX, Tung B, Good WV, et al. Outcome of eyes developing retinal detachment during the Early Treatment for Retinopathy of Prematurity Study (ETROP). *Arch Ophthalmol.* 2006;124:24–30.
2. Roth AM. Retinal vascular development in premature infants. *Am J Ophthalmol.* 1977;84:636–640.
3. Chen J, Smith LE. Retinopathy of prematurity. *Angiogenesis.* 2007;10:133–140.
4. Aiello LP, Avery RL, Arrigg PG, et al. Vascular endothelial growth factor in ocular fluid of patients with diabetic retinopathy and other retinal disorders. *N Engl J Med.* 1994;331:1480–1487.
5. Sonmez K, Drenser KA, Capone A Jr, et al. Vitreous levels of stromal cell-derived factor 1 and vascular endothelial growth factor in patients with retinopathy of prematurity. *Ophthalmology.* 2008;115:1065–1070.
6. International Committee for the Classification of Retinopathy of Prematurity. *Arch Ophthalmol.* 2005;123:991–999.
7. Good WV, Hardy RJ, Dobson V, et al. The incidence and course of retinopathy of prematurity: findings from the early treatment for retinopathy of prematurity study. *Pediatrics.* 2005;116:15–23.
8. The STOP-ROP Multicenter Study Group. Supplemental Therapeutic Oxygen for Prethreshold Retinopathy of Prematurity, a randomized, controlled trial. I: primary outcomes. *Pediatrics.* 2000;105:295–310.
9. Palmer EA, Flynn JT, Hardy RJ, et al. Incidence and early course of retinopathy of prematurity. The Cryotherapy for Retinopathy of Prematurity Cooperative Group. *Ophthalmology.* 1991;98:1628–1640.
10. Schaffer DB, Palmer EA, Plotsky DF, et al. Prognostic factors in the natural course of retinopathy of prematurity. The Cryotherapy for Retinopathy of Prematurity Cooperative Group. *Ophthalmology.* 1993;100:230–237.
11. Reynolds JD, Dobson V, Quinn GE, et al. Evidence-based screening criteria for retinopathy of prematurity: natural history data from the CRYO-ROP and LIGHT-ROP studies. *Arch Ophthalmol.* 2002;120:1470–1476.
12. National Eye Institute. Early Treatment of Blinding Eye Disease in Infants Can Prevent Severe Vision Loss, 2003: Press Release.
13. Good WV. Final results of the Early Treatment for Retinopathy of Prematurity (ETROP) randomized trial. *Trans Am Ophthalmol Soc.* 2004;102:233–248; discussion 248–250.
14. Connolly BP, Ng EY, McNamara JA, et al. A comparison of laser photocoagulation with cryotherapy for threshold retinopathy of prematurity at 10 years: part 2. Refractive outcome. *Ophthalmology.* 2002;109:936–941.
15. Ng EY, Connolly BP, McNamara JA, et al. A comparison of laser photocoagulation with cryotherapy for threshold retinopathy of prematurity at 10 years: part 1. Visual function and structural outcome. *Ophthalmology.* 2002;109:928–934; discussion 935.
16. Shaikh S, Capone A Jr, Schwartz SD, et al. Inadvertent skip areas in treatment of zone 1 retinopathy of prematurity. *Retina.* 2003;23:128–131.
17. Capone A Jr, Trese MT. Lens-sparing vitreous surgery for tractional stage 4A retinopathy of prematurity retinal detachments. *Ophthalmology.* 2001;108:2068–2070.
18. Hubbard GB III, Cherwick DH, Burian G. Lens-sparing vitrectomy for stage 4 retinopathy of prematurity. *Ophthalmology.* 2004;111:2274–2277.
19. McLoone E, O'Keefe M, McLoone S, et al. Long term functional and structural outcomes of laser therapy for retinopathy of prematurity. *Br J Ophthalmol.* 2006;90:754–759.
20. Young TL, Anthony DC, Pierce E, et al. Histopathology and vascular endothelial growth factor in untreated and diode laser-treated retinopathy of prematurity. *J Aapos.* 1997;1:105–110.
21. Lutty GA, Chan-Ling T, Phelps DL, et al. Proceedings of the Third International Symposium on Retinopathy of Prematurity: an update on ROP from the lab to the nursery (November 2003, Anaheim, California). *Mol Vis.* 2006; 12:532–580.
22. Pierce EA, Avery RL, Foley ED, et al. Vascular endothelial growth factor/vascular permeability factor expression in a mouse model of retinal neovascularization. *Proc Natl Acad Sci USA.* 1995;92:905–909.
23. Pierce EA, Foley ED, Smith LE. Regulation of vascular endothelial growth factor by oxygen in a model of retinopathy of prematurity. *Arch Ophthalmol.* 1996;114:1219–1228.

24. Geisen P, Peterson LJ, Martiniuk D, et al. Neutralizing antibody to VEGF reduces intravitreous neovascularization and may not interfere with ongoing intraretinal vascularization in a rat model of retinopathy of prematurity. *Mol Vis.* 2008;14:345–357.
25. Kinsey VE, Hemphill FM. Etiology of retrolental fibroplasia and preliminary report of cooperative study of retrolental fibroplasia. *Trans Am Acad Ophthalmol Otolaryngol.* 1955;59:15–24.
26. Chow LC, Wright KW, Sola A. Can changes in clinical practice decrease the incidence of severe retinopathy of prematurity in very low birth weight infants? *Pediatrics.* 2003;111:339–345.
27. Tokuhiro Y, Yoshida T, Nakabayashi Y, et al. Reduced oxygen protocol decreases the incidence of threshold retinopathy of prematurity (ROP) in infants of less than 33 weeks gestation. *Pediatr Int.* 2009;51:804–806.
28. Wright KW, Sami D, Thompson L, et al. A physiologic reduced oxygen protocol decreases the incidence of threshold retinopathy of prematurity. *Trans Am Ophthalmol Soc.* 2006;104:78–84.
29. Sears JE, Pietz J, Sonnie C, et al. A change in oxygen supplementation can decrease the incidence of retinopathy of prematurity. *Ophthalmology.* 2009;116:513–518.
30. Chen J, Connor KM, Aderman CM, et al. Erythropoietin deficiency decreases vascular stability in mice. *J Clin Invest.* 2008;118:526–533.
31. Suk KK, Dunbar JA, Liu A, et al. Human recombinant erythropoietin and the incidence of retinopathy of prematurity: a multiple regression model. *J Aapos.* 2008;12:233–238.
32. Hellstrom A, Perruzzi C, Ju M, et al. Low IGF-I suppresses VEGF-survival signaling in retinal endothelial cells: direct correlation with clinical retinopathy of prematurity. *Proc Natl Acad Sci USA.* 2001;98:5804–5808.
33. Smith LE, Kopchick JJ, Chen W, et al. Essential role of growth hormone in ischemia-induced retinal neovascularization. *Science.* 1997;276:1706–1709.
34. Chen J, Smith LE. A double-edged sword: erythropoietin eyed in retinopathy of prematurity. *J Aapos.* 2008;12:221–222.
35. Kusaka S, Shima C, Wada K, et al. Efficacy of intravitreal injection of bevacizumab for severe retinopathy of prematurity: a pilot study. *Br J Ophthalmol.* 2008;92:1450–1455.
36. Nazari H, Parvaresh MM, Hashemi M, et al. Intravitreal bevacizumab for the treatment of Aggressive Posterior Retinopathy of Prematurity unresponsive to conventional laser therapy. *Retina.* 2010. In press.
37. Chung EJ, Kim JH, Ahn HS, et al. Combination of laser photocoagulation and intravitreal bevacizumab (Avastin) for aggressive zone 1 retinopathy of prematurity. *Graefes Arch Clin Exp Ophthalmol.* 2007;245:1727–1730.
38. Mintz-Hittner HA, Kuffel RR Jr. Intravitreal injection of bevacizumab (avastin) for treatment of stage 3 retinopathy of prematurity in zone 1 or posterior zone 2. *Retina.* 2008; 28:831–838.
39. Honda S, Hirabayashi H, Tsukahara Y, et al. Acute contraction of the proliferative membrane after an intravitreal injection of bevacizumab for advanced retinopathy of prematurity. *Graefes Arch Clin Exp Ophthalmol.* 2008;246:1061–1063.
40. Lalwani GA, Berrocal AM, Murray TG, et al. Off-label use of intravitreal bevacizumab (Avastin) for salvage treatment in progressive threshold retinopathy of prematurity. *Retina.* 2008;28:S13–S18.
41. Martinez-Castellanos MA, Domenzain-Afendulis JL, Hernandez-Rojas ML, et al. Safety and efficacy of intravitreal bevacizumab for retinopathy of prematurity. *Invest Ophthalmol Vis Sci.* 2007;48: E-Abstract 85.
42. Quiroz-Mercado H, Martinez-Castellanos MA, Hernandez-Rojas ML, et al. Antiangiogenic therapy with intravitreal bevacizumab for retinopathy of prematurity. *Retina.* 2008;28: S19–S25.
43. Sears JE. Anti-vascular endothelial growth factor and retinopathy of prematurity. *Br J Ophthalmol.* 2008;92:1437–1438.
44. O'Keefe M, Kirwan C. Diode laser versus cryotherapy in treatment of ROP. *Br J Ophthalmol.* 2006;90:402–403.
45. Avery RL, Pearlman J, Pieramici DJ, et al. Intravitreal bevacizumab (Avastin) in the treatment of proliferative diabetic retinopathy. *Ophthalmology.* 2006;113:1695e1–1695e15.
46. Sawada O, Kawamura H, Kakinoki M, et al. Vascular endothelial growth factor in fellow eyes of eyes injected with intravitreal bevacizumab. *Graefes Arch Clin Exp Ophthalmol.* 2008;246:1379–1381.
47. Ferrara N. Role of vascular endothelial growth factor in physiologic and pathologic angiogenesis: therapeutic implications. *Semin Oncol.* 2002;29:10–14.
48. Breier G, Albrecht U, Sterrer S, et al. Expression of vascular endothelial growth factor during embryonic angiogenesis and endothelial cell differentiation. *Development.* 1992;114:521–532.
49. Bizzarro MJ, Hussain N, Jonsson B, et al. Genetic susceptibility to retinopathy of prematurity. *Pediatrics.* 2006;118: 1858–1863.
50. Balogh A, Derzbach L, Vannay A, et al. Lack of association between insulin-like growth factor I receptor G(+3174)A polymorphism and retinopathy of prematurity. *Graefes Arch Clin Exp Ophthalmol.* 2006;244:1035–1038.
51. Cooke RW, Drury JA, Mountford R, et al. Genetic polymorphisms and retinopathy of prematurity. *Invest Ophthalmol Vis Sci.* 2004;45:1712–1715.
52. Dunai G, Vasarhelyi B, Szabo M, et al. Published genetic variants in retinopathy of prematurity: random forest analysis suggests a negligible contribution to risk and severity. *Curr Eye Res.* 2008;33:501–505.
53. Haider MZ, Devarajan LV, Al-Essa M, et al. Missense mutations in norrie disease gene are not associated with advanced stages of retinopathy of prematurity in Kuwaiti arabs. *Biol Neonate.* 2000;77:88–91.
54. Hutcheson KA, Paluru PC, Bernstein SL, et al. Norrie disease gene sequence variants in an ethnically diverse population with retinopathy of prematurity. *Mol Vis.* 2005;11:501–508.
55. Kim JH, Yu YS, Kim J, et al. Mutations of the Norrie gene in Korean ROP infants. *Korean J Ophthalmol.* 2002;16:93–96.
56. Vannay A, Dunai G, Banyasz I, et al. Association of genetic polymorphisms of vascular endothelial growth factor and risk for proliferative retinopathy of prematurity. *Pediatr Res.* 2005;57:396–398.
57. Holmstrom G, van Wijngaarden P, Coster DJ, et al. Genetic susceptibility to retinopathy of prematurity: the evidence from clinical and experimental animal studies. *Br J Ophthalmol.* 2007;91:1704–1708.
58. Nonobe NI, Kachi S, Kondo M, et al. Concentration of vascularendothelial growth factor in aqueous humor of eyes with advanced retinopathy of prematurity before and after intravitreal injection of bevacizumab. *Retina.* 2009;29(5):579–585.

CHAPTER

18

Pharmacotherapy in Retinal Vein Occlusions

Amol D. Kulkarni • Jonathan B. Gunther • Michael S. Ip

INTRODUCTION

Retinal vein occlusion (RVO) is the second most common sight-threatening retinal vascular disease following diabetic retinopathy.[1] There are three distinct types of RVO: branch retinal vein occlusion (BRVO), central retinal vein occlusion (CRVO), and an anatomical variant of CRVO, namely, hemiretinal vein occlusion.[2] Many systemic diseases are risk factors for RVO development.[3,4] In addition to recognition and treatment of the underlying systemic disease, there are various treatment modalities for the RVO. These can be broadly categorized into pharmacotherapy, laser photocoagulation, surgical treatment, and combination therapy.[5] This chapter will review the various pharmacological management options for BRVO and CRVO.

BRANCH RETINAL VEIN OCCLUSION

Pathophysiology

BRVO develops at crossing sites where the artery is passing superficially over the vein. Histological examination has shown that BRVO is associated with arteriosclerotic changes in the retinal arterioles, which could cause compression of the adjacent vein leading to thrombus formation and vein occlusion.[6] Another theory suggests hemodynamic variations due to venous contouring at the site of artery over vein intersections as the inciting cause of BRVO.[7] The development of macular edema (ME) secondary to BRVO has been hypothesized to be caused by breakdown of the blood-retinal barrier, vitreoretinal adhesion, or secretion of vasopermeability factors such as vascular endothelial growth factor (VEGF) and interleukin-6 (IL-6).[8] Furthermore, release of VEGF and IL-6 at the border between perfused and nonperfused retina also leads to formation of retinal neovascularization.

Clinical Features

BRVO is characterized by segmental involvement at the crossing of a retinal artery and vein, the most common location being the superotemporal quadrant of the retina.[9] The involved area is usually wedge shaped with dilated and tortuous vein surrounded by deep and superficial retinal hemorrhages, cotton-wool spots, and retinal edema (Fig. 18.1). Approximately 50% to 60% of untreated patients will have a final visual acuity (VA) of 20/40 or better. However, severe vision loss is not uncommon, with 20% to 25% of patients having a VA of 20/200 or worse.[10]

The visually significant complications include ME (most common), nonperfusion, and vitreous hemorrhage from neovascularization.[5,8,9] In patients with perfused ME, approximately one third will regain some vision spontaneously. However, this becomes less likely the longer the edema persists. Early in the course of BRVO, macular nonperfusion can result in permanent vision loss.[8] Large areas of persistent retinal nonperfusion can lead to neovascularization of the retina or disc and can cause vitreous hemorrhage. In the Branch Vein Occlusion Study (BVOS), retinal neovascularization developed in 36% of eyes with five disc diameters or more of retinal nonperfusion.[11] It is important to recognize that perfused BRVO may progress to the nonperfused type during the ensuing weeks, months, and even years.

Diagnostic Testing

Intravenous fluorescein angiography (FA) and optical coherence tomography (OCT) can assist in the evaluation of BRVO. Angiographic findings reflect changes in vessel permeability, caliber, and patency and assist in identifying areas of ME, neovascularization, and nonperfusion. OCT is a useful tool for the detection and monitoring of ME in BRVO. The findings from the Standard Care versus COrticosteroid for REtinal Vein Occlusion (SCORE) Study revealed a modest correlation between OCT-measured center point thickness and VA.[12]

Treatment

As our understanding of the disease improves, the standard of care is likely to continue to evolve. Available data concerning many of the reported treatment modalities are based on case series without controls or randomization. Initial evaluation may include testing for hypertension, fasting blood glucose level, complete blood count with differential and platelets, coagulation studies, and erythrocyte sedimentation

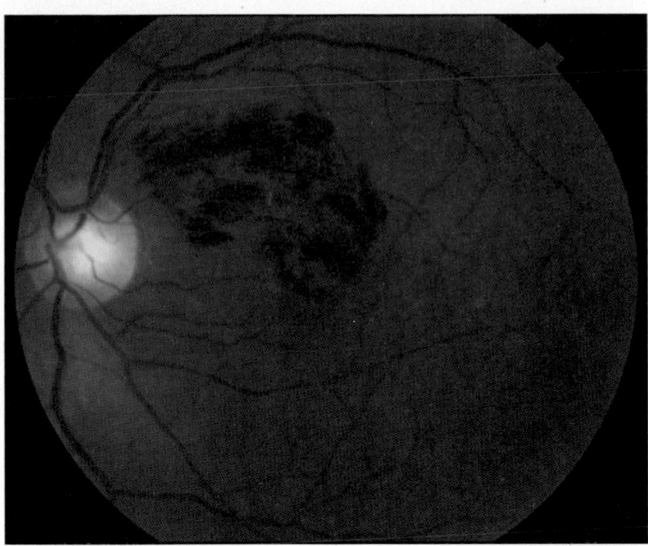

A

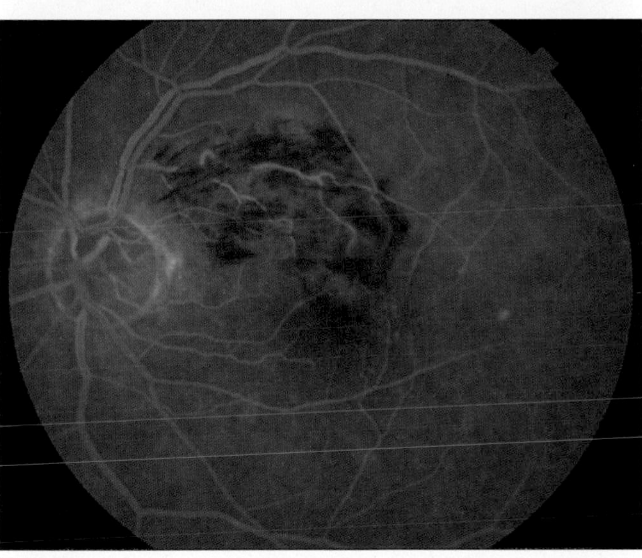

B

FIGURE 18.1. Fundus photo (**A**) and FA (**B**) of acute presentation of BRVO showing dilated and tortuous vein surrounded by wedge-shaped area of deep and superficial retinal hemorrhages and retinal edema. The areas of hyperfluorescence superior to the foveal center are due to ME.

rate. Follow-up generally consists of ophthalmologic evaluation every 1 to 3 months for the first year, followed by every 3 to 12 months thereafter. Grid laser photocoagulation for ME, (BRVO), and scatter laser photocoagulation for retinal or anterior segment neovascularization (BRVO and CRVO) continue to remain the mainstay of treatment.[10,13] Pharmacotherapy is currently used by some clinicians as an adjunct or replacement for laser photocoagulation until data are available from ongoing clinical trials on the use of intravitreal drugs as primary therapy (Figure 18.2).

Intraocular Corticosteroids

Intravitreal triamcinolone acetonide (TA) has been investigated for persistent ME in RVO and has been shown experimentally to reduce the breakdown of the blood-retina barrier by inhibiting factors such as prostaglandins, interleukins, VEGF, and protein kinase C. Small case studies have shown favorable anatomical response to intravitreal injection of TA within several weeks, as demonstrated by OCT images.[14–18] However, a favorable VA response may be more likely in patients with perfused rather than nonperfused ME. Retreatment may also be performed in some patients due to recurrent ME. A human pharmacokinetics study of nonvitrectomized eyes found a single 4-mg intravitreal injection of triamcinolone to have a mean half-life of 18.6 days with measurable concentrations expected to last approximately 3 months.[19] Reported side effects include cataract, increased intraocular pressure (IOP), and injection-related complications including noninfectious and infectious endophthalmitis, retinal detachment, vitreous hemorrhage, and lens injury.[14–18]

The SCORE (**S**tandard care vs. **CO**rticosteroid for **RE**tinal Vein Occlusion) study, a multicenter, randomized, Phase 3 National Eye Institute–sponsored study, elucidated the efficacy and safety of standard care versus intravitreal injection(s) of TA for ME secondary to BRVO and CRVO. Individuals with BRVO or CRVO with associated ME of up to 24 months' duration and best-corrected VA between 19 and 73 ETDRS letters (corresponding to approximately 20/40 to 20/400 Snellen VA) were eligible for participation in the SCORE study.[20] The two primary study objectives of the SCORE-BRVO trial were (a) to determine whether intravitreal TA at 1 and 4-mg doses produces greater visual benefit, with an acceptable safety profile, than grid photocoagulation (standard care), when appropriate, for the treatment of vision loss associated with ME secondary to BRVO and (b) to compare the efficacy and safety of the 1 and 4-mg TA doses. The results of the SCORE-BRVO trial[21] demonstrated no significant differences among the three treatment groups for a gain in VA letter score of 15 or more at 12 months (29%, 26%, and 27% in the standard care, and 1 and 4-mg TA groups, respectively). An early positive treatment response of a gain in VA letter score of 15 or more was observed at month 4 in the 4-mg TA group compared with the 1-mg TA and standard care groups. After month 12 and through month 36, the mean improvement from baseline VA letter score was greatest in the standard care group compared with the two TA groups. With respect to OCT-measured center point thickness, all three groups showed a decrease from baseline to month 12. Analogous to the VA results, only at month 4 did the 4-mg TA group demonstrate a greater treatment effect on center point thickness than the 1-mg and standard care groups; at all other times investigated (months 8–36), the standard care group demonstrated the greatest overall median decrease in center point thickness from baseline. The rates of adverse events were higher in the 4-mg TA group compared with the 1-mg and standard care groups. There was a dose-dependent higher frequency of initiating IOP-lowering medications in the TA groups (41% in 4 mg, and 8% in 1 mg) compared

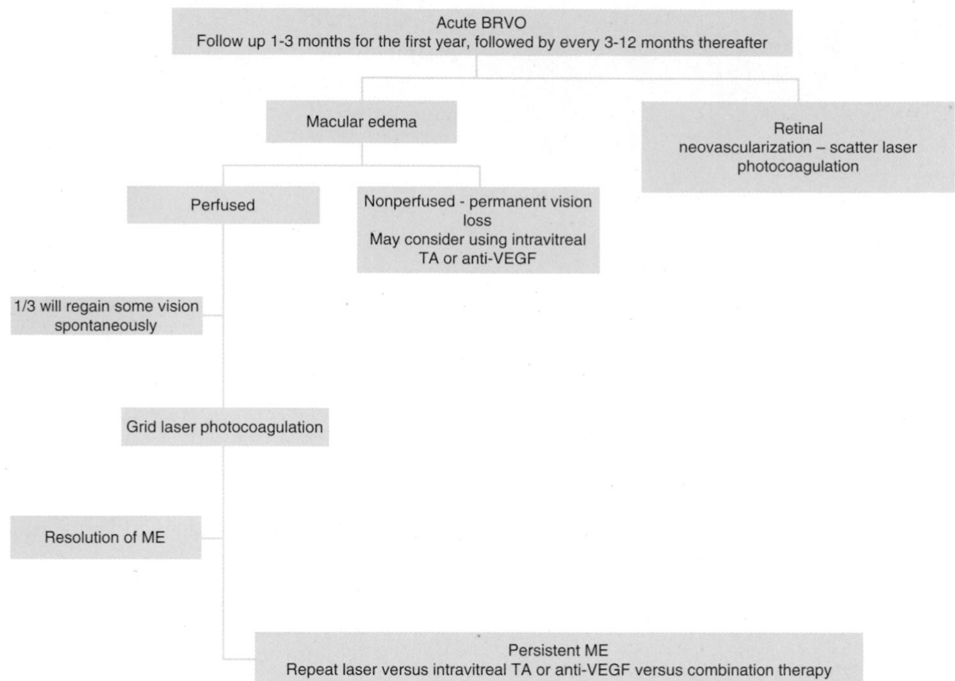

FIGURE 18.2. Stepwise approach for pharmacotherapy of BRVO.

with the standard care group (2%). The proportion of phakic eyes that had new-onset lens opacity or progression of an existing opacity through 12 months based on assessment at the clinical center was greater in the two TA groups (35% in 4 mg, and 25% in 1 mg) compared with the standard care group (13%). Most cataract surgeries were performed during the second year of the study and occurred with the highest frequency in the 4-mg group (n = 35). The rates of adverse events with respect to cataract surgery and elevated IOP were similar between the standard care and 1-mg groups. Thus, the SCORE study results support grid photocoagulation as the continued standard of care for patients with decreased VA associated with ME secondary to BRVO up to 12 months and possibly up to 36 months.[21] Furthermore, the results of this trial also substantiate that grid photocoagulation must be the benchmark against which other treatments for vision loss associated with ME secondary to BRVO should be compared in clinical trials (Box 18.1).

Ozurdex is an extended delivery bioerodable dexamethasone PLGA (polylactic acid polyglycolic acid) copolymer complex, which has been also studied in persistent ME secondary to RVO.[22] The release of dexamethasone depends on the diffusion through the polymer matrix, solubility of the polymer, and rate of degradation of polymer matrix. The drug is released for approximately 35 days, and the polymer matrix is absorbed in 60 to 180 days. A specially designed proprietary instrument is used for the intravitreal injection of the Ozurdex implant, thus obviating the need of surgery.[23] It consist of 22-g hypodermic needle, 1 inch long mounted on a device measuring 165 × 13 mm preloaded with the implantable drug product. The drug is injected at the inferior pars plana by pressing a button. Common adverse events associated with implant procedure include anterior chamber flare, conjunctival hyperemia, conjunctival hemorrhage, eye pain, floaters, IOP increase, vitreous hemorrhage, and vitritis.[23] The efficacy of the Ozurdex implant was tested in a 6-month randomized phase 2 trial for treatment of persistent ME (>90 days) due to various causes including RVO.[22] The VA at entry was 20/40 to 20/200, and the patients were

BOX 18.1 SCORE Trial in BRVO

Purpose: This multicenter, randomized clinical trial compared the efficacy and safety of 1- and 4-mg doses of preservative-free intravitreal triamcinolone with standard care (grid photocoagulation in eyes without dense macular hemorrhage and deferral of photocoagulation until hemorrhage clears in eyes with dense macular hemorrhage) for eyes with vision loss associated with ME secondary to BRVO.

Conclusions: There was no difference identified in VA at 12 months for the standard care group compared with the triamcinolone groups. Rates of adverse events (particularly elevated intraocular pressure and cataract) were highest in the 4-mg group. Grid photocoagulation as applied in the SCORE Study remains the standard care for patients with vision loss associated with ME secondary to BRVO. (SCORE Study Group, *Arch Ophthalmol.* 2009;127:1115).

randomly assigned to one of the three treatment regimens: a single Ozurdex implant containing 350 μg of drug, 700 μg of drug or observation. There was statistically significant improvement in best-corrected VA of 10 letters or more in 35% of patients in the 700-μg dose ($p < 0.001$) at day 90 and the drug was well tolerated for 180 days. There was no cataract progression, and a transient IOP elevation was observed at the different time points, which were readily managed with topical antiglaucoma medications. The dose of 700 μg seemed to be effective and may have potential as new therapy for recalcitrant ME secondary to RVO. A phase 3 clinical trial evaluating the Ozurdex implant for RVO has been completed, and study results are currently pending (Box 18.2).

Periocular Corticosteroids

Periocular application of TA has been also investigated for treatment of ME associated with BRVO. In a randomized study, 60 patients received either a single intravitreal injection (4 mg) or repeated retrobulbar injections (40 mg, three times) of TA, first injection given approximately 1 week after focal laser photocoagulation.[24] The foveal thickness and VA improvements were significantly better after intravitreal injection, and the need for reinjections was significantly greater in the retrobulbar group.

Anti-Vascular Endothelial Growth Factor Antibodies

Intravitreal VEGF levels have been shown to be increased in patients with ME with BRVO and are correlated significantly with the area of nonperfusion and the severity of ME. A number of case reports, small retrospective or prospective noncontrolled studies, describe improved retinal thickness and VA following intravitreal bevacizumab.[25–29] In one series, the best-corrected VA (BCVA) improved from a baseline mean of 20/333 to 20/91 at 4 weeks after one injection of bevacizumab. However, the effect was not sustained, and at 12 weeks, the VA was reduced to 20/126.[30] A recent prospective clinical trial showed an increase in mean VA from 50 letters (20/100) at baseline to 66 letters (20/50+1; +16 letters; $p < 0.001$) at month 12 and central retinal thickness (CRT) decreased from 558 μm at baseline to 309 μm at month 12 (−249 μm; $p < 0.001$) in 21 eyes with persistent ME (>3 months) treated with three initial intravitreal bevacizumab injections of 1 mg at a monthly interval.[31] In this study, retreatment was based on CRT, and if continuous injections were needed up to month 6, the dose was increased to 2.5 mg. However, the ME had not resolved completely in 86.2% of all patients after three initial injections. Furthermore, the retreatment rate was high with a mean of 8 out of 13 possible injections over 12 months. There was recurrence of ME after initial

BOX 18.2 OZURDEX in Retinal Vein Occlusions

Ozurdex (dexamethasone intravitreal implant), 0.7 mg (Allergan), has been approved by the U.S. FDA as the first drug therapy for ME in BRVO or CRVO. It is administered via intravitreal injection via an innovative NOVADUR solid polymer delivery system. The dexamethasone drug delivery system (DDS) is composed of a biodegradable copolymer of lactic acid and glycolic acid. The polymer slowly biodegrades into carbon dioxide and water, as dexamethasone is released. Since the implant eventually dissolves completely, there is no need for surgical removal. Two multicenter, double-masked, randomized clinical trials showed that the time to achieve a ≥15 letter (3-line) improvement in best-corrected visual acuity (BCVA) cumulative response rate curves was significantly faster with the Ozurdex implant compared to sham ($p < 0.01$) with Ozurdex-treated patients achieving a 3-line improvement in BCVA earlier than sham-treated patients. The onset of effect with Ozurdex, defined as a ≥15 letter (3-line) improvement in BCVA, occurred within the first 2 months after implantation in approximately 20% to 30% of subjects. The duration of effect persisted approximately 1 to 3 months after onset. The most common ocular adverse reactions reported by >2% of the patients in the first 6 months included increased intraocular pressure (25%), conjunctival hemorrhage (20%), eye pain (7%), conjunctival hyperemia (7%), ocular hypertension (4%), cataract (4%), and vitreous detachment (3%), and headache (3%).

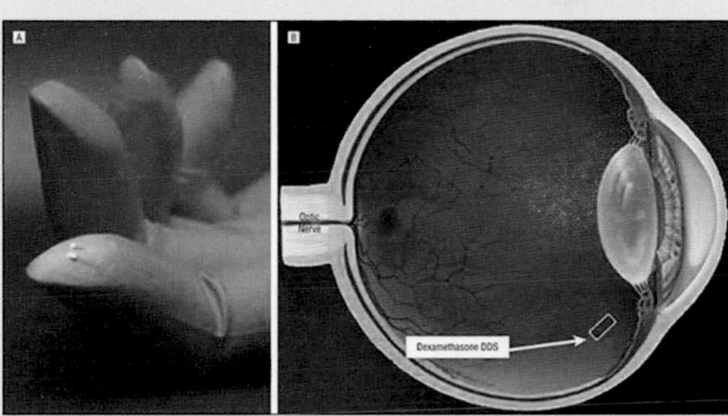

Dexamethasone drug delivery system (DDS). **A:** Dexamethasone DDS implants. The larger implant is the 700-μg dose, and the smaller implant is the 350-μg dose. **B:** Approximate location of the dexamethasone DDS (indicated with the *arrow*; shown larger than actual size for illustrative purposes) after insertion into the eye. (Reproduced from Kuppermann BD, Blumenkranz MS, Haller JA, et al. Randomized controlled study of an intravitreous dexamethasone drug delivery system in patients with persistent macular edema. *Arch Ophthalmol.* 2007;125(3):309–317, with permission.)

improvement in many patients, and 20.7% of all patients showed no complete resorption of ME despite continuous treatment for up to 1 year and an increase of the dose to 2.5 mg after month 6. A 12-month randomized double-masked, sham injection–controlled Phase 3 study (BRAVO) of 397 patients designed to assess the safety and efficacy profile of ranibizumab (Lucentis) in ME secondary to BRVO is currently underway. It consists of a 6-month, sham-controlled treatment period, followed by a 6-month observation period (during which all participants are eligible to receive Lucentis as needed). During the first 6-month period, participants received monthly injections of either 0.3 or 0.5 mg of Lucentis or monthly sham injections. All participants who met prespecified criteria were eligible to receive rescue laser treatment during the first 6-month period. Results at 6 months showed 55.2 percent of patients who received 0.3 mg of Lucentis, and 61.1% who received 0.5 mg of Lucentis had their vision improved by 15 letters or more on the study eye chart compared to 28.8% of patients receiving sham injections (data obtained from Genentech press release on October 4, 2009). Mean gain in BCVA was observed beginning at day 7 with a 7.6- and 7.4-letter gain in the 0.3 and 0.5 mg study arms of Lucentis, respectively, compared with 1.9 letters in the sham injection arm (Box 18.3).

Thus, the role of antivascular endothelial growth factor (anti-VEGF) agents in the treatment of BRVO has yet to be determined. Long-term results and the number of treatments required are unknown. A definitive comparative study of focal laser versus anti-VEGF agents is yet to be performed. Anti-VEGF agents may be a reasonable treatment option when the ME is refractory to laser treatment (Box 18.4) and (Fig. 18.3).

Recombinant Tissue Plasminogen Activator

The pathophysiologic basis for using recombinant tissue plasminogen activator (r-tPA) in BRVO is related to its thrombolytic effects. The additional effects caused by r-tPA include induction of posterior vitreous detachment (PVD) and development of collateral vessels. In a retrospective interventional case series, seventeen eyes presenting with ME caused by BRVO were treated with an intravitreal r-tPA injection.[32] The mean logMAR VA significantly improved from 0.603 ± 0.327 at baseline to 0.388 ± 0.248 ($p < 0.01$) at

BOX 18.3 Anti-VEGF Trials in BRVO and CRVO

The US FDA has approved ranibizumab for treatment of macular edema to retinal vein occlusions based on data from the BRAVO and CRUISE trials.

BRAVO Trial

Purpose: A 12-month randomized double-masked, sham injection-controlled Phase 3 study designed to assess the safety and efficacy profile of ranibizumab in ME secondary to BRVO is ongoing. During the first 6-month period, participants received monthly injections of either 0.3 or 0.5 mg of ranibizumab or monthly sham injections.

Results: Results at 6 months showed 55.2% of patients who received 0.3 mg of ranibizumab and 61.1% who received 0.5 mg of ranibizumab had their vision improved by 15 letters or more on the study eye chart compared to 28.8% of patients receiving sham injections. (Data obtained from Genentech press release on October 4, 2009.)

CRUISE Trial

Purpose: A randomized clinical trial to substantiate the effect and safety of ranibizumab in patients with ME due to CRVO is ongoing. Patients received monthly injections of either 0.3 or 0.5 mg of ranibizumab or monthly sham injections for a 6-month period, followed by a 6-month observation period (during which all participants are eligible to receive ranibizumab as needed).

Results: At 6 months, 46.2% of patients given 0.3 mg of ranibizumab and 47.7% given 0.5 mg of ranibizumab had their vision improved by 15 letters or more compared to 16.9% of patients receiving sham injections. (Data obtained from Genentech press release on October 4, 2009.)

BOX 18.4 Other Clinical Trials in Retinal Vein Occlusions

COPERNICUS Trial: Vascular Endothelial Growth Factor (VEGF) Trap Eye: Investigation of Efficacy and Safety in CRVO

Purpose: A randomized, double-masked, controlled Phase 3 study of the efficacy of VEGF Trap-Eye (Regeneron) injected into the eye on vision function in subjects with ME as a consequence of CRVO. *Arm 1*: Monthly IVT injection of VEGF Trap-Eye 2.0 mg until Week 24 Primary Endpoint. *Arm 2*: Monthly Sham IVT injection until week 24 Primary Endpoint.

Status: Recruitment phase.

GALILEO Trial: Vascular Endothelial Growth Factor (VEGF) Trap-Eye: Investigation of Efficacy and Safety in CRVO

Purpose: A randomized, double-masked, sham-controlled Phase 3 Study of the efficacy of repeated intravitreal administration of VEGF Trap-Eye in subjects with ME due to CRVO. *Arm 1*: Intravitreal injection. Weeks 0 to 20 injection of VEGF Trap-Eye every 4 weeks; weeks 24 to 48 every 4 weeks reassessment and either (PRN) injection of VEGF Trap-Eye or sham injection; weeks 52 to 100 safety follow-up. *Arm 2 Control:* Sham treatment. Weeks 0 to 20 sham treatment every 4 weeks; weeks 24 to 48 every 4 weeks reassessment and sham injection; weeks 52 to 100 safety follow-up.

Status: Recruitment phase.

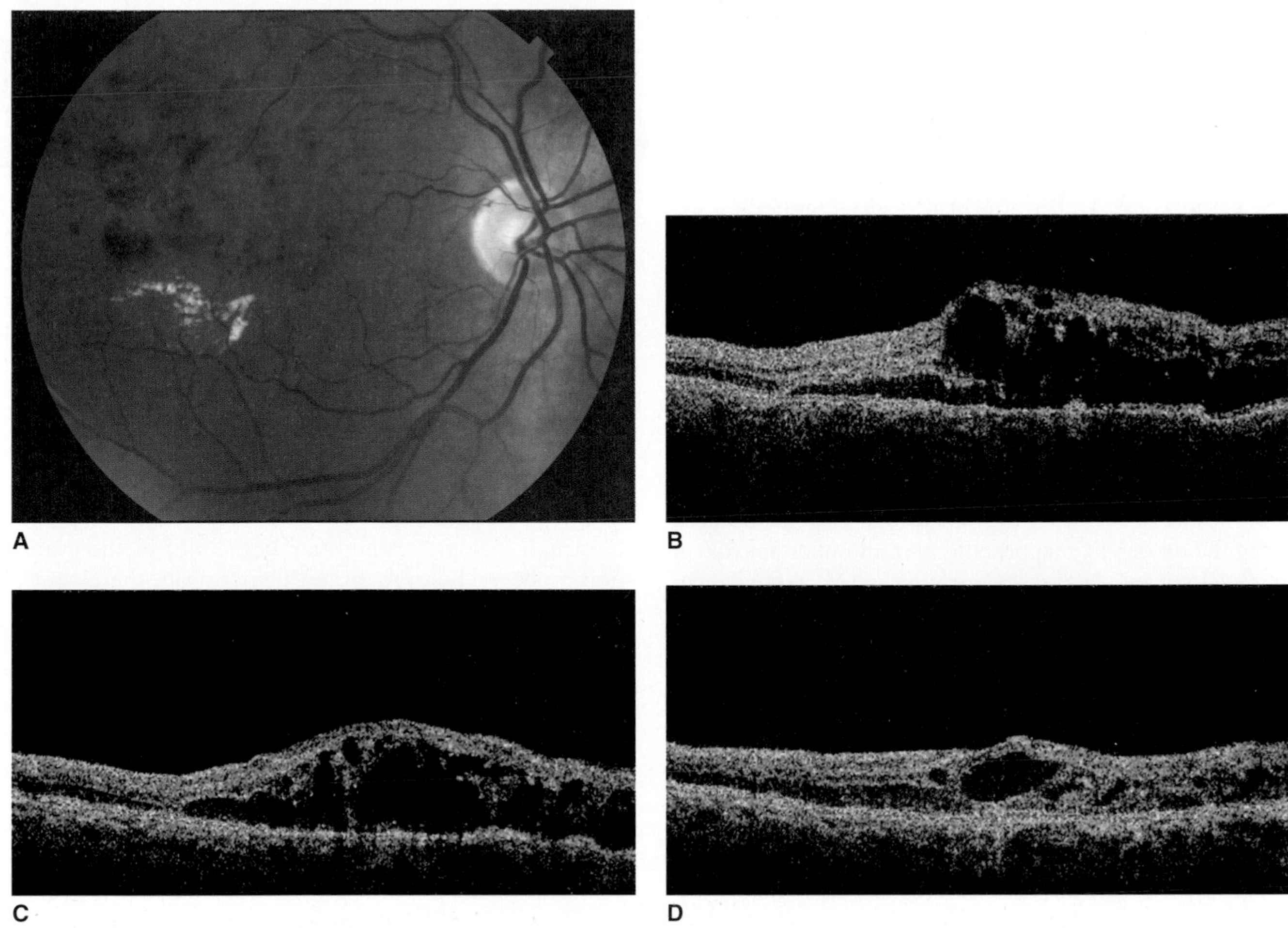

FIGURE 18.3. Fundus photo (**A**) and baseline OCT (**B**) of patient with chronic BRVO and ME. The patient underwent laser photocoagulation; however, there was no resolution of ME as noted in follow-up OCT (**C**). Hence, the patient received intravitreal injection of bevacizumab at 8 months after laser and a second injection 6 weeks after the first injection. There was a considerable resolution of ME as noted on OCT (**D**) following the two injections.

1 month and 0.359 ± 0.319 ($p < 0.05$) at 6 months. The mean foveal thickness significantly decreased from 738 ± 156 μm at baseline to 454 ± 213 μm ($p < 0.001$) at 1 month and 253 ± 164 μm ($p < 0.001$) 6 months. The complications noted in this study were a focal pigmentary alteration sparing the macula in one case and a retinal hole after PVD induced by r-tPA in another case. The efficacy of r-tPA in treatment of BRVO is still unclear, given the absence of randomized trial comparing it with grid laser photocoagulation.

Systemic Therapies

Systemic anticoagulation

Systemic anticoagulation including oral acetylsalicylic acid, subcutaneous heparin, or intravenous thrombolysis has not been shown to be of ocular benefit in patients with BRVO and may potentially worsen concurrent or future intraretinal hemorrhage. Troxerutin has been studied in double-blind randomized study of 26 patients with BRVO <5 months.[33] This drug acts by inhibiting erythrocyte and platelet aggregation and improves erythrocyte deformability, and thereby retinal microcirculation. In this study, baseline visual acuities were well matched, and patients receiving Troxerutin treatment had a mean VA of 20/40 or better than the placebo group, although this difference was not found to be statistically significant. This study was limited by a small sample size, a short randomized, controlled, and masked follow-up period (4 months). Ticlopidine is an inhibitor of platelet aggregation and was compared with placebo in treating patients within 3 weeks from the onset of symptoms for BRVO. At 6-month follow-up, there was a significant difference between the Ticlopidine treatment and placebo groups for VA.[33] However, the Ticlopidine treatment group was associated with gastrointestinal symptoms and skin reactions.

Isovolemic Hemodilution

BRVO has been reported to be associated with hyperviscosity due to higher hematocrit and plasma viscosity. Studies have demonstrated that hypervolemic or isovolemic hemodilution, commenced within 3 months of the onset of symptoms of a BRVO, accelerates the rate of visual recovery and also has a positive effect on the final VA at

1 year.[34] However, reported complications of hemodilution include deep vein thrombosis and hypotension.

CENTRAL RETINAL VEIN OCCLUSION

Pathophysiology

The pathogenesis and treatment of CRVO continue to be highly debated. Hayreh has suggested that perfused CRVO occurs after occlusion of retinal venous flow, while nonperfused CRVO develops after occlusion of venous and arterial flow at their entry into the optic nerve based on animal models.[35] A histopathologic study noted fresh or a recanalized thrombus in enucleated eyes with chronic, nonperfused CRVO, and neovascular glaucoma.[36] Furthermore, vasculitis, thrombophilic factors, and hyperviscous states have been associated with CRVO.[37] An increased risk of CRVO has been noted in eyes with open-angle glaucoma. Hypoxia-induced upregulation of VEGF appears to play an important role in the development of neovascularization and ME secondary to CRVO.[38] Inhibition of VEGF in a nonhuman primate model of CRVO can prevent the development of iris and angle neovascularization.[39] VEGF induces expression of thromboplastin, a potent procoagulant tissue factor that may aggravate the retinal ischemia induced by the CRVO.[40] Furthermore, VEGF induces retinal endothelial swelling, which may lead to further capillary nonperfusion.[41]

Clinical Features

Classically, a CRVO presents with marked dilation and tortuosity of the retinal veins, extensive retinal edema, pronounced superficial and deep retinal hemorrhages radiating outward from the optic disc in all quadrants, cotton-wool spots, and optic disc swelling. Typically, two thirds of all CRVOs are perfused, while the remaining one third are nonperfused.[42] Nonperfused CRVO is often more dramatic in its presentation and is often associated with a relative afferent pupillary defect, and VA worse than 20/400. Overlying retinal hemorrhage may impede the ability to evaluate the underlying capillary perfusion status. One third of perfused CRVOs progress to nonperfused over the course of the disease. Risk factors for progression include worse presenting VA, severe ME, and progressive intraretinal hemorrhage.

The clinical course after a CRVO is highly variable.[42] The retinal hemorrhages may resolve over weeks or may persist for years. The venous dilatation and tortuosity typically resolve with time, and marked fibrous sheathing of the retinal veins and arteries may develop. The disc swelling slowly resolves and may develop disc pallor in nonperfused cases. Optociliary shunt vessels develop commonly following CRVO and may be associated with a decreased risk of developing anterior segment neovascularization. Microaneurysms are a frequent finding following CRVO, whereas macroaneurysms and hard exudates are less common. ME is common following CRVO and may resolve quickly, persist chronically, vary intermittently, or develop late in the course of the disease. Neovascularization typically occurs on the iris in CRVO; however, neovascularization may develop on the disc and/or retina. If neovascularization develops, it usually is present within the first 7 months of the CRVO. The rate of iris neovascularization is 10% in perfused eyes and is 45% to 80% in nonperfused eyes. Of eyes that develop iris neovascularization, approximately two thirds will develop neovascular glaucoma without treatment.[13,43]

Diagnostic Testing

Clinical examination combined with FA is most commonly used to determine perfusion characteristics. The CVOS used 10 disc areas of nonperfusion as its cutoff for predicting risk.[13] In ME, FA shows parafoveal and paramacular capillary leakage that appears as hyperfluorescence that increases in size and intensity with time, often in a petalloid type pattern, and is a risk factor for progression of perfused CRVO to nonperfused CRVO. Nonperfusion near the fovea is associated with worse visual prognosis. Electrophysiologic testing may be helpful in the evaluation process when FA cannot demonstrate the extent of nonperfusion (e.g., in cases with extensive intraretinal hemorrhage). ERG b/a-wave amplitude ratios, photopic and scotopic b-wave amplitudes, and flicker amplitudes were significantly smaller in eyes with extensive capillary nonperfusion than in perfused eyes.[44] The OCT can aid the clinician in evaluating ME, epiretinal membrane formation, and subretinal fluid accumulation following CRVO.

Treatment

While early diagnosis of a CRVO may not require much effort on the part of the clinician, predicting the clinical course and choosing treatment options can be much more difficult and challenging (Figure 18.4). A complete ocular examination, including IOP measurement, slit-lamp biomicroscopy, gonioscopy to rule out neovascularization of the iris or angle, and a dilated fundus examination, is recommended at the initial presentation and at monthly follow-up examinations during the first 9 months. The Central Vein Occlusion Study (CVOS) was a landmark study that recommended prompt application of panretinal photocoagulation after the development of iris or angle neovascularization in eyes with nonperfused CRVO. However, the study showed no benefit from grid laser photocoagulation for CRVO-associated ME.[13] Laser-induced chorioretinal venous anastomosis and radial optic neurotomy have also been shown to improve visual status, but they may be associated with potentially serious complications and have not been evaluated in controlled randomized trials. Various pharmacologic agents have been used as solo or as combination therapies primarily for management of macula edema.

Intraocular Corticosteroids

Small case studies have suggested that there may be a transient benefit from intravitreal injection of steroids for ME associated with CRVO. One such study treated 13 eyes with ME associated with CRVO with an injection of intravitreal TA (4 mg) (Figs. 18.5–18.7).[45] The median duration of symptoms before injection was 8 months (interquartile

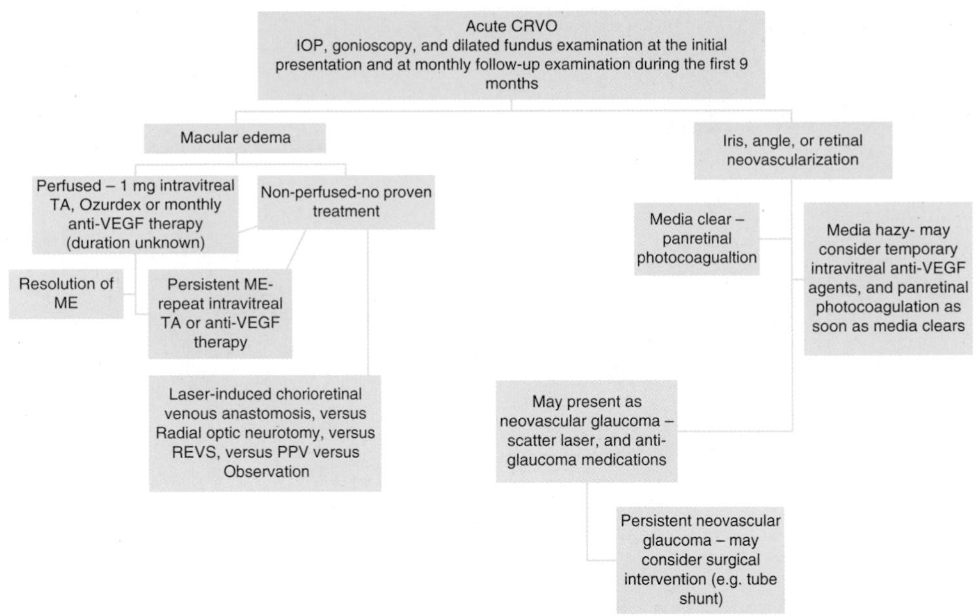

FIGURE 18.4. Stepwise approach for pharmacotherapy of CRVO.

range, 4–9 months), and the mean baseline VA was 20/500 in the affected eye. Mean VA at the 6-month follow-up examination was 20/180 in the affected eye. Eyes with perfused CRVO (n = 5) demonstrated a significant improvement in VA, whereas eyes with nonperfused CRVO (n = 8) demonstrated a nonsignificant VA improvement. Mean baseline foveal thickness as measured by OCT was 590 μm. Mean foveal thickness as measured by OCT at the 1-month follow-up examination in 12 patients was 212 μm. Between the 3- and 6-month follow-up examinations, four patients developed a recurrence of ME. Three of the four patients were retreated with a second injection of TA. Two of these three patients experienced an improvement in VA following retreatment. At the 6-month follow-up examination, mean foveal thickness as measured by OCT for 13 patients was 281 μm. Thus, most patients with CRVO, both nonperfused and perfused, may have a favorable anatomical response to this treatment as demonstrated by OCT images within several weeks of injection; however, a favorable VA response appears more likely in patients with perfused CRVO. Retreatment may also be necessary in some patients due to the recurrence of ME. There may be intravitreal steroid-related adverse events (including cataract and increased IOP) and injection-related adverse events (including noninfectious and infectious endophthalmitis, retinal detachment, vitreous hemorrhage, and lens injury) that could negate the benefit of reduction in ME (Box 18.5).

To address the role of steroids, the SCORE study compared 1- and 4-mg doses of intravitreal TA with standard care (observation) for treatment of vision loss associated with ME secondary to perfused CRVO. It also evaluated the efficacy and safety of the 1- and 4-mg TA doses. The primary outcome of the SCORE-CRVO trial,[46] the percentage of participants with a gain in VA letter score of 15 or more from baseline to month 12, was 6.8%, 26.5%, and 25.6% for the observation, 1-mg, and 4-mg groups, respectively (Fig. 18.8). More eyes in the 4-mg TA group (35%) initiated IOP-lowering medication through 12 months compared with the 1-mg TA (20%) and observation groups (8%). During the first 12 months of the study, two participants in the 1-mg TA group received tube shunt surgery and, between 12 and 24 months, two participants in the 4-mg TA group received tube shunt surgery; the surgery in all participants was deemed by the investigator to be necessary because of the underlying disease (neovascular glaucoma) rather than steroid-related IOP elevation. Among eyes that were phakic at baseline, the estimate through month 12 of new-onset lens opacity or progression of an existing opacity in the observation group, based on assessment at the clinical center, was 18% compared with 26% and 33% for the 1- and 4-mg TA groups, respectively. While no eyes in the observation or 1-mg TA groups had cataract surgery through month 12, four eyes in the 4-mg group received cataract surgery. Similarly, cataract surgery was more frequent between months 12 and 24 in the 4-mg group, with 21 eyes receiving cataract surgery compared with 3 in the 1-mg group and 0 in the observation group. Through month 12, there were no reports of infectious or noninfectious endophthalmitis or retinal detachment in any of the three study groups. In summary, intravitreal TA in both a 1- and 4-mg dose had better VA outcomes over 1 year, and possibly 2 years, than the untreated natural history of ME secondary to perfused CRVO. The superior safety profile of the 1-mg dose compared with the 4-mg dose, particularly with respect to glaucoma and cataract, makes it the preferred dose.

Ozurdex, as discussed in BRVO, in a dose of 700 μg is also being evaluated and may also have potential as a new therapy for ME secondary to CRVO.[22]

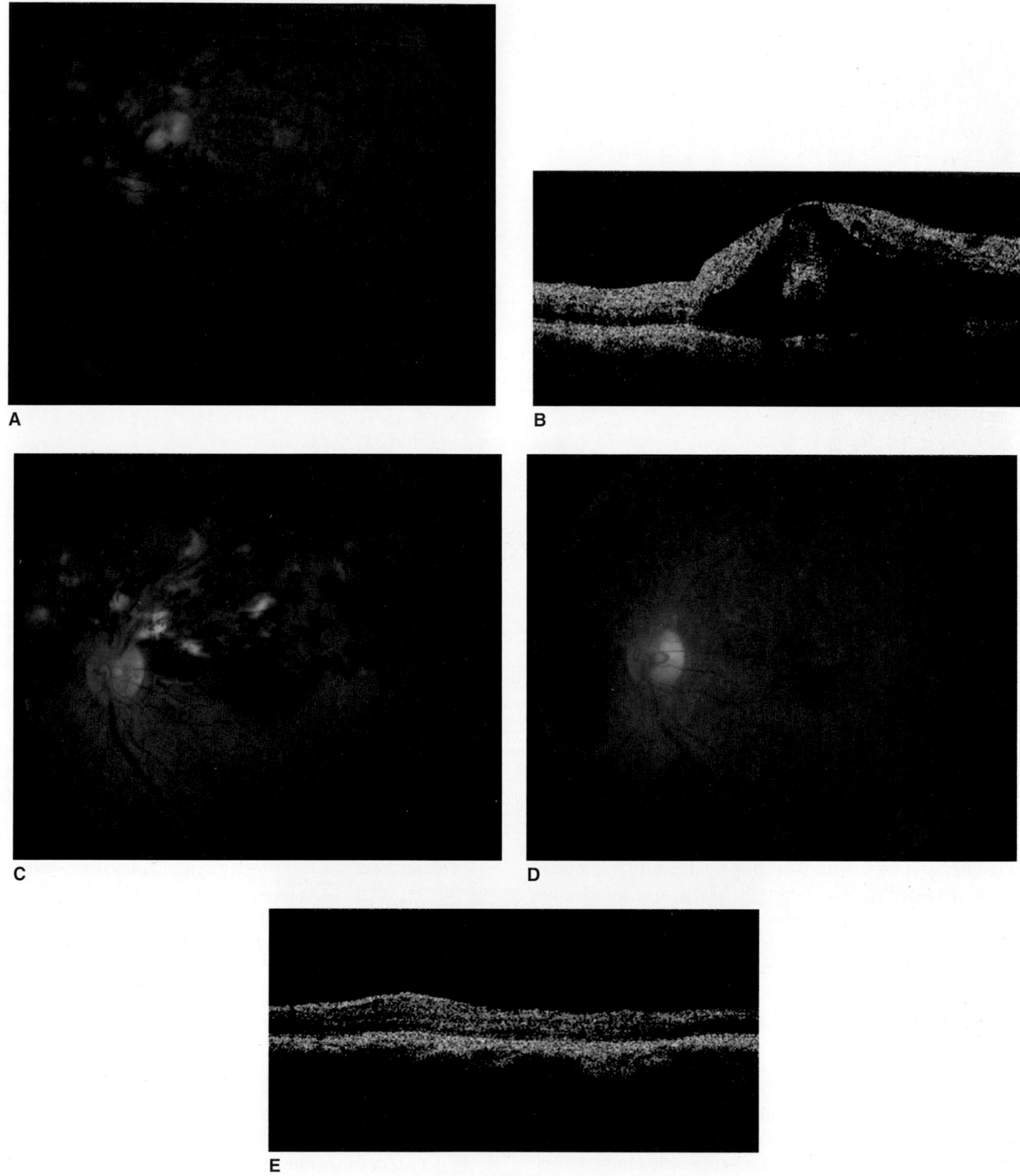

FIGURE 18.5. Fundus photo (**A**) and baseline OCT (**B**) of patient with ischemic CRVO and ME. The patient underwent one intravitreal injection of bevacizumab at 2-month follow-up in view of persisting ME (**C**). There was a considerable resolution of ME (**D, E**) at 3 months following the single bevacizumab injection.

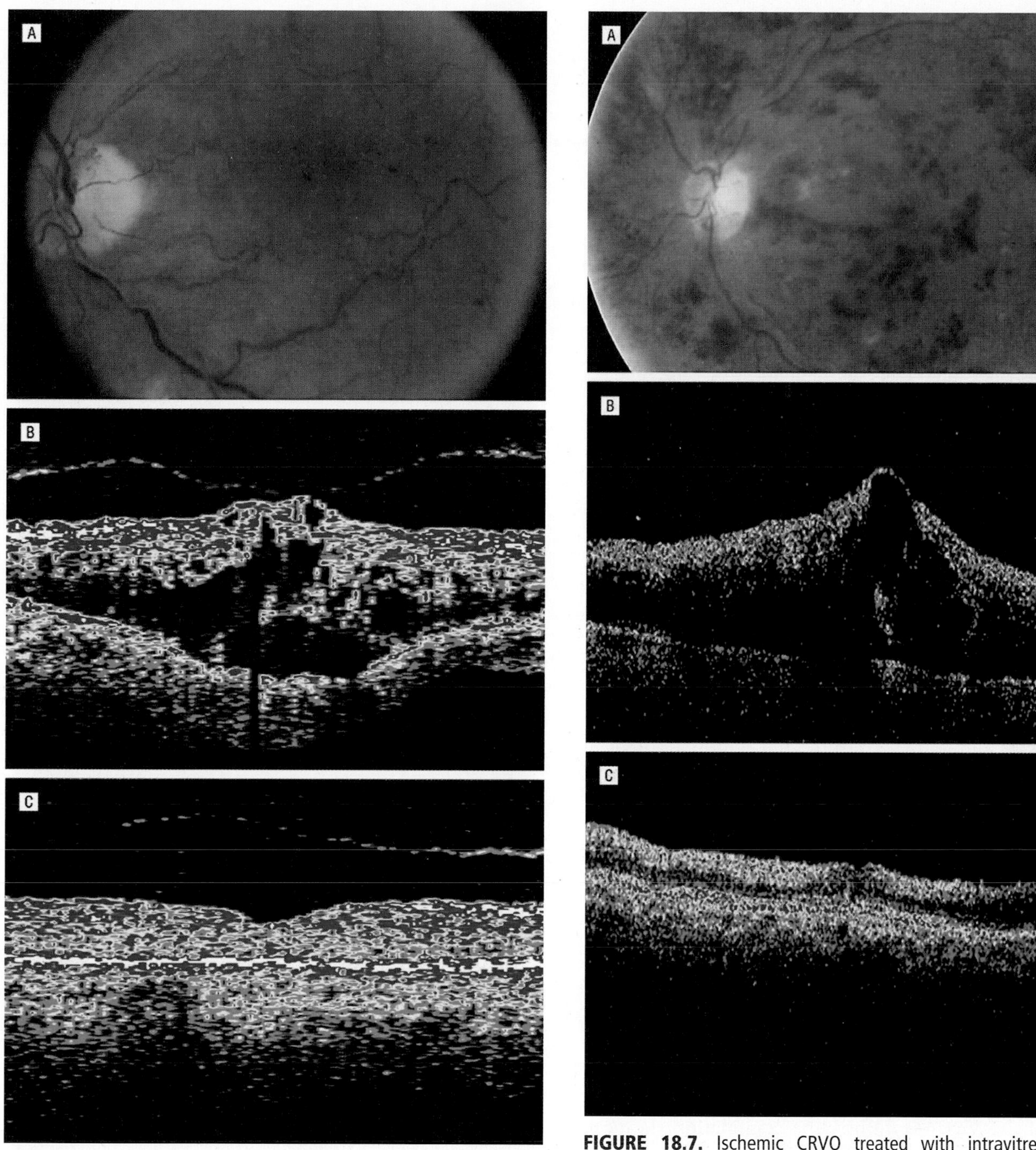

FIGURE 18.6. Nonischemic CRVO treated with intravitreal triamcinolone. **A:** Fundus photograph obtained prior to the initiation of therapy. **B:** Optical coherence tomogram obtained before therapy. **C:** Optical coherence tomogram obtained 1 month after triamcinolone injection. The VA improved along with the resolution of ME. (Reproduced from Ip, et al. *Arch Ophthalmol.* 2004;122:1131, with permission.)

FIGURE 18.7. Ischemic CRVO treated with intravitreal triamcinolone. **A:** Fundus photograph obtained prior to the initiation of therapy. **B:** Optical coherence tomogram obtained before therapy. **C:** Optical coherence tomogram obtained 6 months after triamcinolone injection. Although retinal edema resolved following treatment, VA remained unchanged. (Reproduced from Ip, et al. *Arch Ophthalmol.* 2004;122:1131, with permission.)

Antivascular Endothelial Growth Factor Antibodies

Various anti-VEGF agents are being used in off-label settings in the treatment of CRVO. These include pegaptanib (Macugen), ranibizumab (Lucentis), and bevacizumab (Avastin).

Pegaptanib

Pegaptanib sodium is a 40-kDa RNA aptamer, which binds to VEGF165, the predominant pathological isoform in ischemia-mediated ocular neovascularization. The use of intravitreal pegaptanib (0.3 m and 1 mg) in a phase 2,

BOX 18.5 SCORE Trial in CRVO

Purpose: This multicenter, randomized, clinical trial compared the efficacy and safety of 1- and 4-mg doses of preservative-free intravitreal triamcinolone with observation for eyes with vision loss associated with ME secondary to perfused CRVO.

Conclusions: Intravitreal triamcinolone is superior to observation for treating vision loss associated with ME secondary to CRVO. There was no difference identified between the 1- and 4-mg groups. The rates of elevated intraocular pressure and cataract were similar for the observation and 1-mg groups but higher in the 4-mg group. Intravitreal triamcinolone in a 1-mg dose, following the retreatment criteria applied in the SCORE Study, should be considered for up to 1 year, and possibly 2 years, for patients with characteristics similar to those in the SCORE-CRVO trial. (SCORE Study Research Group, *Arch Ophthalmol.* 2009;127:1101.)

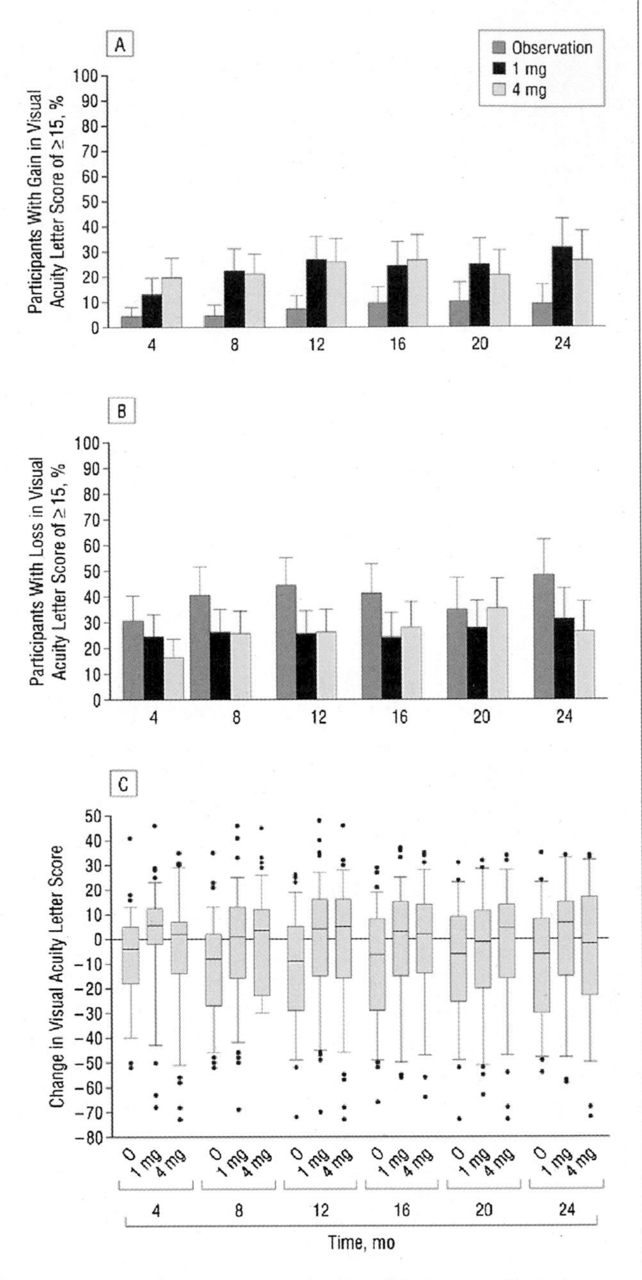

FIGURE 18.8. Change from baseline in electronic Early Treatment Diabetic Retinopathy Study VA letter score at each 4-month follow-up visit. The histograms show the percentages of participants with a gain (**A**) or loss (**B**) in VA letter score of 15 or more from baseline. The dashed line from each bar represents the upper 95% confidence limit. **C:** Box plot with whiskers represents the 5th and 95th percentiles; the line in the box represents the median; dots, values outside the whiskers; O, observation; 1 mg and 4 mg, doses of intravitreal triamcinolone acetonide. (SCORE Study Research Group, *Arch Ophthalmol.* 2009;127:1101.)

randomized, controlled trial given every 6 weeks for a total of five injections for subjects with ME secondary to CRVO revealed 15 letters or more gain of VA measured at the 30-week follow-up visit, although without statistical significance compared with the placebo group.[47] However, a secondary analysis showed a significant reduction in the percentage of subjects losing 15 or more letters and a lower incidence of retinal or iris neovascularization in the groups treated with pegaptanib. No serious ocular and systemic adverse events related to VEGF inhibition were detected.

Bevacizumab

Bevacizumab is a full-length humanized monoclonal antibody to VEGF, which is being used for the treatment of ME secondary to CRVO (see Fig. 18.5). One case series evaluated seven eyes with ischemic CRVO with a mean duration of 7 months prior to treatment with intravitreal bevacizumab (IVB).[48] At the baseline examination, the mean BCVA was 20/320 and the CRT was 730 μm. IVB treatments were administered every 12 weeks if ME persisted. After a single injection, the mean BCVA had improved by 3.34 lines at 12 weeks. Four of the seven eyes had improved by three or more lines. At the final 25-week follow-up, the mean CRT had improved from 730 to 260 μm. A prospective case series studied 14 patients with ME due to CRVO and evaluated ETDRS VA as well as CRT.[49] After a single IVB injection, all patients had improved VA by more than two lines at 3 to 6 weeks of follow-up, with a corresponding decrease in CRT from a mean of 614 to 229 μm ($p = 0.03$). However, between weeks 6 and 9 of follow-up, the retinal thickness increased and VA decreased. A separate retrospective study found that 4 to 10 IVB treatments were required to maintain the benefit over a 1-year period.[50] The optimal timing to initiate treatment with IVB is another issue requiring further study. One retrospective series studied 23 eyes treated with IVB within 3 months of diagnosis compared to another 23 eyes treated after 3 months of diagnosis.[51] The study showed no statistical significant difference in the mean number of ETDRS letters gained between the two groups at 6 months (<3 months = 15.8, >3 months = 13.4 letters). However, the <3-month group had a better baseline VA and posttreatment outcome. Thus, several case series indicate that IVB may be beneficial in the treatment of ME caused by CRVO without the risks of increased IOP and cataract formation. However, the effect is often transient and most case reports lack controls and in some cases, improvement in VA may be due to the natural course of the disease. The timing of initial treatment and the duration of treatment required to achieve long-term results require further evaluation. Multiple consecutive treatments may be required, and ischemic damage may preclude VA improvement in some cases even if the ME responds. Furthermore, numerous reports describe successful treatment of CRVO-induced neovascular glaucoma with regression of neovascular vessels and improvement in IOP as early as 48 hours after the administration of IVB.[52–55] However, the standard treatment for neovascular glaucoma remains PRP with IOP lowering medications as needed. Intravitreal bevacizumab is useful in those who are unable to undergo PRP or as bridge therapy until PRP can be performed (e.g., media opacities).[56] In cases of severe pressure elevation despite maximal medical therapy, IVB may be administered in conjunction with PRP in an attempt to achieve rapid regression of neovascularization, thereby preventing permanent angle synechiae and more quickly achieving pressure control.

Ranibizumab

Ranibizumab is a Fab fragment that binds and neutralizes all isoforms of VEGF-A. Moreover, it has potentially increased retinal penetration because of a smaller molecular size and a higher binding affinity for VEGF than bevacizumab. In a prospective study, 20 eyes with ME secondary to CRVO were treated with intravitreal ranibizumab 0.5 mg administered at baseline, and monthly for two more doses. Additional doses were given if there was evidence of ME by OCT or new intraretinal hemorrhage on examination.[57] A week following the first injection, the mean VA improved 8.3 letters and the CRT decreased by a mean of 349.2 to 225.4 μm of thickness. There was VA improvement of 6.2 letters over baseline and a CRT of 273 μm at 1 month, but at 3-month follow-up, the VA again showed a mean improvement of 10.4 letters over baseline, and there was a decrease of the CRT to 199 μm. The mean VA improved to 64.3 letters, and the CRT decreased to 186 μm at 12 months of follow-up (Fig. 18.9). The patients received a mean number of 8.5 injections. The study had several limitations including small sample size, no control group, nonmasked, and early exit of four patients from the study. To substantiate the effect and safety of ranibizumab in patients with ME due to CRVO, the CRUISE phase 3 trials are underway. The study includes 392 patients with ME secondary to CRVO receiving monthly injections of either 0.3 or 0.5 mg of Lucentis or monthly sham injections for a 6-month period, followed by a 6-month observation period (during which all participants are eligible to receive Lucentis as needed). At 6 months, 46.2% (61/132) of patients given 0.3 mg of Lucentis and 47.7% (62/130) given 0.5 mg of Lucentis had their vision improved by 15 letters or more compared to 16.9% (22/130) of patients receiving sham injections (data obtained from Genentech press release on October 4, 2009). Mean gain in BCVA was observed beginning at day 7 with an 8.8 and 9.3 letter gain in the 0.3 and 0.5 mg study arms of Lucentis, respectively compared with 1.1 letters in the sham injection arm. Thus, the role of anti-VEGF agents in the treatment of CRVO has yet to be determined. Long-term results and the number of treatments required are unknown.

Recombinant Tissue Plasminogen Activator

r-tPA is a synthetic fibrinolytic agent that converts plasminogen to plasmin and destabilizes intravascular thrombi. As therapy for CRVO, r-tPA has been administered by several routes: systemic, intravitreal, subretinal, and via endovascular cannulation of retinal vessels.

Systemic administration of low-dose (50 mg) r-tPA has been associated with serious complications, including patient mortality. Intravitreal delivery of r-tPA has potential advantages including directed delivery to the retinal vessels as well as decreased risk of ocular and systemic complications. Of 47 persons in three studies of intravitreal r-tPA for both ischemic and nonischemic CRVO of <21 days duration, 28% to 44% experienced three lines of VA improvement with 6 months follow-up.[58–60] However, another study showed use of intravitreal r-tPA within 3 days of diagnosis of acute nonperfused CRVO did not significantly alter final perfusion status.[61] These reports suggest prompt use of intravitreal r-tPA, especially in perfused CRVO, may provide visual improvement, although study limitations, such as the lack of a control group, preclude definitive conclusions. A subretinal peripapillary tPA injection in a patient with unresolved CRVO at 4 months with a modest improvement of VA from finger counting to 20/400 has been also described.[62] Retinal endovascular surgery (REVS) is a novel approach involving insertion of a microcannula into branches of the retinal vasculature for delivery of tPA. In a study of 28 eyes with CRVO of >1 month duration and preoperative acuity worse than 20/400, 50% recovered more than 3 lines of acuity with a mean follow-up of 12 months after REVS.[63] There was also a trend toward increased perfusion on FA; however, seven eyes developed vitreous hemorrhage and one eye had retinal detachment.

Systemic Therapies

The role of systemic anticoagulation in CRVO is unclear as there is no evidence that agents such as aspirin, heparin, or warfarin prevent or alter the natural history of CRVO. Patients taking warfarin have been reported to develop CRVO despite maintaining therapeutic levels of anticoagulation.[64] Limited data suggest that systemic hemodilution and/or pentoxifylline (lowers blood viscosity) may be beneficial in improving VA and ME and reducing the risk of progression to ischemic CRVO.[65]

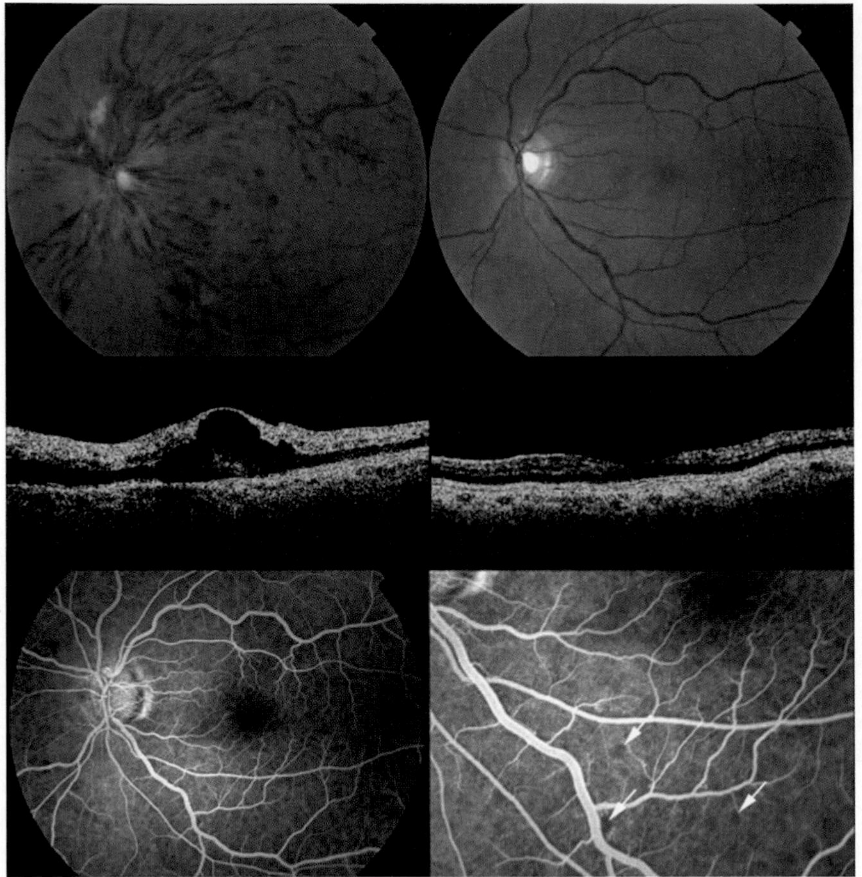

FIGURE 18.9. Images obtained from a 53-year-old male with a 1-day history of CRVO. (**Top left**) Fundus photograph showing optic nerve head hyperemia and swelling, dilated tortuous veins, intraretinal hemorrhage, and foveal pseudocyst. The patient received intravitreal ranibizumab 0.5 mg at baseline and monthly for two additional doses. (**Top right**) Fundus photograph obtained at the 1-year follow-up showing the manifestations of the CRVO resolved. (**Middle left and right**) OCT images obtained at baseline and at the 1-year of follow-up showing dramatic resolution of the ME. (**Bottom left**) Midphase FA showing a normal appearance grossly. (**Bottom right**) However, on closer examination, there was a moth-eaten appearance of the capillary bed with very small areas of nonperfusion (*arrows*). The patient's VA improved 22 letters. (Reproduced from Spaide, et al. *Am J Ophthalmol.* 2009;147:298, with permission.)

KEY POINTS

BRVO

- Most studies evaluating pharmacological interventions have the following characteristics:
  - Lack of sufficient sample size and power
  - Lack of an adequate control using placebo or best practice intervention
  - Combined one interventional therapy with another making it difficult to determine treatment effect
  - Insufficient follow-up times for long-term assessment of outcomes
  - Lack of masking potentially resulting in observer and responder bias
- The SCORE study results substantiate the use of grid photocoagulation as the continued standard of care for patients with ME secondary to BRVO and that it must be the benchmark against which other treatments should be compared in clinical trials.
- The results of several ongoing randomized controlled trials into the use of anti-VEGF agents, and slow-release intravitreal dexamethasone implants are awaited.

CRVO

- The SCORE study results substantiate the use of intravitreal triamcinolone in the 1-mg dose for patients similar to those enrolled in the SCORE-CRVO trial for up to 12 months and possibly 2 years.
- The results of ongoing randomized controlled trials into the use of anti-VEGF agents and slow-release intravitreal dexamethasone implants are awaited.
- Until the results of long-term, randomized studies are available, the optimal management of CRVO will remain unclear, and hence ophthalmologists should exercise caution in recommending unproven treatments.

REFERENCES

1. Orth DH, Patz A. Retinal branch vein occlusion. *Surv Ophthalmol.* 1978;22:357–376.
2. Hayreh SS, Zimmerman MB, Podhajsky P. Incidence of various types of retinal vein occlusion and their recurrence and demographic characteristics. *Am J Ophthalmol.* 1994;117:429–441.
3. The Eye Disease Case-control Study Group. Risk factors for branch retinal vein occlusion. *Am J Ophthalmol.* 1993; 116:286–296.
4. The Eye Disease Case-control Study Group. Risk factors for central retinal vein occlusion. *Arch Ophthalmol.* 1996; 114:545–554.
5. Ai E, Yang SS. Venous occlusive disease: the latest in current management. *Retina.* 2006;26(6 Suppl):S63–S64.
6. Bowers DK, Finkelstein D, Wolff SM, et al. Branch retinal vein occlusion. A clinicopathologic case report. *Retina.* 1987; 7:252–259.
7. Jefferies P, Clemett R, Day T. An anatomical study of retinal arteriovenous crossings and their role in the pathogenesis of retinal branch vein occlusions. *Aust N Z J Ophthalmol.* 1993;21:213–217.
8. Rehak J, Rehak M. Branch retinal vein occlusion: pathogenesis, visual prognosis, and treatment modalities. *Curr Eye Res.* 2008;33(2):111–131.
9. Battaglia-Parodi M, Bandello F. Branch retinal vein occlusion: classification and treatment. *Ophthalmologica.* 2009;223(5): 298–305.
10. Branch Vein Occlusion Study Group. Argon laser photocoagulation for macular edema in branch vein occlusion. *Am J Ophthalmol.* 1984;98:271–282.
11. Branch Vein Occlusion Study Group. Argon laser scatter photocoagulation for prevention of neovascularization and vitreous hemorrhage in branch vein occlusion. A randomized clinical trial. *Arch Ophthalmol.* 1986;104:34–41.
12. Scott IU, VanVeldhuisen PC, Oden NL, et al. SCORE Study report 1: baseline associations between central retinal thickness and visual acuity in patients with retinal vein occlusion. *Ophthalmology.* 2009;116(3):504–512.
13. Central Vein Occlusion Study Group. A randomized clinical trial of early panretinal photocoagulation for ischemic central vein occlusion. The central vein occlusion study group N report. *Ophthalmology.* 1995;102:1434–1444.
14. Lee H, Shah GK. Intravitreal TA as primary treatment of cystoid macular edema secondary to branch retinal vein occlusion. *Retina.* 2005;25:551–555.
15. Yepremyan M, Wertz FD, Tivnan T, et al. Early treatment of cystoid macular edema secondary to branch retinal vein occlusion with intravitreal triamcinolone acetonide. *Ophthalmic Surg Lasers Imaging.* 2005;36:30–36.
16. Ozkiris A, Evereklioglu C, Erkilic K, et al. The efficacy of intravitreal triamcinolone acetonide on macular edema in branch retinal vein occlusion. *Eur J Ophthalmol.* 2005;15: 96–101.
17. Jonas JB, Akkoyun I, Kamppeter B, et al. Branch retinal vein occlusion treated by intravitreal triamcinolone acetonide. *Eye.* 2005;19:65–71.
18. Chen SD, Sundaram V, Lochhead J, et al. Intravitreal triamcinolone for the treatment of ischemic macular edema associated with branch retinal vein occlusion. *Am J Ophthalmol.* 2006;141:876–883.
19. Beer PM, Bakri SJ, Singh RJ, et al. Intraocular concentration and pharmacokinetics of triamcinolone acetonide after a single intravitreal injection. *Ophthalmology.* 2003;110:681–686.
20. Scott IU, Ip MS. It's time for a clinical trial to investigate intravitreal triamcinolone for macular edema due to retinal vein occlusion: The SCORE study. *Arch Ophthalmol.* 2005; 123:581–582.
21. Scott IU, Ip MS, VanVeldhuisen PC, et al. A randomized trial comparing the efficacy and safety of intravitreal triamcinolone with standard care to treat vision loss associated with macular edema secondary to branch retinal vein occlusion: the Standard Care vs Corticosteroid for Retinal Vein Occlusion (SCORE) study report 6. *Arch Ophthalmol.* 2009;127(9):1115–11128.
22. Kuppermann BD, Blumenkranz MS, Haller JA, et al. Randomized controlled study of an intravitreous dexamethasone drug delivery system in patients with persistent macular edema. *Arch Ophthalmol.* 2007;125(3):309–317.
23. Haller JA, Dugel P, Weinberg DV, et al. Evaluation of the safety and performance of an applicator for a novel intravitreal dexamethasone drug delivery system for the treatment of macular edema. *Retina.* 2009;29(1):46–51.
24. Hayashi K, Hayashi H. Intravitreal versus retrobulbar injections of triamcinolone for macular edema associated with branch retinal vein occlusion. *Am J Ophthalmol.* 2005; 139:972–982.
25. Kreutzer TC, Alge CS, Wolf AH, et al. Intravitreal bevacizumab for the treatment of macular oedema secondary to branch retinal vein occlusion. *Br J Ophthalmol.* 2008; 92(3):351–355.
26. Wu L, Arevalo JF, Roca JA, et al. Comparison of two doses of intravitreal bevacizumab (Avastin) for treatment of macular edema secondary to branch retinal vein occlusion: results from the Pan-American Collaborative Retina Study Group at 6 months of follow-up. *Retina.* 2008;28(2):212–219.
27. Gündüz K, Bakri SJ. Intravitreal bevacizumab for macular oedema secondary to branch retinal vein occlusion. *Eye.* 2008 22(9):1168–1171.
28. Jaissle GB, Leitritz M, Gelisken F, et al. One-year results after intravitreal bevacizumab therapy for macular edema secondary to branch retinal vein occlusion. *Graefes Arch Clin Exp Ophthalmol.* 2009;247(1):27–33.
29. Rabena MD, Pieramici DJ, Castellarin AA, et al. Intravitreal bevacizumab (Avastin) in the treatment of macular edema secondary to branch retinal vein occlusion. *Retina.* 2007;27(4):419–425.
30. Pai SA, Shetty R, Vijayan PB, et al. Clinical, anatomic, and electrophysiologic evaluation following intravitreal bevacizumab for macular edema in retinal vein occlusion. *Am J Ophthalmol.* 2007;143(4):601–606.
31. Prager F, Michels S, Kriechbaum K, et al. Intravitreal bevacizumab (Avastin) for macular oedema secondary to retinal vein occlusion: 12-month results of a prospective clinical trial. *Br J Ophthalmol.* 2009;93(4):452–456.
32. Murakami T, Takagi H, Kita M, et al. Intravitreal tissue plasminogen activator to treat macular edema associated with branch retinal vein occlusion. *Am J Ophthalmol.* 2006;142(2):318–320.
33. McIntosh RL, Mohamed Q, Saw SM, et al. Interventions for branch retinal vein occlusion: an evidence-based systematic review. *Ophthalmology.* 2007;114(5):835–838.

34. Chen HC, Wiek J, Gupta A, et al. Effect of isovolaemic haemodilution on visual outcome in branch retinal vein occlusion. *Br J Ophthalmol.* 1998;82:162–167.
35. Hayreh SS. Prevalent misconceptions about acute retinal vascular occlusive disorders. *Prog Retin Eye Res.* 2005;24: 493–519.
36. Green WR, Chan CC, Hutchins GM, et al. Central retinal vein occlusion: a prospective histopathologic study of 29 eyes in 28 cases. *Trans Am Ophthalmol Soc.* 1981;79:371–422.
37. Marcucci R, Bertini L, Giusti B, et al. Thrombophilic risk factors in patients with central retinal vein occlusion. *Thromb Haemost.* 2001;86:772–776.
38. Boyd SR, Zachary I, Chakravarthy U, et al. Correlation of increased vascular endothelial growth factor with neovascularization and permeability in ischemic central vein occlusion. *Arch Ophthalmol.* 2002;120:1644–1650.
39. Adamis AP, Shima DT, Tolentino MJ, et al. Inhibition of vascular endothelial growth factor prevents retinal ischemia-associated iris neovascularization in a nonhuman primate. *Arch Ophthalmol.* 1996;114(1):66–71.
40. Sassa Y, Hata Y, Murata T, et al. Functional role of Egr-1 mediating VEGF-induced tissue factor expression in the retinal capillary endothelium. *Graefes Arch Clin Exp Ophthalmol.* 2002;240(12):1003–1010.
41. Hofman P, van Blijswijk BC, Gaillard PJ, et al. Endothelial cell hypertrophy induced by vascular endothelial growth factor in the retina: new insights into the pathogenesis of capillary nonperfusion. *Arch Ophthalmol.* 2001;119(6):861–866.
42. Quinlan PM, Elman MJ, Bhatt AK, et al. The natural course of central retinal vein occlusion. *Am J Ophthalmol.* 1990;110:118–123.
43. Magargal LE, Donoso LA, Sanborn GE. Retinal ischemia and risk of neovascularization following central retinal vein obstruction. *Ophthalmology.* 1982;89:1241–1245.
44. Matsui Y, Katsumi O, Mehta MC, et al. Correlation of electroretinographic and fluorescein angiographic findings in unilateral central retinal vein obstruction. *Graefes Arch Clin Exp Ophthalmol.* 1994;232:449–457.
45. Ip MS, Gottlieb JL, Kahana A, et al. Intravitreal triamcinolone for the treatment of macular edema associated with central retinal vein occlusion. *Arch Ophthalmol.* 2004;122:1131–1136.
46. Ip MS, Scott IU, VanVeldhuisen PC, et al. A randomized trial comparing the efficacy and safety of intravitreal triamcinolone with observation to treat vision loss associated with macular edema secondary to central retinal vein occlusion: the Standard Care vs Corticosteroid for Retinal Vein Occlusion (SCORE) study report 5. *Arch Ophthalmol.* 2009;127(9):1101–1114.
47. Wroblewski JJ, Wells JA III, Adamis AP, et al. Pegaptanib sodium for macular edema secondary to central retinal vein occlusion. *Arch Ophthalmol.* 2009;127(4):374–380.
48. Costa RA, Jorge R, Calucci D, et al. Intravitreal bevacizumab (avastin) for central and hemicentral retinal vein occlusions: IBeVO study. *Retina.* 2007;27(2):141–149.
49. Stahl A, Agostini H, Hansen LL, et al. Bevacizumab in retinal vein occlusion-results of a prospective case series. *Graefes Arch Clin Exp Ophthalmol.* 2007;245(10):1429–1436.
50. Ferrara DC, Koizumi H, Spaide RF. Early bevacizumab treatment of central retinal vein occlusion. *Am J Ophthalmol.* 2007; 144(6):864–871.
51. Priglinger SG, Wolf AH, Kreutzer TC, et al. Intravitreal bevacizumab injections for treatment of central retinal vein occlusion: six-month results of a prospective trial. *Retina.* 2007; 27(8):1004–1012.
52. Batioglu F, Astam N, Ozmert E. Rapid improvement of retinal and iris neovascularization after a single intravitreal bevacizumab injection in a patient with central retinal vein occlusion and neovascular glaucoma. *Int Ophthalmol.* 2008;28(1):59–61.
53. Kahook MY, Schuman JS, Noecker RJ. Intravitreal bevacizumab in a patient with neovascular glaucoma. *Ophthalmic Surg Lasers Imaging.* 2006;37(2):144–146.
54. Iliev ME, Domig D, Wolf-Schnurrbursch U, et al. Intravitreal bevacizumab (Avastin) in the treatment of neovascular glaucoma. *Am J Ophthalmol.* 2006;142(6):1054–1056.
55. Davidorf FH, Mouser JG, Derick RJ. Rapid improvement of rubeosis iridis from a single bevacizumab (Avastin) injection. *Retina.* 2006;26(3):354–356.
56. Ehlers JP, Spirn MJ, Lam A, et al. Combination intravitreal bevacizumab/panretinal photocoagulation versus panretinal photocoagulation alone in the treatment of neovascular glaucoma. *Retina.* 2008;28(5):696–702.
57. Spaide RF, Chang LK, Klancnik JM, et al. Prospective study of intravitreal ranibizumab as a treatment for decreased visual acuity secondary to central retinal vein occlusion. *Am J Ophthalmol.* 2009;147(2):298–306.
58. Lahey JM, Fong DS, Kearney J. Intravitreal tissue plasminogen activator for acute central retinal vein occlusion. *Ophthalmic Surg Lasers.* 1999;30:427–434.
59. Glacet-Bernard A, Kuhn D, Vine AK, et al. Treatment of recent onset central retinal vein occlusion with intravitreal tissue plasminogen activator: A pilot study. *Br J Ophthalmol.* 2000;84:609–613.
60. Elman MJ, Raden RZ, Carrigan A. Intravitreal injection of tissue plasminogen activator for central retinal vein occlusion. *Trans Am Ophthalmol Soc.* 2001;99:219–221.
61. Ghazi NG, Noureddine B, Haddad RS, et al. Intravitreal tissue plasminogen activator in the management of central retinal vein occlusion. *Retina.* 2003;23:780–784.
62. Lam HD, Blumenkranz MS. Treatment of central retinal vein occlusion by vitrectomy with lysis of vitreopapillary and epipapillary adhesions, subretinal peripapillary tissue plasminogen activator injection, and photocoagulation. *Am J Ophthalmol.* 2002;134:609–611.
63. Weiss JN, Bynoe LA. Injection of tissue plasminogen activator into a branch retinal vein in eyes with central retinal vein occlusion. *Ophthalmology.* 2001;108:2249–2257.
64. Mruthyunjaya P, Wirostko WJ, Chandrashekhar R, et al. Central retinal vein occlusion in patients treated with long-term warfarin sodium (coumadin) for anticoagulation. *Retina.* 2006;26:285–291.
65. Mohamed Q, McIntosh RL, Saw SM, et al. Interventions for central retinal vein occlusion: an evidence-based systematic review. *Ophthalmology.* 2007;114(3):507–519, 524.

CHAPTER

19

Intravitreal Injection: Technique and Complications

Elias Reichel

INTRODUCTION

Intravitreal injections are becoming an increasingly common part of clinical practice. In the past, indications for injection of substances into the vitreous cavity were relatively limited. The advent of new therapies targeting the posterior pole has resulted in an exponential rise in the number of injections performed. As the number of these procedures increases, careful technique becomes a more important part of producing safe and effective results.

Today, there are a host of pharmaceuticals used to treat retinal diseases via intravitreal injection, with many more under investigation. The most commonly injected medications are those used to treat exudative macular degeneration. Ranibizumab (Lucentis, Genentech, San Francisco, CA) has been the subject of large clinic trials and may be administered at a minimum interval of 4 weeks. The use of bevacizumab (Avastin, Genentech) has also been well studied. In addition, bevacizumab is also used to treat other forms of retinal neovascularization as well as macular edema. Trials for use of ranibizumab for a number of these conditions are currently under way.

Another commonly injected medication is triamcinolone acetate (Kenalog, Bristol Myers Squibb, New York, NY). Used off label, this steroid preparation has been used for treating macular edema, uveitis, and as an adjunct to macular degeneration therapy. Other applications of intravitreal injections include antiviral medications of cytomegalovirus (CMV) or herpetic infections, antibiotics for endophthalmitis, and tissue plasminogen activator for submacular hemorrhage. In-office injections of intravitreal gas are also used to treat retinal detachments with pneumatic retinopexy.

As the role of intravitreal injections in office-based practice has expanded, basic guidelines for the technique have been discussed.[1] Since then, our knowledge of the risks and complications of injections have also expanded. While intravitreal injections are most often safe and relatively pain-free procedures, they are still associated with risk, while rare, serious complications such as endophthalmitis, retinal detachment, traumatic cataract, and vitreous hemorrhage have been reported. This chapter discusses injection protocol and issues related to peri-injection management.

Injection Protocol

While injection protocol is subject to minor variation between clinicians, the general technique remains the same.

Preinjection

1. Prior to the day of the injection, some clinicians elect to pretreat the affected eye with a topical antibiotic, usually for a period of 3 days.

Injection

1. The patient is examined. Injection is contraindicated in the presence of active ocular or periocular infection.
2. Informed consent is obtained, and the eye to be injected is verified.
3. The eye to be injected is dilated.
4. The lid and eyelashes are cleaned with 5% povidone-iodine.
5. Five percent povidone-iodine is placed on the conjunctiva prior to subconjunctival injection of anesthetic.
6. If T/topical anesthesia is administered, the conjunctiva is then flushed with 5% povidone-iodine to clean the conjunctiva and remove any anesthetic vehicle that may be on the ocular surface.
7. Some clinicians elect to use a sterile drape, use of gloves is recommended.
8. A sterile lid speculum is placed.
9. The injection site is marked 3.5 mm posterior to limbus in pseudophakic eyes and 4.0 mm posterior to limbus in phakic eyes.
10. Five percent povidone iodine is instilled into the eye at the injection site, most commonly inferotemporally.
11. The drug is injected using either a 30- or 27-gauge needle directed toward the center of the vitreous cavity. Care is taken to avoid contact with the eyelashes or lid margin.

12. The injection is performed slowly, but firmly.
13. A cotton-tipped applicator is used to apply brief pressure at the injection site to prevent reflux.
14. The lid speculum is removed and topical antibiotic is administered.
15. The patient's vision is checked to confirm hand motions.
16. Perfusion of the optic nerve is confirmed using indirect ophthalmoscopy.
17. The intraocular pressure is checked 10 minutes following the injection and the patient is discharged if the IOP is within safe levels, usually 35 mm Hg or below.
18. If the intraocular pressure is high, topical glaucoma drops are administered and the pressure is rechecked. Rarely, an anterior chamber paracentesis may be required.

Postinjection

1. The patient is instructed to use topical antibiotics for 3 to 7 days following the injection.
2. A telephone follow-up is usually done the week following the injection. The patient should be examined if there is significant pain or decrease in vision.

Techniques

Although the rate of complications following intravitreal injections is low, meticulous antisepsis should be maintained to minimize serious sequelae such as endophthalmitis.

Gloves and Draping

Prior to the procedure, it is common practice to wear gloves. While the gloves need not be sterile, they are a part of universal safety precautions. Some physicians also drape the eyelids and lashes prior to the injection. Draping may help to prevent contamination of the needle with eyelid flora but is optional.

Eyelid Speculum and Povidone Iodine

Possible sources for bacterial contamination of the needle include the eyelashes and the conjunctiva. To minimize contact with the eyelashes, the use of a sterile eyelid speculum is recommended. In addition, the application of 5% to 10% povidone iodine to the periorbita and 5% to the injection site itself is critical. The use of povidone iodine has been shown to reduce the number of conjunctival bacteria.[2] Furthermore, the application of povidone iodine reduces the risk of endophthalmitis following cataract surgery.[3–7] Just prior to the injection, the povidone iodine may be applied as drops, a swab, or an irrigating flush.[5]

Antibiotic Prophylaxis

Many clinicians also choose to use preinjection and/or postinjection antibiotics for prophylaxis. The role of preinjection antibiotics remains controversial. Previous studies have shown that, prior to cataract surgery, a 3-day course of topical antibiotics provides a further decrease in bacterial colonization than povidone iodine prep. alone.[2] However, recent data suggest that a fourth-generation fluoroquinolone does not provide additional benefit over povidone iodine alone.[14] For cataract surgery, preoperative antibiotics are possibly relevant but do not definitely alter clinical outcomes.[7] Preinjection antibiotics were not used in the SCORE of DRCRnet clinical trials and a low incidence of endophthalmitis was observed,[3] suggesting that they may not be necessary. In contrast, most clinicians prescribe topical antibiotic prophylaxis following an injection. However, there have been reported case series with a low incidence of endophthalmitis in which a significant portion of patients were not given postinjection antibiotics.[11]

Anesthesia

A variety of methods are employed to provide anesthesia for intravitreal injections. The most common method is to employ a topical anesthetic. Some clinicians elect to apply proparacaine- or tetracaine-soaked pledgets to the injection site prior to delivery of the medication. An alternative is to use viscous tetracaine or 2% lidocaine jelly.[6] Our current practice is to use two administrations of 3.5% lidocaine gel,[10] separated by a 5-minute interval, which provides adequate anesthesia. Subconjunctival injection of 2% lidocaine solution is less commonly employed and may be associated with more chemosis, hemorrhage, and accidental perforation of the eye wall.

Complications

In general, intravitreal injections are well tolerated and rates of complications are low. In large studies, the most common adverse events were benign and included subconjunctival hemorrhage and keratoconjunctivitis sicca. However, serious adverse events such as endophthalmitis, retinal detachment, vitreous hemorrhage, and traumatic cataract can occur. Anticoagulation or the use of platelet inhibitors does not appear to increase the risk of vitreous hemorrhage in conjunction with intravitreal injections. Table 19.1 summarizes the complication rates seen during several large clinical trials of anti-VEGF agents.

While infrequent, endophthalmitis remains the most serious potential complication of an intravitreal injection. Reported rates of endophthalmitis per injection vary. As shown in Table 19.1, large clinical trials of anti-VEGF agents have found a very low rate of endophthalmitis. Large retrospective reviews have also described low rates of infection for both ranibizumab and bevacizumab.[8–15] In clinical trials using triamcinolone, the rate of infectious endophthalmitis was also very low.[3] Some reviews have quoted higher rates of endophthalmitis following intravitreal triamcinolone that may have been related to multiuse vials, filtering blebs, or diabetes mellitus.[13] In cases of culture positive endophthalmitis, eyelid or conjunctival flora

Table 19.1.

Complication rates in several clinical trials of anti-VEGF agents

Study	Endophthalmitis (%)	Vitreous Hemorrhage (%)	Traumatic Cataract (%)	Retinal Detachment (%)	Retinal Tear (%)
ANCHOR	0.05	0.03	0	0.03	0.01
MARINA	0.05	0.02	0	0	0.02
PIER	0	0	0	0	0
PrONTO	0	0	0	0	0
SCORE/DRCRnet	0.05				

such as *Streptococcus* or *Staphylococcus* species are often isolated. Many cases respond to injection of intravitreal antibiotics, but vitrectomy may be necessary. Prophylaxis with povidone-iodine, and antibiotics, along with meticulous antiseptic technique may minimize the risk of post-injection endophthalmitis.[16–18]

KEY POINTS

- Intravitreal injection is a safe and effective means of drug delivery to the posterior pole.
- Meticulous antiseptic technique should be used including a lid speculum and povidone iodine.
- Postinjection antibiotic drops are used by most clinicians.

REFERENCES

1. Aiello LP, Brucker AJ, Chang S, et al. Evolving guidelines for intravitreous injections. *Retina*. 2004;24(5 Suppl):S3–S19.
2. Apt L, Isenberg SJ, Yoshimori R, et al. Outpatient topical use of povidone-iodine in preparing the eye for surgery. *Ophthalmology*. 1989;96(3):289–292.
3. Bhavsar AR, Ip MS, Glassman AR, et al. The risk of endophthalmitis following intravitreal triamcinolone injection in the DRCRnet and SCORE clinical trials. *Am J Ophthalmol*. 2007;144(3):454–456.
4. Brown DM, Kaiser PK, Michels M, et al. Ranibizumab versus verteporfin for neovascular age-related macular degeneration. ANCHOR Study Group. *N Engl J Med*. 2006;355(14):1432–1444.
5. Brown DM, Michels M, Kaiser PK, et al. Ranibizumab versus verteporfin photodynamic therapy for neovascular age-related macular degeneration: Two-year results of the ANCHOR study. *Ophthalmology*. 2009;116(1):57–65.
6. Busbee BG, Alam A, Reichel E. Lidocaine hydrochloride gel for ocular anesthesia: results of a prospective, randomized study. *Ophthalmic Surg Lasers Imaging*. 2008;39(5):386–390.
7. Ciulla TA, Starr MB, Masket S. Bacterial endophthalmitis prophylaxis for cataract surgery: an evidence-based update. *Ophthalmology*. 2002;109(1):13–24.
8. Fintak DR, Shah GK, Blinder KJ, et al. Incidence of endophthalmitis related to intravitreal injection of bevacizumab and ranibizumab. *Retina*. 2008;28(10):1395–1399.
9. Jonas JB, Spandau UH, Schlichtenbrede F. Short-term complications of intravitreal injections of triamcinolone and bevacizumab. *Eye*. 2008;22(4):590–591.
10. Kozak I, Cheng L, Freeman WR. Lidocaine gel anesthesia for intravitreal drug administration. *Retina*. 2005;25(8):994–998.
11. Diago T, McCannel CA, Bakri SJ, et al. Infectious endophthalmitis after intravitreal injection of antiangiogenic agents. *Retina*. 2009;29(5):601–605.
12. Lalwani GA, Rosenfeld PJ, Fung AE, et al. A variable-dosing regimen with intravitreal ranibizumab for neovascular age-related macular degeneration: year 2 of the PrONTO Study. *Am J Ophthalmol*. 2009;148(1):43–58.
13. Moshfeghi DM, Kaiser PK, Scott IU, et al. Acute endophthalmitis following intravitreal triamcinolone acetonide injection. *Am J Ophthalmol*. 2003;136(5):791–796.
14. Moss JM, Sanislo SR, Ta CN. A prospective randomized evaluation of topical gatifloxacin on conjunctival flora in patients undergoing intravitreal injections. *Ophthalmology*. 2009;116:1498–1501.
15. Pilli S, Kotsolis A, Spaide RF, et al. Endophthalmitis associated with intravitreal anti-vascular endothelial growth factor therapy injections in an office setting. *Am J Ophthalmol*. 2008;145(5):879–882.
16. Regillo CD, Brown DM, Abraham P, et al. Randomized, double-masked, sham-controlled trial of ranibizumab for neovascular age-related macular degeneration: PIER Study year 1. *Am J Ophthalmol*. 2008;145(2):239–248.
17. Speaker MG, Menikoff JA. Prophylaxis of endophthalmitis with topical povidone-iodine. *Ophthalmology*. 1991;98(12):1769–1775.
18. Ta CN. Minimizing the risk of endophthalmitis following intravitreous injections. *Retina*. 2004;24(5):699–705.

CHAPTER

20

The Role of Optical Coherence Tomography in the Management of Age-Related Macular Degeneration and Macular Edema

Pearse A. Keane • Srinivas R. Sadda

INTRODUCTION TO OPTICAL COHERENCE TOMOGRAPHY

Optical coherence tomography (OCT), first described by Huang et al.[1] in 1991, allows high-resolution cross-sectional (tomographic) images of the neurosensory retina to be obtained in a noninvasive manner. Commercially available OCT systems are now capable of obtaining retinal images with an axial resolution of approximately 5 to 8 μm, and a transverse resolution of approximately 15 to 20 μm.[2] As a result, OCT has been characterized as in vivo "clinical biopsy" and has transformed the diagnosis and management of vitreoretinal disorders.[3]

BASIC PRINCIPLES

OCT works by measuring the properties of light waves reflected from, and scattered by, tissue (analogous to ultrasonography).[4] The use of light waves in OCT results in images with much greater resolution than ultrasonography as the wavelength of light is many times less than that of sound. However, the use of light instead of sound is challenging as the speed of light exceeds the speed of sound by a factor of 150,000 times, making direct measurements of optical "echoes" impossible over small distances. OCT instruments employ a number of the distinctive physical properties of light waves to overcome this technological hurdle, in particular the principle of interference.

Interference is a phenomenon that occurs when two light waves meet each other and are superimposed. The resulting waveform depends on the wavelength, amplitude, and relative phase of the two waves. Interferometry uses the principle of interference to deduce the original state of waves by analyzing the result of their combination.[4] In interferometers, a single beam of light is split into two identical beams—each beam travels a separate path before being recombined together at a single detector. The combination of light reflected from the tissue of interest, and light reflected from a reference mirror, produces characteristic patterns of interference that are diagnostic of the mismatch between the reflected waves. In the earliest OCT systems, these interference patterns were assessed as a function of time—"time domain" OCT.

TIME DOMAIN OCT

In 1993, the first time domain OCT device capable of in vivo use in humans was developed.[5] This technology was acquired by Humphrey Instruments (a division of Carl Zeiss Meditec, Dublin, California), who subsequently developed the first commercial devices—OCT1 and OCT2. Improvements in the technology led to the development of OCT3—termed StratusOCT, currently the most commonly used OCT system worldwide. Although time domain OCT systems are capable of generating high-resolution images (8–10 μm for StratusOCT), they require the use of a mobile reference mirror for the assessment of interference patterns—a requirement that limits their image acquisition speed (400 A-scans per second for StratusOCT).[4] This is a major restriction for clinical practice as only sparse coverage of the macular area is possible when acquiring any given image set.[6] Fortunately, this technological hurdle has been overcome in recent years with the introduction of "spectral domain" OCT—a technology that removes the requirement for a mobile reference mirror by the assessment of interference patterns as a function of frequency rather than of time.[7]

SPECTRAL DOMAIN OCT

Spectral domain OCT systems use spectral interferometry and a mathematical function (Fourier transformation) to assess interference patterns as a function of frequency.[8,9] Thus, light scattered from different depths within the tissue can be measured simultaneously, and images can be acquired 50 to 100 times more quickly than in time domain systems (typically over 20,000 A-scans per second).

The first in vivo imaging of the human retina using spectral domain OCT was reported in 2002.[10] More recently, a number of commercial OCT systems, which incorporate spectral domain technology, have been released. These devices include Cirrus HD-OCT (Carl Zeiss Meditec, Dublin, CA), 3D OCT-1000 (Topcon Medical Systems, Japan), Spectralis OCT (Heidelberg Engineering, Germany), RTVue-100 (Optovue Corporation, Fremont, CA), Spectral OCT SLO (Opko Instrumentation/OTI, Canada), SOCT Copernicus HR (Reichert Ophthalmic Instruments, New York, NY), and 3D SDOCT (Bioptigen, NC). In addition to their increased speed and sensitivity, many of these instruments offer incremental improvements in axial resolution through the use of improved light sources.

Each of the recently introduced commercial spectral domain OCT systems is capable of acquiring sizable image sets over short time periods. As a result, new methods of utilizing these image sets have evolved, significantly enhancing the evaluation of vitreoretinal disorders.

RETINAL IMAGING WITH SPECTRAL DOMAIN TECHNOLOGY

Raster Scanning

The high speed of spectral domain OCT facilitates significantly greater sampling of the macular area via the use of raster scanning protocols.[11–13] Raster scans consist of a rectangular pattern of horizontal line scans that run in parallel across the macula (e.g., 128 B-scans, with each B-scan consisting of 512 A-scans). The greater retinal sampling density of spectral domain raster scans may facilitate early detection of morphologic changes in disease states, as well as allowing these changes to be more accurately followed over time.

When dense raster scanning is performed, spectral domain OCT systems have the ability to perform volumetric rendering of the OCT images (rendering is the processing of OCT images to make them appear solid and three dimensional [3D]). Volumetric rendering allows enhanced visualization of the retina, which may take place from any direction, and which may be useful in disorders such as epiretinal membrane (ERM), or vitreomacular traction.[14]

OCT Fundus Images

Another important feature of spectral domain OCT is the ability to generate "OCT fundus images" that mimic the images obtained from standard fundus photography.[12,13] These images are generated from the raster scan OCT data by summing the intensity of pixels in the axial direction, resulting in a pixel brightness value for each axial scan position. OCT fundus images show a direct view of the macula in which the retinal vascular arcades may be clearly visible and spatially consistent with the vasculature on color photographic, or angiographic, images. OCT fundus images are useful in the clinical setting as they can facilitate registration of any point on an OCT image with a corresponding point on the retinal surface. OCT fundus images also permit the acquisition of images in the same location over time, although this is not always possible in the setting of severe disease (where the vascular pattern and other landmarks may be less apparent) or in patients with poor fixation.

Other Features

Although it is possible to generate large 3D data stacks with spectral domain OCT, motion artifacts (e.g., vertical microsaccades) remain a problem when very high sampling density is required. Many spectral domain OCT systems address this problem by sacrificing sampling density along one axis of the raster scan; however, some commercially available OCT instruments (e.g., Spectralis, Heidelberg Engineering, Germany) also provide real-time eye motion tracking with the potential for longer acquisition times and higher density data sets.[2]

The rapid scanning of spectral domain OCT also allows multiple B-scans to be averaged, which reduces speckle noise and allows detailed visualization of fine structures—in many cases B-scan averaging results in images that rival or surpass prototype "ultrahigh resolution" systems.[15]

IMAGE INTERPRETATION IN NORMAL EYES

The high axial resolution offered by OCT is particularly well suited to assessment of the multilayered retinal structure (Fig. 20.1).[4] On OCT false-color B-scans, highly reflective tissue is reddish-white in color, while hyporeflective

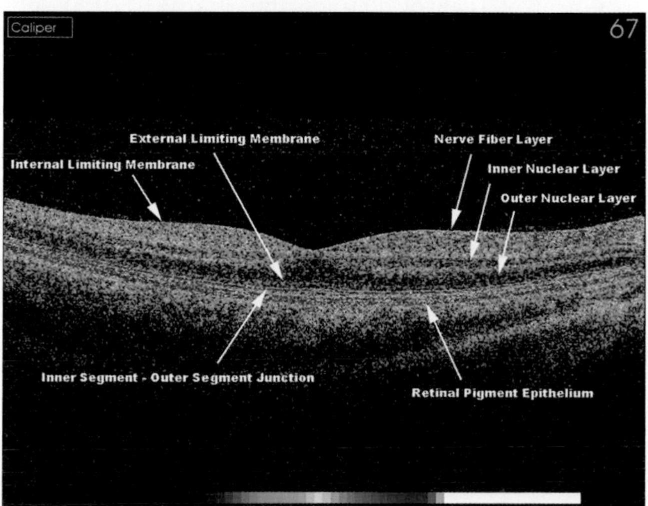

FIGURE 20.1. Optical coherence tomography B-scan produced using the 3D-OCT 1000 system (Topcon Medical Systems, Japan). The high axial resolution offered by OCT is well suited to providing information regarding the multilayered structure of the retina.

tissue is blue-black in color.[16] In most scans, the first hyperreflective layer detected is the internal limiting membrane (ILM) at the vitreoretinal interface. In a subset of the population, the posterior hyaloid may be seen as a thin hyperreflective layer above the ILM. Within the retina, the ganglion cell layer and both the inner and outer plexiform layers are seen as hyperreflective layers while the inner and outer nuclear layers are hyporeflective.

Correlation of OCT images with the microstructure of the outer retina is less well defined.[17] The first continuous hyperreflective line typically seen in the outer retina corresponds to the junction of the inner and outer segments of the photoreceptors (IS-OS junction). A faint, less continuous hyperreflective line may be present above this line and is thought to represent the external limiting membrane (ELM). Beneath the IS-OS junction, the interdigitations of the photoreceptor outer segments and apical microvilli of the retinal pigment epithelium (RPE) may be visible with high-resolution OCT systems. Finally, a wide, hyperreflective line corresponding to the RPE-Bruch membrane-choriocapillaris complex lies at the outermost extent of these tissue layers. Using spectral domain OCT, larger choroidal vessels, the suprachoroidal space, and the choroidal-scleral junction may also be seen in good quality images.[18,19]

Quantitative Image Analysis

The high axial resolution offered by OCT is also well suited to the objective, accurate measurement of retinal thickness. StratusOCT uses image processing techniques to automatically detect the inner and outer retinal boundaries on OCT B-scans (segmentation) and thus provide measurements of retinal thickness.[4] Using these techniques, it is possible to measure retinal thickness at multiple locations and to construct retinal thickness maps corresponding to the Early Treatment of Diabetic Retinopathy Study (ETDRS) subfields. Caution is required in the use of this information as errors in retinal segmentation are known to occur, and these errors are often severe in macular disorders such as neovascular age-related macular degeneration (AMD).[20–29]

As with StratusOCT, spectral domain OCT systems include image analysis software that provides measurements of retinal thickness. The speed and image resolution advantages of these systems may facilitate improved accuracy of retinal segmentation; however, further improvement in image processing algorithms may be required before segmentation errors can be eliminated entirely, particularly for disorders with complex morphology.[30,31]

AGE-RELATED MACULAR DEGENERATION

AMD is the leading cause of irreversible visual loss in people aged 50 years or older in the developed world.[32] The clinical hallmark of AMD is the deposition of acellular, polymorphous material, termed drusen, between the RPE and Bruch membrane.[33] In early AMD, drusen are often accompanied by focal retinal pigmentary abnormalities. As AMD progresses, alterations in the RPE often accumulate, resulting in the loss of large areas of RPE and outer retina, a phenomenon termed geographic atrophy (GA). In some patients with AMD, the abnormalities in the outer retina, Bruch membrane, and choroid may also result in the development of choroidal neovascularization (CNV), the characteristic feature of neovascular AMD.

In neovascular AMD, abnormal blood vessels develop from the choroidal circulation, pass anteriorly through breaks in Bruch membrane, and then proliferate in the sub-RPE or subretinal space.[34] CNV lesions may thus result in pigment epithelium detachment (PED), fluid exudation, lipid deposition, subretinal hemorrhage, and ultimately fibrotic scar formation with irreversible visual loss. For many years, fluorescein angiography (FA) was the cornerstone of neovascular AMD treatment. However, with the recent introduction of antiangiogenic agents, e.g., ranibizumab (Lucentis; Genentech, South San Francisco, CA) and the need for frequent monitoring of patients receiving these treatments, OCT has emerged as an essential tool in the follow-up of patients with AMD.[35,36]

FEATURES OF AGE-RELATED MACULAR DEGENERATION ON OCT

Pigment Epithelium Detachment

In neovascular AMD, growth of CNV in the sub-RPE space produces an elevated lesion that is often visible on clinical examination and is termed a fibrovascular PED.[34,37] Lesion growth is often accompanied by leakage of serous fluid, or frank hemorrhage, leading to the formation of serous or hemorrhagic PEDs. On OCT, PEDs appear as broad elevations of the RPE band relative to Bruch membrane (Fig. 20.2A).[38] The boundaries of a PED may be either gently sloped (as with some fibrovascular PEDs) or steeply sloped (as with many serous PEDs), although it is often not possible to distinguish between PED subtypes with confidence using OCT. In serous PEDs, Bruch membrane is often visible as a thin hyperreflective line at the outer aspect of the PED; Bruch membrane is less commonly seen in hemorrhagic PEDs, where there is often dramatic posterior shadowing below the RPE.

The detailed structural characteristics and precise mechanisms of PED formation have not been completely resolved—in part due to the relative inability of conventional OCT devices to visualize the areas underneath the highly reflective RPE. Recent studies have utilized enhanced spectral domain OCT imaging to aid visualization of the sub-RPE space.[18,19,39] Using this method, many fibrovascular PEDs appear to be filled with solid layers of material of medium reflectivity, separated by hyporeflective clefts—a finding consistent with previous histopathologic reports.[40,41] In many serous PEDs, collections of solid material—the apparent fibrovascular proliferation—can

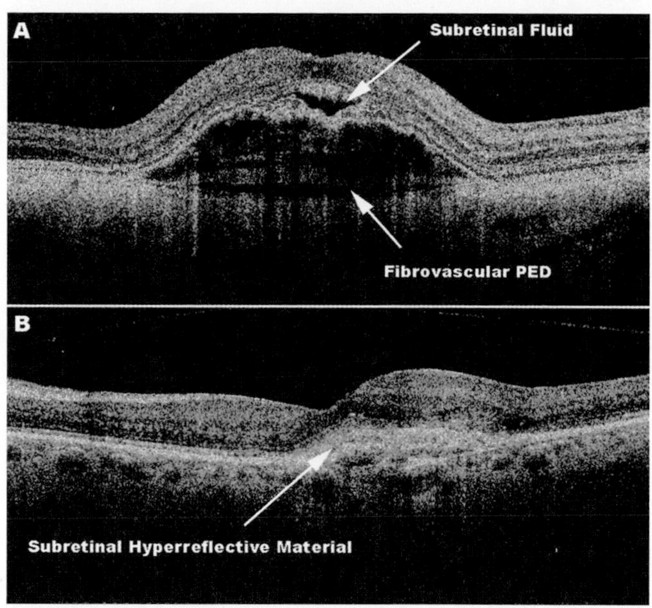

FIGURE 20.2. Optical coherence tomography B-scans (Cirrus HD-OCT, Carl Zeiss Meditec, Dublin, CA) demonstrating fibrovascular pigment epithelial detachment (PED) **(A)** and subretinal hyperreflective material **(B)**.

be seen adherent to the outer surface of the RPE, and associated with an underlying hyporeflective space—the serous fluid compartment. Following treatment with antiangiogenic agents, these supposed areas of sub-RPE CNV can be seen to contract and separate from the RPE, with flattening of the PED, resulting in RPE tear formation in a minority of cases (see below).[39]

Subretinal Hyperreflective Material

In many cases of neovascular AMD, the abnormal blood vessels may pass directly into the subretinal space after their initial penetration of Bruch membrane.[34] In these initial growth phases, the CNV membrane is often highly vascular and appears on OCT as an amorphous lesion of medium- to high-reflectivity above the RPE (Fig. 20.2B).[42,43] As the CNV lesion becomes less active over time, the vascular component typically regresses, while the fibrous component increases, resulting in disciform scar formation that appears on OCT as a well-demarcated highly hyperreflective lesion. Scar formation may be associated with loss of the overlying photoreceptor layer and irreversible reduction in visual acuity—this may often be seen on OCT as disruption of the IS-OS junction.[44,45] Hemorrhage, lipid, or thick fibrin may also appear as hyperreflective material in the subretinal space but should not be mistaken for the fibrovascular lesion.

Subretinal Fluid

As the choroidal neovascular membrane grows, it is often accompanied by profuse leakage from its immature blood vessels. Consequently, pockets of fluid commonly accumulate between the neurosensory retina and the RPE; and these areas may be seen on OCT as hyporeflective spaces (Fig. 20.2A).[42] CNV lesions growing in the subretinal space are typically associated with the greatest volume of subretinal fluid; however, sub-RPE lesions may also result in subretinal fluid when there is sufficient dysfunction of the outer blood-retinal barrier.[46] When fluid exudation is serous in nature, subretinal fluid pockets are seen on OCT as homogenous hyporeflective spaces; when the exudate contains fibrin or red blood cells, the area of subretinal fluid may by sparsely hyperreflective. Profuse fibrinous exudation in neovascular AMD, seen after PDT or in particularly active classic CNV lesions, may result in the formation of distinct subretinal fluid compartments separated by fibrinous membranes—these compartments may sometimes be seen on FA as areas of loculated fluid.[47] Spectral domain OCT allows enhanced visualization of the subretinal space, and assessment of the optical density of subretinal fluid compartments may have value for the differentiation of macular disorders associated with subretinal accumulation.[48]

Intraretinal Fluid

Disruption of the ELM-photoreceptor complex in the outer retina, by the active CNV membrane, may result in the accumulation of fluid in the neurosensory retina.[49] Initially, this fluid collection manifests as diffuse thickening of the outer nuclear layer.[50] Severe outer nuclear layer swelling may sometimes be mistaken for subretinal fluid—the distinction can usually be made by the presence of an intact IS-OS junction at the outer aspect of outer nuclear layer thickening. With more severe fluid exudation, cystoid spaces may form and can be seen on OCT as round or oval hyporeflective areas (Fig. 20.3).[50,51] Larger cystoid spaces often contain tissue septae and may involve all layers of the retina. Treatment with antiangiogenic agents often leads to cessation of CNV leakage with consequent resolution of these cystoid spaces. In severe cases, however, cystoid spaces may persist even in the absence of leakage, and these areas have been termed "cystoid macular degeneration."[52]

Drusen and Retinal Pigment Abnormalities

Drusen may sometimes be difficult to assess on time domain OCT images, where undulation of the RPE baseline due to motion artifact may mimic the appearance of drusen.[53–55] On spectral domain OCT, small and intermediate size drusen may be more clearly seen as discrete areas of RPE elevation with variable reflectivity, reflecting the variable composition of the underlying material (Fig. 20.4A).[56,57] In large drusen, or drusenoid PED, greater elevation of the RPE may be seen, often dome shaped, with a hyporeflective or medium-reflective material separating the RPE from the underlying Bruch membrane.[54] Disruption of the IS-OS junction and ELM, as well as significant thinning of the outer nuclear layer, may often be seen

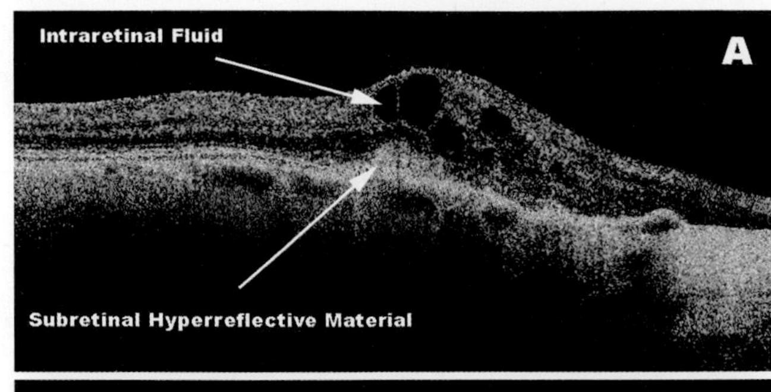

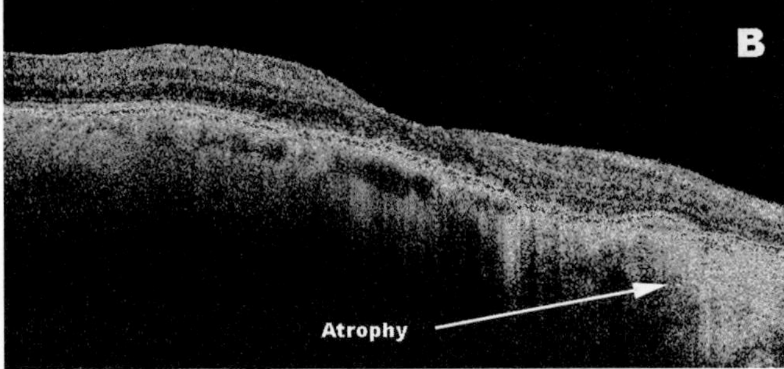

FIGURE 20.3. Optical coherence tomography B-scans (Cirrus HD-OCT, Carl Zeiss Meditec, Dublin, CA), demonstrating resolution of intraretinal fluid following treatment with ranibizumab (Lucentis, Genentech, South San Francisco, CA), in a patient with neovascular AMD. Pretreatment **(A)**, posttreatment .

overlying drusen.[57] In patients with extensive drusen, apparent thickening of the photoreceptor outer segments may sometimes be seen—the accumulation of material in this area may represent incomplete phagocytosis of the outer segment material.[58]

Drusen are often accompanied by RPE abnormalities that can be visualized on OCT.[57] In particular, pigment migration and clumping may be seen as discrete areas of hyperreflectivity in the outer nuclear layer with underlying shadowing. Focal areas of RPE loss may result in increased reflectivity of the underlying choroidal vessels. A recent study has also shown that drusen may be associated with a diffuse hyperreflective haze at the inner boundary of the outer nuclear layer, although the origin and significance of this finding remain uncertain.[59]

Geographic Atrophy

In GA, confluent areas of RPE atrophy are accompanied by loss of the overlying photoreceptors.[60] On OCT, GA appears as areas of sharply demarcated choroidal hyperreflectivity due to loss of the overlying RPE (Fig. 20.4B).[61] GA is also accompanied by thinning of the overlying neurosensory retina that can be seen on spectral domain OCT as absence of the outer nuclear layer, ELM, and IS-OS junctions (these layers may be seen to taper off in the junctional zone surrounding GA).[58] Islands of preserved outer retina may sometimes be identified in areas of GA, as can regressing drusenoid material, seen as hyperreflective plaques at the level of the RPE.[58] Preliminary OCT evidence also suggests that mild retinal swelling in areas of foveal sparing may represent a preapoptotic stage of neuronal cellular elements indicative of imminent atrophy.[62]

The OCT fundus images provided by spectral domain OCT devices show an increased total signal in areas where GA is apparent on clinical examination.[63] As a result, it is possible to manually quantify areas of GA by registering these images to fundus photographs and delineating the GA boundaries with imaging software. This approach may allow more accurate and reproducible measurements of GA progression in future clinical trials of this disorder.

Abnormalities of the Vitreomacular Interface

Retinal imaging with OCT allows detailed evaluation of the structural features of the vitreomacular interface. On OCT, vitreomacular traction may be seen when a thickened, taut, posterior hyaloid causes deformation of the inner retinal surface, which may often be accompanied by cystoid macular edema (CME).[64] ERMs are often seen on OCT as hyperreflective bands anterior to the inner retinal surface, with distortion of the underlying anatomy (Fig. 20.5).[65] In recent years, it has been suggested that abnormalities of this interface may play a role in CNV pathogenesis.[66] A number of studies, employing both time domain and spectral domain OCT, have reported a higher prevalence of vitreomacular adhesion in patients

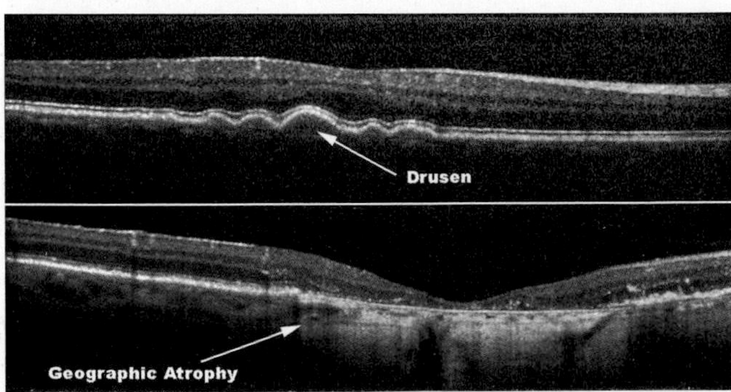

FIGURE 20.4. Optical coherence tomography B-scans (Spectralis, Heidelberg Engineering, Germany) demonstrating drusen **(A)** and geographic atrophy **(B)**.

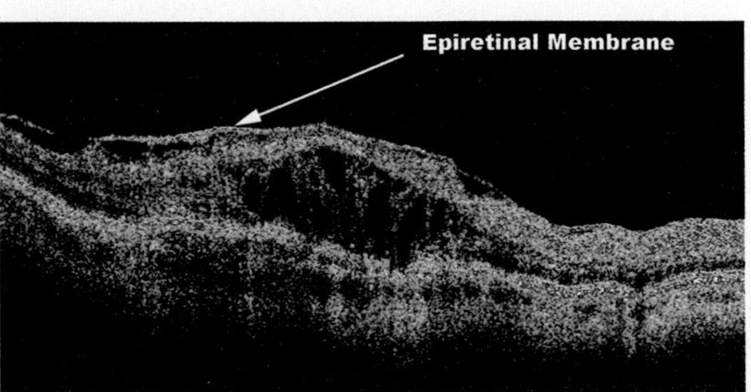

FIGURE 20.5. Evidence of dense ERM formation in a patient receiving treatment for neovascular AMD (Stratus OCT, Carl Zeiss Meditec, Dublin, CA).

with neovascular AMD.[67–70] Further study is required to confirm this association and to determine whether it has any prognostic or patient management implications.

CLINICAL APPLICATIONS OF OCT IN AGE-RELATED MACULAR DEGENERATION

Diagnosis

In elderly patients complaining of acute or subacute unilateral visual loss, the combination of biomicroscopic (e.g., drusen, macular hemorrhage, subretinal fibrosis) and tomographic (e.g., PED, subretinal hyperreflective material, subretinal fluid) findings often allows a diagnosis of neovascular AMD to be made with confidence.[71] This is particularly the case with the advent of spectral domain OCT, where areas of focal macular pathology are less likely to be missed with raster scanning of the macula. However, clinical studies have not yet adequately addressed this issue, and FA is still regarded by most retinal specialists as mandatory for the initial diagnosis of neovascular AMD.[35] Aside from its emerging diagnostic role, OCT allows assessment of disease activity and, in this context, has become essential in guiding the treatment of patients with neovascular AMD.

Role in Retreatment Protocols

In 2006, the MARINA and ANCHOR phase III clinical trials demonstrated that treatment with ranibizumab was capable of improving visual acuity in many patients with neovascular AMD.[72,73] In parallel with this, use of OCT had become widespread among retinal specialists for the management of neovascular AMD. Consequently, OCT measurements were soon adopted as anatomic outcome parameters, and as a means of guiding retreatment, in clinical trials. In the PrONTO study, an OCT-guided variable dosing regimen was assessed for the treatment of neovascular AMD with ranibizumab.[74] In this study, ranibizumab re-treatment was performed, in part, based on OCT criteria: a loss of five letters of visual acuity in conjunction with fluid on OCT, an increase of OCT central retinal thickness of at least 100 μm, or the persistence of fluid on OCT 1 month after previous treatment. In the second year of this study, these criteria were amended so that any qualitative OCT changes suggestive of recurrent fluid in the macula (e.g., the appearance of retinal cysts or subretinal fluid or enlargement of a PED) were indications for re-treatment.[75] The results of this study suggested that an OCT-guided re-treatment regimen could result in visual outcomes comparable to those from clinical trials with fixed monthly dosing. The efficacy of this approach is now being evaluated in large-scale clinical trials—in particular, the CATT (Comparison of Age-Related Macular Degeneration Treatments Trials) and the SUSTAIN (Study of Ranibizumab in Patients With Subfoveal Choroidal Neovascularization Secondary to Age-Related Macular Degeneration) trials.

Correlations with Visual Acuity

Many clinical trials have demonstrated substantial changes in retinal thickness in response to antiangiogenic therapies.[76–78] However, many of these studies have failed to find a significant correlation between OCT-derived retinal thickness and visual acuity.[77,79] This failure may be due, at least in part, to the frequent inaccuracy of retinal thickness measurements provided by OCT image analysis software.[28] Manual segmentation of OCT images allows accurate measurement of retinal thickness, as well as allowing quantification of any morphologic space of interest in the retina (e.g., intraretinal cysts, subretinal hyperreflective material, subretinal fluid, or PED).[80,81] Using this approach, modest correlations have been found between the volume of subretinal hyperreflective material, the thickness of the neurosensory retina, and visual acuity in patients newly diagnosed with neovascular AMD.[46] Manual grading has also shown that regression of any anatomic improvement gained after treatment with ranibizumab is strongly associated with reduction in visual acuity.[82] Manual segmentation has usually been performed using custom software, although OCT image analysis software from certain vendors has begun to offer this facility (e.g., Stratus OCT v5.0). Spectral domain OCT may allow more accurate quantification of retinal pathology, although manual grading of these images may not be feasible for large studies.[48,83–85]

Correlation with Fluorescein Angiography

CNV lesions in neovascular AMD are commonly described as "classic" or "occult", depending on their leakage characteristics on FA.[86] Classic CNV is believed to correspond to fibrovascular proliferation in the subretinal space, while occult CNV is believed to correspond to fibrovascular proliferation beneath the RPE.[34,87] This classification may have clinical significance in terms of disease progression over time and impact on visual function. A number of studies have examined the relationship between OCT findings and FA in neovascular AMD.[38,88,89] In these studies, classic lesions are associated with significantly greater volumes of subretinal hyperreflective material than occult lesions, while occult lesions are more commonly associated with PED. Studies of this manner are first steps toward development of hybrid OCT-FA classifications systems for neovascular AMD—the development of such systems may allow clinicians to identify those patients most likely to respond to any given therapeutic intervention and thus improve clinical outcomes.

OTHER FEATURES OF AGE-RELATED MACULAR DEGENERATION ON OCT

Retinal Angiomatous Proliferation

Although neovascular AMD is predominantly a disorder of the choroidal vasculature, the retinal circulation may also be involved in some patients, and retinochoroidal anastomoses may form in advanced disease.[90] In 2001, Yannuzzi et al.[91] suggested that the initial event in the development of retinochoroidal anastomosis was intraretinal neovascularization and coined the term retinal angiomatous proliferation (RAP). Conversely, Gass et al.[92] suggested that the initial event in retinal involvement was the development of occult anastomosis at the site of a sub-RPE CNV lesion. A recent histopathologic study has provided evidence supportive of an intraretinal origin for the neovascular process in these patients.[93] However, recent OCT studies suggest that the earliest change visible in these patients is the development of fibrovascular PED—a feature more consistent with the Gass theory of occult chorioretinal anastomosis.[94,95] Thus, it has been suggested that retinal involvement in neovascular AMD may incorporate both sub-RPE and intraretinal origins ("the expanded spectrum of RAP").[95] On OCT, active RAP lesions have a characteristic appearance, typified by frank CME overlying a serous PED, and accompanied by subretinal fluid.[96,97] In some cases, the retinochoroidal anastomosis may be seen on OCT as a discrete hyperreflective area extending through the retina.

Polypoidal Choroidal Vasculopathy

In 1990, Yannuzzi et al.[98] suggested the term "idiopathic polypoidal choroidal vasculopathy" for a disorder characterized by multiple serosanguineous PEDs, commonly seen in black and Asian populations. This disorder was initially felt to be a distinct entity with its own risk factors and clinical course; however, in recent years, the disease spectrum has been greatly expanded, with many authorities now considering PCV to be an important form of neovascular AMD.[99] On indocyanine green (ICG) angiography, PCV appears as a branching vascular network below the RPE that ends in reddish-orange polypoidal lesions and is often associated with serosanguineous PEDs.[100] On Stratus OCT, and more recently with spectral domain OCT, the branching vascular network appears as a shallow elevation of the RPE, while the polypoidal lesions appear as sharper protuberances (Fig. 20.6).[101–107] As the exudative complications of these lesions evolve, large serosanguineous PEDs develop adjacent to the polypoidal bulges, creating a tomographic notch. With continued exudation, these polypoidal lesions remain adherent to the RPE and are lifted away from Bruch membrane.[107] ICG angiography is still considered essential for the diagnosis of PCV, although OCT is likely to play a greater role as the technology improves and the awareness of this disorder grows.

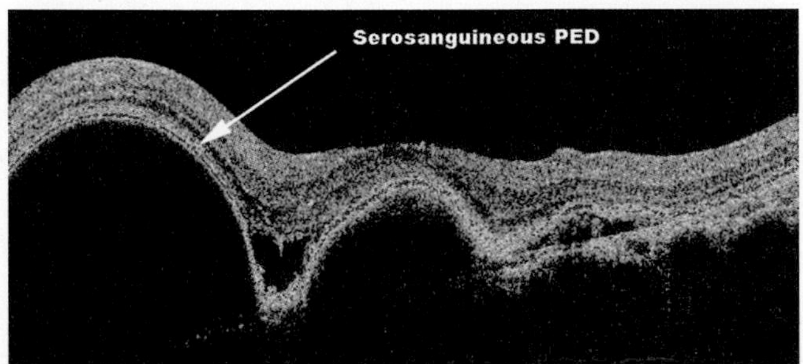

FIGURE 20.6. Optical coherence tomography B-scan (Cirrus HD-OCT, Carl Zeiss Meditec, Dublin, CA), demonstrating serosanguineous pigment epithelium detachments (PEDs) in a patient with polypoidal choroidal vasculopathy.

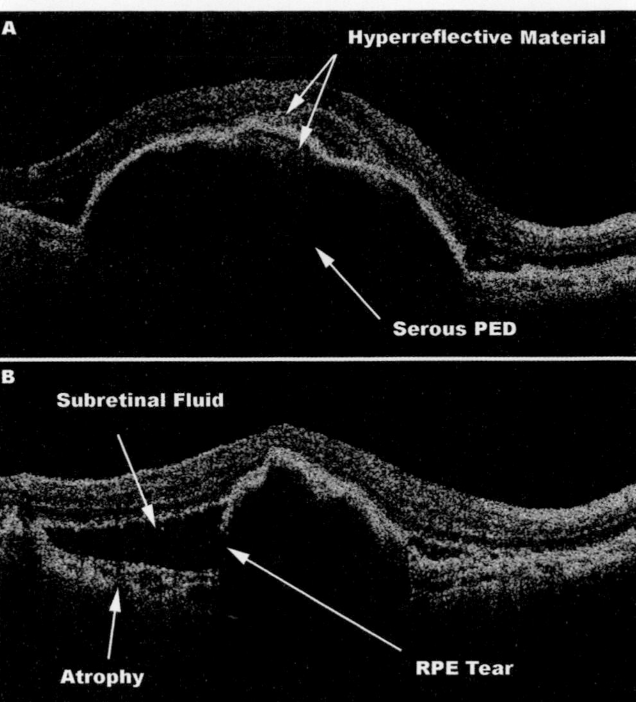

FIGURE 20.7. Optical coherence tomography B-scans (Stratus OCT, Carl Zeiss Meditec, Dublin, California), obtained before **(A)** and after **(B)** the development of a retinal pigment epithelium (RPE) tear.

Retinal Pigment Epithelium Tears

RPE tears, a well-described complication of neovascular AMD, have achieved a new prominence with the introduction of new pharmacotherapies for this disorder.[108] On OCT, RPE tears are typically seen as an area of discontinuity in a large PED, with the free edge of the RPE often curled under the PED creating a corrugated appearance.[109–111] Adjacent to the tear, an area of atrophy can usually be seen as increased reflectivity of the choroidal vessels. The overlying retina is typically intact but may be separated from the area of atrophy by subretinal fluid (Fig. 20.7). In the long term, the area of the tear is usually covered by disciform scar formation and the visual outcome is poor if the fovea is involved.[112]

MACULAR EDEMA

Macular edema may be defined as abnormal thickening of the neurosensory retina that occurs as a result of excess fluid accumulation in the extracellular space of the retina.[113] CME is said to occur when extracellular fluid

Table 20.1.

Macular edema—etiologies

Retinal Vascular Disease
Diabetic retinopathy
Retinal vein occlusion
Hypertensive retinopathy
Radiation retinopathy
Retinal artery macroaneurysm
Choroidal Vascular Disease
Choroidal neovascularization
Inflammatory Disease
Uveitic syndromes
Postsurgical
Postlaser
Inherited Retinal Dystrophies
Retinitis pigmentosa
Drug Reactions
Nicotinic acid
Prostaglandin analogues
Tractional Maculopathies
Vitreomacular traction
Epiretinal membrane
Optic Nerve Head Abnormalities
Intraocular Tumors

accumulation leads to the formation of cyst-like spaces in the retina; these spaces can often be visualized on biomicroscopic examination or with retinal imaging techniques such as FA. Macular edema has a large number of potential etiologies (Table 20.1).[114] Despite this, there is considerable overlap in the pathophysiologic mechanisms that underlie these disorders, and the associated OCT features are often similar. Consequently, many of the OCT studies evaluating the structural characteristics of macular edema have focused on a single, prototypical disorder—diabetic macular edema.

DIABETIC MACULAR EDEMA

Breakdown of the inner blood-retinal barrier in diabetic retinopathy leads to extravasation of blood, serous fluid, and lipoproteinaceous fluid. DME is the abnormal thickening of the macula that occurs as a result of this fluid accumulation.[114] Another term, clinically significant macular edema (CSME) was coined in the Early Treatment of Diabetic Retinopathy Study (ETDRS) to describe a subset of patients with DME who were deemed to be at greater risk of visual loss without treatment.[115] As DME progresses, cystoid spaces may occur—these spaces are initially restricted to the outer nuclear layer and the outer plexiform layer of Henle but may subsequently extend to the inner retina. In severe cases, the supporting glial cells of the retina (Muller cells) may develop intracellular edema and undergo secondary degeneration, leading to further disorganization of retinal structure.[116] DME may also be accompanied by serous detachment of the neurosensory retina, although the pathophysiology of this process is incompletely understood.

Of note, the vitreous may also play a significant role in the pathogenesis of macular edema. Evidence suggests that the vitreous structure is altered in patients with diabetes, and that stronger, more persistent, vitreoretinal interactions may occur.[117] Thus, by exerting mechanical traction on the inner retina, or by acting as a reservoir for growth factors, the vitreous of diabetic patients may contribute to the progression of DME.

FEATURES OF DIABETIC MACULAR EDEMA ON OCT

On OCT, DME is generally seen as an area of retinal thickening that is often accompanied by loss of the foveal depression.[118] In areas of long-standing edema, lipid and protein may precipitate in the outer retina, forming hard exudates that appear as focal areas of hyperreflectivity with posterior shadowing (Fig. 20.8).[119,120]

Approximately 90% of patients with DME show evidence of sponge-like retinal thickening associated with decreased optical backscattering on OCT—this thickening may be localized to the outer nuclear layer or extend diffusely to involve the entire retina.[121,122] Sponge-like retinal

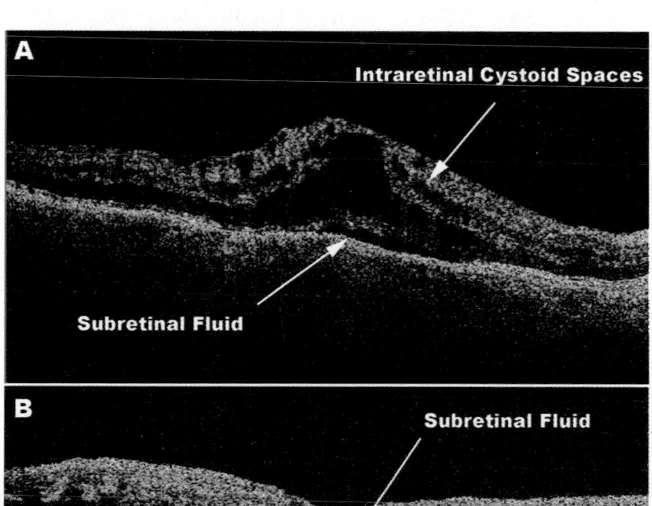

FIGURE 20.8. Patterns of structural change on optical coherence tomography (OCT) in patients with diabetic macular edema. OCT B-scans demonstrate cystoid macular edema **(A)**, lipid exudates **(B)**, and subretinal fluid **(A, B)**.

thickening is often seen in association with both CME and serous retinal detachment; however, it may also occur in isolation, particularly in patients with mild-to-moderate nonproliferative diabetic retinopathy, and in this context, it is associated with less severe visual loss.[123]

Approximately 50% of patients with DME demonstrate evidence of round or oval hyporeflective areas on OCT that are consistent with intraretinal cystoid space formation.[121,122] On FA, leakage into cystoid spaces may result in a "petalloid" or "honeycomb" appearance. On OCT, petalloid hyperfluorescence is associated with cystoid space formation in the radially arranged outer plexiform layer of Henle, while honeycomb hyperfluorescence correlates with cystoid space in the vertically arranged inner nuclear layer.[124] Detection of CME on OCT is associated with a more severe reduction in visual acuity and a poorer response to treatment than OCTs displaying sponge-like retinal thickening alone.[125]

Approximately 15% to 30% of patients with DME demonstrate evidence of serous retinal detachment on OCT.[121,122,126–129] Serous retinal detachment occurs when fluid accumulation leads to separation of the neurosensory retina and the RPE and is seen on OCT as a hyporeflective space. Serous retinal detachment is not easily seen on clinical examination and does not appear to correlate with specific patterns of fluorescein angiographic leakage.[130,131] The presence of a serous retinal detachment may represent a specific feature of a severe stage of DME,[121,123] although this feature may occur even when the central retinal thickness above the detachment is within the normal range.[127] Furthermore, serous retinal detachment may resolve despite worsening of DME, and the presence of this feature on OCT does not appear indicative of a poor prognosis.[127,129]

Abnormalities of the vitreomacular interface are also commonly seen in DME.[121,132] On OCT, the posterior hyaloid may be seen as a thin hyperreflective membrane with a broad or focal adhesion to the retinal surface. This membrane may be thickened and taut, exerting obvious traction on the retina and resulting in a characteristic peaked appearance.[133] ERMs commonly form in patients with DME and may be clearly seen on OCT. Elucidation of these findings has clinical implications (see below) and evaluation of the vitreomacular interface should always be performed in patients with DME, particularly when retinal thickening is present on clinical examination but FA discloses no significant leakage or ischemia.[134]

CLINICAL APPLICATIONS OF OCT IN DIABETIC MACULAR EDEMA

In general, patients presenting with CSME are initially treated with an application of focal/grid laser photocoagulation to the macula.[135] Pharmacotherapies such as corticosteroids or antiangiogenic agents are commonly used in cases of DME that prove refractory to laser treatment. In more severe or persistent cases, particularly with evidence of an abnormal vitreo-retinal interface, surgical intervention in the form of pars plana vitrectomy is often considered. Measurements of retinal thickness obtained from OCT now play a key role in assessing the anatomic response to each of these treatments.[136]

Correlation with Visual Acuity

Numerous studies have also examined the correlation between retinal parameters derived from OCT and visual acuity. Initial studies found evidence of a strong correlation, although many involved small sample sizes and lacked best-corrected ETDRS visual acuities.[120,122,126,129,137,138] The evidence from more recent studies is less clear. The most comprehensive data currently available come from the DRCR network: in an initial study, network investigators found a modest correlation between OCT-measured foveal center point thickness and visual acuity ($r = 0.52$) and a modest correlation between changes in retinal thickening and visual acuity after laser treatment for DME ($r = 0.44$).[139] The strength of the observed correlations may be treatment dependent—in a recent randomized controlled trial assessing the efficacy of intravitreal triamcinolone, no statistically significant correlation was detected between changes in retinal thickness and visual acuity in treated patients.[140] It is likely that visual acuity is also determined by functional parameters not evaluated by OCT, including the perfusion status of the foveal capillaries, and the degree of photoreceptor and RPE dysfunction. The duration of time for which macular edema is present may also be a key determinant of these parameters.

Screening

A number of studies have shown that OCT is more sensitive than clinical examination or stereoscopic fundus photography for the detection of retinal thickening and CSME.[136,141] Retinal thickening detectable only with OCT has been termed *subclinical diabetic macular edema*.[141] The prevalence of DME is known to increase as the severity of diabetic retinopathy increases.[142] However, it is not clear at what retinopathy level OCT should be performed to detect subclinical DME, and whether treatment of subclinical DME would improve the prognosis of patients with diabetic retinopathy. A recent report suggests that routine screening of patients with OCT is unlikely to be of benefit in those with diabetes and no retinopathy, or with mild to moderate retinopathy, when clinical examination fails to detect macular edema.[143] In the future, the point at which medical or surgical intervention is appropriate in DME is likely to be determined by objective criteria on OCT rather than on subjective criteria determined solely on clinical examination.

OTHER CAUSES OF MACULAR EDEMA

Histopathologic reports suggest that the features of macular edema may vary according to its underlying etiology (e.g., intraretinal cyst location and extent; serous retinal detachment frequency and severity).[116] Despite the widespread adoption of OCT for the evaluation of treatment effects, differences in the tomographic features of these disorders have been less well defined.

Retinal Vein Occlusion

Both central retinal vein occlusion (CRVO) and branch retinal vein occlusion (BRVO) are common causes of macular edema.[114] In these disorders, acute extravasation of fluid into the extracellular space of the retina results from increased hydrostatic pressure in retinal veins distal to their point of occlusion. In addition, growth factors released in response to hypoxia (e.g., vascular endothelial growth factor [VEGF]) may lead to breakdown of the inner blood-retinal barrier, thus greatly facilitating fluid extravasation. Macular edema in retinal vein occlusion appears similar to that in DME, although in BRVO, the observed changes on OCT are usually restricted to either the superior or inferior aspects of the macula.[144] In addition, serous detachment of the retina is more commonly seen in retinal vein occlusions than from other etiologies, although the presence of serous macular detachments is not in itself associated with worse visual outcomes.[126] A number of studies have evaluated the correlation between OCT-derived retinal thickness parameters and visual acuity but have only identified moderate correlations.[126,145] More recently, studies have shown that the integrity of the ELM, and photoreceptor IS-OS junction, appears to correlate with visual acuity in both forms of retinal vein occlusion.[146–149] While there is no proven treatment for macular edema complicating CRVO, grid laser photocoagulation may be effective for treatment of persistent macular edema associated with BRVO—changes in retinal thickness following this treatment modality have been well described with OCT.[150]

Uveitic Syndromes

Macular edema typically develops in patients with intermediate and posterior uveitis but may also be seen in cases of isolated anterior uveitis and is a common cause of visual loss.[151,152] Many of the edematous change seen on OCT in DME may also be seen in chronic uveitis. As with DME, OCT plays a crucial role in the monitoring of treatment in patients with macular edema secondary to uveitis.

Radiation Retinopathy

Radiotherapy is an effective treatment for uveal melanoma, although loss of vision from radiation retinopathy is a relatively frequent occurrence. Many of the clinical and histopathologic findings of radiation retinopathy are similar to those of diabetic retinopathy.[114] Thus, OCT has been used to characterize the macular edema in radiation retinopathy and to monitor the effects of treatment with laser photocoagulation, intravitreal triamcinolone, and anti-VEGF agents.[153,154]

CONCLUSIONS

It is clear that OCT plays a critical role in the management of both AMD and macular edema—in the future, advances in OCT technology, and in our ability to interpret OCT images, may provide guidance on a number of unresolved questions related to these disorders. In macular edema, improved characterization of structural changes on OCT may allow the clinician to determine when irreversible structural damage has occurred and, therefore, the point at which further treatment is unlikely to be of benefit. In AMD, improved understanding of OCT images may change the manner in which neovascular AMD is diagnosed. Neovascular AMD is clearly an anatomically heterogeneous disorder, and a more nuanced classification system may become a necessity as the range of available therapies rapidly grows. The development of hybrid OCT-FA classification systems may determine which lesions are suitable for treatment, and their optimum retreatment regimens. In the short term, much of this information may emerge from the large clinical trials that have already begun to incorporate spectral domain OCT imaging. In the longer term, the role of OCT is likely to evolve in other, potentially unforeseen ways, as functional extensions of OCT (e.g., Doppler OCT) provide additional insights into the pathogenesis of these disorders.

REFERENCES

1. Huang D, Swanson EA, Lin CP, et al. Optical coherence tomography. *Science*. 1991;254:1178–1181.
2. Drexler W, Fujimoto JG. State-of-the-art retinal optical coherence tomography. *Prog Ret Eye Res*. 2008;27:45–88.
3. Voo I, Mavrofrides EC, Puliafito CA. Clinical applications of optical coherence tomography for the diagnosis and management of macular diseases. *Ophthalmol Clin North Am*. 2004;17:21–31.
4. Schuman JS, Puliafito CA, Fujimoto JG. *Optical Coherence Tomography of Ocular Diseases*, 2nd ed. Thorofare, NJ: Slack Inc.; 2004.
5. Swanson E, Izatt J, Hee M, et al. In vivo retinal imaging by optical coherence tomography. *Opt Lett*. 1993;18:1864–1866.
6. Keane PA, Bhatti RA, Brubaker JW, et al. Comparison of clinically relevant findings from high-speed fourier-domain and conventional time-domain optical coherence tomography. *Am J Ophthalmol*. 2009;148:242–248.
7. van Velthoven ME, Faber DJ, Verbraak FD, et al. Recent developments in optical coherence tomography for imaging the retina. *Prog Ret Eye Res*. 2007;26:57–77.
8. Wojtkowski M, Bajraszewski T, Gorczyńska I, et al. Ophthalmic imaging by spectral optical coherence tomography. *Am J Ophthalmol* 2004;138:412–419.
9. Chen TC, Cense B, Pierce MC, et al. Spectral domain optical coherence tomography: ultra-high speed, ultra-high resolution ophthalmic imaging. *Arch Ophthalmol*. 2005;123:1715–1720.
10. Wojtkowski M, Leitgeb R, Kowalczyk A, et al. In vivo human retinal imaging by Fourier domain optical coherence tomography. *J Biomed Opt*. 2002;7:457–463.

11. Srinivasan VJ, Wojtkowski M, Witkin AJ, et al. High-definition and 3-dimensional imaging of macular pathologies with high-speed ultrahigh-resolution optical coherence tomography. *Ophthalmology*. 2006;113:2054.e1–2054.e14.
12. Wojtkowski M, Srinivasan V, Fujimoto JG, et al. Three-dimensional retinal imaging with high-speed ultrahigh-resolution optical coherence tomography. *Ophthalmology*. 2005;112:1734–1746.
13. Schmidt-Erfurth U, Leitgeb RA, Michels S, et al. Three-dimensional ultrahigh-resolution optical coherence tomography of macular diseases. *Invest Ophthalmol Vis Sci*. 2005; 46:3393–3402.
14. Koizumi H, Spaide RF, Fisher YL, et al. Three-dimensional evaluation of vitreomacular traction and epiretinal membrane using spectral-domain optical coherence tomography. *Am J Ophthalmol*. 2008;145:509–517.
15. Sakamoto A, Hangai M, Yoshimura N. Spectral-domain optical coherence tomography with multiple B-scan averaging for enhanced imaging of retinal diseases. *Ophthalmology*. 2008;115:1071–1078.
16. Brar M, Bartsch DU, Nigam N, et al. Colour versus grey-scale display of images on high-resolution spectral OCT. *Br J Ophthalmol*. 2009;93:597–602.
17. Srinivasan VJ, Monson BK, Wojtkowski M, et al. Characterization of outer retinal morphology with high-speed, ultrahigh-resolution optical coherence tomography. *Invest Ophthalmol Vis Sci*. 2008;49:1571–1579.
18. Spaide RF. Age-related choroidal atrophy. *Am J Ophthalmol*. 2009;147:801–810.
19. Spaide RF, Koizumi H, Pozonni MC. Enhanced depth imaging spectral-domain optical coherence tomography. *Am J Ophthalmol*. 2008;146:496–500.
20. Domalpally A, Danis R, Zhang B, et al. Quality issues in interpretation of optical coherence tomograms in macular diseases. *Retina*. 2009;29:775–781.
21. Ghazi N, Kirk T, Allam S, et al. Quantification of error in optical coherence tomography central macular thickness measurement in wet age-related macular degeneration. *Am J Ophthalmol*. 2009;148:90–96.
22. Karam EZ, Ramirez E, Arreaza PL, et al. Optical coherence tomographic artifacts in diseases of the retinal pigment epithelium. *Br J Ophthalmol*. 2007;91:1139–1142.
23. Keane PA, Liakopoulos S, Jivrajka RV, et al. Evaluation of optical coherence tomography central retinal thickness parameters for use as anatomic outcomes in clinical trials for neovascular age-related macular degeneration. *Invest Ophthalmol Vis Sci*. 2009;50:3378–3385.
24. Keane PA, Liakopoulos S, Walsh AC, et al. Limits of the retinal-mapping program in age-related macular degeneration. *Br J Ophthalmol*. 2009;93:274–275.
25. Krebs I, Haas P, Zeiler F, et al. Optical coherence tomography: limits of the retinal-mapping program in age-related macular degeneration. *Br J Ophthalmol*. 2008;92:933–935.
26. Patel PJ, Chen FK, da Cruz L, et al. Segmentation error in Stratus optical coherence tomography for neovascular age-related macular degeneration. *Invest Ophthalmol Vis Sci*. 2009;50:399–404.
27. Ray R, Stinnett SS, Jaffe GJ. Evaluation of image artifact produced by optical coherence tomography of retinal pathology. *Am J Ophthalmol*. 2005;139:18–29.
28. Sadda SR, Wu Z, Walsh AC, et al. Errors in retinal thickness measurements obtained by optical coherence tomography. *Ophthalmology*. 2006;113:285–293.
29. Taban M, Sharma S, Williams DR, et al. Comparing retinal thickness measurements using automated fast macular thickness map versus six-radial line scans with manual measurements. *Ophthalmology*. 2009;116:964–970.
30. Keane PA, Mand PS, Liakopoulos S, et al. Accuracy of retinal thickness measurements obtained with cirrus optical coherence tomography. *Br J Ophthalmol*. 2009;93:1461–1467.
31. Krebs I, Falkner-Radler C, Hagen S, et al. Quality of the threshold algorithm in age-related macular degeneration: stratus versus cirrus OCT. *Invest Ophthalmol Vis Sci*. 2009;50:995.
32. Pascolini D, Mariotti SP, Pokharel GP, et al. 2002 global update of available data on visual impairment: a compilation of population-based prevalence studies. *Ophthalmic Epidemiol*. 2004;11:67–115.
33. Jager RD, Mieler WF, Miller JW. Age-related macular degeneration. *N Engl J Med*. 2008;358:2606–2617.
34. Grossniklaus HE, Green WR. Choroidal neovascularization. *Am J Ophthalmol*. 2004;137:496–503.
35. Mitchell P, Korobelnik J, Lanzetta P, et al. Ranibizumab (Lucentis) in neovascular age-related macular degeneration: evidence from clinical trials. *Br J Ophthalmol*. 2010;94:2–13.
36. Schmidt-Erfurth UM, Richard G, Augustin A, et al. Guidance for the treatment of neovascular age-related macular degeneration. *Acta Ophthalmol Scand*. 2007;85:486–494.
37. Macular Photocoagulation Study Group. Subfoveal neovascular lesions in age-related macular degeneration. Guidelines for evaluation and treatment in the macular photocoagulation study. *Arch Ophthalmol*. 1991;109:1242–1257.
38. Coscas F, Coscas G, Souied E, et al. Optical coherence tomography identification of occult choroidal neovascularization in age-related macular degeneration. *Am J Ophthalmol*. 2007;144:592–599.
39. Spaide RF. Enhanced depth imaging optical coherence tomography of retinal pigment epithelial detachment in age-related macular degeneration. *Am J Ophthalmol*. 2009;147:644–652.
40. Green WR, Enger C. Age-related macular degeneration histopathologic studies. The 1992 Lorenz E. Zimmerman Lecture. *Ophthalmology*. 1993;100:1519–1535.
41. Green WR, McDonnell PJ, Yeo JH. Pathologic features of senile macular degeneration. *Ophthalmology*. 1985;92: 615–627.
42. Joeres S, Tsong JW, Updike PG, et al. Reproducibility of quantitative optical coherence tomography subanalysis in neovascular age-related macular degeneration. *Invest Ophthalmol Vis Sci*. 2007;48:4300–4307.
43. Keane PA, Liakopoulos S, Chang KT, et al. Comparison of the optical coherence tomographic features of choroidal neovascular membranes in pathological myopia versus age-related macular degeneration, using quantitative subanalysis. *Br J Ophthalmol*. 2008;92:1081–1085.
44. Hayashi H, Yamashiro K, Tsujikawa A, et al. Association between foveal photoreceptor integrity and visual outcome in neovascular age-related macular degeneration. *Am J Ophthalmol*. 2009;148:83–89.

45. Sayanagi K, Sharma S, Kaiser PK. Photoreceptor status after antivascular endothelial growth factor therapy in exudative age-related macular degeneration. *Br J Ophthalmol.* 2009;93:622–626.
46. Keane PA, Liakopoulos S, Chang KT, et al. Relationship between optical coherence tomography retinal parameters and visual acuity in neovascular age-related macular degeneration. *Ophthalmology*. 2008;115:2206–2214.
47. Bressler NM, Bressler SB, Alexander J, et al. Loculated fluid. A previously undescribed fluorescein angiographic finding in choroidal neovascularization associated with macular degeneration. Macular Photocoagulation Study Reading Center. *Arch Ophthalmol.* 1991;109:211–215.
48. Ahlers C, Golbaz I, Einwallner E, et al. Identification of optical density ratios in subretinal fluid as a clinically relevant biomarker in exudative macular disease. *Invest Ophthalmol Vis Sci.* 2009;50:3417–3424.
49. Gass JD. *Stereoscopic Atlas of Macular Diseases: Diagnosis and Treatment*, Vol 1, Chap 2, 4th ed. St Louis: CV Mosby; 1997.
50. Kashani AH, Keane P, Dustin L, et al. Quantitative subanalysis of intraretinal cystoid spaces and outer nuclear layer using optical coherence tomography in neovascular age-related macular degeneration. *Invest Ophthalmol Vis Sci.* 2009;50:3366–3373.
51. Ting TD, Oh M, Cox TA, et al. Decreased visual acuity associated with cystoid macular edema in neovascular age-related macular degeneration. *Arch Ophthalmol.* 2002;120:731–737.
52. Iida T, Yannuzzi LA, Spaide RF, et al. Cystoid macular degeneration in chronic central serous chorioretinopathy. *Retina.* 2003;23:1–7; quiz 137–138.
53. Hee MR, Baumal CR, Puliafito CA, et al. Optical coherence tomography of age-related macular degeneration and choroidal neovascularization. *Ophthalmology*. 1996;103:1260–1270.
54. Roquet W, Roudot-Thoraval F, Coscas G, et al. Clinical features of drusenoid pigment epithelial detachment in age related macular degeneration. *Br J Ophthalmol.* 2004;88:638–642.
55. Pieroni CG, Witkin AJ, Ko TH, et al. Ultrahigh resolution optical coherence tomography in non-exudative age related macular degeneration. *Br J Ophthalmol.* 2006;90:191–197.
56. Khanifar AA, Koreishi AF, Izatt JA, et al. Drusen ultrastructure imaging with spectral domain optical coherence tomography in age-related macular degeneration. *Ophthalmology*. 2008;115:1883–1890.
57. Gorczynska I, Srinivasan VJ, Vuong LN, et al. Projection OCT fundus imaging for visualising outer retinal pathology in non-exudative age-related macular degeneration. *Br J Ophthalmol.* 2009;93:603–609.
58. Fleckenstein M, Charbel Issa P, Helb HM, et al. High-resolution spectral domain-OCT imaging in geographic atrophy associated with age-related macular degeneration. *Invest Ophthalmol Vis Sci.* 2008;49:4137–4144.
59. Schuman SG, Koreishi AF, Farsiu S, et al. Photoreceptor layer thinning over drusen in eyes with age-related macular degeneration imaged in vivo with spectral-domain optical coherence tomography. *Ophthalmology*. 2009;116:488.e2–496.e2.
60. Holz FG, Pauleikhoff D, Klein R, et al. Pathogenesis of lesions in late age-related macular disease. *Am J Ophthalmol.* 2004;137:504–510.
61. Wolf-Schnurrbusch UE, Enzmann V, Brinkmann CK, et al. Morphologic changes in patients with geographic atrophy assessed with a novel spectral OCT-SLO combination. *Invest Ophthalmol Vis Sci.* 2008;49:3095–3099.
62. Schmitz-Valckenberg S, Fleckenstein M, Helb HM, et al. In-vivo imaging of foveal sparing in geographic atrophy secondary to age-related macular degeneration. *Invest Ophthalmol Vis Sci.* 2009;50:3915–3921.
63. Lujan BJ, Rosenfeld PJ, Gregori G, et al. Spectral domain optical coherence tomographic imaging of geographic atrophy. *Ophthalmic Surg Laser Imaging.* 2009;40:96–101.
64. Chang LK, Fine HF, Spaide RF, et al. Ultrastructural correlation of spectral-domain optical coherence tomographic findings in vitreomacular traction syndrome. *Am J Ophthalmol.* 2008;146:121–127.
65. Legarreta JE, Gregori G, Knighton RW, et al. Three-dimensional spectral-domain optical coherence tomography images of the retina in the presence of epiretinal membranes. *Am J Ophthalmol.* 2008;145:1023–1030.
66. Schulze S, Hoerle S, Mennel S, et al. Vitreomacular traction and exudative age-related macular degeneration. *Acta Ophthalmol.* 2008;86:470–481.
67. Krebs I, Brannath W, Glittenberg C, et al. Posterior vitreomacular adhesion: a potential risk factor for exudative age-related macular degeneration? *Am J Ophthalmol.* 2007;144:741–746.
68. Lee S, Lee C, Koh H. Posterior vitreomacular adhesion and risk of exudative age-related macular degeneration: paired eye study. *Am J Ophthalmol.* 2009;147:621.e1–626.e1.
69. Mojana F, Cheng L, Bartsch DU, et al. The role of abnormal vitreomacular adhesion in age-related macular degeneration: spectral optical coherence tomography and surgical results. *Am J Ophthalmol.* 2008;146:218–227.
70. Robison CD, Krebs I, Binder S, et al. Vitreomacular adhesion in active and end-stage age-related macular degeneration. *Am J Ophthalmol.* 2009;149:79–82.
71. Talks J, Koshy Z, Chatzinikolas K. Use of optical coherence tomography, fluorescein angiography and indocyanine green angiography in a screening clinic for wet age-related macular degeneration. *Br J Ophthalmol.* 2007;91:600–601.
72. Brown DM, Kaiser PK, Michels M, et al. Ranibizumab versus verteporfin for neovascular age-related macular degeneration. *N Engl J Med.* 2006;355:1432–1444.
73. Rosenfeld PJ, Brown DM, Heier JS, et al. Ranibizumab for neovascular age-related macular degeneration. *N Engl J Med.* 2006;355:1419–1431.
74. Fung AE, Lalwani GA, Rosenfeld PJ, et al. An optical coherence tomography-guided, variable dosing regimen with intravitreal ranibizumab (Lucentis) for neovascular age-related macular degeneration. *Am J Ophthalmol.* 2007;143:566–583.
75. Lalwani GA, Rosenfeld PJ, Fung AE, et al. A variable-dosing regimen with intravitreal ranibizumab for neovascular age-related macular degeneration: year 2 of the PrONTO study. *Am J Ophthalmol.* 2009;148:43–58.

76. Kaiser PK, Blodi BA, Shapiro H, et al. Angiographic and optical coherence tomographic results of the MARINA study of ranibizumab in neovascular age-related macular degeneration. *Ophthalmology*. 2007;114:1868–1875.
77. Spaide RF, Fisher YL. Intravitreal bevacizumab (Avastin) treatment of proliferative diabetic retinopathy complicated by vitreous hemorrhage. *Retina*. 2006;26:275–278.
78. Keane PA, Liakopoulos S, Ongchin SC, et al. Quantitative subanalysis of optical coherence tomography after treatment with ranibizumab for neovascular age-related macular degeneration. *Invest Ophthalmol Vis Sci*. 2008;49: 3115–3120.
79. Moutray T, Alarbi M, Mahon G, et al. Relationships between clinical measures of visual function, fluorescein angiographic and optical coherence tomography features in patients with subfoveal choroidal neovascularisation. *Br J Ophthalmol*. 2008;92:361–364.
80. Joeres S, Kaplowitz K, Brubaker JW, et al. Quantitative comparison of optical coherence tomography after pegaptanib or bevacizumab in neovascular age-related macular degeneration. *Ophthalmology*. 2008;115:347.e2–354.e2.
81. Sadda SR, Joeres S, Wu Z, et al. Error correction and quantitative subanalysis of optical coherence tomography data using computer-assisted grading. *Invest Ophthalmol Vis Sci*. 2007;48:839–848.
82. Keane PA, Chang KT, Liakopoulos S, et al. Effect of ranibizumab retreatment frequency on neurosensory retinal volume in neovascular AMD. *Retina*. 2009;29:592–600.
83. Ahlers C, Golbaz I, Stock G, et al. Time course of morphologic effects on different retinal compartments after ranibizumab therapy in age-related macular degeneration. *Ophthalmology*. 2008;115:e39–e46.
84. Kiss C, Geitzenauer W, Simader C, et al. Evaluation of ranibizumab-induced changes of high-resolution optical coherence tomographic retinal morphology and their impact on visual function. *Invest Ophthalmol Vis Sci*. 2009;50:2376–2383.
85. Witkin AJ, Vuong LN, Srinivasan VJ, et al. High-speed ultrahigh resolution optical coherence tomography before and after ranibizumab for age-related macular degeneration. *Ophthalmology*. 2009;116:956–963.
86. Barbazetto I, Burdan A, Bressler NM, et al. Photodynamic therapy of subfoveal choroidal neovascularization with verteporfin: fluorescein angiographic guidelines for evaluation and treatment–TAP and VIP report No. 2. *Arch Ophthalmol*. 2003;121(9):1253–1268.
87. Lafaut BA, Bartz-Schmidt KU, Vanden Broecke C, et al. Clinicopathological correlation in exudative age related macular degeneration: histological differentiation between classic and occult choroidal neovascularisation. *Br J Ophthalmol*. 2000;84:239–243.
88. Liakopoulos S, Ongchin SC, Bansal A, et al. Quantitative optical coherence tomography findings in various subtypes of neovascular age-related macular degeneration. *Invest Ophthalmol Vis Sci*. 2008;49:5048–5054.
89. Krebs I, Ansari-Shahrezaei S, Goll A, et al. Activity of neovascular lesions treated with bevacizumab: comparison between optical coherence tomography and fluorescein angiography. *Graefes Arch Clin Exp Ophthalmol*. 2008;246:811–815.
90. Green WR, Gass JD. Senile disciform degeneration of the macula. Retinal arterialization of the fibrous plaque demonstrated clinically and histopathologically. *Arch Ophthalmol*. 1971;86:487–494.
91. Yannuzzi LA, Negrão S, Iida T, et al. Retinal angiomatous proliferation in age-related macular degeneration. *Retina*. 2001;21:416–434.
92. Gass JD, Agarwal A, Lavina AM, et al. Focal inner retinal hemorrhages in patients with drusen: an early sign of occult choroidal neovascularization and chorioretinal anastomosis. *Retina*. 2003;23:741–751.
93. Monson DM, Smith JR, Klein ML, et al. Clinicopathologic correlation of retinal angiomatous proliferation. *Arch Ophthalmol*. 2008;126:1664–1668.
94. Costa RA, Calucci D, Paccola L, et al. Occult chorioretinal anastomosis in age-related macular degeneration: a prospective study by optical coherence tomography. *Am J Ophthalmol*. 2005;140:107–116.
95. Freund KB, Ho IV, Barbazetto IA, et al. Type 3 neovascularization: the expanded spectrum of retinal angiomatous proliferation. *Retina*. 2008;28:201–211.
96. Truong SN, Alam S, Zawadzki RJ, et al. High resolution Fourier-domain optical coherence tomography of retinal angiomatous proliferation. *Retina*. 2007;27:915–925.
97. Krebs I, Glittenberg C, Hagen S, et al. Retinal angiomatous proliferation: morphological changes assessed by stratus and cirrus OCT. *Ophthalmic Surg Lasers Imaging*. 2009;40:285–289.
98. Yannuzzi LA, Sorenson J, Spaide RF, et al. Idiopathic polypoidal choroidal vasculopathy (IPCV). *Retina*. 1990;10:1–8.
99. Ciardella AP, Donsoff IM, Huang SJ, et al. Polypoidal choroidal vasculopathy. *Surv Ophthalmol*. 2004;49:25–37.
100. Costa RA, Navajas EV, Farah ME, et al. Polypoidal choroidal vasculopathy: angiographic characterization of the network vascular elements and a new treatment paradigm. *Prog Ret Eye Res*. 2005;24:560–586.
101. Iijima H, Iida T, Imai M, et al. Optical coherence tomography of orange-red subretinal lesions in eyes with idiopathic polypoidal choroidal vasculopathy. *Am J Ophthalmol*. 2000;129:21–26.
102. Iijima H, Imai M, Gohdo T, et al. Optical coherence tomography of idiopathic polypoidal choroidal vasculopathy. *Am J Ophthalmol*. 1999;127:301–305.
103. Ojima Y, Hangai M, Sakamoto A, et al. Improved visualization of polypoidal choroidal vasculopathy lesions using spectral-domain optical coherence tomography. *Retina*. 2009;29:52–59.
104. Otsuji T, Takahashi K, Fukushima I, et al. Optical coherence tomographic findings of idiopathic polypoidal choroidal vasculopathy. *Ophthalmic Surgery Lasers*. 2000;31: 210–214.
105. Saito M, Iida T, Nagayama D. Cross-sectional and en face optical coherence tomographic features of polypoidal choroidal vasculopathy. *Retina*. 2008;28:459–464.
106. Sato T, Kishi S, Watanabe G, et al. Tomographic features of branching vascular networks in polypoidal choroidal vasculopathy. *Retina*. 2007;27:589–594.
107. Tsujikawa A, Sasahara M, Otani A, et al. Pigment epithelial detachment in polypoidal choroidal vasculopathy. *Am J Ophthalmol*. 2007;143:102–111.

108. Chang LK, Sarraf D. Tears of the retinal pigment epithelium: an old problem in a new era. *Retina*. 2007; 27:523–534.
109. Chiang A, Chang LK, Yu F, et al. Predictors of Anti-VEGF-associated retinal pigment epithelial tear using FA and OCT analysis. *Retina*. 2008;28:1265–1269.
110. Giovannini A, Amato G, Mariotti C, et al. Optical coherence tomography in the assessment of retinal pigment epithelial tear. *Retina*. 2000;20:37–40.
111. Leitritz M, Gelisken F, Inhoffen W, et al. Can the risk of retinal pigment epithelium tears after bevacizumab treatment be predicted? An optical coherence tomography study. *Eye*. 2008;22:1504–1507.
112. Hoskin A, Bird AC, Sehmi K. Tears of detached retinal pigment epithelium. *Br J Ophthalmol*. 1981;65:417–422.
113. Tranos PG, Wickremasinghe SS, Stangos NT, et al. Macular edema. *Surv Ophthalmol*. 2004;49:470–490.
114. Johnson MW. Etiology and treatment of macular edema. *Am J Ophthalmol*. 2009;147:11.e1–21.e1.
115. Early Treatment Diabetic Retinopathy Study Research Group. Early photocoagulation for diabetic retinopathy. ETDRS report number 9. *Ophthalmology*. 1991;98: 766–785.
116. Tso MO. Pathology of cystoid macular edema. *Ophthalmology*. 1982;89:902–915.
117. Sebag J, Balazs EA. Pathogenesis of cystoid macular edema: an anatomic consideration of vitreoretinal adhesions. *Surv Ophthalmol*. 1984;28 Suppl:493–498.
118. Massin P, Girach A, Erginay A, et al. Optical coherence tomography: a key to the future management of patients with diabetic macular oedema. *Acta Ophthalmol Scand*. 2006;84:466–474.
119. Bolz M, Schmidt-Erfurth U, Deak G, et al. Optical coherence tomographic hyperreflective foci: a morphologic sign of lipid extravasation in diabetic macular edema. *Ophthalmology*. 2009;116:914–920.
120. Otani T, Kishi S. Tomographic findings of foveal hard exudates in diabetic macular edema. *Am J Ophthalmol*. 2001;131:50–54.
121. Kim BY, Smith SD, Kaiser PK. Optical coherence tomographic patterns of diabetic macular edema. *Am J Ophthalmol*. 2006;142:405–412.
122. Otani T, Kishi S, Maruyama Y. Patterns of diabetic macular edema with optical coherence tomography. *Am J Ophthalmol*. 1999;127:688–693.
123. Alkuraya H, Kangave D, Abu El-Asrar AM. The correlation between optical coherence tomographic features and severity of retinopathy, macular thickness and visual acuity in diabetic macular edema. *Int Ophthalmol*. 2005;26:93–99.
124. Otani T, Kishi S. Correlation between optical coherence tomography and fluorescein angiography findings in diabetic macular edema. *Ophthalmology*. 2007;114:104–107.
125. Brasil OF, Smith SD, Galor A, et al. Predictive factors for short-term visual outcome after intravitreal triamcinolone acetonide injection for diabetic macular oedema: an optical coherence tomography study. *Br J Ophthalmol*. 2007;91:761–765.
126. Catier A, Tadayoni R, Paques M, et al. Characterization of macular edema from various etiologies by optical coherence tomography. *Am J Ophthalmol*. 2005;140:200–206.
127. Gaucher D, Sebah C, Erginay A, et al. Optical coherence tomography features during the evolution of serous retinal detachment in patients with diabetic macular edema. *Am J Ophthalmol*. 2008;145:289–296.
128. Ozdemir H, Karacorlu M, Karacorlu S. Serous macular detachment in diabetic cystoid macular oedema. *Acta Ophthalmol Scand*. 2005;83:63–66.
129. Ozdemir H, Karacorlu M, Karacorlu SA. Regression of serous macular detachment after intravitreal triamcinolone acetonide in patients with diabetic macular edema. *Am J Ophthalmol*. 2005;140:251–255.
130. Soliman W, Sander B, Hasler PW, et al. Correlation between intraretinal changes in diabetic macular oedema seen in fluorescein angiography and optical coherence tomography. *Acta Ophthalmol*. 2008;86:34–39.
131. Soliman W, Sander B, Jørgensen TM. Enhanced optical coherence patterns of diabetic macular oedema and their correlation with the pathophysiology. *Acta Ophthalmol Scand*. 2007;85:613–617.
132. Gaucher D, Tadayoni R, Erginay A, et al. Optical coherence tomography assessment of the vitreoretinal relationship in diabetic macular edema. *Am J Ophthalmol*. 2005;139:807–813.
133. Thomas D, Bunce C, Moorman C, et al. Frequency and associations of a taut thickened posterior hyaloid, partial vitreomacular separation, and subretinal fluid in patients with diabetic macular edema. *Retina*. 2005;25:883–888.
134. Ghazi NG, Ciralsky JB, Shah SM, et al. Optical coherence tomography findings in persistent diabetic macular edema: the vitreomacular interface. *Am J Ophthalmol*. 2007;144:747–754.
135. Mohamed Q, Gillies MC, Wong TY. Management of diabetic retinopathy: a systematic review. *JAMA*. 2007;298:902–916.
136. Browning DJ, Fraser CM, Powers ME. Comparison of the magnitude and time course of macular thinning induced by different interventions for diabetic macular edema: implications for sequence of application. *Ophthalmology*. 2006;113:1713–1719.
137. Goebel W, Kretzchmar-Gross T. Retinal thickness in diabetic retinopathy: a study using optical coherence tomography (OCT). *Retina*. 2002;22:759–767.
138. Hee MR, Puliafito CA, Duker JS, et al. Topography of diabetic macular edema with optical coherence tomography. *Ophthalmology*. 1998;105:360–370.
139. Diabetic Retinopathy Clinical Research Network. Relationship between optical coherence tomography-measured central retinal thickness and visual acuity in diabetic macular edema. *Ophthalmology*. 2007;114:525–536.
140. Larsson J, Zhu M, Sutter F, et al. Relation between reduction of foveal thickness and visual acuity in diabetic macular edema treated with intravitreal triamcinolone. *Am J Ophthalmol*. 2005;139:802–806.
141. Brown JC, Solomon SD, Bressler SB, Set al. Detection of diabetic foveal edema: contact lens biomicroscopy compared with optical coherence tomography. *Arch Ophthalmol*. 2004;122:330–335.
142. Klein R, Klein BE, Moss SE, et al. The Wisconsin Epidemiologic Study of Diabetic Retinopathy: XVII. The 14-year incidence and progression of diabetic retinopathy and associated risk factors in type 1 diabetes. *Ophthalmology*. 1998;105:1801–1815.

143. Browning DJ, Fraser CM, Clark S. The relationship of macular thickness to clinically graded diabetic retinopathy severity in eyes without clinically detected diabetic macular edema. *Ophthalmology*. 2008;115:533.e2–539.e2.
144. Spaide RF, Lee JK, Klancnik JK, et al. Optical coherence tomography of branch retinal vein occlusion. *Retina*. 2003;23:343–347.
145. Scott IU, Blodi BA, Ip M, et al. SCORE Study Report 2: interobserver agreement between investigator and reading center classification of retinal vein occlusion type. *Ophthalmology*. 2009;116:756–761.
146. Ota M, Tsujikawa A, Kita M, et al. Integrity of foveal photoreceptor layer in central retinal vein occlusion. *Retina*. 2008;28:1502–1508.
147. Ota M, Tsujikawa A, Murakami T, et al. Association between integrity of foveal photoreceptor layer and visual acuity in branch retinal vein occlusion. *Br J Ophthalmol*. 2007;91:1644–1649.
148. Ota M, Tsujikawa A, Murakami T, et al. Foveal photoreceptor layer in eyes with persistent cystoid macular edema associated with branch retinal vein occlusion. *Am J Ophthalmol*. 2008;145:273–280.
149. Yamaike N, Tsujikawa A, Ota M, et al. Three-dimensional imaging of cystoid macular edema in retinal vein occlusion. *Ophthalmology*. 2008;115:355.e2–362.e2.
150. Russo V, Barone A, Conte E, et al. Bevacizumab compared with macular laser grid photocoagulation for cystoid macular edema in branch retinal vein occlusion. *Retina*. 2009;29:511–515.
151. Gallagher MJ, Yilmaz T, Cervantes-Castañeda RA, et al. The characteristic features of optical coherence tomography in posterior uveitis. *Br J Ophthalmol*. 2007;91:1680–1685.
152. Tran TH, de Smet MD, Bodaghi B, et al. Uveitic macular oedema: correlation between optical coherence tomography patterns with visual acuity and fluorescein angiography. *Br J Ophthalmol*. 2008;92:922–927.
153. Horgan N, Shields CL, Mashayekhi A, et al. Periocular triamcinolone for prevention of macular edema after plaque radiotherapy of uveal melanoma. *Ophthalmology*. 2009;116:1383–1390.
154. Horgan N, Shields CL, Mashayekhi A, et al. Early macular morphological changes following plaque radiotherapy for uveal melanoma. *Retina*. 2008;28:263–273.

CHAPTER 21

Role of Laser in the Era of Pharmacotherapy

Thomas R. Friberg • Peter M. Brennen

INTRODUCTION

Laser treatment to the human retina was pioneered in the late 1960s and early 1970s by Zweng, Little, and Peabody, using a ruby laser to produce a lesion in the retina, a process now referred to as photocoagulation. Later, they popularized the use of the argon wavelengths (488/512 nm), which had distinct advantages over the longer wavelength emitted by the ruby crystal[1,2] and used an articulated slit lamp delivery system to perform photocoagulation in a controlled, noninvasive manner. Hundreds of patients with diabetic retinopathy and retinal vascular disease underwent photocoagulation using both focal lesions and lesions in a panretinal scatter pattern. Photocoagulation was tried in many retinal disorders and showed efficacy in the treatment of retinal breaks, proliferative and nonproliferative diabetic retinopathy, and vascular retinal diseases. Laser photocoagulation was also recommended for eyes that developed rubeosis iridis,[3] eyes with central serous retinopathy,[4] and a host of other choroidal and retinal abnormalities. Panretinal photocoagulation for proliferative diabetic retinopathy was rapidly embraced on the west coast of the United States and was subsequently proven to be efficacious in a randomized clinical study.

Diabetic Retinopathy Study

The Diabetic Retinopathy Study (DRS) established efficacy of peripheral retinal ablation using either xenon arc or argon laser spots (Box 21.1). In eyes of patients meeting the entry criteria, which hinged on the features of proliferative disease, the approach reduced the chance of poor vision in treated versus untreated eyes and the treatment was ultimately embraced. More than 1,700 subjects were included in the DRS, and 5-year results demonstrated a 20% absolute risk reduction for severe visual loss when comparing control and treated eyes. Of note, the treatment effect was deemed so successful, especially in eyes with neovascularization of the optic disc, that at 2 years, the study protocol was changed to allow treatment of control eyes. The 5-year analysis of severe visual loss kept those control eyes that were later treated in the control group, and it is reasonable to assume the true magnitude of risk reduction is in fact higher than the results suggest.[5] However, the laser settings used for such early historic treatment included the use of large, intense burns, and the treatment sometimes induced macular edema. Wide angle imaging[6] of such eye emphasizes the degree of peripheral ablation that can result (Fig. 21.1). To avoid this, it was suggested that laser applications be performed in divided sessions.

Early Treatment Diabetic Retinopathy Study

Similarly, treatment for diabetic macular edema was also established as efficacious. The Early Treatment Diabetic Retinopathy Study (ETDRS) established that focal photocoagulation for diabetic macular edema was effective in preventing visual loss, and the study provided guidelines for treatment including spot size, placement of applications, and ablation of microaneurysms.[7] The results showed that such treatment not only reduced the risk of progressive visual loss but also increased the chance of visual recovery, and it was recommended that all eyes with clinically significant macular edema be at least considered for treatment as defined by the ETDRS protocol. It is important to note that this therapy was recommended for those eyes in which vision had not yet been affected but had impending macular involvement based on stereo fundus photography. Visual field loss was found to be minimal with focal photocoagulation (Box 21.2).

Panretinal photocoagulation is effective ostensibly by ablating the photoreceptors and deeper retinal layers in areas of ischemia, thereby decreasing the vascular endothelial growth factor (VEGF) load in the eye, which in turn induces involution of existing retinal neovascular fronds. For eyes with very advanced proliferative diabetic retinopathy and in eyes with tractional retinal detachment, the panretinal approach is much less effective.

As described in the preceding chapters, VEGF is a potent vasodilator and causes exudation as well as angiogenesis, or the growth of new blood vessels. Interestingly, panretinal photocoagulation may promote retinal edema,

BOX 21.1 DRS: Diabetic Retinopathy Study

Purpose: Could photocoagulation prevent severe vision loss in eyes with PDR? Is there a difference in safety and efficacy between xenon arc and argon laser? Is there a difference in response to treatment depending on the stage of retinopathy?
Results: Photocoagulation prevented severe vision loss by 50% in PDR patients (at 4 years, 20% risk in treated eyes versus 44% risk in untreated eyes with HRC). The beneficial effect was seen in either xenon arc or laser modality. However, the xenon group showed more decreased visual acuity and constricted visual field. The DRS identified four retinopathy risk factors: (a) presence of new vessels, (b) new vessels on/within 1 disc diameter of the optic nerve (NVD), (c) NVD equal or greater than one fourth to one third disc area, or NVE (new vessels elsewhere) equal or greater than half disc area. (d) preretinal or vitreous hemorrhage.
Conclusions: Prompt photocoagulation prevents severe vision loss and is recommended in PDR eyes with HRC. Because of side effects, argon laser was recommended over xenon arc. The DRS identified four retinopathy risk factors for severe visual loss in eyes with PDR.

swelling, and inflammation, probably by promoting the additional release of VEGF in the areas of treatment, a consequence contrary to the theoretical goal of treatment. Indeed, marked edema is considered a potential complication of panretinal photocoagulation. On the other hand, when laser applications are performed in a less intense and gentler manner, efficacy can typically be achieved without inducing or exacerbating macular edema. Gentle panretinal treatment as a therapy controlled and titrated for the prevention of macular edema has been described.[8] In experienced hands, panretinal photocoagulation seldom, if ever, exacerbates diabetic macular edema if the laser lesions are less intense. Use of indirect laser delivery systems can make the performance of panretinal laser photocoagulation much easier to achieve (Fig. 21.2).[9,10] Furthermore, continued application of panretinal photocoagulation after a certain point is not in the patient's best interest, as it creates night-vision difficulties and results in marked changes to the visual field. Severe loss of visual field can easily be demonstrated when patients have undergone confluent, intent panretinal photocoagulation. This approach, thus, does the patient a disservice and we need to improve our outcomes of this disease using alternatives.

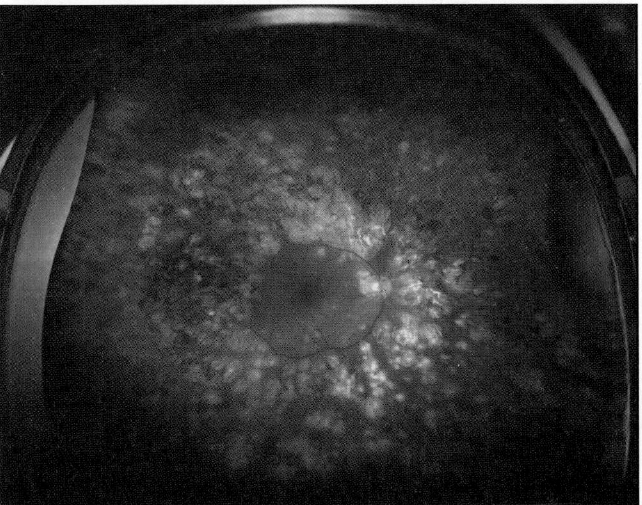

FIGURE 21.1. In this ultrawide angle fundus photograph, multiple laser scars from panretinal laser photocoagulation can be seen. The peripheral retina is largely ablated here, but efficacy of treatment may often be achieved by using less intense, less destructive laser lesions.

While the DRS and ETDRS were scientifically sound and pivotal in their scope, many clinicians unfortunately consider the laser treatment parameters used in the context of these studies as the only ones that have been proven, despite the fact that the investigators intended to establish efficacy, while the side effects of some treatments were not highlighted. Many have not modified their approach as technology has advanced and have assumed that laser treatment is a method where modifications and nuances do not matter. This leads to the belief that laser treatment implies a generic approach to retinal disorders despite the fact that careful selection of laser parameters is essential both to induce a therapeutic effect and to prevent avoidable complications.

With the advent of anti-VEGF approaches over the past several years, there has been a distinct shift away from laser photocoagulation as a primary treatment. Intravitreal injections, on the other hand, have been advocated or attempted for virtually all disease previously treated by retinal photocoagulation, except perhaps for the treatment of retinal tears or retinal detachment. In the wake of the success of anti-VEGF agents, laser treatment has waned in popularity much like the production of black and white movies, hardwired telephones, and print newspapers. To the lay public, the term "laser treatment" conjures up refractive surgery as they have much greater exposure to advertisements for LASIK and other procedures.

For wet macular degeneration, destructive laser photocoagulation was effective for limiting the overall extent of the neovascular lesion. The treatment effect, however, was preceded by an immediate reduction in visual acuity secondary to nonselective laser damage in the fovea. In essence, the patient traded off some of this immediate

BOX 21.2 ETDRS: Early Treatment Diabetic Retinopathy Study

Purpose:

(a) Is focal photocoagulation beneficial in management of diabetic macular edema?
(b) When scatter photocoagulation should be initiated to be most effective in management of diabetic retinopathy?
(c) Is aspirin effective in altering the course of diabetic retinopathy?

Results:

(a) Focal photocoagulation reduced the risk of moderate vision loss by 50% in diabetic macular edema (12% risk in treated eyes vs. 24% risk in untreated eyes). The benefit was more apparent in patients with "clinically significant diabetic macular edema" (CSDME) (13% risk in treated eyes vs. 33% risk in untreated eyes).
(b) In severe and very severe NPDR, there is a much higher risk of progression to high-risk PDR (15% risk of developing high-risk characteristics, HRC at 1 year and 56% risk at 5 years in severe NPDR, and 45% risk at 1 year and 71% risk at 5 years in very severe NPDR).
(c) Aspirin did not have any effect on the progression to high-risk retinopathy, development of vitreous hemorrhage, or risk of visual loss.

Conclusions:

(a) The ETDRS recommended prompt focal laser photocoagulation in eyes with CSDME to prevent vision loss.
(b) Early photocoagulation should be considered in eyes with severe or very severe NPDR and in those with early PDR.
(c) There is no contraindication to aspirin use in NPDR or early PDR.

visual function for long-term security and gain by limiting the size of the central scotoma caused by a neovascular process. Side effects of retinal photocoagulation are multiple, but arguably, the most important are the creation of small central scotomata, difficulty fixating, and worsening of night vision due to disruption of the outer retina (Box 21.3). Later, verteporfin dye was introduced to make laser treatment for macular degeneration more tissue selective. The dye was administered intravenously after which the neovascular lesion was irradiated with a photosensitizing wavelength to induce localized tissue destruction. Verteporfin binds to lipoproteins and accumulates preferentially in areas of choroidal neovascularization. A 10-minute washout period is allowed for the dye to clear from the normal retinal vasculature. The laser energy by itself is not sufficient to cause denaturation of proteins or retinal photocoagulation. With dye present, occasionally retinal scarring and even frank photocoagulation may occur, though infrequently. In any case, the use of a pharmacologic agent for treatment became commonplace.

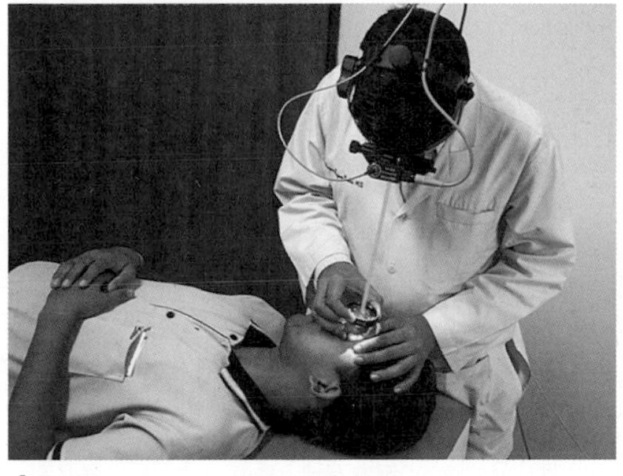
A

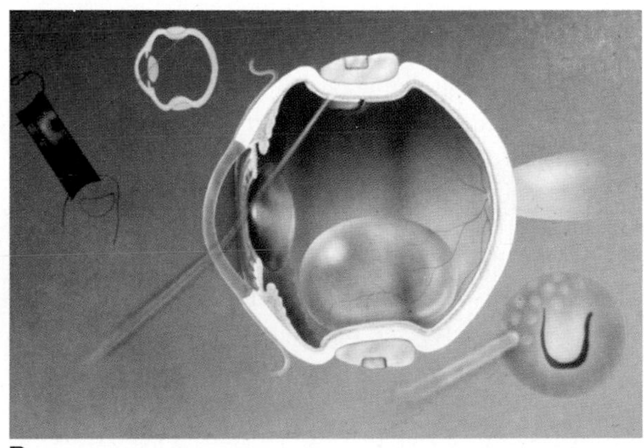
B

FIGURE 21.2. Laser delivery via an indirect ophthalmoscopy and hand-held lens (**A**) facilitates rapid panretinal photocoagulation. No contact lens is used, (**B**) and topical anesthesia is all that is required for the procedure. Retrobulbar anesthesia is seldom necessary. The patient is typically much more comfortable using this method as compared to slit lamp systems where the patient's position must be more rigid. (Courtesy of LV Prasad Eye Institute, Hyderabad, India.)

BOX 21.3 MPS: Macular Photocoagulation Study

Purpose: To examine whether direct laser photocoagulation of a choroidal neovascular membrane due to ARMD prevents vision loss as compared to observation alone.

Results:

(a) **Extrafoveal CNV Study:** At 6 months, severe vision loss was reduced significantly by laser treatment (25% risk in treated eyes vs. 60% risk in untreated eyes). There was recurrence of CNV in 54% treated eyes after 5 years.

(b) **Juxtafoveal Krypton Laser Study:** At 3 years, severe vision loss was reduced by laser treatment, and the benefit was high in normotensive patients (49% risk in treated eyes vs. 58% risk in untreated eyes).

(c) **Subfoveal Argon or Krypton Laser Study:** Although there was an immediate severe vision loss in treated eyes, long-term results showed a more stable vision. At 4 years, severe vision loss was seen in 22% of treated eyes versus 47% of untreated eyes.

(d) **Recurrent Subfoveal CNV Study:** At 3 years, severe vision loss occurred in 12% of treated eyes versus 36% of untreated eyes.

Conclusions: Direct laser treatment of choroidal neovascular membrane prevented severe vision loss, and the benefit was most apparent in extrafoveal lesions. Only a small percentage of patients with neovascular ARMD qualified for laser treatment as laser was indicated for an angiographically well-defined membrane.

Another reason why laser treatment for macular edema might be regulated to a second-line strategy for some is that it is more difficult to properly perform laser photocoagulation in a grid, in a panretinal fashion, or focally, than to inject a drug intravitreally. Maintaining proper patient positioning and the placement of a handheld lens on the cornea during a laser procedure require considerable skill. This difficulty is reflected in the relatively higher value placed on the performance of laser by insurers versus an intravitreal injection. Patient positioning, time to set up the laser, a patient's ability to sit correctly at the slit lamp, and placement of a contact lens all add to the time required to treat a patient with retinal vascular disease. For these reasons, at least one of us prefers to use the indirect laser delivery system to perform panretinal photocoagulation in virtually every patient needed to be treated in an outpatient setting. The reason for this is that setup time is virtually nonexistent. Similarly, some patients who could not be treated at the slit lamp but have macular disease can also be treated with the indirect laser delivery systems if due care is exercised and the laser surgeon is experienced.[11]

The introduction of better laser delivery systems such as the OptiMedica PASCAL unit[12] was a leap forward or at least a step forward (Fig. 21.3). Its Star Wars feel and video game–like interface made laser treatment now fun to do once again and gave the retinal photocoagulator camp some much needed ammunition against those advocating anti-VEGF strategies for virtually everything. The system's customizable grid patterns allow delivery of multiple laser applications simultaneously, decreasing treatment time and patient discomfort. Preliminary studies have demonstrated equal efficacy for focal and panretinal photocoagulation and when comparing the PASCAL system to traditional laser delivery systems.

While laser strategies and anti-VEGF therapy may seem to be unrelated, they are indeed interconnected. Some 50 years ago, Wise observed the development of rubeosis iridis in eyes with severe diabetic retinopathy.[13] He postulated a diffusible factor *x* was present and must migrate from the posterior segment into the anterior segment. Factor *x* ultimately became known as VEGF and is now believed to be expressed by the retina in conditions with a component of retinal ischemia. When laser photocoagulation became available, it was proposed as treatment in a wide variety of retinal disease. One reason for

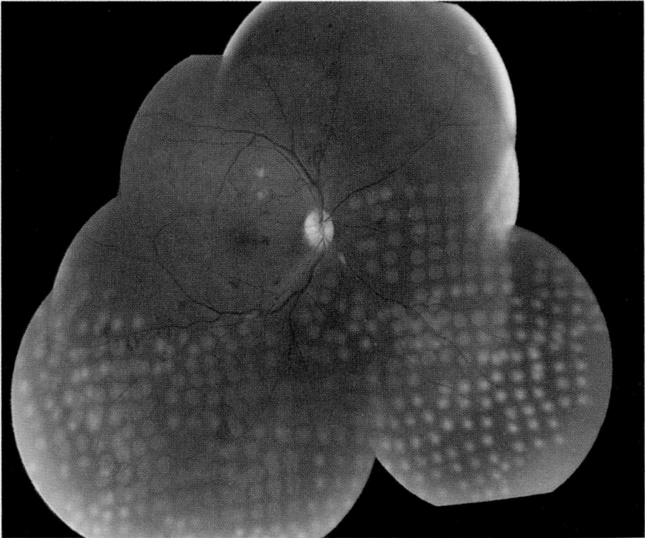

FIGURE 21.3. Automated laser delivery systems such as the PASCAL laser shown here can put in a pattern of laser spots more efficiently and with more flexibility than other slit lamp–based delivery systems. (Courtesy of Harry Flynn, MD.)

this was that few other modalities existed that were relatively noninvasive. Similarly, when pharmacotherapy was available, virtually all available anti-VEGF drugs were used for multiple disease states in pioneering efforts. Prior to the introduction of anti-VEGF therapy, steroid preparations administered either sub-Tenon's or intravitreally were occasionally used in the treatment of macular edema. However, the safety profile of intravitreal steroids was later found to be unfavorable, since repeated injections lead to cataract formation and intractable glaucoma ultimately requiring surgery. Nevertheless, when macular edema responded, many clinicians took this approach in preference to applying additional laser treatment. Despite the safety profiles of such injections, they were a legitimate off-label strategy. Many clinicians were convinced of the efficacy of such a treatment and the safety issues became secondary as it provided some relief for their patients.

Interestingly, the Standard Care versus Corticosteroid for Retinal Vein Occlusion (SCORE) study investigated the usefulness of intravitreal steroids in the treatment of retinal vascular disease, particularly venous occlusion, and compared this to laser treatment head to head. Many clinicians were, thus, quite surprised when after a 2-year follow-up, the planned endpoint, laser photocoagulation produced a result superior to the use of intravitreal steroid injections for branch retinal vein occlusion (BRVO), with a mean VA improvement from baseline of 11.3 letters for laser compared with 6.3 and 4.0 letters for 1 and 4 mg of triamcinolone, respectively.[14] Data extending from 12 to 36 months also favored laser treatment when evaluating mean improvement from baseline visual acuity for BRVO.

New systems for intravitreal steroid delivery have recently been introduced. These systems aim to reduce the frequency of intravitreal injection for steroid therapy by using implants that slowly diffuse drugs with short half-lives over a period of weeks. Preliminary studies with the Posurdex dexamethasone drug delivery system (DDS) have demonstrated a benefit with respect to visual acuity in patients with macular edema due to diabetic retinopathy and vein occlusion when compared to observation. While traditional steroid therapy has not been proven superior for BRVO, future studies will assess the performance of these alternative drug delivery approaches compared to the current gold standard laser therapy.

There are a few controlled studies where anti-VEGF treatments have been given for macular edema or retinal vascular disease. Ranizumab and pegaptanib were initially approved for age-related macular degeneration, and of this writing, the approval process for a drug agent for diabetic retinopathy is much more arduous than for wet AMD. There is evidence, however, that anti-VEGF treatment is valuable in retinal vascular disease. Regarding pegaptanib, surprisingly proliferative diabetic retinopathy responded quite well to injections, dramatic amelioration of the disease has been reported by Victor Gonzalez.[15] In another study, intravitreal pegaptanib improved the mean visual acuity in eyes with diabetic macular edema and was superior to laser treatment in a 6-month follow-up study.[16] Larger studies regarding the relative efficacy of laser versus anti-VEGF treatment have not been reported to date, although some are presently underway (Box 21.4).

BOX 21.4 Is Focal Laser the Gold Standard Treatment in Diabetic Macular Edema?

Three randomized clinical trials compared the role of focal laser with intravitreal drug therapies.

Focal Laser Versus Steroid? A randomized trial evaluating 1- and 4-mg doses of preservative-free intravitreal triamcinolone compared with focal/grid photocoagulation for treatment of diabetic macular edema. Results do not indicate a long-term benefit of intravitreal triamcinolone relative to focal/grid photocoagulation in patients with diabetic macular edema. Most eyes receiving 4 mg of triamcinolone are likely to require cataract surgery. (DRCR Network. *Arch Ophthalmol.* 2009;127:245.)

Focal Laser Versus Bevacizumab? A randomized phase 2 clinical trial in patients with diabetic macular edema randomly assigned to one of five groups: (a) focal photocoagulation at baseline, (b) intravitreal injection of 1.25 mg of bevacizumab at baseline and 6 weeks, (c) intravitreal injection of 2.5 mg of bevacizumab at baseline and 6 weeks, (d) intravitreal injection of 1.25 mg of bevacizumab at baseline and sham injection at 6 weeks, or (e) intravitreal injection of 1.25 mg of bevacizumab at baseline and 6 weeks with photocoagulation at 3 weeks. There were no meaningful differences in CST observed for bevacizumab relative to photocoagulation after the 3-week time point. Combining focal photocoagulation with bevacizumab resulted in no apparent short-term benefit or adverse outcomes. These results demonstrate that intravitreal bevacizumab can reduce DME in some eyes, but a phase 3 clinical trial is needed to explore the clinical benefits further. (DRCR Network. *Ophthalmology.* 2007;114:1860.)

Focal Laser Versus Ranibizumab? The READ-2 Trial, a prospective, randomized, interventional, multicenter clinical trial, compared ranibizumab with focal/grid laser or a combination of both in diabetic macular edema (DME). During a span of 6 months, ranibizumab injections by the study protocol had a significantly better visual outcome than focal/grid laser treatment in patients with DME. Long-term results are awaited to explore the benefits of intravitreal ranibizumab. (READ-2 Study Group. *Ophthalmology.* 2009;11:2175).

KEY POINTS

- Large clinical trials have shown that laser treatment is efficacious for diabetic macular edema and proliferative diabetic retinopathy.
- With the advent of anti-VEGF drugs that have been shown to be effective in wet macular degeneration, laser photocoagulation is now reserved only for selective cases.
- A careful selection of laser parameters is essential both to induce a therapeutic effect and to prevent avoidable complications.
- The new PASCAL system's customizable grid patterns allow delivery of multiple laser applications simultaneously, decreasing treatment time and patient discomfort.
- The SCORE study has shown that laser photocoagulation produced a result superior to the use of intravitreal steroid injections for BRVO, with a mean VA improvement from baseline of 11.3 letters for laser compared with 6.3 and 4.0 letters for 1 and 4 mg of triamcinolone, respectively.
- Laser treatment adds durability to treatment with anti-VEGF drugs, and probably a combination approach of laser and anti-VEGF therapy will be the new strategy for the future.

CONCLUSION

In our opinion, treatment of retinal vascular disease and edema is aided by anti-VEGF agents. However, laser treatment adds durability to such treatment, and newer strategies will probably incorporate a combination of laser and the use of anti-VEGF therapy, with the latter potentially being given as a booster therapy.

REFERENCES

1. Zweng HC, Little HL, Peabody RR. Laser photocoagulation of macular lesions. *Trans Am Acad Ophthalmol Otolaryngol.* 1968;72(3):377–388.
2. Little HL, Zweng HC, Peabody RR. Argon laser slit-lamp retinal photocoagulation. *Trans Am Acad Ophthalmol Otolaryngol.* 1970;74(1):85–97.
3. Peabody RR, Zweng HC, Little HL. Treatment of retinal vascular disease with argon laser slit lamp photocoagulation. *Trans Pac Coast Otoophthalmol Soc Annu Meet.* 1970;51:307–326.
4. Zweng HC, Little HL, Peabody RR. Argon laser photocoagulation of diabetic retinopathy. *Arch Ophthalmol.* 1971;86(4):395–400.
5. Zweng HC, Fahrenbruch RC, Little HL. Argon laser photocoagulation in the treatment of retinal vein occlusions. *Mod Probl Ophthalmol.* 1974;12:261–270.
6. Friberg TR, Pandya A, Eller AW. Non-mydriatic panoramic fundus imaging using a non-contact scanning laser based system (Optos Panoramic 200). *Ophth Surg Lasers Imaging.* 2003;34(6):488–497.
7. The Diabetic Retinopathy Study Research Group. Preliminary report on effects of photocoagulation therapy. *Am J Ophthalmol.* 1976;81(4):383–396.
8. The Diabetic Retinopathy Study Research Group. Photocoagulation treatment of proliferative diabetic retinopathy. Clinical application of Diabetic Retinopathy Study (DRS) findings, DRS Report Number 8. *Ophthalmology.* 1981;88(7):583–600.
9. Friberg TR. Principles of photocoagulation using binocular indirect ophthalmoscope laser delivery system. *Int Ophthalmol Clin.* 1990;30:89–94.
10. Friberg TR. Laser photocoagulation using binocular indirect ophthalmoscope laser delivery systems. *Ophthal Surg Lasers.* 1996;28:78–87.
11. Early Treatment Diabetic Retinopathy Study research group. Photocoagulation for diabetic macular edema. Early Treatment Diabetic Retinopathy Study report number 1. *Arch Ophthalmol.* 1985;103(12):1796–1806.
12. Blumenkranz MS, Yellachich D, Andersen DE, et al. Semiautomated pattern scanning laser for photocoagulation. *Retina.* 2006;26(3):370–376.
13. Little HL, Rosenthal AR, Dellaporta A, et al. The effect of pan-retinal photo-coagulation on rubeosis iridis. *Am J Ophthalmol.* 1976;81(6):804–809.
14. Peabody RR, Zweng HC, Little HL. Treatment of persistent central serous retinopathy. *Arch Ophthalmol.* 1968;79(2):166–169.
15. González VH, Giuliari GP, Banda RM, et al. Intravitreal injection of pegaptanib sodium for proliferative diabetic retinopathy. *Br J Ophthalmol.* 2009;93:1474–1478.
16. Cunningham ET Jr, Adamis AP, Altaweel M, et al. A phase 1 randomized double-masked trial of pegaptanib, an anti-vascular endothelial growth factor aptamer, for diabetic macular edema. *Ophthalmology.* 2005;112:1747–1757.

CHAPTER 22

PDT—Still An Option?

Albert Augustin

INTRODUCTION

As more people live longer, choroidal neovascularization (CNV) secondary to age-related macular degeneration (AMD) represents a substantial and growing cause of vision loss. AMD was the most common cause of 5-year incident legal blindness in a recent study of a middle-aged and elderly Icelandic population.[1] The overall prevalence of AMD in Europe ranges from 9% to 25%; it increases with age and varies by country, with highest rates in Western Europe (35% in the United Kingdom, 36% in the Netherlands, 39% in Germany, and 40% in France).[2] In the United States, AMD is the leading cause of blindness among white adults,[3] affects women more than men,[4] and reaches a prevalence of 15% among white women 80 years and older.[5] In countries with rapidly aging populations, these numbers will undoubtedly increase. By 2020, Friedman et al.[5] estimate that almost 3 million people in the United States will have AMD.

TREATMENT OVERVIEW

Fortunately, over the past decade or so, treatment options have expanded considerably. Indeed, in our ability to select among therapeutic options and to devise combination therapies, retina specialists are now somewhat akin to medical oncologists. As an example, medical oncologists until recently had to rely almost solely on 5-fluorouracil to treat metastatic colorectal cancer. With the availability of additional cytotoxic agents and the targeted biologic agents that inhibit angiogenesis (e.g., bevacizumab), they can now offer several different first-, second-, and third-line therapies.[6] These additional treatment options, although highly welcome, are accompanied by additional challenges. As no single regimen has yet emerged as the standard of care for metastatic colorectal cancer, oncologists face the challenge of developing optimal combinations and sequencing to improve outcomes for each individual patient.

Similarly, retina specialists can now consider several different treatments for patients with CNV secondary to AMD, and these expanded therapeutic options bring with them the challenge of devising optimal individual treatment plans. In concert, evidence has accumulated that inflammation, proliferation of vascular endothelial growth factor (VEGF), and vascular components are three key contributors to the disease process.

With different therapies available to target these different components of the disease and no single treatment able to address the multifactorial pathogenesis of CNV secondary to AMD, combination therapy is now of intense interest. Combination therapies will be increasingly used to treat ocular angiogenesis that is due to AMD as their different mechanisms of action have more potential to successfully treat the various pathogenetic factors contributing to CNV than any single therapy approach.

As a component of combination therapies, verteporfin photodynamic therapy (PDT) continues to be a viable treatment option. This chapter summarizes the current treatment approaches to CNV secondary to AMD with emphasis on PDT-containing therapies, and in particular, on triple therapy—a combination of verteporfin PDT and the intravitreal application of a steroid and an anti-VEGF drug.

CURRENT THERAPEUTIC OPTIONS

Intravitreal corticosteroids are used because of their efficacy in treating and preventing inflammation, a significant pathogenetic factor in AMD. Corticosteroids also block the upregulation of VEGF, which is produced by all inflammatory cells,[7] narrow the gaps between endothelial cells in the capillary walls, and limit fibrosis, which decreases retina scarring.[8] Triamcinolone acetonide has been shown to improve visual acuity when administered intravitreally,[9–11] but its use as monotherapy has largely been abandoned in favor of combination therapy.

Verteporfin PDT, a two-stage process involving administration of verteporfin for injection and nonthermal red light, targets the vascular component of CNV secondary to AMD by producing local damage to neovascular endothelium, which results in vessel occlusion.[12] It has been shown to reduce the risk of further vision loss in patients

BOX 22.1 PDT Trials

TAP Study

Purpose: A randomized, double-blind trial in patients with subfoveal CNV secondary to ARMD examined the efficacy of verteporfin treatment every 3 months versus sham treatment (intravenous dextrose followed by light treatment).

Results: At the month 24 examination for the primary outcome, 53% of verteporfin-treated patients compared with 38% placebo-treated patients lost fewer than 15 letters. In subgroup analyses for predominantly classic lesions at baseline, 59% of verteporfin-treated patients compared with 31% placebo-treated patients lost fewer than 15 letters at the month 24 examination. For minimally classic lesions at baseline, no statistically significant differences in visual acuity were noted.

Conclusions: The visual acuity benefits of verteporfin therapy for AMD patients with predominantly classic CNV subfoveal lesions are safely sustained for 2 years. For minimally classic lesions, there is insufficient evidence to warrant routine use of verteporfin therapy (Bressler et al., *Arch Ophthalmol.* 2001;119:198).

VIP Study

Purpose: A randomized trial in patients with occult CNV secondary to ARMD and pathological myopia examined the efficacy of verteporfin treatment every 3 months versus sham treatment.

Results: At 12 months, there was no difference between two groups in terms of the primary outcome. At 24 months, a significant treatment benefit was seen in verteporfin treated eyes. About 54% of verteporfin treated eyes compared with 67% of placebo-treated patients lost at least 15 letters. About 4.4% of verteporfin treated eyes and none of the placebo-treated patients had a severe decrease of vision of 20 letters or more within 7 days of treatment, and this was attributed to the result of the development of subretinal pigment epithelial blood, marked subretinal fluid associated with choroidal hypofluorescence, or no obvious cause.

Conclusions: In patients with occult CNV, verteporfin therapy significantly reduced the risk of moderate and severe visual acuity loss. The VIP Study Group recommends that this therapy should be considered for the treatment of patients with AMD with subfoveal lesions composed of occult with no classic CNV who are presumed to have recent disease progression (VIP Study Group, *Am J Ophthalmol.* 2001;131:541).

VALIO Study: Verteporfin with Altered Light in Occult CNV

Purpose: A Phase 2, multicenter, masked, randomized clinical trial to compare PDT therapy with verteporfin using either standard or delayed light application after the start of the infusion.

Conclusions: There were no significant differences between verteporfin therapy using the delayed light application regimen of 30 minutes or the standard light regimen of 15 minutes in eyes with occult with no classic CNV (Rosenfeld et al., *Am J Ophthalmol.* 2007;144:970).

VIM Study: Verteporfin in Minimally Classic CNV

Purpose: A Phase 2, multicenter, double-masked, placebo-controlled, randomized clinical trial to compare the treatment effect and safety of PDT using a standard (SF) or reduced (RF) light fluence rate with that of placebo therapy in patients with subfoveal minimally classic CNV with ARMD.

Conclusions: Verteporfin therapy safely reduced the risks of losing at least 15 letters (≥3 lines) of visual acuity and progression to predominantly classic CNV for at least 2 years in individuals with subfoveal minimally classic lesions due to AMD measuring 6 MPS disc areas or less. The VIM Study Group recommends verteporfin therapy for relatively small minimally classic lesions as were enrolled in the VIM Trial. There was no conclusive evidence of differences between the two verteporfin regimens identified (Azab et al., *Arch Ophthalmol.* 2005;123:448).

with predominantly classic subfoveal CNV secondary to AMD,[13] with beneficial outcomes sustained at 2[14] and 5 years.[15] Visual acuity improved in a small minority of patients at 1- and 2-year examinations (Box 22.1).[16]

The current therapeutic gold standard is the anti-VEGF agent ranibizumab, a recombinant, humanized monoclonal antibody fragment that binds and inhibits the biologic activity of VEGF A.[17] The rationale for the use of anti-VEGF drugs stems from the identification of angiogenesis as a leading culprit in neovascular and exudative eye diseases.[18] In pivotal clinical trials, ranibizumab, given as a monthly intravitreal injection, was shown to improve visual acuity,[19,20] with benefit in visual acuity maintained at 24 months.[20]

These results, showing the first meaningful vision improvement in significant numbers of patients with AMD treated with ranibizumab, also generated considerable off-label use of intravitreal bevacizumab.[21–23] Bevacizumab is derived from the same recombinant humanized monoclonal antibody as ranibizumab, and is indicated for use in treating metastatic colorectal cancer, lung cancer, and breast cancer, because of demonstrated efficacy in inhibiting metastatic angiogenesis.[24] Pegaptanib, the first anti-VEGF agent approved to treat CNV secondary to AMD,[25] has largely been replaced by ranibizumab and bevacizumab as monotherapy with this class of drugs.

Other therapies, that is, laser photocoagulation and anecortave acetate, an indirect angiogenesis inhibitor, are appropriate in only a small minority of patients[26] or are not available for use in North America and Europe, respectively. Their limited use precludes further discussion here.

As monotherapy, neither a steroid, verteporfin PDT, nor an anti-VEGF agent is able to treat the multifactorial pathogenesis of CNV. No single agent can reduce inflammation, eradicate existing CNV and inhibit further CNV, and limit VEGF expression. Thus, dual- and triple-combination therapies are being intensively investigated and increasingly used. Combination therapies with a verteporfin PDT component are the focus of this chapter.

VERTEPORFIN PDT IN DUAL COMBINATION THERAPIES

Verteporfin PDT and Triamcinolone

Among dual combinations, we have the most experience with verteporfin PDT plus intravitreal triamcinolone. In a prospective, comparative, nonrandomized trial, Chan et al. reported that a significantly higher proportion of patients treated with verteporfin PDT + triamcinolone did not develop moderate visual loss at 1 year compared with the PDT monotherapy group (71% vs. 33%, respectively, $p = 0.009$). Eyes treated with combination therapy had significantly fewer lines lost than eyes treated with monotherapy (0.7 vs. 3.5 lines, respectively, $p = 0.015$). None of the 48 trial participants developed ocular or systemic complications related to PDT. With combination therapy, there were transient increases in intraocular pressure but no serious complications such as endophthalmitis and retinal detachment.[27]

In a prospective randomized study involving 61 patients, verteporfin PDT + triamcinolone combination therapy was significantly better than PDT monotherapy in maintaining visual acuity ($p = 0.001$) and reducing lesion size ($p = 0.001$) and foveal thickness ($p = 0.03$). Combination therapy was also associated with a significantly lower retreatment rate ($p = 0.04$). Common ocular events included glaucoma (26%) and cataract progression (32%) and were considered triamcinolone-related.[28] Case series have also reported good results for this combination, but glaucoma, cataract formation, and increased intraocular pressure have been noted.[29–33] A representative case of a serous retinal pigment epithelium detachment and a small extrafoveal classic CNV treated with verteporfin PDT and triamcinolone dual combination therapy is shown in Figure 22.1.

Verteporfin PDT and Anti-VEGF Agents

Dual combinations of PDT + anti-VEGF therapy are also of great interest. There is in vivo evidence from an animal model that PDT + ranibizumab may have synergistic effects. Real-time monitoring of angio-occlusion in the chick chorioallantoic membrane under conditions similar to clinical settings showed selective vascular closure with PDT and prevention of reperfusion of occluded vessels with topical application of the anti-VEGF agent.[34]

In clinical trials, the multicenter, randomized, single-masked, controlled FOCUS study found that PDT + ranibizumab was more efficacious than PDT alone in treating neovascular AMD. At 12 months, 95 of the 105 (91%) PDT + ranibizumab-treated patients and 38 of the 56 (68%) PDT monotherapy patients had lost fewer than 15 letters from baseline visual acuity ($p < 0.001$). PDT retreatment occurred significantly less in the combined therapy group. Ranibizumab treatment was associated with an increased risk of serious intraocular inflammation, possibly related to the trial's use of an early formulation of this agent; nevertheless, affected patients on average still experienced visual acuity benefit.[35]

Clinical trial evidence also supports the administration of dual-combination therapy on the same day. Using PDT + bevacizumab, Lazic et al. showed increased visual acuity and fewer retreatments with combination therapy than with either agent alone after 1 month, with maintenance of these benefits at 3 months. Each therapy was given once on the same day in this randomized, controlled, open-label pilot trial ($n = 165$). Significant reductions in central foveal thickness occurred with all three treatments ($p < 0.0001$ for all 3-month vs. baseline comparisons). Three pigment epithelial tears (all in the bevacizumab group), 12 posterior vitreous detachments (4 in the combination group and 8 in the bevacizumab group), and 7 cataract progressions (3 in the combination group and 4 in the bevacizumab group) were observed.[36]

Same-day administration of verteporfin PDT + ranibizumab is also feasible, per the prospective, multicenter PROTECT study ($N = 32$). Standard verteporfin therapy was administered at baseline and, if fluorescein leakage was present, at months 3, 6, and 9. Ranibizumab was administered at baseline and months 1, 2, and 3. There were no reports of severe vision loss due to ocular inflammation or uveitis. There was one case of moderate vision loss, three of mild/moderate uveitis, and one retinal pigment epithelial tear. At 9 months, all lesions were inactive with no recurrent leakage on fluorescein angiography and optical coherence tomography (OCT), and all cases of macular edema and subretinal fluid had resolved. The investigators concluded that same-day administration of verteporfin and ranibizumab was safe and not associated with severe vision loss or severe ocular inflammation.[37]

Same-day combination therapy might lower the risk of retinal toxicity. In a subanalysis of the PROTECT trial, Kiss et al. evaluated the effects of the above-described regimen on retinal anatomy, choroidal perfusion, and visual function. The vascular effects of same-day combination therapy were immediate photothrombosis of CNV and surrounding choroid. Retinal sensitivity also improved

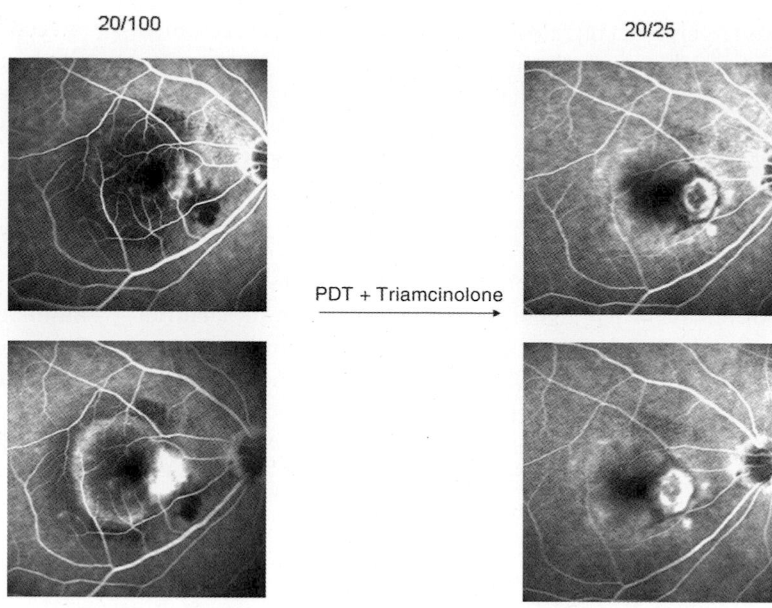

FIGURE 22.1. Early and late phase angiography in a patient with a serous RPE detachment, small extrafoveal classic CNV, and basline visual acuity of 20/100. Following one administration of dual combination therapy, consisting of verteporfin PDT followed by 25 mg of crystalline triamcinolone acetonide injected intravitreally 16 hours later (Arias, et al. *Ophthalmology.* 2006;113:2243–2250), the lesion was dry and visual acuity increased to 20/25. At 24-month follow-up, the lesion remained dry. *Note*: At the time of treatment this was not an indication for PDT monotherapy according to TAP criteria. (*Arch Ophthalmol.* 1999;117:1329–1345) because the neovascular component covered less than half of the lesion area.

immediately and continued over time, despite lingering choroidal malperfusion. Although the study was small in size and lacked a comparison group, the vascular effects were apparently substantial and long-lasting.[38]

In the prospective, randomized, double-masked, multicenter VERITAS trial, verteporfin PDT + pegaptanib was compared with verteporfin PDT + triamcinolone given as either 1- or 4- mg.[39] Interim 6-month results showed equivalent efficacy among the three treatments in the percentage of patients who lost fewer than 15 letters of visual acuity, the study's primary endpoint. Verteporfin PDT + triamcinolone (at both doses) was significantly more effective than verteporfin + pegaptanib in reducing the total CNV area. No serious ocular adverse events were reported.[40]

In the randomized, double-masked, 2-year Mont Blanc trial, PDT + ranibizumab is being compared with ranibizumab alone in 257 patients. Standard fluence verteporfin PDT is administered on the same day as ranibizumab. Thereafter, PDT is given as needed at >90 day intervals, and ranibizumab at 1 and 2 months and as needed thereafter. Monthly follow-up will consist of visual acuity and OCT assessments, with 1-year results expected in 2009.[41]

Also currently under way is DENALI, a 2-year, multicenter controlled trial of dual combination therapy in which approximately 300 patients were randomized to receive ranibizumab + standard fluence PDT, ranibizumab + reduced fluence PDT, or ranibizumab monotherapy. Patients receiving combination therapy will receive it on the same day. In the first two treatment groups, ranibizumab will be given at baseline, months 1 and 2, and then as needed; in the third group, ranibizumab will be administered monthly for the first year and as needed for the second year. Verteporfin PDT will be administered at baseline and every 3 months after as needed. Monthly follow-up will consist of visual acuity and OCT assessments, with retreatment based on OCT findings. One-year results are expected in 2010.[42]

Reduced fluence PDT may have effects on CNV closure that are equivalent to standard fluence therapy, but with less detrimental effect on the choroidal vasculature. Michels et al. compared the effects of standard and reduced fluence PDT on the CNV and the choroidal vasculature. Reduced fluence PDT was administered as either reduced treatment time (600 mW/cm^2 over 42 seconds for a dose of 25 J/cm^2) or reduced fluence rate (300 mW/cm^2 over 83 seconds for a dose of 25 J/cm^2). Using sensitive angiographic techniques, they noted minimal choroidal hypoperfusion in eyes treated with 25 J/cm^2; in contrast, eyes treated with standard fluence (50 J/cm^2) showed significant choriocapillary nonperfusion at week 1, which continued for as long as 3 months in some. Standard fluence PDT also produced a more extensive, although transient, increase in leakage area shown on fluorescein angiography at day 1.[43] In a 40-patient comparison of standard versus reduced fluence PDT + same-day triamcinolone, the reduced fluence group showed significantly better visual outcome, less choroidal alteration, and a trend toward lower recurrence rate than the standard fluence group at 3 months.[44] A trend toward better visual outcome with reduced fluence PDT was observed in the 117-patient VIM Trial, which compared reduced fluence PDT, standard fluence PDT, and placebo.[45]

Dual therapy with a verteporfin PDT component continues to be intensively explored. Numerous trials involving PDT at standard or reduced fluence in combination with ranibizumab, bevacizumab, pegaptanib, or triamcinolone acetonide are now either recruiting patients or under way.[46]

THE EMERGING OPTION OF TRIPLE COMBINATION THERAPY

Rationale

We are increasingly appreciating that CNV, once considered to be primarily a vascular disease arising from angiogenesis, is actually a complex multifactorial disease that involves nonvascular components. It may be helpful to view CNV as a two-compartment model, as Spaide has proposed: a vascular component consisting of endothelial cells, circulating endothelial progenitor cells, and pericytes, and an extravascular component consisting of inflammatory cells, such as retinal pigment epithelial cells, macrophages, lymphocytes, and granulocytes, which contribute to broad-spectrum inflammation.[47] A nonspecific granulation tissue response involving inflammation, angiogenesis, and fibrosis, key components of the wound-healing response, has also been implicated in CNV.[48–50] Wound healing involves a series of events beginning with the release of inflammatory cytokines that interact with target cells involved in a continually evolving extracellular matrix. Angiogenesis, matrix deposition, remodeling, and fibrosis accompany the inflammation.[50]

The progression of CNV can be viewed as a cascade that starts with oxidative stress of the RPE followed by RPE dysfunction; release of inflammatory mediators and proangiogenic factors, notably VEGF; inappropriate growth of new vessels, which can penetrate Bruch membrane and grow into the RPE and subretinal space; exudation and hemorrhage; and ultimately formation of disciform scars (Fig. 22.2).[48,51–54] To treat this complex, multifactorial disease process, triple combination therapy is being intensely explored. The goal is to provide different and quite possibly complementary or synergistic mechanisms of action to lessen inflammation, eradicate existing and prevent new CNV, and inhibit VEGF proliferation.

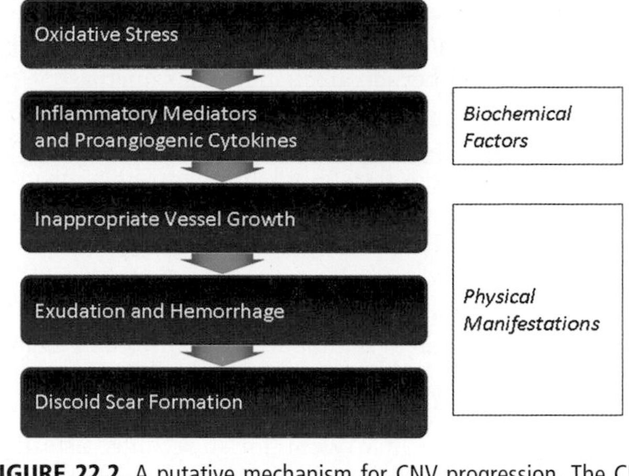

FIGURE 22.2. A putative mechanism for CNV progression. The CNV cascade begins with oxidative stress of the retinal pigment epithelium (RPE), where drusen accumulate between Bruch membrane and RPE, leading to hypoxia, oxidative and inflammatory processes, and an altered balance of proangiogenic and antiangiogenic factors. RPE dysfunction results in release of inflammatory mediators and proangiogenic factors, notably VEGF, with inward migration of macrophages. The release of proangiogenic factors leads to inappropriate growth of new vessels, which can penetrate Bruch membrane and grow into the subretinal space and leak blood and fluid, ultimately resulting in development of disciform scars. (Bainbridge. *Clin Sci (Lond)*. 2003; Schlingemann. *Graefes Arch Clin Exp Ophthalmology*. 2004; Ambati. *Surv Ophthalmology*. 2003; Grossniklaus. *Am J Ophthalmol*. 2004]).

Clinical Findings

One potential approach to triple combination therapies is verteporfin PDT, a steroid, and an antiangiogenic/anti-VEGF agent. Verteporfin PDT eradicates existing neovasculature, but it may also induce an inflammatory reaction that affects adjoining tissues and triggers new expression of VEGF. Giving it in combination with a steroid and an anti-VEGF drug reduces inflammation and prevents formation of new vasculature, respectively (Fig. 22.3).

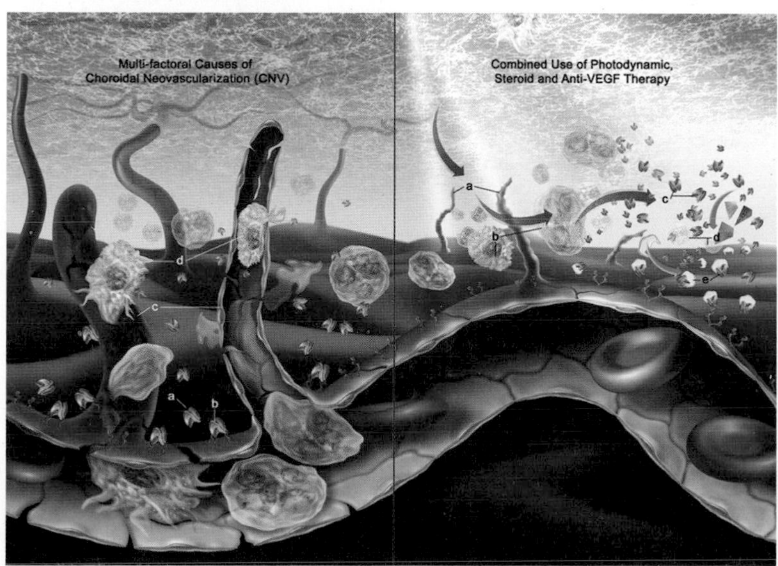

FIGURE 22.3. Left, the multifactorial causes of CNV: **A:** VEGF; **B:** VEGF bound to VEGF receptor; **C:** formation of neovasculature; **D:** extravasation of inflammatory cells. **Right,** triple combination therapy with verteporfin PDT, a steroid, and an anti-VEGF agent provides different mechanisms of action to treat several pathogenetic factors: **A:** PDT eradicates neovasculature; **B:** PDT causes an inflammatory reaction that affects adjoining tissues; **C:** inflammation triggers new additional expression of VEGF; **D:** steroid therapy reduces the inflammation; **E:** anti-VEGF competitively inhibits the binding of VEGF, thus preventing formation of new vasculature.

In a prospective, noncomparative, interventional case series, we administered triple combination therapy with verteporfin PDT, bevacizumab, and dexamethasone to 104 patients.[55] We selected bevacizumab as the anti-VEGF therapy (ranibizumab was not available for use at the time) and dexamethasone as the steroid for its anti-inflammatory as well as its antifibrotic, antiproliferative, and antimigratory effects.[56–59] Other factors influencing our use of dexamethasone instead of triamcinolone acetonide are its availability as a transparent formulation, shorter half-life, lower risk of elevated intraocular pressure, and higher anti-inflammatory potency. To lessen the potential for choroidal damage, we administered verteporfin PDT at a reduced light dose, 600 mW/cm^2 for 70 seconds instead of 83 seconds, which is about 84% of the standard light dose. After verteporfin PDT was administered, dexamethasone and bevacizumab were intravitreally injected approximately 16 hours later. At 6-week follow-up visits, patients had visual acuity and intraocular pressure measurement, slit-lamp and ophthalmoscopic examination, and OCT. Fluorescein angiography was performed every 3 months or earlier if OCT showed significant edema.[55]

Over a mean follow-up period of 40 weeks (range, 22–60 weeks), visual acuity increased by a mean of 1.8 lines and retinal thickness decreased by a mean of 182 μm ($p < 0.01$ for both comparisons vs. baseline). In addition to significant and sustained visual acuity improvement after only one cycle of treatment, no serious adverse events and no ocular events were noted. Notably, 81 of the 104 patients (78%) had a satisfactory response to one course of triple therapy.[54] In another prospective interventional case series, Veritti et al. recently reported results of verteporfin PDT + modified juxtascleral triamcinolone + ranibizumab in 30 patients with CNV secondary to AMD. PDT was given as standard fluence/standard irradiance PDT (50 J/cm^2, 600 mW/cm^2), reduced fluence/standard irradiance PDT (25 J/cm^2, 600 mW/cm^2), or reduced fluence/reduced irradiance PDT (25 J/cm^2, 300 mW/cm^2). Over 6 months of follow-up, no angiographic leakage occurred in any treatment group, leading the investigators to conclude that reduced fluence PDT is safe and may reduce treatment frequency. The investigators also note that a hypofluorescent area corresponding to the laser spot was visible on both fluorescein and indocianine green angiography at 6 months in 90% of eyes treated with standard PDT compared with 40% and 30% of eyes treated with reduced fluence/standard irradiance PDT and reduced fluence/reduced irradiance PDT, respectively.[60]

Same-day triple therapy has also been reported with good results in a retrospective case series (n = 31) by Bakri et al. One administration of reduced fluence PDT, dexamethasone, and bevacizumab on the same day maintained visual acuity and decreased macular thickness in all patients over a mean follow-up of 13.7 months. Both treatment-naïve patients and those previously treated with an anti-VEGF agent benefited, with the same mean number of repeat triple therapy treatments, 0.3, in both groups, and no adverse effects noted at 1 year of follow-up.[61] The investigators noted that most patients were offered same-day triple therapy because they wanted to avoid prolonged, monthly follow-up.

Representative case series of triple combination therapy with verteporfin PDT, bevacizumab and dexamethasone are shown in Figures 22.4 and 22.5.

Ongoing Triple-combination Clinical Trials

Among ongoing randomized clinical trials, the multicenter, single-masked RADICAL study is assessing whether triple-combination therapy reduces retreatment rates compared with ranibizumab alone with similar vision outcomes and tolerability profiles. In RADICAL, 162 patients were

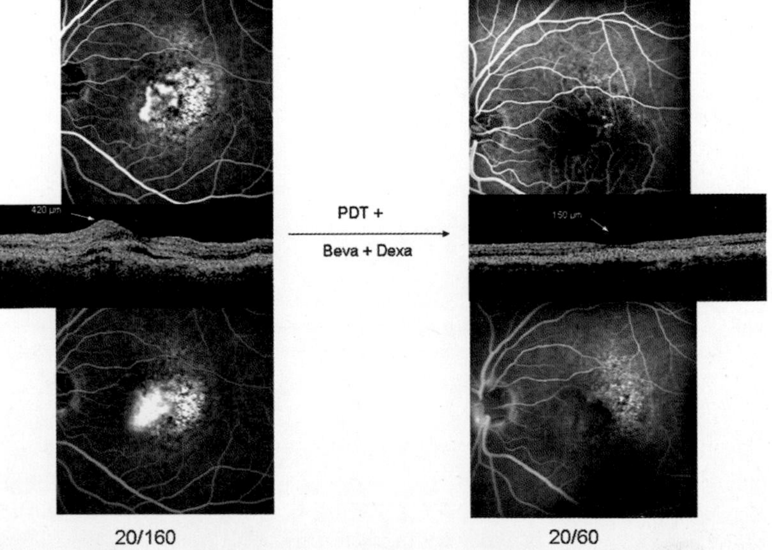

FIGURE 22.4. Early and late phase angiography and OCT of a minimally classic lesion with some fibrosis and baseline visual acuity of 20/160. After one administration of triple therapy, consisting of verteporfin PDT, bevacizumab, and dexamethasone, visual acuity improved to 20/60. Over 14 months of follow-up, no further retreatment was required.

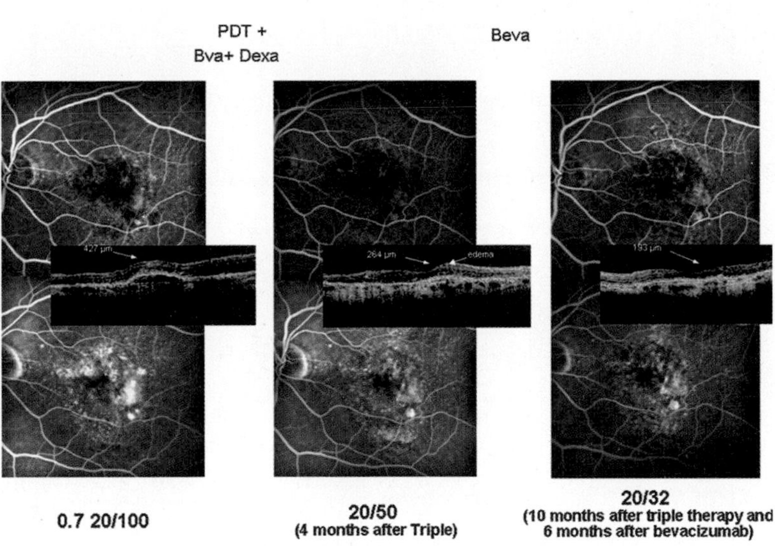

FIGURE 22.5. Early and late phase angiography and OCT in a patient who received triple therapy, consisting of verteporin PDT, bevacizumab, and dexamethasone, with bevacizumab retreatment required 4 months later to treat remaining edema and some metamorphopsia. Visual acuity increased from 20/100 to 20/50. After bevacizumab retreatment, visual acuity further improved 20/32 and both metamorphopsia and edema disappeared. Vision remains stable with approximately 12 months of follow-up.

randomized to one of four treatment groups: (a) reduced fluence PDT (300 mW/cm^2 for 83 seconds to deliver 25 J/cm^2) followed within 2 hours by ranibizumab; (b) reduced fluence PDT + ranibizumab + dexamethasone; (c) very low fluence PDT (180 mW/cm^2 for 83 seconds to deliver 15 J/cm^2) + ranibizumab + dexamethasone; and (d) ranibizumab monotherapy at baseline, months 1 and 2, and as needed thereafter.[62]

At ARVO 2009, Hughes and Sang reported interim results of a randomized controlled clinical trial to determine if triple therapy with verteporfin/reduced duration PDT + dexamethasone + ranibizumab, with ranibizumab booster given 1 month later, would reduce the number of treatments required compared with monthly ranibizumab alone in 60 patients with CNV secondary to AMD. The triple regimen reduced the number of ranibizumab retreatments required over 9 months compared with monthly ranibizumab monotherapy, with favorable final visual acuities.[63] Sheidow et al. presented 6-month interim results of a prospective randomized clinical trial comparing triple therapy with low fluence PDT + bevacizumab + triamcinolone versus PDT + bevacizumab versus bevacizumab alone. The mean number of treatments at the interim analysis was lowest with triple therapy with similar effects on visual acuity with all treatments.[64]

Ongoing trials of dual and triple therapy studies containing verteporfin PDT are listed in Table 22.1.[39–42,62–70] We await final results before drawing any conclusions.

Possible Additional Advantages of Triple Combination Therapy

Triple therapy may offer benefits in terms of safety, cost, and convenience for many patients with CNV secondary to AMD. By decreasing the need for retreatment, triple therapy may result in an improved safety profile by reducing the risks associated with repeated intravitreal injections, including the potential for arterial thromboembolic events, retinal detachment, and endophthalmitis.[17,19,20]

The Registry of Visudyne AMD Therapy recently reported real-world practice patterns that showed low overall rates of retreatment with verteporfin PDT and bevacizumab combination therapy. This was a retrospective analysis of a database of 1,073 patients with CNV due to AMD; all received intravitreal bevacizumab within 14 days of verteporfin PDT and were followed up for at least 6 months. Patients were retreated according to investigator discretion and retreatments did not have to be combination therapy. After baseline combination treatment, patients received a mean of 0.6 verteporfin PDT and 2.2 bevacizumab retreatments over the mean follow-up period of 15 months. It is of interest that 27% (284/1,073) of patients required no additional treatment during follow-up. The mean time to first retreatment was 6.3 months for verteporfin PDT and 4.4 months for bevacizumab, with no substantial differences in retreatment rates between treatment-naïve and previously treated patients.[71] A smaller (N = 539) registry in the same database assessed retreatments in patients who received either dual combination, verteporfin PDT + ranibizumab, or triple combination therapy, PDT + ranibizumab or bevacizumab + a corticosteroid. Rates of retreatment were low and similar to those reported in the larger registry.[72]

If repeat treatments can be lessened, overall costs of combination treatment would likely decrease, as well. At present, the manufacturer recommends monthly injection of ranibizumab on a continuing basis,[17] and per-labeling use of ranibizumab is costly. Smiddy recently measured cost versus benefit of various AMD therapies in US dollars per line-year. Using hospital-based practice modeling that included costs of clinical examinations, imaging, and treatments, pharmaceuticals accounted for the highest proportion of treatment costs, and per-protocol use of ranibizumab was the most costly drug, accounting for 83% of total costs of a ranibizumab-containing regimen. The cost per line-year for 1 year of treatment ranged from $84 with as-needed bevacizumab to $766 for protocol-style

Table 22.1.

Ongoing randomized controlled clinical trials of dual and triple combination therapy with a PDT component

Trial (Ref.) (Clinical Trial Identifier)	Study Design	Patients (*N*)	Treatments	Schedules	Primary Outcome Measure	Date of Completion
Dual combination						
VERITAS[39,40,65] [NCT00242580]	2-y, double masked, multicenter	111	PDT + pegaptanib or PDT + triamcinolone 1 mg or PDT + triamcinolone 4 mg	vPDT at baseline, prn thereafter pegaptanib at baseline, every 6 wk thereafter triamcinolone at baseline, every 3 mo thereafter	% of patients losing <15 letters of VA at month 12	Spring 2009
Mont Blanc[41] [CVT00433017]	2-y, double-masked, multicenter	257	sfPDT + ranibizumab or sham PDT + ranibizumab	vPDT at baseline and every 3 mo prn thereafter ranibizumab at baseline, at months 1 and 2, and prn thereafter	BCVA at 12 mo	June 2009 (12-mo data)
DENALI[42,66] [NCT00436553]	2-y, double-masked, multicenter;	318	rf vPDT + ranibizumab prn or sf vPDT + ranibizumab prn or sham vPDT + ranibizumab	vPDT at baseline and every 3 mo prn thereafter + ranibizumab at baseline, at months 1 and 2, and prn thereafter; ranibizumab alone = monthly during year 1; prn thereafter	BCVA at 12 mo and treatment-free interval	January 2010 (12-mo data)
Triple combination						
PDEX II[67] [NCT00390208]	1-y, single-masked	60	vPDT + ranibizumab + dexamethasone or ranibizumab monotherapy	PDT + dexamethasone + ranibizumab at baseline, thereafter each prn; ranibizumab monotherapy = monthly on a fixed schedule until week 48	Change in visual acuity by 15 or more ETDRS letters at 6 and 12 mo	December 2009
RADICAL[62,68,69] [NCT00492284]	2-y, single-masked, multicenter,	162	rfPDT + ranibizumab or rfPDT + ranibizumab + dexamethasone or very low fluence PDT + ranibizumab + dexamethasone or ranibizumab monotherapy	Combination therapy at baseline, then every 2 mo prn; ranibizumab monotherapy at baseline, months 1 and 2, then monthly prn	Mean change in BCVA at 12 mo and mean number of retreatments	June 2010
Hughes and Sang[63] [NCT00794923]	Multicenter	60	rdPDT + ranibizumab + dexamethasone or ranibizumab monotherapy	In combination therapy, ranibizumab every 4 wk prn; all three therapies repeated prn at month 3 followed by ranibizumab booster 1 mo later; ranibizumab monotherapy = monthly	Intervention rates with double- and triple therapies vs. monotherapy	NA
Sheidow et al.[64,70] [NCT00376701]	1-y multi-center, open-label	106	rfPDT + bevacizumab + triamcinolone or rfPDT + bevacizumab or bevacizumab monotherapy	NA	Intervention rates with combination therapies vs. monotherapy	March 2009

BCVA, best corrected visual acuity; NA, not available; prn, as needed; rd, reduced duration; RF, reduced fluence; SF, standard fluence; vPDT, verteporfin photodynamic therapy .

use of ranibizumab. Combination treatments ranged from $71 to $269 in cost per line-year. Notably, the lowest cost per line-year, $71, was achieved with triple therapy with PDT + dexamethasone + bevacizumab.[73]

Thus, several strategies are available to lower the treatment burden for both patients and health care systems. These include same-day treatment, fewer repeat treatments with an anti-VEGF agent, and one cycle of triple therapy. Besides potential cost-savings, such strategies may be more convenient to patients. Patients who live in rural areas, for whom visits to a treatment center involve extensive travel and caregiver considerations, might especially benefit from combination therapy that lessens the need for retreatments and follow-up visits.

COMBINATION THERAPY: CHALLENGES TO OVERCOME

The biggest challenge to treating CNV with combination therapy is devising a treatment plan that addresses each treatable component of the disease with optimal drugs, doses, and dosing schedules in each patient. Therapy that would improve vision with as few administrations as possible, ideally in one cycle, while maintaining efficacy and tolerability is the goal. Triple combination therapy now appears most capable of achieving it.

The number of variables involved in combination therapy, that is, the different agents, dosings, timing and sequences, makes it difficult to carry out large randomized clinical trials that would provide definitive, conclusive answers to what constitutes the triple combination therapy that is the standard of care for every patient.[74] Expert opinion and consensus guidelines might be a more practical way to address this rapidly changing environment.

Another unanswered question is whether different patient characteristics, such as disease stage, vision status, previous treatments, and lesion characteristics and location, affect safety profiles and treatment results. Further, all currently available therapies and combinations may limit or destroy CNV, but the underlying cause remains. It is possible that CNV could manifest in another way at a later time despite apparently successful treatment. Whether there are long-term sequelae of any of these therapies is also not yet known.[74]

The optimal dosing schedule for ranibizumab also remains to be determined. As noted, there are real world database findings showing vision benefit with reduced rates of retreatment with both dual and triple therapies.[71,72] There is also clinical trial evidence favoring per-label, monthly injection. In the multicenter, randomized, double-masked, sham injection-controlled PIER trial, ranibizumab, 0.3 or 0.5 mg, was administered monthly for 3 months and then quarterly. After 12 months, ranibizumab provided significant visual acuity benefit and was well tolerated. However, the PIER investigators noted that outcomes were more robust in the pivotal clinical trials, ANCHOR and MARINA, which used fixed monthly dosing of ranibizumab.[75] Monthly dosing may be necessary in some patients for maximal treatment benefit. The Comparison of Age-Related Macular Degeneration Treatments Trials: Lucentis-Avastin Trial (CATT) is a large randomized clinical trial now under way to directly compare the efficacy and safety of bevacizumab and ranibizumab. It is also evaluating whether variable dosing is as effective as a fixed monthly schedule. Results, expected in 2011, will further inform the use of reduced dosing schedules of anti-VEGF agents in treating CNV.[76]

Lastly, is there an optimal sequence of drug administration? As noted, there is evidence from an animal study that PDT + ranibizumab given in that order has synergistic effects,[34] but clinical data would be welcome.

CONCLUSIONS

With different therapies available to target the different components of CNV secondary to AMD and no single treatment able to address its complex multifactorial pathogenesis, combination therapies are now of intense interest. They will be increasingly used to treat ocular angiogenesis that is due to AMD as their different mechanisms of action have a greater potential to successfully treat the various pathogenetic factors contributing to CNV than any single therapy. As a component of dual or preferably triple combination therapies, verteporfin PDT remains an option in treating ocular angiogenesis. Triple therapy with verteporfin PDT, a steroid, and an anti-VEGF agent provides three different and quite possibly synergistic mechanisms of action to lessen inflammation, eradicate existing CNV, prevent formation of new CNV, and inhibit VEGF proliferation. Triple therapy may also result in less need for

KEY POINTS

- As a component of combination therapies, verteporfin PDT continues to be a viable treatment option.
- Verteporfin PDT, a two-stage process involving administration of verteporfin for injection and nonthermal red light, targets the vascular component of CNV by producing vessel occlusion.
- Triple therapy with verteporfin PDT, a steroid, and an anti-VEGF agent provides three different synergistic mechanisms of action to lessen inflammation, regress existing CNV, prevent formation of new CNV, and inhibit VEGF-dependent cell proliferation.
- Numerous variables to be assessed when treating CNV underscore the need for individualized therapy for each patient.

retreatments, yielding such benefits as an improved safety profile, cost savings, and greater patient convenience.

The numerous variables to be assessed when treating CNV, including disease characteristics, treatment selection, retreatment, and patient factors and preferences, underscore the need for individualized therapy for each patient. Multiple therapeutic options will continue to be available, and customizing therapy for each patient remains essential.

DISCLOSURES

QLT Inc. supported the preparation of this chapter.

ACKNOWLEDGMENT

The author wishes to thank Margaret Phelan for her assistance in preparing this chapter for publication.

REFERENCES

1. Gunnlaugsdottir E, Arnarsson A, Jonasson F. Five-year incidence of visual impairment and blindness in older Icelanders: the Reykjavik Eye Study. *Acta Ophthalmol.* 2010; 88:358–366.
2. Prokofyeva E, Wilke R, Zrenner E. Prevalence and incidence of age-related macular degeneration in Europe: meta-analysis based on a systematic literature review [Abstract A367]. Presented at the Annual Meeting of the Association for Research in Vision and Ophthalmology. May 3, 2009. Fort Lauderdale, FL.
3. Congdon N, O'Colmain B, Klaver CC, et al. Causes and prevalence of visual impairment among adults in the United States. *Arch Ophthalmol.* 2004;122:477–485.
4. Javitt JC, Zhou Z, Maguire MG, et al. Incidence of exudative age-related macular degeneration among elderly Americans. *Ophthalmology.* 2003;110:1534–1539.
5. Friedman DS, O'Colmain BJ, Muñoz B, et al. Prevalence of age-related macular degeneration in the United States. *Arch Ophthalmol.* 2004;122:564–572.
6. National Cancer Comprehensive Cancer Network. *NCCN Clinical Practice Guidelines in Oncology. Colon Cancer.* V.2.2009. Available at: www.nccn.org. Accessed March 1, 2009.
7. Möhle R, Green D, Moore MA. Constitutive production and thrombin-induced release of vascular endothelial growth factor by human mega-karyocytes and platelets. *PNAS.* 1997;94:663–668.
8. Augustin AJ, Scholl S, Kirchoff J. Treatment of neovascular age-related macular degeneration: current therapies. *Clin Ophthalmol.* 2009;3:175–182.
9. Danis RP, Ciulla TA, Pratt LM. Intravitreal triamcinolone aceotonide in exudative age-related macular degeneration. *Retina.* 2000;20:244–250.
10. Challa JK, Gillies MC, Penfold PL, et al. Exudative macular degeneration and intravitreal triamcinolone: 18 month follow up. *Aust N Z J Ophthalmol.* 1998;26:277–281.
11. Penfold PL, Gyory JF, Hunyor AB. Exudative macular degeneration and intravitreal triamcinolone. A pilot study. *Aust N Z J Ophthalmol.* 1995;23:293–298.
12. Visudyne [package insert]. East Hanover, NJ: Novartis Pharmaceuticals Corp; 2007.
13. Photodynamic therapy of subfoveal choroidal neovascularization in age-related macular degeneration with verteporfin: one-year results of 2 randomized clinical trials—TAP report. Treatment of age-related macular degeneration with photodynamic therapy (TAP) Study Group. *Arch Ophthalmol.* 1999;117:1329–1345.
14. Treatment of Age-Related Macular Degeneration with Photodynamic Therapy (TAP) Study Group. Photodynamic therapy of subfoveal choroidal neovascularization in age-related macular degeneration with verteporfin: two-year results of 2 randomized clinical trials—TAP Report 2. *Arch Ophthalmol.* 2001;119:198–207.
15. Kaiser PK, Treatment of age-related macular degeneration with photodynamic therapy (TAP) Study Group. Verteporfin therapy of subfoveal choroidal neovascularization in age-related macular degeneration: 5-year results of two randomized clinical trials with an open-label extension: TAP report no. 8. *Graefes Arch Clin Exp Ophthalmol.* 2006;244:1132–1142.
16. Anand R, Bressler NM, Bressler SB, et al, Writing Committee for the TAP Study Group. Improvement after verteporfin therapy. *Arch Ophthalmol.* 2003;121:415–416.
17. Lucentis [package insert]. South San Francsico, CA: Genentech, Inc.; 2008.
18. Michels S, Schmidt-Erfurth U, Rosenfeld PJ. Promising new treatments for neovascular age-related macular degeneration. *Expert Opin Investig Drugs.* 2006;15:779–793.
19. Brown MD, Kaiser PK, Michels M, et al; ANCHOR Study Group. Ranibizumab versus verteporfin for neovascular age-related macular degeneration. *N Engl J Med.* 2006;355: 1432– 1444.
20. Rosenfeld PJ, Brown DM, Heier JS, et al. Ranibizumab for neovascular age-related macular degeneration. *N Engl J Med.* 2006;355:1419–1431.
21. Rich RM, Rosenfeld PJ, Puliafito CA, et al. Short-term safety and efficacy of intravitreal bevacizumab (Avastin) for neovascular age-related macular degeneration. *Retina.* 2006;26:495–511.
22. Spaide RF, Laud K, Fine HF, et al. Intravitreal bevacizumab treatment of choroidal neovascularization secondary to age-related macular degeneration. *Retina.* 2006;26:383–390.
23. Bashshur ZF, Bazarbachi A, Schakal A, et al. Intravitreal bevacizumab for the management of choroidal neovascularization in age-related macular degeneration. *Am J Ophthalmol.* 2006;142:1–9.
24. Avastin [package insert]. South San Francisco, CA: Genentech, Inc.; 2008.
25. About Macugen (pegaptanib sodium injection). Available at: www.macugen.com. Accessed April 9, 2009.
26. Freund KB, Yannuzzi LA, Sorenson JA. Age-related macular degeneration and choroidal neovascularization. *Am J Ophthalmol.* 1993;115:786–791.
27. Chan WM, Lai TY, Wong AL, et al. Combined photodynamic therapy and intravitreal triamcinolone injection for the treatment of subfoveal choroidal neovascularisation in age related macular degeneration: a comparative study. *Br J Ophthalmol.* 2006;90:337–341.
28. Arias L, Garcia-Arumi J, Ramon JM, et al. Photodynamic therapy with intravitreal triamcinolone in predominantly classic choroidal neovascularization: one-year results of a randomized study. *Ophthalmology.* 2006;113:2243–2250.
29. Augustin AJ, Schmidt-Erfurth U. Verteporfin and intravitreal triamcinolone acetonide combination therapy for occult

choroidal neovascularization in age-related macular degeneration. *Am J Ophthalmol.* 2006;141:638–645.
30. Augustin AJ, Schmidt-Erfurth U. Verteporfin therapy combined with intravitreal triamcinolone in all types of choroidal neovascularization due to age-related macular degeneration. *Ophthalmology.* 2006;113:14–22.
31. Spaide RF, Sorenson J, Maranan L. Combined photodynamic therapy with verteporfin and intravitreal triamcinolone acetonide for choroidal neovascularization. *Ophthalmology.* 2003;110:1517–1525.
32. Spaide RF, Sorenson J, Maranan L. Photodynamic therapy with verteporfin combined with intravitreal injection of triamcinolone acetonide for choroidal neovascularization. *Ophthalmology.* 2005;112:301–304.
33. Ruiz-Moreno JM, Montero JA, Barile S, et al. Photodynamic therapy and high-dose intravitreal triamcinolone to treat exudative age-related macular degeneration: 1-year outcome. *Retina.* 2006;26:602–612.
34. van den Bergh H, Wagnieres G, Debefve E, et al. Video monitoring of neovessel occlusion induced by photodynamic therapy in combination with anti-VEGF therapy. *Invest Ophthalmol Vis Sci.* 2008;49:E-Abstract 2721.
35. Heier JS, Boyer DS, Ciulla TA, et al. Ranibizumab combined with verteporfin photodynamic therapy in neovascular age-related macular degeneration: year 1 results of the FOCUS Study. *Arch Ophthalmol.* 2006;124:1532–1542.
36. Lazic R, Gabric N. Verteporfin therapy and intravitreal bevacizumab combined and alone in choroidal neovascularization due to age-related macular degeneration. *Ophthalmology.* 2007;114:1179–1185.
37. Schmidt-Erfurth U, Wolf S, PROTECT Study Group. Same-day administration of verteporfin and ranibizumab 0.5 mg in patients with choroidal neovascularisation due to age-related macular degeneration. *Br J Ophthalmol.* 2008;92:1628–1635.
38. Kiss CG, Simader C, Michels S, et al. Combination of verteporfin photodynamic therapy and ranibizumab: effects on retinal anatomy, choroidal perfusion and visual function in the PROTECT study. *Br J Ophthalmol.* 2008;92:1620–1627.
39. Kaiser PK, VERITAS Study Group. Verteporfin therapy in combination with pegaptanib or triamcinolone for wet AMD: 6-month results of the VERITAS trial [Abstract 2870]. Presented at the Annual Meeting of the Association for Research in Vision and Ophthalmology. May 8, 2007. Fort Lauderdale, FL.
40. Kaiser PK, for the VERITAS Study Group. VERITAS 6-month interim analysis. Presented at the Annual Meeting of the Association for Research in Vision and Ophthalmology. May 8, 2007. Fort Lauderdale, FL.
41. Mont Blanc Trial. Data on file, QLT and Novartis.
42. DENALI Trial. Data on file, QLT and Novartis.
43. Michels S, Hansmann F, Geitzenauer W, Schmidt-Erfurth U. Influence of treatment parameters on selectivity of verteporfin therapy. *Invest Ophthalmol Vis Sci.* 2006;47:371–376.
44. Sacu S, Varga A, Michels S, et al. Reduced fluence versus standard photodynamic therapy in combination with intravitreal triamcinolone: short-term results of a randomised study. *Br J Ophthalmol.* 2008;92:1347–1351.
45. Visudyne in Minimally Classic Choroidal Neovascularization Study Group. Verteporfin therapy of subfoveal minimally classic choroidal neovascularization in age-related macular degeneration: 2-year results of a randomized clinical trial. *Arch Ophthalmol.* 2005;123:448–457.
46. NIH. Clinical Trials Registry. Available at: http://clinicaltrials.gov/. Accessed March 27, 2009.
47. Spaide RF. Perspectives: rationale for combination therapies for choroidal neovascularization. *Am J Ophthalmol.* 2006;141:149–156.
48. Schlingemann RO. Role of growth factors and the wound healing response in age-related macular degeneration. *Graefes Arch Clin Exp Ophthalmology.* 2004;242:91–101.
49. Grossniklaus HE, Miskala PH, Green WR, et al. Histopathologic and ultrastructural features of surgically excised subfoveal choroidal neovascular lesions: submacular surgery trials report no. 7. *Arch Ophthalmol.* 2005;123:914–921.
50. Kent D, Sheridan C. Choroidal neovascularization: a wound healing perspective. *Mol Vis.* 2003;9:747–755.
51. Kannan R, Zhang N, Sreekumar PG, et al. Stimulation of apical and basolateral VEGF-A and VEGF-C secretion by oxidative stress in polarized retinal pigment epithelial cells. *Mol Vis.* 2006;12:1649–1659.
52. Bainbridge JW, Mistry AR, Thrasher AJ, et al. Gene therapy for ocular angiogenesis. *Clin Sci (Lond).* 2003;104:561–575.
53. Ambati J, Ambati BK, Yoo SH, et al. Age-related macular degeneration: etiology, pathogenesis, and therapeutic strategies. *Surv Ophthalmol.* 2003;48:257–293.
54. Grossniklaus HE, Green WR. Choroidal neovascularization. *Am J Ophthalmol.* 2004;137:496–503.
55. Augustin AJ, Puls S, Offermann I. Triple therapy for choroidal neovascularization due to age-related macular degeneration: verteporfin PDT, bevacizumab, and dexamethasone. *Retina.* 2007;27:113–140.
56. Chen F, Gong L, Zhang L, et al. Short courses of low dose dexamethasone delay bleomycin-induced lung fibrosis in rats. *Eur J Pharmacol.* 2006;536:287–295.
57. Voisard R, Seitzer U, Baur R, et al. Corticosteroid agents inhibit proliferation of smooth muscle cells from human atherosclerotic arteries in vitro. *Int J Cardiol.* 1994;43:257–267.
58. Reil TD, Kashyap VS, Sarkar R, et al. Dexamethasone inhibits the phosphorylation of retinoblastoma protein in the suppression of human vascular smooth muscle cell proliferation. *J Surg Res.* 2000;92:108–113.
59. Pross C, Farooq MM, Angle N, et al. Dexamethasone inhibits vascular smooth muscle cell migration via modulation of matrix metalloproteinase activity. *J Surg Res.* 2002;102:57–62.
60. Veritti D, Lanzetta P, Cascavill ML, et al. Triple therapy for choroidal neovascularization due to age-related macular degeneration. ranibizumab, modified juxtascleral triamcinolone acetonide, and verteporfin PDT [Abstract A598]. Presented at the Annual Meeting of the Association for Research in Vision and Ophthalmology. May 4, 2009. Fort Lauderdale, FL.
61. Bakri SJ, Couch SM, McCannel CA, et al. Same-day triple therapy with photodynamic therapy, intravitreal dexamethasone, and bevacizumab in wet age-related macular degeneration. *Retina.* 2009;29:573–578.
62. QLT announces interim results of RADICAL study. December 16, 2008, QLT Inc. press release.
63. Hughes MS, Sang DN. Triple plus therapy compared with monthly ranibizumab reduces the retreatment rate in a randomized study in age-related macular degeneration [Abstract A593]. Presented at the Annual Meeting of the Association for Research in Vision and Ophthalmology. May 4, 2009. Fort Lauderdale, FL.
64. Sheidow TG, Hooper PL, Kertes PJ, et al. Combination therapy in neovascular age-related macular degeneration (AMD):

a three-armed, randomized, prospective clinical trial of low fluence photodynamic therapy (rPDT) with adjunctive Avastin and triamcinolone acetonide (Kenalog) (triple therapy) versus rpdt with adjunctive Avastin (double therapy) versus monotherapy with Avastin [Abstract A612]. Presented at the Annual Meeting of the Association for Research in Vision and Ophthalmology. May 4, 2009. Fort Lauderdale, FL.

65. A safety and efficacy study comparing the combination treatments of verteporfin therapy plus one of two different doses of intravitreal triamcinolone acetonide and the verteporfin therapy plus intravitreal pegaptanib (VERITAS). Available at: http://clinicaltrials.gov/ct/show/NCT00242580. Accessed April 15, 2009.
66. Efficacy/safety of verteporfin photodynamic therapy and ranibizumab compared with ranibizumab in patients with subfoveal choroidal neovascularization [DENALI]. Available at: http://clinicaltrials.gov/ct/show/NCT436553. Accessed April 15, 2009.
67. Triple therapy—PDT plus IVD and intravitreal ranibizumab versus Lucentis monotherapy to treat age-related macular degeneration (PDEX). Available at: http://clinicaltrials.gov/ct/show/NCT00390208. Accessed April 8, 2009.
68. RADICAL Trial. Data on file, QLT and Novartis.
69. Reduced fluence Visudyne-anti-VEGF-dexamethasone in combination for AMD lesions (RADICAL). Available at: http://clinicaltrials.gov/ct/show/NCT00492284. Accessed April 15, 2009.
70. Combination Therapy for Age-Related Macular Degeneration. Available at: http://clinicaltrials.gov/ct/show/NCT00376701. Accessed April 16, 2009.
71. Kaiser PK, for the Registry of Visudyne AMD Therapy Writing Committee. Verteporfin photodynamic therapy combined with intravitreal bevacizumab for neovascular age-related macular degeneration. *Ophthalmology.* 2009;116:747–755.
72. Small KW, Silva-Garcia R, Registry Investigator Groups. Treating wet AMD with verteporfin PDT in triple or double combination therapy: results of two Visudyne registry databases [Abstract A615]. Presented at the Annual Meeting of the Association for Research in Vision and Ophthalmology. May 4, 2009. Fort Lauderdale, FL.
73. Smiddy WE. Economic implications of current age-related macular degeneration treatments. *Ophthalmology.* 2009;116:481–487.
74. Augustin AJ, Offermann I. Combination therapy for choroidal neovascularisation. *Drugs Aging.* 2007;24:979–990.
75. Regillo CD, Brown DM, Abraham P, et al. Randomized, double-masked, sham-controlled trial of ranibizumab for neovascular age-related macular degeneration: PIER study year 1. *Am J Ophthalmol.* 2008;145:239–248.
76. Comparison of age-related macular degeneration treatments trials: Lucentis-Avastin trial [CATT]. Available at: http://clinicaltrials.gov/ct/show/NCT00593450. Accessed March 16, 2009.

CHAPTER

23

Combination Therapy for Age-Related Macular Degeneration

Michael Engelbert • Richard F. Spaide

GROWTH OF NEW VESSELS

Choroidal neovascularization (CNV) is the anatomical endpoint of a complex pathogenic cascade that likely receives input from a multitude of sources, both genetic and environmental. Consequently, the respective contribution of these influences is probably different from patient to patient, based on the individual genetic background and environment. It is easy to imagine that this will have a therapeutic target, and its respective importance in the individual pathogenic cascade. This should be kept in mind while reviewing the following pathogenic model of age-related macular degeneration (AMD).

A genetic contribution to AMD was always surmised based on the differential incidences in various ethnicities and concordant phenotypes in twins. Several recent discoveries highlight the importance of the immune system in the pathogenesis of AMD. In particular, susceptibility alleles encoding variants of complement factor H (CFH)[1,2] and other components of the complement cascade such as complement 2 (C2) and/or complement factor B (CFB),[3] complement 3 (C3)[4] and complement factor I (CFI)[5] have been identified. Protective alleles, such as CFHR1 and CFHR3 convey a decreased susceptibility to AMD.[6,7]

Angiogenic stimuli activate vascular endothelial cells, which allow gaps to form between their adjacent capillary walls.[8,9] Capillaries also become more permeable, and plasma proteins such as fibrinogen extravasate, which aids in forming a provisional matrix to support the newly growing vessels. This matrix in turn is degraded by matrix metalloproteinase expressed by the advancing edge of the neovascular bud, which also expresses integrins, which guide the interaction of the neovessel with the surrounding tissue components it encounters.[10] A single point mutation in HTRA1, a gene believed to regulate extracellular matrix degradation and inhibit transforming growth factor-β, has been shown to confer an increased risk of advanced AMD, possibly by facilitating permeation of Bruch membrane by choroidal neovascular vessels.[11] The advancing neovessel grows away from the preexisting vessel toward the angiogenic stimulus. The endothelial cells in the vascular sprout proliferate, and additional bone-marrow derived endothelial progenitor cells are recruited from the circulation to the site of angiogenesis, where they assume the phenotype of a vascular endothelial cell.[12,13] After capillary formation of a lumen, neighboring sprouts anastomose and form capillary loops. At this stage, the neovessels only possess a thin, pericyte-poor wall, but mural cell precursors are subsequently recruited and lend support to the vascular endothelial cells through several mechanisms, including paracrine secretion of growth factors.[14,15,16]

CANCER, ANGIOGENESIS, AND ANTIANGIOGENIC THERAPY

Angiogenesis has been most intensively studied in the context of cancer. While treatment of cancer first relied on surgical extrication of neoplastic tissue, subsequent attempts selectively inhibited or attacked the cancer cells with radiation or drugs. Since the growing cancer depends on a vascular network that can meet its growing metabolic needs, inhibition of the concomitantly growing tumor vasculature may limit the growth potential of the cancer itself. Proof of this principle was provided when it was shown in animal models that endostatin and angiostatin lead to vascular regression and tumor death.[17,18] This led to grand expectations, including immediate curing of cancer in humans,[19] but early results of endostatin and angiostatin could not be replicated in many instances, and tumor eradication was not seen even in responsive neoplasms.[20] This was possibly due to the fact that partial sequences within endostatin may have not only antiangiogenic but also proangiogenic effects, which was not discovered until later.[21] Another important proangiogenic factor, vascular endothelial growth factor (VEGF), was inhibited through monoclonal antibodies and this proved to limit the growth of human tumor xenografts in animal models of cancer.[22] This lead to the development of bevacizumab (Avastin, Genentech, South San Francisco, CA) a monoclonal antibody directed against VEGF.

Bevacizumab was then tested in several cancer trials, with ambivalent results. While a clinical trial examining the effects of bevacizumab in breast cancer patients already under chemotherapy showed no prolongation of life,[23] patients with advanced colon cancer being treated with chemotherapy showed a statistically remarkable prolongation of life from a mean of 15.6 to 20.3 months.[24] This difference in the therapeutic response may at least in part be due to different angiogenic proteins elaborated by the tumors. Colon cancer is a more aggressive tumor and may rely predominantly on VEGF for angiogenesis, while breast carcinoma cells express multiple angiogenic molecules, including VEGF, fibroblast growth factor, placental growth factor, and transforming growth factor-β. Furthermore, the proportion of these mediators constituting this "angiogenic cocktail" may shift with the stage of the cancer.[19,25] In a later study of patients previously untreated for breast cancer,[26] patients treated with a combination of bevacizumab and paclitaxel had an increase in response rate (28%) compared with paclitaxel alone (14%), but clearly most patients did not respond in either case. More recently, a randomized phase 3 trial investigated the combination of bevacizumab with carboplatin versus carboplatin alone in the treatment of advanced nonsquamous Non-small cell lung cancer (NSCLC), and combination therapy achieved both statistically increased survival and progression-free survival compared to monotherapy, with a response rate of 35% in the combination therapy group and only 15% in the monotherapy group.[27] It appears therefore that incremental improvements in outcome may be achieved for several types of cancer in certain developmental stages, but only when anti-VEGF treatment is used in combination with chemotherapeutic agents.[28–31]

In the context of breast cancer, angiogenesis arises from multiple stimuli and blocking a single molecule may not suffice to inhibit vascular development due to the inherent redundancy of the pathogenic cascade.[32] In biologic systems, the output of a process often acts as a feedback to modulate or control the process in a form of self-correction. It is possible that varying degrees of inhibition of one pathway for angiogenesis will upregulate alternate pathways that will accomplish the same result.

Not only may the angiogenic profile of a tumor vary with the stage of the cancer, but the responsiveness of the neovessel to angiogenic inhibition may vary according to its developmental stage as well. While VEGF inhibition may lead to regression of new vessels, if they do not have periendothelial support cells such as pericytes or smooth muscle cells,[32,33] blocking VEGF/VEGFR-2 signaling did not cause vascular regression in a C6 tumor angiogenesis model among vessels with pericytes, apparently because of Ang-1/Tie2 signaling between the pericytes and the endothelial cells.[33] However, if both neovessels and their supporting pericytes were targeted by combined blockade of platelet derived growth factor receptor and the VEGFR-2 receptor, vascular regression in the newly developed tumor vessels ensued.[33] Interestingly, simultaneous blockade did not have an effect on the normal vessels of the host tissue, indicating that newly developed vessels have a plasticity not found in older, established vessels (Fig. 23.1).[30]

NORMALIZATION OF TUMOR VASCULATURE

The early vessels in angiogenesis do not organize graceful filigrees with the sequential hierarchy of arterioles, capillaries, and venules; instead, they form a relatively chaotic network of loops, shunts, and saccular dilations. The wall structure of these early vessels is abnormal, with large inter-endothelial junctions, more fenestrations, vesicles, and lack of a normal basement membrane.[34] The surrounding perivascular cells are equally abnormal. As a result of this defective vascular organization, leakage occurs and increases tissue hydrostatic pressure, which may alter blood flow as well.[35] The resultant local differences in blood flow may lead to inadequate delivery of O_2 and metabolites in certain areas of the tumor. The resultant imbalance of proangiogenic and antiangiogenic factors is presumably key to theses vascular anomalies and their improper maturation.[36] Antiangiogenic treatment can effectively prune the more immature, poorly formed vessels from the vascular complexes, and leave vessels that adopt a more normal phenotype. This process has

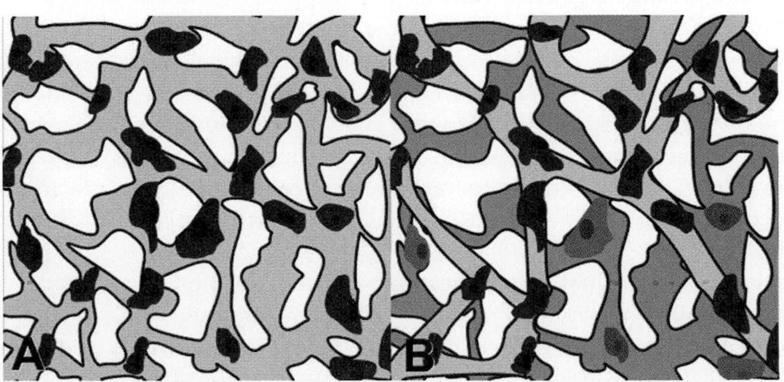

FIGURE 23.1. A: Intense angiogenesis leads to a plexus of vessels with shunts and saccular dilations. **B:** Antiangiogenic therapy can lead to a pruning of vessels, particularly those that are relatively poor in pericyte coverage. The remaining vessels adopt a more ordinary phenotype **(B)** in a process known as vascular normalization. (Reproduced from Spaide. *Am J Ophthalmol.* 2006;141:149–156, with permission.)

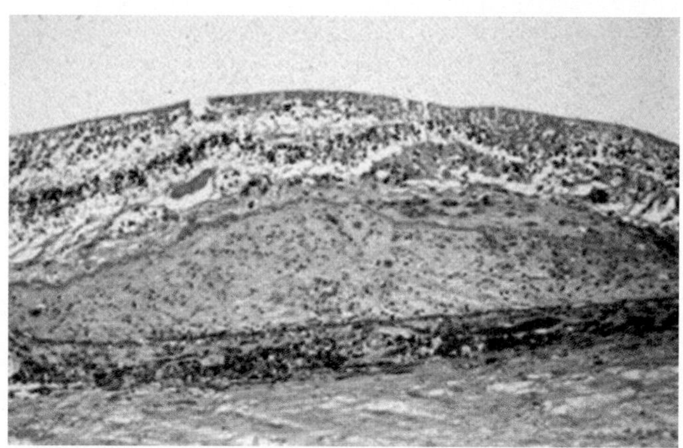

FIGURE 23.2. Choroidal neovascularization secondary to AMD is a tissue invasion of a multitude of cells, many of which are inflammatory. The actual vascular component is a small minority of the lesion and grows into in with and to an extent because of, the extravascular component. (Reproduced from Spaide. *Am J Ophthalmol.* 2006;141:149–156, with permission; Photograph courtesy of Hans Grossniklaus, MD.)

been called vascular normalization.[37,38] This outcome may occur because more mature vessels with pericyte coverage are protected through pericyte mediated survival mechanisms, which involve Ang-1/Tie2 signaling between the pericytes and the endothelial cells.[7,8] Vascular normalization has been associated with improved outcomes, partly because tumor-associated edema is relieved,[39] but possibly also because of improved delivery of chemotherapeutic agents through improved blood flow to and decreased interstitial fluid pressure within the tumor.[34] The effect of bevacizumab in colon cancer could have been attributable to the improved delivery of chemotherapeutic agents rather than direct antiangiogenic induced tumor regression in one study.[40] Interestingly, the effect of radiation also appeared to be enhanced when combined with anti-VEGF treatment in human glioma xenografts,[34] and this synergy could only be observed during a time window, when "normalized" vessels were present (Fig. 23.2).

TWO-COMPONENT MODEL OF CNV

Cancer is constituted of two principle components, tumor cells and vascular cells. Proof of the principle has been provided that treatment of both components may be more efficacious compared with treatment of either component alone.[41,42] CNV is a condition commonly referred to as "neovascularization" because of its angiographic appearance. This neglects the fact that histopathologically, CNV is really a tissue invasion of vascular cells and extravascular cells.[43,44] In analogy to solid cancers, CNV can be thought of as a two-component system as well. Just as we described for cancers, the vascular CNV component consists of endothelial cells, circulating endothelial progenitor cells, and pericytes. The extravascular component is composed of invading inflammatory cells such as macrophages, lymphocytes, granulocytes, foreign body giant cells, as well as fibrocytes, myofibroblasts, retinal pigment epithelial cells, and glial cells.[44–47] In pathologic angiogenesis, resident cells recruit vessel progenitors, and vessels themselves enhance further growth. For example, stromal fibroblasts colocalize with the tumor vasculature even deep inside the tumor,[48] and this has been shown to be tumorigenic in and in-vivo model of breast cancer.[49] The same appears to be true for inflammatory cells in cancer, where they may counterintuitively stimulate angiogenesis and tumor growth, rather than combat it.[50,51] In particular, macrophages can have either proangiogenic or antiangiogenic functions, depending on their phenotypes.[52] While classical, or M1 macrophages have cytotoxic activity, M2 macrophages suppress the immune response, promote wound healing, angiogenesis (by secretion of factors such as VEGF) and tissue remodeling, and thus are thought to aid in tumor progression. The important role of inflammatory cells in neovascularization that has been demonstrated in tumor angiogenesis appears to apply to CNV as well, where the amount of VEGF expressed is proportional to the number of inflammatory cells present and VEGF in CNV colocalizes with the inflammatory cells.[44,53] This may be further amplified by VEGF induced expression of cellular adhesion molecules in vessels, thus recruiting more inflammatory cells.[54] Further, supportive evidence for a crucial role that inflammatory cells have in pathogenesis of CNV comes from animal experiments in which depletion of monocytes inhibits the formation of CNV.[55] Even in health, hypoxia prevails in the outer retina, and this may be a further stimulus for invading cells to produce angiogenic factors.[56,57] Over the course of the disease process CNV produces vascular invasion, proliferation, matrix formation with or without hemorrhage, remodeling of the tissue, and eventual vascular regression in involutional lesions.[58] This is more consistent with a wound healing response than growth of vessels in response to ischemia alone, where the invading vessels would attempt to recapitulate the organization of the choriocapillaris.[43,58,59]

TWO-COMPONENT MODEL AND COMBINATION THERAPY

Therapy for CNV is aimed at the vascular component, the extravascular component, or potentially both simultaneously. Inhibiting the vascular component addresses the neovessels but does not directly affect the extravascular component, although it is possible, that reduced blood supply may lead to reduction of the extravascular component through ischemia. Conversely, ischemia, and resultant tissue damage may lead to increased elaboration of angiogenic and proinflammatory factors.

Limitations of Monotherapies

Several monotherapies directed predominantly against the vascular component have been developed and tested in large clinical trials. They include photodynamic therapy (PDT) with 689 nm wavelength laser-activated verteporforin (Visudyne, Novartis Pharmaceuticals Corporation, Hanover, NJ) and pharmacological approaches such as pegaptanib (Macugen, Eyetech Pharmaceuticals, New York, NY), ranibizumab (Lucentis, Genentech, South San Francisco, CA) and bevacizumab (Avastin, Genentech, South San Francisco, CA). Initial data from studies examining pegaptanib have shown continued growth and leakage, not shrinkage, of the neovascular lesions. This may suggest a process like vascular normalization may be occurring, possibly related to incomplete inhibition of possible mediators of angiogenesis.[60]

Ranibizumab was tested in two large randomized clinical trials: ANCHOR (predominantly classic lesions treated with either PDT or ranibizumab)[61] and MARINA (predominantly occult lesions randomized to ranibizumab or sham injections).[62] Both trials demonstrated mean visual gains after 24 months, and the 24 month ANCHOR trial data demonstrated that monthly injections of ranibizumab provided patients who had angiographically predominantly classic CNV lesions with better visual outcomes than the previous standard of care, PDT. For the first time did a therapy for wet AMD result in improved vision, not just long-term stabilization at the cost of initial visual loss. Similar results appear to be achieved with bevacizumab,[63,64] which is frequently used in an off-label fashion for the same indication[65–67] and its equivalence is the subject of an ongoing NIH sponsored trial (http://www.nei.nih.gov/CATT).

However, this therapeutic paradigm shift now commits the patient to monthly office visits and invasive treatment, arguably because not all pathogenetic components are addressed, thus maintaining a chronic disease state. While inhibition of VEGF also may decrease the inflammatory effects of induced cellular adhesion molecule expression and inflammatory cell recruitment to the lesion, administration of anti-VEGF agents may induce intraocular inflammation as well, so the net anti-inflammatory effect is not known.

As a case in point, the PIER trial attempted to induce with three monthly injections, followed by quarterly injections, with only about 13% of patients gaining more than 15 letters compared to 33% to 40% of patients receiving monthly injections in the ANCHOR and MARINA trial, demonstrating that the vast majority of patients needed more frequent injections. While several dosing regimens have been designed to tailor a schedule to the individual patient by OCT guidance,[68,69] thus reducing the need for injections, more or less regular injections are still required. No matter which regimen is used, it has become clear that patients will depend on long-term, and possibly lifelong injections, as demonstrated in the HORIZON[70] and other trials examining the longterm outcomes of AMD treated with anti-angiogenic drugs.[68,69]

The strategy of inhibiting the extravascular component would include targeting the action of the extravascular cells or important cytokines (such as with immunomodulators or biologicals),[71] thus hopefully addressing all factors that maintain the pathogenic process and consequently lead to chronicity of disease. In cancer, the large variety of possible cancer cells, their potential to secrete inappropriate cytokines, and their genetic instability make such an indirect approach difficult.[72] In CNV, however, the makeup of invading cells is fairly consistent from patient to patient, and these cells are genetically stable. There are no published reports of pure inhibitors of the extravascular cellular component of CNV at present, although corticosteroids inhibit many aspects of the extravascular component. Some therapies, such as thermal laser, radiation,[73] and the combination of PDT and intravitreal triamcinolone[74] inhibit both components (Fig. 23.3). Due to its indiscriminate action not only on the vascular and extravascular component, but also innocent neuroretina, thermal laser has been essentially abandoned for the treatment of subfoveal and most other CNV. Therefore, we will focus on current attempts to halt CNV with radiation, PDT, anti-inflammatory agents, or a combination of them.

Radiation Therapy for AMD

Ionizing radiation has widespread cellular effects, affecting neovascularization, inflammation and tissue remodeling,

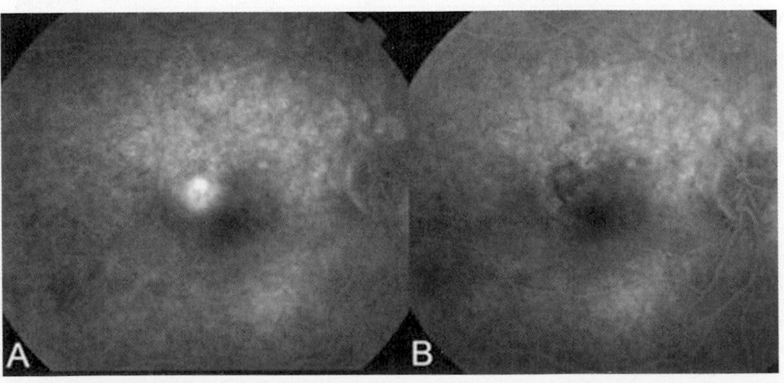

FIGURE 23.3. **A:** At presentation, visual acuity was 20/40. The patient had one combined treatment of intravitreal triamcinolone and PDT. **B:** One year later, there was resolution of the leakage but some persistent staining. Visual acuity was 20/20. (Reproduced from Spaide, et al. *Retina.* 2005;25:685–690, with permission.)

depending on the type, dose and delivery time of radiation, as well as the target tissue. Since the biological effect of ionizing radiation is mediated by breaking double-stranded DNA, it is more effective on rapidly dividing cells, such as lymphomas and carcinomas, less effective on fibroblasts, and least effective on mature cells, such as mature endothelial cells.[75] Theoretically, this could target all components simultaneously, both active vascular and extravascular while sparing mature neighboring cells. Various treatment strategies have been explored and are evaluated in a major review by the Cochrane Collaboration, with variable results.[76] Several approaches are currently under investigation. One employs a beta-radiation strontium-90 applicator (EpiRad, NeoVista, Fremont, California), which is inserted into the eye after a limited vitrectomy and held over the macula to deliver 24 Gy of radiation (Fig. 23.4). This epimacular low-dose mono-brachytherapy had promising preliminary results[77] and its safety and efficacy is currently being evaluated in the **CABERNET** (CNV Secondary to AMD Treated with Beta RadiatioN Epiretinal Therapy) phase 3 clinical trial in combination with ranibizumab and compared to ranibizumab alone. The **MERITAGE** (Macular EpiRetinal Brachytherapy in Treated Age Related Macular Degeneration Patients) trial will examine whether the treatment burden can be alleviated in patients who are unable to maintain vision without regular anti-VEGF injections (Box 23.1).

It is possible that normalization of the vascular organization by VEGF inhibition prior to radiation, an approach which has been reported in combination with ionizing radiation of solid tumors, would lead to better responses. In the case of PDT, one retrospective study demonstrated that only 48% of patients receiving a single intravitreal injection of 1.25 mg bevacizumab 2 weeks prior to PDT required retreatment, which is much lower than previously reported.[78]

While radiation therapy promises long-term control of wet AMD through addressing both the neovascular and extravascular components of the disease, it is unclear what the longterm effects on the vasculature, as well as "innocent" bystander cells are. Radiation associated choroidal neovasculopathy (RACN) has been described as a late sequel of external beam radiation.[79] Another concern is that the retinal pigment epithelium (RPE) may suffer as well and that wet AMD might turn into geographic atrophy, for which no effective treatment is available to date.

BOX 23.1 Ranibizumab + Radiation

CABERNET Trial: CNV Secondary to AMD Treated with Beta RadiatioN Epiretinal Therapy (NeoVista) (Radiation + Ranibizumab vs. Ranibizumab alone)

Purpose: A Phase 2, randomized, prospective trial using the Epi-Rad90 (beta radiation strontium 90) Ophthalmic System to evaluate the safety and efficacy of focal delivery of radiation for the treatment of subfoveal CNV associated with wet AMD. The Epi-Rad90 Ophthalmic System treats neovascularization of retinal tissue by means of a focal, directional delivery of radiation to the target tissues in the retina. **Arm 1:** A single procedure using the Epi-Rad90 Ophthalmic System plus two injections of Lucentis administered 1 month apart, **Arm 2:** Lucentis injection administered monthly for the first three injections followed by quarterly injections.

Status: Ongoing.

MERITAGE Trial: Macular EpiRetinal Brachytherapy in Treated Age Related Macular Degeneration Patients (NeoVista)

Purpose: A Phase 1/2 nonrandomized, open-label, uncontrolled trial to evaluate strontium 90 beta radiation in neovascular ARMD patients who require persistent anti-VEGF therapies. The treatment involves a single procedure with the NeoVista Ophthalmic System, with Lucentis (0.5 mg) or Avastin (1.25 mg) administered on an as needed basis for 3 years.

Status: Ongoing.

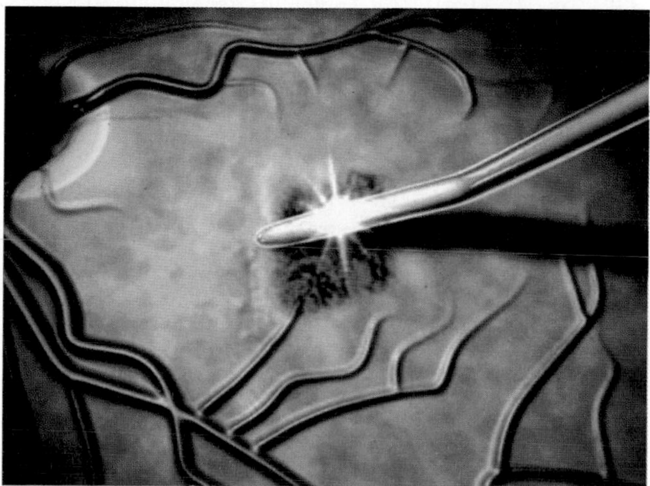

FIGURE 23.4. An illustration of the intraocular, epiretinal beta radiation (strontium-90) delivery device placed in proximity to the CNV complex. (Reproduced from Avila, et al. *Retina.* 2009;29:157, with permission.)

Combination Therapy with PDT and Anti-VEGF agents

PDT with Verteporforin was the first FDA approved treatment for neovascular AMD. Few patients actually experienced visual improvement, but rather stabilization of vision and lesion regression in the pre-pharmacological era.[80–82] Lipophilic verteporforin is taken up by neovascular endothelial cells through the Low density lipoprotein (LDL)-receptor, which isoverexpressed by cells undergoing rapid division.[83] Subsequent activation with a nonthermal laser generates reactive oxygen species, which damage the neovascular endothelial cells, leading to platelet binding, aggregation, and vascular occlusion.[84] However, this effect is not as specific as desired, and reduction of blood flow in physiologic choriocapillaris has been demonstrated in multiple instances after PDT.[85,86] This leads to varying degrees of outer retinal ischemia as well as inflammation, stimulating regrowth of new vessels, apparently mediated in part by VEGF.[87] To antagonize this, double and triple combinations of all permutations of PDT, an anti-inflammatory and/or an angiogenic drug have been proposed. Posterior sub-Tenon injection of triamcinolone combined with PDT lead to decreased choriocapillaris ischemia at 3 months compared to PDT alone, but no difference at 12 months.[88] However, there was a decreased need for retreatment, indicating that the short-term effect on choroidal perfusion may indeed be biologically relevant. However, despite encouraging results from several prior studies, the **VERITAS** trial, which compared the visual acuity response of PDT with verteporforin as compared with PDT and two different doses of triamcinolone, did not show any significant benefit in the triamcinolone groups.[89]

The multicenter **FOCUS** trial, examined the efficacy and toxicities of combined PDT and ranibizumab in patients with neovascular AMD over the course of 2 years.[90] PDT was administered at baseline and then as needed every 3 months to all 162 patients. In addition to obligatory treatment with PDT, 106 patients received monthly injections of 0.5 mg ranibizumab and 56 received sham injections. At the end of 24 months, 88% of those on the combination versus 75% of those on PDT alone had lost <15 letters in visual acuity, while 25% of the combination versus 7% of the PDT-alone patients had gained at least 15 letters ($p < 0.05$ for both outcomes). Interestingly, serious intraocular inflammation occurred in 12% of those on the combination versus none of those on PDT alone, but it was concluded that this risk was outweighed by the improved efficacy. This is a contentious issue, and the cause for this phenomenon is not certain (Box 23.2).

BOX 23.2 Ranibizumab + PDT

FOCUS Trial: RhuFab V2 Ocular Treatment Combining the Use of Visudyne to Evaluate Safety

Purpose: A 2-year, multicenter, randomized, single-masked, controlled study to compare the safety, tolerability, and efficacy of ranibizumab treatment in conjunction with PDT versus PDT alone in patients with subfoveal, predominantly classic CNV secondary to AMD.

Results: At month 24, 88% of ranibizumab + PDT patients had lost <15 letters from baseline VA (vs. 75% for PDT alone), 25% had gained ≥15 letters (vs. 7% for PDT alone), and the two treatment arms differed by 12.4 letters in mean VA change. On average, ranibizumab + PDT patients exhibited less lesion growth and greater reduction of CNV leakage and subretinal fluid accumulation, and required fewer PDT retreatments, than PDT-alone patients (mean = 0.4 vs. 3.0 PDT retreatments). However, endophthalmitis occurred in 12% of the combination group.

Conclusions: Ranibizumab + PDT was more effective than PDT alone and had a low rate of associated adverse events. (Antoszyk AN, Tuomi L, Chung CY, et al. Ranibizumab combined with verteporfin photodynamic therapy in neovascular age-related macular degeneration (FOCUS): year 2 results. *Am J Ophthalmol.* 2008;145:863.)

SUMMIT Trial (Novartis)

Randomized trials comparing the efficacy between PDT and Ranibizumab versus Ranibizumab alone: The SUMMIT clinical trial program consists of three trials: (a) **DENALI** in USA and Canada, (b) **MONT BLANC** in Europe, and (c) **EVEREST** in Asia.

DENALI Trial: Efficacy/Safety of Verteporfin PDT and Ranibizumab Compared With Ranibizumab in Patients With Subfoveal Choroidal Neovascularization

Purpose: A Phase 2/3 trial to compare three groups: ranibizumab alone, ranibizumab with full light-dose PDT, and ranibizumab with half light-dose PDT.

Conclusions: Ongoing.

MONT BLANC Trial

Purpose: A Phase 2/3 24-month randomized, double-masked, multicenter trial in patients with subfoveal CNV due to ARMD to compare PDT and Ranibizumab versus Ranibizumab monotherapy. **Arm 1:** Standard-fluence Visudyne (600 mW/cm^2 for 83 seconds to deliver 50 J/cm^2) followed by same day intravitreal Ranibizumab (0.5 mg), **Arm 2:** Ranibizumab monotherapy (0.5 mg). The Ranibizumab monotherapy group received sham Visudyne treatment to maintain masking.

Conclusions: Twelve-month results show that combining standard-fluence Visudyne with Lucentis 0.5 mg can deliver VA improvements that are noninferior to a Lucentis monotherapy regimen with three Lucentis loading doses followed by injections on a monthly as-needed basis (noninferiority margin of seven letters). There was no significant difference between the combination and monotherapy groups with regard to proportion of patients with a treatment-free interval of at least 3 months duration after month 2. (QLT Press release, June 15, 2009.)

Unfortunately, it is thus far impossible to titrate a treatment precisely enough to allow for recanalization of physiological choriocapillaris with restoration of physiological choroidal flow on the one hand, but avoid regrowth of the CNV.

Combination Therapy with Anti-inflammatory Agents

Corticosteroids may inhibit vascular proliferation indirectly by affecting the extravascular component through their anti-inflammatory properties. Triamcinolone has been shown to inhibit ocular neovascularization in a variety of models.[91–93] Corticosteroids decrease platelet-derived growth factor (PDGF)-induced VEGF secretion[94] and in models of oxidative stress,[94,95] and strongly inhibit VEGF production by macrophages.[96,97] Intravitreal injections of triamcinolone showed 100% reduction in CNV in laser induced models of CNV.[98] In contrast, nonselective cyclooxygenase (COX) inhibition, selective COX-1, or selective COX-2 inhibition did suppress laser induced CNV.[99] Interestingly, corneal cautery-induced neovascularization was inhibited by corticosteroids despite a decrease in VEGF upregulation by only 27%, which suggests that corticosteroids can modulate downstream signaling by VEGF, or antagonize other important proangiogenic pathways.[100] Many cytokine and cellular effects related to inflammation and the breakdown of the blood-ocular barrier are attenuated by corticosteroids.[101–107] For example, triamcinolone inhibits VEGF-induced breakdown of the blood-retina barrier,[108] decreases basic fibroblast growth factor (bFGF) proliferation of retinal vascular endothelial cells in a dose dependent fashion[109] and reduces bFGF induced migration and tube formation in choroidal vascular endothelial cells.[110] While there was no benefit in terms of immediate occlusion of lesions in response to the combination of PDT and dexamethasone in a rodent model of laser-induced CNV, 6 days after treatment, only 10% of the lesions treated with monotherapy remained closed versus 31% of the lesions receiving combination therapy.[111] Interestingly, this effect was accompanied by less photoreceptor apoptosis (Box 23.3).

Some of these findings could be reproduced in small human trials with patients affected by CNV secondary to AMD.[112–114] One randomized clinical trial of a single dose of 4 mg intravitreal triamcinolone demonstrated decreased lesion growth at 3 months in treated patients. However, there was no significant difference in visual acuity at 1 year.[115] But another nonrandomized comparative series was able to show that patients with intravitreal triamcinolone had visual acuity improvement compared with control patients who did not receive a corticosteroid injection.[116]

However, corticosteroids have well-known vision-threatening ocular side-effects, and other immunosuppressive drugs are therefore currently being investigated.

The pleiotropic cytokine TNF-alpha has been demonstrated in CNV specimens[117] and intravitreal injection of infliximab, a monoclonal antibody to TNF-alpha has recently been examined prospectively and promising visual outcomes were recorded in this small cohort comprising three patients who were unresponsive to consecutive monthly injections of ranibizumab.[118]

BOX 23.3 PDT + Triamcinolone Acetonide

VISTA Trial: Study of combined Visudyne therapy with Kenalog in CNV secondary to AMD

Purpose: To determine the effect of PDT therapy in combination with 1 or 4 mg intravitreal triamcinolone on the mean change in BCVA at month 12.

Status: Ongoing.

PDT + Triamcinolone Acetonide Versus PDT + Pegaptanib

VERITAS Trial: Verteporfin Intravitreal Triamcinolone Acetonide Study

Purpose: To compare combination treatment with PDT plus pegaptanib to that of combination treatment with PDT plus triamcinolone acetonide in two different doses (1 and 4 mg).

Conclusions: At 6 months, all three groups lost vision and there was no difference between the three groups.

Rapamycin (Sirolimus) is a widely used immunosuppressive agent. It inhibits mammalian target of rapamycin (mTOR); it achieves a myriad of cellular effects, ranging from anti-inflammatory (reducing COX-1, IL-8, GCP-2, EMAP-11, and blocking activation of cells of the innate and adaptive immune response), to antiangiogenic (reducing VEGF, TGF-beta, and HIF-1 alpha), anti-proliferative (blocking FGF-1) and anti-fibrotic effects.[119] Rapamaycin reduced VEGF expression in cultured RPE cells and endothelial cell sprouting in vitro.[120] It has been shown to inhibit retinal and choroidal neovascularization in vivo when administered systemically in murine models of hypoxia/hyperoxia ROP and laser-induced CNV.[121] This makes it a true combination therapeutic agent, which is currently being investigated as an intravitreal or subconjunctival agent in a phase 2 clinical trial for the treatment of CNV.

Fluocinolone is a more traditional immunosuppressive agent of the steroid class and manufactured as a slow release implant form (Medidur, Alimera Inc., Atlanta, GA). It is currently being investigated in combination with ranibizumab for the treatment of wet AMD in the Medidur FA for AMD Pilot (**MAP**) pilot study.

There exists ample evidence that the complement cascade plays an important role in the pathogenesis of AMD, and probably at all stages, that is, from drusen formation to geographic atrophy, or CNV and eventual cicatrization. This has lead to the development of a myriad of complement inhibitors which could potentially work for patients with early as well as advanced AMD. Whether it is advantageous to inhibit upstream or downstream in the complement cascade is up to debate since the current rationale for tackling complement at this point relies on strong epidemiological evidence, rather than a detailed understanding of the molecular mechanisms.

POT-4 (Potentia Pharmaceuticals Inc., Louisville, KT) is a cyclic 13 amino acid peptide, which interferes with the cleavage of C3, the component all three pathways of complement activation converge on. It was the first complement inhibitor to be studied in patients with AMD. It forms an intravitreal gel deposit that functions as a depot for the drug, and preliminary phase 1 data suggest that it may be safe and well tolerated at the doses studied in a limited number of patients. Other compounds target the terminal complement component C5, which is critical for membrane attack complex formation and production of the highly proinflammatory molecule C5a. Eculizumab (Alexion Pharmaceuticals Inc., Cheshire, CT) is a humanized monoclonal antibody to C5. It is FDA approved for the treatment of paroxysmal nocturnal hemoglobinuria. The COMPLETE (*COMPL*ement inhibition with *E*culizumab for the *T*reatment of Non-*E*xudative Age-Related Macular Degeneration) study is randomizing patients with dry AMD to Eculizumab or Placebo, with the hope of reducing both the growth rate of geographic atrophy and high risk drusen area and volume. Another agent targeting C5 is ARC 1905 (Ophthotech, Princeton, New Jersey), a pegylated aptamer that inhibits the complement component C5; phase 1 trials for dry AMD and CNV (in combination with an anti-VEGF agent) are currently underway. JPE1375 (Jerini Ophthalmic Inc., New York, NY) is a peptidomimetic small molecule that targets the receptor for C5a on inflammatory cells. It is a biodegradable injectable designed to last for 6 months.

One concern that has been raised is that complement inhibition may decrease the eye's ability to fight iatrogenically induced pathogens, thus potentially increasing the incidence or aggravating the outcome of injection-related endophthalmitis. Complement, however, is present in the vitreous only in minute quantities, and while important in the pathogenesis of AMD, it may play less of a role in the defense against intraocular pathogens than was previously thought.[122] However, repeated intravitreal injections of any drug place the eye undoubtedly at risk for developing endophthalmitis. The combination of corticosteroids and PDT affect the vascular component twice and the extravascular component as well.[123] Pilot studies of PDT and intravitreal triamcinolone suggest most patients have improved or stabilized acuity at 1 year.[124]

Some pilot studies on triple therapy with PDT, antiangiogenic, and anti-inflammatory agents have demonstrated promising results (Fig. 23.5).[125] Positive 12-month primary analysis results from the Phase 2 **RADICAL** study (*R*educed Fluence Visudyne *A*nti-VEGF-*D*examethasone

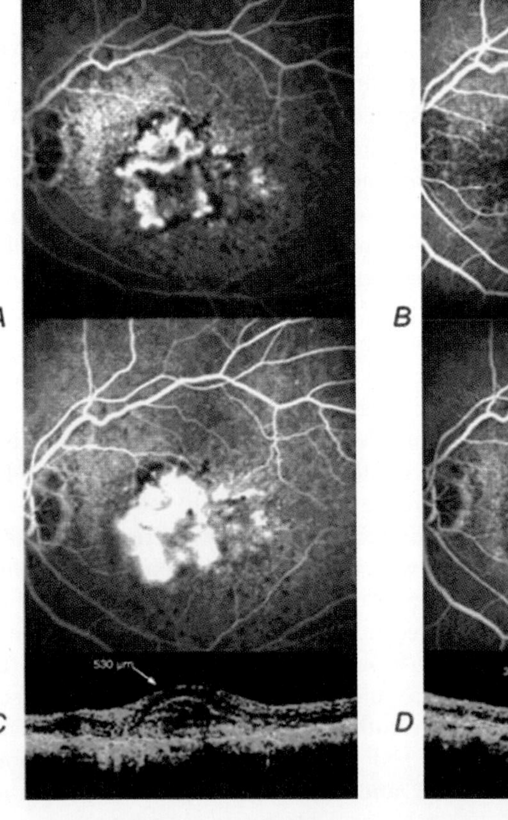

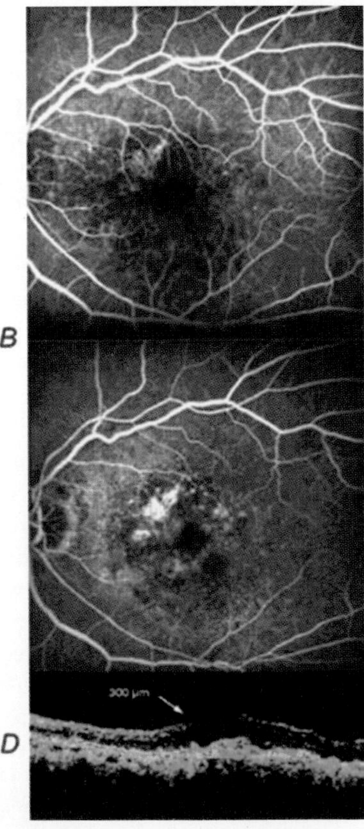

FIGURE 23.5. A minimally classic CNV lesion, for which the patient received one triple therapy cycle (reduced light verteporfin PDT followed 16 hours later by intravitreal injections of dexamethasone and bevacizumab) and no further treatment. Pretreatment early and late phase fluorescein angiography (FA) show the lesion **(A)**. FA after 24 weeks shows no CNV activity **(B)**. Pretreatment optical coherence tomography shows central retinal thickness of 530 µm **(C)**. After 24 weeks the retinal thickness decreased to 300 µm **(D)**. Visual acuity improved by one line. (Reproduced from Augustin, et al. *Retina.* 2007;27:133, with permission.)

In Combination for AMD Lesions) in patients with wet age-related macular degeneration ("wet AMD") have just been released (http://www.qltinc.com/newsCenter/2009/090602.htm). The purpose of this multicenter, randomized, single-masked study was to determine if Visudyne combined with Lucentis reduces retreatment rates compared with Lucentis monotherapy, while maintaining similar vision outcomes and an acceptable safety profile (Box 23.4). Three Visudyne-Lucentis-Dexamethasone combination therapies were evaluated against Lucentis monotherapy. The overall results showed that fewer retreatment visits were required with the combination therapies than with Lucentis monotherapy, and the differences were statistically significant, with the triple therapy half-fluence group demonstrating the best results, with the fewest retreatment visits and mean VA improvement.

Extracellular Matrix Modulators

As already mentioned, a point mutation in HTRA1, a regulator of extracellular matrix degradation and inhibitor of transforming growth factor-β, was associated with an increased risk of advanced AMD, possibly by facilitating permeation of Bruch membrane by choroidal neovascular vessels.[126] It is intuitive that modulating the extracellular matrix may be beneficial in controlling the extravascular component of CNV, and possibly preventing fibrosis. Several other agents are being investigated.

Integrins play a role in a variety of proliferative processes as mediators of adhesion both between cells and between cells and extracellular matrix. Integrin $\alpha5\beta1$ is one of the best characterized, and has been shown to be upregulated in AMD and tumor angiogenesis, but not in normal vasculature.[127] Increased cell surface expression was found on endothelial cells, RPE cells, macrophages, and fibroblasts.[128] It could be involved in multiple pathogenic pathways in AMD, including neovascularization, vascular leakage, inflammation, and fibrosis. Volociximab (M200) is a chimeric monoclonal antibody that targets integrin $\alpha5\beta1$ to block its ligation with fibronectin, thus inhibiting neovascularization in primate choroid tissue and tumor angiogenesis in rabbits.[129,130] Preclinical safety studies are nearing completion, and clinical trials have begun in November, 2008.

Another therapeutic target is the protein kinase mTOR. Its proinflammatory properties have already been discussed, but it has also been implicated in a number of proliferative processes.[131] Its role in fibrosis has been demonstrated in studies with palomid 529, an mTOR inhibitor with strong anti-fibrotic effect in animal models of retinal fibrosis. Clinical studies have not yet been initiated but clinical development is being pursued.

Antiangiogenic Biologicals

VEGF Trap-Eye is a novel, and possibly the most potent extracellular VEGF inhibitor. VEGF Trap-Eye is made from two different domains of VEGF receptors 1 and 2, which are linked to a human Fc fragment, and jointly creating a receptor decoy. VEGF Trap-Eye has greater VEGF avidity than the physiological receptor and a greater affinity than either ranibizumab or bevacizumab.[132] More importantly, its duration of activity may be up to three times greater, thus potentially dramatically decreasing the need for frequent dosing. A phase 2 study has been completed with encouraging results,[133] and phase 3 testing is currently underway.

Other potential targets are the many tyrosine kinases activated by VEGF. This is supported by promising work in animal models of ocular neovascularization.[134,135] Tyrosine kinase inhibitors are of great interest to the field of oncology and developments in this active field might benefit treatment of AMD. Although one would intuitively expect upstream VEGF inhibition to have a greater effect on angiogenesis than further downstream inhibition, one has to keep in mind that redundancy in the signaling cascade probably exists and that inhibition of several components of this cascade may lead to a more profound effect.

Another novel agent, the small interfering RNA agent bevasiranib was designed to work upstream of VEGF signaling by blocking the production of VEGF directly through messenger RNA inhibition. Proof of principle has been provided in a randomized phase 2 trial, and phase 3 testing of bevasirinab in combination with

BOX 23.4 Triple Therapy (PDT + Ranibizumab + Dexamethasone) Versus Ranibizumab Alone

RADICAL Trial: *R*educed Fluence Visudyne *A*nti-VEGF-*D*examethasone *I*n Combination for *A*MD *L*esions

Purpose: A Phase 2 randomized, single-masked study to compare reduced-fluence Visudyne-Lucentis combination therapies (with or without dexamethasone) to Lucentis monotherapy in neovascular ARMD. Four treatment groups: (a) Quarter-fluence Visudyne followed within 2 hours by intravitreal Lucentis (0.5 mg) and then intravitreal dexamethasone (0.5 mg); (b) Half-fluence Visudyne followed within two hours by intravitreal Lucentis (0.5 mg) and then intravitreal dexamethasone (0.5 mg); (c) Half-fluence Visudyne followed within two hours by intravitreal Lucentis (0.5 mg); or (d) Lucentis monotherapy (0.5 mg).

Conclusions: Fewer re-treatment visits were required with the combination therapies than with Lucentis monotherapy, and the differences were statistically significant, with the triple therapy half-fluence group demons (triple therapy with half-fluence Visudyne followed by Lucentis and then dexamethsone) presenting the best results, with the fewer retreatment visits and mean VA improvement.

ranibizumab is underway. While small interfering RNA agents theoretically appear to work through turning off target genes, some of their effects appear to be rather nonspecific. A recent study demonstrated a potent antiangiogenetic effect of any 21-nucleotide or longer small interfering RNA administered to mice regardless of the target gene.[136]

VEGF is only one of many proangiogenic factors that may play a role in CNV. Antagonization of the VEGF mediated angiogenic pathway might well upregulate alternate, compensatory pathways. For example, in addition to VEGF, bFGF, and hepatocyte growth factor (HGF), have been implicated in an animal model of CNV.[137] Also, VEGF might not be the most upstream molecule in the angiogenic cascade of CNV. Intriguingly, monoclonal blockade of human epidermal growth factor signaling in an experimental model of breast cancer not only downregulated multiple angiogenic factors, such as VEGF, TGF-α, Ang1 and PAI-1, and induced the antiangiogenic factor thrombospondin-1, thus killing multiple birds with one stone.[138] Another promising approach may be inhibition of intracellular signaling rather than extracellular messengers. For example, the tyrosine kinase activities of VEGF-receptors 1 and 2, as well as platelet derived growth factor and others that converge on the proangiogenic Raf/MEK/ERK signaling pathway, can be inhibited by sorafenib, an agent that has been approved by the FDA for the treatment of renal cell carcinoma. Proof of principle in a laser-induced paradigm of rat CNV was recently provided.[139] It is thus likely, that intervening further upstream in the vasogenic cascade or targeting multiple receptor tyrosine kinase downstream, thus antagonizing multiple molecular targets, or adding other recombinant antiangiogenic factors into the mix would improve on the current pharmacological treatment of CNV.

Inhibitors of the already mentioned mTOR, such as sirolimus, have demonstrated good antiangiogenic, anti-inflammatory, and anti-fibrotic effects, making it a true combination therapeutic agent. It is currently under investigation in neovascular AMD when administered subconjunctivally.[140] RTP-801i, a RNA interfering molecule targets upstream activators of mTOR, and has also completed phase 1 trials.[141]

Additional possibilities include application of cancer chemotherapeutic agents, which may affect the vascular component, the extravascular component, or both. For example, chemotherapy has the potential to affect the extravascular component, while low dose chemotherapy (also known as metronomic chemotherapy) may affect vascular endothelial cells.[41]

Rational combination of therapeutics for CNV relies on the understanding of the physiology of CNV, the mechanisms and effects of each therapeutic agent, and how the combinatorial approach may modify disease progression. While single-agent anti-VEGF inhibition has provided unprecedented visual outcomes it is likely that some of the novel combinatorial approaches discussed above will improve on these outcomes, decrease the need for frequent dosing and the risk of untoward side effects.

KEY POINTS

- Neovascular AMD is the result of a complex pathogenic cascade involving proangiogenic and antiangiogenic stimuli, cells, proteases, and rheological factors.
- Monotherapy with monthly injections of ranibizumab, an antiangiogenic agent targeting one important proangiogenic cytokine, VEGF, has become the gold standard in the treatment of CNV. But, VEGF is only one of many proangiogenic factors that may play a role in CNV.
- Combining monotherapeutic approaches into a combination therapy may offer the possibility of improved outcome, need for less frequent intervention, or decreased side-effects.
- Intervening further upstream in the vasogenic cascade or targeting multiple receptor tyrosine kinase downstream, thus antagonizing multiple molecular targets, or adding other recombinant antiangiogenic factors into the mix would improve on the current pharmacological treatment of CNV.

REFERENCES

1. Edwards AO, Ritter R III, Abel KJ, et al. Complement factor H polymorphism and age-related macular degeneration. *Science*. 2005;308(5720):421–424.
2. Hageman GS, Anderson DH, Johnson LV, et al. A common haplotype in the complement regulatory gene factor H (HF1/CFH) predisposes individuals to age-related macular degeneration. *Proc Natl Acad Sci USA*. 2005;102(20):7227–7232.
3. Sepp T, Khan JC, Thurlby DA, et al. Complement factor H variant Y402H is a major risk determinant for geographic atrophy and choroidal neovascularization in smokers and nonsmokers. *Invest Ophthalmol Vis Sci*. 2006;47(2):536–540.
4. Yates JR, Sepp T, Matharu BK, et al. Complement C3 variant and the risk of age-related macular degeneration. *N Engl J Med*. 2007;357(6):553–561.
5. Fagerness JA, Maller JB, Neale BM, et al. Variation near complement factor I is associated with risk of advanced AMD. *Eur J Hum Genet*. 2009;17(1):100–104.
6. Hughes AE, Orr N, Esfandiary H, et al. A common CFH haplotype, with deletion of CFHR1 and CFHR3, is associated with lower risk of age-related macular degeneration. *Nat Genet*. 2006;38(10):1173–1177.
7. Spencer KL, Hauser MA, Olson LM, et al. Deletion of CFHR3 and CFHR1 genes in age-related macular degeneration. *Hum Mol Genet*. 2008;17(7):971–977 [Epub 2007 Dec 15].
8. Dvorak HF, Brown LF, Detmar M, et al. Vascular permeability factor/vascular endothelial growth factor, microvascular hyperpermeability, and angiogenesis. *Am J Pathol*. 1995;146:1029–1039.

9. Roberts WG, Palade GE. Increased microvascular permeability and endothelial fenestration induced by vascular endothelial growth factor. *J Cell Sci.* 1995;108:2369–2379.
10. Silletti S, Kessler T, Goldberg J, et al. Disruption of matrix metalloproteinase 2 binding to alpha(v)beta3 by an organic molecule inhibits angiogenesis and tumor growth in vivo. *Proc Natl Acad Sci USA.* 2001;98:119–124.
11. Yang Z, Camp NJ, Sun H, et al. A variant of the HTRA1 gene increases susceptibility to age-related macular degeneration. *Science.* 2006;314(5801):992–993.
12. Asahara T, Masuda H, Takahashi T, et al. Bone marrow origin of endothelial progenitor cells responsible for postnatal vasculogenesis in physiological and pathological neovascularization. *Circ Res.* 1999;85:221–228.
13. Lyden D, Hattori K, Dias S, et al. Impaired recruitment of bone marrow-derived endothelial and hematopoietic precursor cells blocks tumor angiogenesis and growth. *Nat Med.* 2001;7:1194–1201.
14. Hirschi KK, Rohovsky SA, Beck LH, et al. Endothelial cells modulate the proliferation of mural cell precursors via platelet-derived growth factor-BB and heterotypic cell contact. *Circ Res.* 1999;84:298–305.
15. Darland DC, Massingham LJ, Smith SR, et al. Pericyte production of cell-associated VEGF is differentiation-dependent and is associated with endothelial survival. *Dev Biol.* 2003;264:275–288.
16. Abramsson A, Lindblom P, Betsholtz C. Endothelial and nonendothelial sources of PDGF-B regulate pericyte recruitment and influence vascular pattern formation in tumors. *J Clin Invest.* 2003;112:1142–1151.
17. O'Reilly MS, Boehm T, Shing Y, et al. Endostatin: an endogenous inhibitor of angiogenesis and tumor growth. *Cell.* 1997; 88:277–285.
18. O'Reilly MS, Holmgren L, Shing Y, et al. Angiostatin: a novel angiogenesis inhibitor that mediates the suppression of metastases by a Lewis lung carcinoma. *Cell.* 1994;79:315–328.
19. Marx J. Angiogenesis: a boost for tumor starvation. *Science.* 2003;301:452–454.
20. Marshall E. Cancer therapy: setbacks for endostatin. *Science.* 2002;295:2198–2199.
21. Morbidelli L, Donnini S, Chillemi F, et al. Angiosuppressive and angiostimulatory effects exerted by synthetic partial sequences of endostatin. *Clin Cancer Res.* 2003;9: 5358–5369.
22. Kim KJ, Li B, Winer J, et al. Inhibition of vascular endothelial growth factor-induced angiogenesis suppresses tumor growth in vivo. *Nature.* 1993;362:841–844.
23. Miller KD, Chap LI, Holmes FA, et al. Randomized phase 3 trial of capecitabine compared with bevacizumab plus capecitabine in patients with previously treated metastatic breast cancer. *J Clin Oncol.* 2005;23:792–799.
24. Hurwitz H, Fehrenbacher L, Novotny W, et al. Bevacizumab plus irinotecan, fluorouracil, and leucovorin for metastatic colorectal cancer. *N Engl J Med.* 2004;350:2335–2342.
25. Relf M, LeJeune S, Scott PA, et al. Expression of the angiogenic factors vascular endothelial cell growth factor, acidic and basic fibroblast growth factor, tumor growth factor β-1, platelet-derived endothelial cell growth factor, placenta growth factor, and pleiotrophin in human primary breast cancer and its relation to angiogenesis. *Cancer Res.* 1997;57:963–969.
26. Hampton T. Monoclonal antibody therapies shine in breast cancer clinical trials. *JAMA.* 2005;293:2985–2989.
27. Di Costanzo F, Mazzoni F, Micol Mela M, et al. Bevacizumab in non-small cell lung cancer. *Drugs.* 2008;68:737–746.
28. Wagner AD, Arnold D, Grothey AA, et al. Anti-angiogenic therapies for metastatic colorectal cancer. *Cochrane Database Syst Rev.* 2009;(3):CD005392 (Review).
29. Rini BI. Vascular endothelial growth factor-targeted therapy in metastatic renal cell carcinoma. *Cancer.* 2009;115 (10 Suppl):2306–2312 (Review).
30. Marneros AG. Tumor angiogenesis in melanoma. *Hematol Oncol Clin North Am.* 2009;23(3):431–446; vii–viii.
31. Timke C, Zieher H, Roth A, et al. Combination of vascular endothelial growth factor receptor/platelet-derived growth factor receptor inhibition markedly improves radiation tumor therapy. *Clin Cancer Res.* 2008;14(7):2210–2219.
32. Bergers G, Song S, Meyer-Morse N, et al. Benefits of targeting both pericytes and endothelial cells in the tumor vasculature with kinase inhibitors. *J Clin Invest.* 2003;111:1287–1295.
33. Erber R, Thurnher A, Katsen AD, et al. Combined inhibition of VEGF and PDGF signaling enforces tumor vessel regression by interfering with pericyte-mediated endothelial cell survival mechanisms. *FASEB J.* 2004;18:338–340.
34. Winkler F, Kozin SV, Tong RT, et al. Kinetics of vascular normalization by VEGFR2 blockade governs brain tumor response to radiation: role of oxygenation, angiopoietin-1, and matrix metalloproteinases. *Cancer Cell.* 2004;6:553–563.
35. Carmeliet P, Jain RK. Angiogenesis in cancer and other diseases. *Nature.* 2000;407:249–257.
36. Jain RK. A new target for tumor therapy. *N Engl J Med.* 2009;360(25):2669–2671.
37. Jain RK. Normalizing tumor vasculature with anti-angiogenic therapy: a new paradigm for combination therapy. *Nature Med.* 2001;7:987–989.
38. Jain RK. Normalization of tumor vasculature: an emerging concept in antiangiogenic therapy. *Science.* 2005;307:58–62.
39. Kamoun WS, Ley CD, Farrar C, et al. Edema control by cediranib, a vascular endothelial growth factor receptor-targeted kinase inhibitor, prolongs survival despite persistent brain tumor growth in mice. *J Clin Oncol.* 2009;27: 2542–2552.
40. Mayer RJ. Two steps forward in the treatment of colorectal cancer. *N Engl J Med.* 2004;350:2406–2408.
41. Gasparini G, Longo R, Fanelli M, et al. Combination of anti-angiogenic therapy with other anticancer therapies: results, challenges, and open questions. *J Clin Oncol.* 2005;23; 1295–1311.
42. Abdollahi A, Lipson KE, Sckell A, et al. Combined therapy with direct and indirect angiogenesis inhibition results in enhanced antiangiogenic and antitumor effects. *Cancer Res.* 2003;63:8890–8898.
43. Grossniklaus HE, Green WR. Choroidal neovascularization. *Am J Ophthalmol.* 2004;137:496–503.
44. Grossniklaus HE, Ling JX, Wallace TM, et al. Macrophage and retinal pigment epithelium expression of angiogenic cytokines in choroidal neovascularization. *Mol Vis.* 2002;8: 119–126.
45. Tsutsumi-Miyahara C, Sonoda KH, Egashira K, et al. The relative contributions of each subset of ocular infiltrated cells in experimental choroidal neovascularization. *Br J Ophthalmol.* 2004;88:1217–1222.

46. Espinosa-Heidmann DG, Reinoso MA, Pina Y, et al. Quantitative enumeration of vascular smooth muscle cells and endothelial cells derived from bone marrow precursors in experimental choroidal neovascularization. *Exp Eye Res.* 2005;80:369–378.
47. Killingsworth MC. Angiogenesis in early choroidal neovascularization secondary to age-related macular degeneration. *Graefes Arch Clin Exp Ophthalmol.* 1995;233:313–323.
48. Brown EB, Campbell RB, Tsuzuki Y, et al. In vivo measurements of gene expression, antiogenesis, and physiological function in tumors using multiphoton laser scanning microscopy. *Nat Med.* 2001;7(9):864–868.
49. Noel A. Enhancement of tumorigenicity of human breast adenocarcinoma cells in nume mice by matrigel and fibroblasts. *Br J Cancer.* 1993;68:909–915.
50. De Visser KE. Paradoxical roles of the immune system during cancer development. *Nat Rev Cancer.* 2006;6:24–37.
51. Pollard JW. Tumour-educated macrophages promote tumour progression and metastasis. *Nat Rev Cancer.* 2004;4:71–78.
52. Allavena P, Sica A, Garlandea C, et al. The Yin-Yang of tumor-associated macrophages in neoplastic progression and immune surveillance. *Immunol Rev.* 2008;222:155–161.
53. Oh H, Takagi H, Takagi C, et al. The potential angiogenic role of macrophages in the formation of choroidal neovascular membranes. *Invest Ophthalmol Vis Sci.* 1999; 40:1891–1898.
54. Cursiefen C, Chen L, Borges LP, et al. VEGF-A stimulates lymphangiogenesis and hemangiogenesis in inflammatory neovascularization via macrophage recruitment. *J Clin Invest.* 2004;113:1040–1050.
55. Espinosa-Heidmann DG, Suner IJ, Hernandez EP, et al. Macrophage depletion diminishes lesion size and severity in experimental choroidal neovascularization. *Invest Ophthalmol Vis Sci.* 2003;44:3586–3592.
56. Ahmed J, Braun RD, Dunn R, et al. Oxygen distribution in the macaque retina. *Invest Ophthalmol Vis Sci.* 1993;34:516–521.
57. Spaide RF. Etiology of late-age-related macular disease. In: *Medical Retina.* Holz F, Spaide RF, eds. New York, NY: Springer-Verlag; 2005.
58. Spaide RF. Rationale for combination therapies for choroidal neovascularization. *Am J Ophthalmol.* 2006;141(1):149–156.
59. Kent D, Sheridan C. Choroidal neovascularization: a wound healing perspective. *Mol Vis.* 2003;9:747–755.
60. Rakic JM, Lambert V, Devy L, et al. Placental growth factor, a member of the VEGF family, contributes to the development of choroidal neovascularization. *Invest Ophthalmol Vis Sci.* 2003;44:3186–3193.
61. Brown DM, Kaiser PK, Michels M, et al. Ranibizumab versus verteporfin for neovascular age-related macular degeneration. *N Engl J Med.* 2006;355(14):1432–1444.
62. Rosenfeld PJ, Brown DM, Heier JS, et al. Ranibizumab for neovascular age-related macular degeneration. *N Engl J Med.* 2006;355(14):1419–1431.
63. Ip MS, Scott IU, Brown GC, et al. Anti-vascular endothelial growth factor pharmacotherapy for age-related macular degeneration: a report by the American Academy of Ophthalmology. *Ophthalmology.* 2008;115(10):1837–1846.
64. Schouten JS, La Heij EC, Webers CA, et al. A systematic review on the effect of bevacizumab in exudative age-related macular degeneration. *Graefes Arch Clin Exp Ophthalmol.* 2009;247(1):1–11.
65. Michels S, Rosenfeld PJ, Puliafito CA, et al. Systemic bevacizumab (Avastin) therapy for neovascular age-related macular degeneration twelve-week results of an uncontrolled open-label clinical study. *Ophthalmology.* 2005;112(6): 1035–1047.
66. Avery RL, Pieramici DJ, Rabena MD, et al. Intravitreal bevacizumab (Avastin) for neovascular age-related macular degeneration. *Ophthalmology.* 2006;113(3):363–372 [Epub 2006 Feb 3].
67. Spaide RF, Laud K, Fine HF, et al. Intravitreal bevacizumab treatment of choroidal neovascularization secondary to age-related macular degeneration. *Retina.* 2006;26(4):383–390.
68. Fung AE, Lalwani GA, Rosenfeld PJ, et al. An optical coherence tomography-guided, variable dosing regimen with intravitreal ranibizumab (Lucentis) for neovascular age-related macular degeneration. *Am J Ophthalmol.* 2007; 143(4):566–583.
69. Lalwani GA, Rosenfeld PJ, Fung AE, et al. A variable-dosing regimen with intravitreal ranibizumab for neovascular age-related macular degeneration: year 2 of the PrONTO Study. *Am J Ophthalmol.* 2009;148(1):43–58.
70. Awh C. An extension treial of ranibizumab for neovascular age-related maculat degeneration: first-year safety and efficacy results. Paper presented at: 26th Annual Meeting of the American Society of Retina Specialists; October 11–15. 2008; Maui, HI.
71. Markomichelakis NN, Theodossiadis PG, Sfikakis PP. Regression of neovascular age-related macular degeneration following infliximab therapy. *Am J Ophthalmol.* 2005; 139:537–540.
72. Gasparini G. Metronomic scheduling: the future of chemotherapy? *Lancet Oncol.* 2001;2:733–740.
73. Hori K, Saito S, Tamai M. Effect of irradiation on neovascularization in rat skinfold chambers: implications for clinical trials of low-dose radiotherapy for wet-type age-related macular degeneration. *Int J Radiat Oncol Biol Phys.* 2004; 60:1564–1571.
74. Spaide RF, Sorenson J, Maranan L. Combined photodynamic therapy and intravitreal triamcinolone for nonsubfovel choroidal neovascularization. *Retina.* 2005;25(6):685–690.
75. Seiwert TY, Salama JK, Voleks EE. The concurrent chemoradiation paradigm—general principles. *Nat Clin Pract Oncol.* 2007;4:86–100.
76. Sivagnanavel V, Evans JR, Ockrim Z, et al. Radiotherapy for neovascular age-related macular degeneration. *Cochrane Database Sys Rev.* 2004;4:CD004004.
77. Avila MP, Farah ME, Santos A, et al. Twelve-month safety and visual acuity results from a feasibility study of intraocular, epiretinal radiation therapy for the treatment of subfoveal CNV secondary to AMD. *Retina.* 2009;29:157–169.
78. Smith BT, Dhalla MS, Shah GK, et al. Intravitreal injection of bevacizumab combined with verteporfin photodynamic therapy for choroidal neovascularization in age-related macular degeneration. *Retina.* 2008;28:675–681.
79. Spaide RF, Guyer DR, McCormick B, et al. External beam radiation therapy for choroidal neovascularization. *Ophthalmology.* 1998;105(1):24–30.
80. Treatment of Age-Related Macular Degeneration with Photodynamic Therapy (TAP) Study Group. Photodynamic Therapy of subfoveal choroidal neovascularization in age-related macular degeneration with verteporforin: two-year

results of 2 randomized clinical trials—TAP report 2. *Arch Ophthalmol.* 2001;119:198–207.

81. Verteporforin in Photodynamic Therapy (VIP) Study Group. Verteporforin therapy of subfoveal choroidal neovascularization in age-related macular degenertion: two-year results of a randomized clinical trial including lesions with occult with no classic choroidal neovascularization—verteporforin in photodynamic therapy report 2. *Am J Ophthalmol.* 2001; 131:541–560.
82. Visudyne in Minimally Classic CNV (VIM) Study Group. Verteporforin therapy of subfoveal minimally classic choroidal neovascularization in age-related macular degeneration: 2-year results of a randomized clinical trial. *Arch Ophthalmol.* 2005;123:448–457.
83. Fogelman AM, Berliner JA, Van Lenten BJ, et al. Lipoprotein receptors and endothelial cells. *Semin Thromb Hemost.* 1988;14:206–209.
84. Schmidt-Erfurth U, Hasan T. Mechanisms of action of photodynamic therapy with verteporforin for the treatment of age-related macular degeneration. *Surv Ophthalmol.* 2000; 45:195–214.
85. Michels S, Schmidt-Erfurth U. Sequence of early vascular events after photodynamic therapy. *Invest Ophthalmol Vis Sci.* 2003;44:2147–2154.
86. Recchia PM, Greenbaum S, Recchia CA, et al. Self-reported acute decrease in visual acuity after photodynamic therapy for age-related macular degeneration. *Retina.* 2006;26: 1042–1048.
87. Schmidt-Erfurth U, Schlotzer-Schrehard U, Cursiefen C, et al. Influence of photodynamic therapy on expression of vascular endothelial growth factor (VEGF), VEGF receptor 3, and pigment epithelium-derived factor. *Invest Ophthalmol Vis Sci.* 2003;44:4473–4480.
88. Iriyama A, Obata R, Inoue Y, et al. Effect of posterior juxtascleral triamcinolone acetonide on the efficacy and choriocapillaris hypoperfusion of photodynamic therapy. *Graefes Arch Clin Exp Ophthalmol.* 2008;246:339–344.
89. Kaiser PK, VERITAS Study Group. Verteporforin therapy in combination with pegaptanib or triamcinolone for wet AMD: 6 month results of the VERITAS trial. *Invest Ophthalmol Vis Sci.* 2007;48[ARVO e-abstract]:2870.
90. Antoszyk AN, Tuomi L, Chung CY, et al. Ranibizumab combined with verteporfin photodynamic therapy in neovascular age-related macular degeneration (FOCUS): year 2 results. *Am J Ophthalmol.* 2008;145:862–874.
91. Ishibashi T, Miki K, Sorgente N, et al. Effects of intravitreal administration of steroids on experimental subretinal neovascularization in the subhuman primate. *Arch Ophthalmol.* 1985;103:708–711.
92. Danis RP, Bingaman DP, Yang Y, et al. Inhibition of preretinal and optic nerve head neovascularization in pigs by intravitreal triamcinolone acetonide. *Ophthalmology.* 1996;103:2099–2104.
93. Antoszyk AN, Gottlieb JL, Machemer R, et al. The effects of intravitreal triamcinolone acetonide on experimental pre-retinal neovascularization. *Graefes Arch Clin Exp Ophthalmol.* 1993;231:34–40.
94. Nauck M, Karakiulakis G, Perruchoud AP, et al. Corticosteroids inhibit the expression of the vascular endothelial growth factor gene in human vascular smooth muscle cells. *Eur J Pharmacol.* 1998;341:309–315.
95. Matsuda S, Gomi F, Oshima Y, et al. Vascular endothelial growth factor reduced and connective tissue growth factor induced by triamcinolone in ARPE19 cells under oxidative stress. *Invest Ophthalmol Vis Sci.* 2005;46:1062–1068.
96. Itaya H, Imaizumi T, Yoshida H, et al. Expression of vascular endothelial growth factor in human monocyte/macrophages stimulated with lipopolysaccharide. *Thromb Haemost.* 2001; 85:171–176.
97. Li YH, Brauner A, Jensen JS, et al. Induction of human macrophage vascular endothelial growth factor and intercellular adhesion molecule-1 by ureaplasma urealyticum and downregulation by steroids. *Biol Neonate.* 2002; 82:22–28.
98. Ciulla TA, Criswell MH, Danis RP, et al. Intravitreal triamcinolone acetonide inhibits choroidal neovascularization in a laser-treated rat model. *Arch Ophthalmol.* 2001; 119:399–404.
99. Castro MR, Lutz D, Edelman JL. Effect of COX inhibitors on VEGF-induced retinal vascular leakage and experimental corneal and choroidal neovascularization. *Exp Eye Res.* 2004;79:275–285.
100. Edelman JL, Castro MR, Wen Y. Correlation of VEGF expression by leukocytes with the growth and regression of blood vessels in the rat cornea. *Invest Ophthalmol Vis Sci.* 1999;40:1112–1123.
101. Bolkenius U, Hahn D, Gressner AM, et al. Glucocorticoids decrease the bioavailability of TGF-β which leads to a reduced TGF-beta signaling in hepatic stellate cells. *Biochem Biophys Res Commun.* 2004;325:1264–1270.
102. Tamura H, Miyamoto K, Kiryu J, et al. Intravitreal injection of corticosteroid attenuates leukostasis and vascular leakage in experimental diabetic retina. *Invest Ophthalmol Vis Sci.* 2005;46:1440–1444.
103. Penfold PL, Wen L, Madigan MC, et al. Triamcinolone acetonide modulates permeability and intercellular adhesion molecule-1 (ICAM-1) expression of the ECV304 cell line: implications for macular degeneration. *Clin Exp Immunol.* 2000;121:458–465.
104. Penfold PL, Wen L, Madigan MC, et al. Modulation of permeability and adhesion molecule expression by human choroidal endothelial cells. *Invest Ophthalmol Vis Sci.* 2002;43:3125–3130.
105. Kang BS, Chung EY, Yun YP, et al. Inhibitory effects of anti-inflammatory drugs on interleukin-6 bioactivity. *Biol Pharm Bull.* 2001;24:701–703.
106. Breuninger LM, Dempsey WL, Uhl J, et al. Hydrocortisone regulation of interleukin-6 protein production by a purified population of human peripheral blood monocytes. *Clin Immunol Immunopathol.* 1993;69:205–214.
107. Antonetti DA, Wolpert EB, DeMaio L, et al. Hydrocortisone decreases retinal endothelial cell water and solute flux coincident with increased content and decreased phosphorylation of occludin. *J Neurochem.* 2002;80:667–677.
108. Edelman JL, Lutz D, Castro MR. Corticosteroids inhibit VEGF-induced vascular leakage in a rabbit model of blood-retinal and blood-aqueous barrier breakdown. *Exp Eye Res.* 2005;80:249–258.
109. Spandau UH, Sauder G, Schubert U, et al. Effect of triamcinolone acetonide on proliferation of retinal endothelial cells in vitro and in vivo. *Br J Ophthalmol.* 2005;89: 745–747.

110. Wang YS, Friedrichs U, Eichler W, et al. Inhibitory effects of triamcinolone acetonide on bFGF-induced migration and tube formation in choroidal microvascular endothelial cells. *Graefes Arch Clin Exp Ophthalmol.* 2002;240:42–48.
111. She H, Nakazawa T, Matsubara A, et al. Photoreceptor protection after photodynamic therapy using dexamethasone in a rat model of choroidal neovascularization. *Invest Ophthalmol Vis Sci.* 2008;49(11):5008–5014.
112. Penfold PL, Gyory JF, Hunyor AB, et al. Exudative macular degeneration and intravitreal triamcinolone: a pilot study. *Aust N Z J Ophthalmol.* 1995;23:293–298.
113. Challa JK, Gillies MC, Penfold PL, et al. Exudative macular degeneration and intravitreal triamcinolone: 18 month follow up. *Aust N Z J Ophthalmol.* 1998;26:277–281.
114. Danis RP, Ciulla TA, Pratt LM, et al. Intravitreal triamcinolone acetonide in exudative age-related macular degeneration. *Retina.* 2000;20:244–250.
115. Gillies MC, Simpson JM, Luo W, et al. A randomized clinical trial of a single dose of intravitreal triamcinolone acetonide for neovascular age-related macular degeneration: one-year results. *Arch Ophthalmol.* 2003;121:667–773.
116. Jonas JB, Kreissig I, Hugger P, et al. Intravitreal triamcinolone acetonide for exudative age related macular degeneration. *Br J Ophthalmol.* 2003;87:462–468.
117. Oh H, Takagi H, Takagi C, et al. The potential angiogenic role of macrophages in the formation of choroidal neovascular membranes. *Invest Opthhalmol Vis Sci.* 1999;40:1891–1898.
118. Theodossiadis PG, Liarakos VS, Sfikakis PP, et al. Intravitreal administration of the anti-tumer necrosis factor agent infliximab for neovascular age-related macular degeneration. *Am J Ophthalmol.* 2009;147:825–830.
119. Thomson AW, Turnquist HR, Raimondi G. Immunoregulatory functions of mTOR inhibition. *Nat Rev Immunol.* 2009;9(5):324–337 (Review).
120. Stahl A, Paschek L, Martin G, et al. Rapamycin reduces VEGF expression in retinal pigment epithelium (RPE) and inhibits RPE-induced sprouting angiogenesis in vitro. *FEBS Lett.* 2008;582(20):3097–3102 [Epub 2008 Aug 12].
121. Dejneka NS, Kuroki AM, Fosnot J, et al. Systemic rapamycin inhibits retinal and choroidal neovascularization in mice. *Mol Vis.* 2004;10:964–972.
122. Engelbert M, Gilmore MS. Fas ligand but not complement is critical for control of experimental *Staphylococcus aureus* endophthalmitis. *Invest Ophthalmol Vis Sci.* 2005; 46(7):2479–2486.
123. Spaide RF, Sorenson J, Maranan L. Combined photodynamic therapy with verteporforin and intravitreal triamcinolone acetonide for choroidal neovacularization. *Ophthalmology.* 2003;110:1517–1525.
124. Tatar O, Shinoda K, Kaiserling E, et al. Early effects of triamcinolone on vascular endothelial growth factor and endostatin in human choroidal neovascularization. *Arch Ophthalmol.* 2008;126:193–199.
125. Augustin AJ, Puls S, Offermann I. Triple therapy for choroidal neovascularization due to age-related macular degeneration: verteporfin PDT, bevacizumab, and dexamethasone. *Retina.* 2007;27:133–140.
126. Yang Z, Camp NJ, Sun H, et al. A variant of the HTRA1 gene increases susceptibility to age-related macular degeneration. *Science.* 2006;314(5801):992–993 [Epub 2006 Oct 19].
127. Kim S, Bell K, Mousa SA, et al. Regulation of angiogenesis in vivo by ligation of integrin alpha5beta1 with the central cell-binding domain of fibronectin. *Am J Pathol.* 2000; 156:1345–1362.
128. Klatt K, et al. Integrin a5b1in preretinal membranes associated with proliferative vitreoretinopathy (PVR). ARVO Annual meeting 2007.
129. Ramakrishnan V, Bhaskar V, Law DA, et al. Preclinical evaluation of an anti-alpha5beta1 integrin antibody as a novel anti-angiogenic agent. *J Exp Ther Oncol.* 2006;5:273–286.
130. Bhaskar V, Fox M, Breinberg D, et al. Volociximab, a chimeric integrin alpha5beta1 antibody, inhibits the growth of VX2 tumors in rabbits. *Invest New Drugs* 2008;26:7–12.
131. Faivre S, Kroemer G, Raymond E. Current development of mTOR inhibitors as anticancer agents. *Nat Rev Drug Disc.* 2006;5:671–688.
132. Steward MW, Rosenfeld PJ. Predicted biological activity of intravitreal VEGF trap. *Br J Ophthalmol.* 2008;92: 667–668.
133. Heier J, et al. Abstract. Retina Society Annual Meeting, September, 2007. Boston.
134. Scheppke L, Aguilar E, Gariano RF, et al. Retinal vascular permeability suppression by topical application of a novel VEGFR2/Src kinase inhibitor in mice and rabbits. *J Clin Invest.* 2008;118:2337–2346.
135. Doukas J, Mahesh S, Umeda N, et al. Topical administration of a multi-targeted kinase inhibitor suppresses choroidal neovascularization and retinal edema. *J Cell Physiol.* 2008;216:29–37.
136. Kleinman ME, Yamada K, Takeda A, et al. Sequence- and target-independent angiogenesis suppression by siRNA via TLR3. *Nature.* 2008;452:591–597.
137. Hu W, Criswell MH, Fong SL, et al. Differences in the temporal expression of regulatory growth factors during choroidal neovascular development. *Exp Eye Res.* 2009;88(1):79–91.
138. Izumi Y, Xu L, di Tomaso E, et al. Tumour biology: herceptin acts as an anti-angiogenic cocktail. *Nature.* 2002; 416(6878):279–280.
139. Chung EJ, Yoo S, Lim HJ, et al. Inhibition of choroidal neovascularization in mice by systemic administration of the multikinase inhibitor, sorafenib. *Br J Ophthalmol.* 2008 [Epub ahead of print].
140. Chiang GG, Abraham RT. Targeting the mTOR signaling network in cancer. *Trends Molec Med.*2007;13:433–442.
141. Chappelow AV, Kaiser PK. Neovascular age-related macular degeneration: potential therapies. *Drugs.* 2008;68: 1029–1036.

CHAPTER 24

Corneal Neovascularization

Salwa Abdel-Aziz • Bryan K. Monson • Derick Holt • Brian Zaugg • Balamurali K. Ambati

INTRODUCTION

Optimal visual acuity relies upon optical clarity along the visual axis, which spans from the tear film to the retina. As the initial "window" into the eye, the cornea must remain transparent and is thus one of the few body tissues that actively maintains an avascular state. When corneal avascularity is compromised, significant visual loss results. The importance of corneal avascularity is underscored by its conservation across nearly all vertebrate species, with the notable exception of certain freshwater mammals that live in environments with a high degree of particulate matter.[1] A recent study examining tissue from stillborn human fetuses suggests that corneal avascularity is maintained throughout intrauterine development.[2] Additional studies in murine models indicate that intact corneal epithelium inhibits angiogenesis.[3] These observations strongly suggest that corneal tissue contains an intrinsic capacity to actively maintain avascularity, and recent work over the last several years has significantly advanced our understanding of the regulatory mechanisms underlying this remarkable property.

The human cornea is approximately 11.5 mm in diameter, with the horizontal diameter slightly larger than the vertical diameter. The peripheral border where the cornea meets the sclera (with its overlying conjunctiva) is known as the corneoscleral limbus. There is considerable clinical and experimental evidence to suggest that this specialized transition zone houses a population of cells possessing stem cell characteristics.[4–11] In addition to its proposed role in replenishing corneal epithelium, there is evidence to suggest that the corneoscleral limbus may participate in the maintenance of corneal avascularity. In a rabbit model of limbal stem cell deficiency, transplantation of limbal epithelial stem cells that were ex-vivo expanded on rabbit amniotic membrane led to better surgical outcomes with higher rates of clear, avascular corneas when compared to transplantation of amniotic membrane alone.[12] This observation suggests that stem cells developing in the corneoscleral transition zone may acquire antiangiogenic properties that are retained through ex-vivo expansion and subsequent transplantation. It will be important to determine which, if any, of the molecular factors outlined below function in this "transplantable corneal protection," and to evaluate whether distinct mechanisms are used in different areas of the cornea to ensure that the requisite transparency is maintained along the optical axis.

CORNEAL ANTIANGIOGENIC HOMEOSTASIS

In order to understand the molecular factors involved in the establishment and active maintenance of corneal avascularity, the first step is to identify which potential regulatory factors are expressed in this specialized tissue. Candidates with the proper expression patterns are then tested using several different corneal neovascularization (KNV) model systems to evaluate if they function in corneal protection. Although the list of potential candidate molecules known to be expressed in the cornea is extensive, this section limits discussion to factors where experimental data reveals some degree of antiangiogenic activity in at least one in vivo KNV model system. To date, such factors roughly fall into two broad groups. First, there are factors that modify or are derived from components of the extracellular matrix (ECM). Secondly, there is a group of endothelial growth factors and other related signaling molecules known to regulate the processes of endothelial cell activation, vessel growth, and angiogenesis.

Matrix Metalloproteinases/Angiostatin/Endostatin

Matrix metalloproteinases (MMPs) are zinc-dependent endopeptidases capable of degrading diverse ECM proteins. Depending upon expression patterns and substrate specificity, MMP activity can be either proangiogenic or antiangiogenic. There are at least 12 MMPs expressed in the cornea[13]; of these, MMP2 and MMP14 (also known as MT1-MMP) are likely the most important proangiogenic MMPs, while MMP3 and MMP7 are important antiangiogenic factors. Antiangiogenic MMPs antagonize vessel growth by cleaving inactive precursor molecules into products that possess intrinsic antiangiogenic activity. Important examples include generation of angiostatin from plasminogen, endostatin derived from collagen XVIII, and restin derived from collagen XV.[13–18]

Experiments in MMP3$^{-/-}$ and MMP7$^{-/-}$ mice have demonstrated that genetic depletion of these factors results in KNV if a portion of the corneoscleral limbus is surgically compromised. In contrast, partial limbal deficiency in wild-type control mice did not lead to KNV.[13] MMP7$^{-/-}$ mice also show increased susceptibility to KNV relative to wild-type controls in a laser-induced corneal injury model.[19] In addition to genetic deletion of MMP enzymes, disruption of MMP cleavage products is also known to affect corneal avascularity. Both MMP3 and MMP7 are able to generate the antiangiogenic peptides angiostatin and endostatin through cleavage of their respective precursor molecules.[13] Angiostatin derived from either tumor implantation or recombinant sources has been shown to both inhibit and regress existing KNV in a mouse corneal injury model.[20] Furthermore, treatment with antiangiostatin antibodies has been shown to enhance KNV in response to laser-induced corneal injury.[16] Finally, endostatin delivered through subconjunctival injection of an adenoassociated viral vector inhibited KNV in mice treated with silver nitrate cautery.[21]

Thrombospondins

Thrombospondins represent another class of ECM proteins with antiangiogenic activity, which are known to be expressed in the cornea.[22–24] Two family members, thrombospondin-1 and -2 (TSP-1, -2), are thought to antagonize vessel growth through multiple mechanisms. TSP-1 and -2 act through the CD36 receptor to induce vascular endothelial cell apoptosis,[25,26] and are also thought to indirectly affect growth factor availability through their interactions with the ECM.[27] Both TSP-1 and TSP-2 protect against basic fibroblast growth factor (bFGF)-induced KNV in mice.[28,29] Furthermore, TSP1$^{-/-}$ and TSP2$^{-/-}$ mice exhibit enhanced KNV in response to corneal injury relative to controls.[23] Loss of the TSP-1 and -2 cognate receptor also compromises corneal avascularity, as CD36$^{-/-}$ mice acquire KNV in old age.[30] Finally, in experiments utilizing antibodies that bind different portions of the CD36 molecule, treatment with neutralizing antibodies led to enhancement of KNV, whereas treatment with activating antibodies had a protective effect in a murine corneal injury model.[31]

Prolactin

Fragments of the prolactin (PRL) hormone family also possess antiangiogenic activity, and treatment with a 16 kDa PRL fragment protected against neovascularization in a rat model of bFGF-induced KNV. The same study also reported that treatment with anti-PRL antibodies induced KNV in rats.[32] While these observations suggest that endogenous PRL-like fragments may exist in the cornea; to date, only PRL receptors have been detected in this tissue.[32] It is thought that antiangiogenic PRL fragments may be generated through proteolytic processing in the pituitary,[33] or following PRL production at other sites such as the lacrimal gland[34] or vascular endothelial cells in retina or other ocular tissues.[35]

Proangiogenic Factors

In additional to the multiple antiangiogenic factors expressed and actively functioning in the cornea, a multitude of proangiogenic factors are also present.[13,36] It is widely believed that a delicate balance between these factors maintains avascularity until circumstances such as injury or inflammation tip the scale in favor of proangiogenic factors and enables growth of new vessels into the cornea. The final common pathway for all new blood vessel growth is vascular endothelial cell activation, and multiple mitogenic growth factors and signaling partners are known to influence endothelial cell survival, growth, and migration. The most notable of these include vascular endothelial growth factor (VEGF), platelet-derived growth factor (PDGF), insulin-like growth factor (IGF), bFGF, integrins, angiopoietins, protein kinase C (PKC), and ephrins. VEGF, acting through one of three tyrosine kinase receptors (VEGFR-1, -2, and -3) is commonly considered the most prominent proangiogenic factor, and many of the other regulators are likely to act indirectly through VEGF-dependent pathways.

Pigment Epithelium–derived Factor

It is not surprising, therefore, that the most important antiangiogenic factors in the cornea act through regulation of VEGF signaling. These include pigment epithelium–derived factor (PEDF), a member of the serine protease inhibitor (Serpin) family[37]; VEGFR-3; and sFlt-1, a soluble isoform of VEGFR-1 generated through alternative splicing. PEDF is expressed in both corneal epithelium and endothelium in adult rats,[38] and treatment of rat corneas with neutralizing anti-PEDF antibodies leads to KNV.[39] PEDF is among the most potent antiangiogenic factors in the body, functions in multiple locations within the eye, and acts at least in part through disrupting VEGFR-1 signaling.[40] However, PEDF$^{-/-}$ mice show no alteration in the development or patterning of ocular vasculature, indicating that PEDF is dispensable as an endogenous inhibitor of angiogenesis.[41]

VEGFR-3

VEGFR-3, a cognate receptor for VEGF-C and VEGF-D isoforms, was recently found to be highly expressed in normal avascular corneal epithelium.[3] In a mouse model of injury-induced KNV, transplantation of control corneal epithelium was protective, whereas epithelium treated with neutralizing VEGFR-3 antibodies prior to transplantation exhibited higher levels of neovascularization. Finally, the same study reported that treatment with a VEGFR-3 chimeric protein was protective against KNV when compared to treatment with Fc fragment alone.[3] These observations are supportive of a model in which VEGFR-3 expressed at high levels in nonendothelial corneal cells acts as a "decoy receptor" for VEGF-C and VEGF-D isoforms, thus promoting corneal avascularity. While these observations represent significant new insight into yet another antiangiogenic protective mechanism in the cornea, the effects are only observed in the setting of corneal injury and involve a receptor that is unable to bind and neutralize VEGF-A, which is widely thought to be the most important VEGF isoform involved in mediating KNV.[42–44]

VEGFR-1

VEGFR-1 (also known as Flt-1) is a cognate receptor for VEGF-A. Alternative splicing of Flt-1 pre-mRNA can lead to expression of a soluble isoform (denoted sFlt-1) that retains VEGF binding ability but lacks the transmembrane domain found in the full-length protein. Both VEGF-A and sFlt-1 are expressed at high levels in normal avascular corneal tissue, and native protein electrophoresis experiments revealed that the vast majority of corneal VEGF-A is not free but instead is bound to another protein[1] (Fig. 24.1). Co-immunoprecipitation experiments suggested that this partner protein was sFlt-1, and subsequent disruption of sFlt-1 expression at the genetic, pre-mRNA, and protein levels resulted in marked KNV.[1] Furthermore, $Pax6^{+/-}$ and *corn-1* mice, which develop spontaneous KNV, were found to have undetectable levels of sFlt-1 in corneal tissue. Analysis of corneal specimens from human patients suffering from KNV revealed similarly low levels of sFlt-1 expression. Finally, examination of diverse species revealed that sFlt-1–mediated corneal protection is evolutionarily conserved, as only those vertebrates with natural vascularized corneas (such as the Florida manatee) lack high corneal expression of sFlt-1.[1]

In a recent report, mouse corneas were treated with a novel tetrameric tripeptide to interrupt sFlt-1 binding to VEGF-A. As in prior experiments, where different strategies were used to disrupt sFlt-1 function, these treatments resulted in significant KNV.[45] Examination of several human subjects using immunohistochemistry and immunoprecipitation techniques revealed that normal avascular human corneal tissue contains high levels of sFlt-1, which normally binds and sequesters VEGF. In contrast, corneal tissue from subjects with KNV resulting from diverse etiologies including alkali burns, aniridia, ocular cicatricial pemphigoid, and interstitial keratitis contained low levels of sFlt-1 with correspondingly higher levels of free VEGF.[46] These finding are an important extension to the initial discovery outlined above and demonstrate that the model of sFlt-1–dependent VEGF sequestration is likely to be important in a wide variety of corneal disease states involving neovascularization.

For many years, it was thought that a collection of redundant mechanisms, rather than a single molecular factor, was responsible for the preservation of corneal avascularity. While the data summarized above indicate that several biologic pathways are involved in corneal protection, it is now clear that sFlt-1–dependent binding and sequestration of VEGF-A is the dominant mechanism. Thus, although it is critically important for the field to consider multiple targets in the development of future strategies to combat KNV, the sFlt-1 pathway is certainly the single most attractive candidate at this time. Of even greater significance is the prospect of leveraging this regulatory system to treat other common disease states where stimulation or inhibition of angiogenesis may be beneficial.

CAUSES OF CORNEAL NEOVASCULARIZATION

It is estimated that 1.4 million people in the United States develop KNV in a given year and that 4% of the US population has KNV.[47] In simple terms, the overall cause of KNV is a loss of balance between angiogenic and antiangiogenic growth factors.[48] When extensive KNV develops, corneal and visual clarity declines. Any surface ocular disease involving inflammation predisposes a patient to developing KNV. Chronic infections are more likely to cause KNV because of the associated macrophage infiltration. Many causes associated with KNV will be described in four categories: inflammatory, infectious, traumatic injury, and models used for research (Fig. 24.2).

Inflammatory

Inflammatory causes of KNV vary from iatrogenic in surgery to graft rejection to aberrant immune diseases. Associated conditions discussed here include graft rejection, optimizing surgical technique, ocular cicatricial pemphigoid, Stevens-Johnson, and conjunctivitis.

KNV in graft rejection occurs in many cases of keratoplasty. One study showed the incidence of KNV in corneal buttons analyzed after keratoplasty at almost 20%.[49] Many different risk factors have been identified to help minimize the probability of graft rejection. Graft rejection has been associated with host corneas with more than two quadrants of prior neovascularization, herpes simplex keratitis, uveitis, silicone oil keratopathy, previous rejected grafts, young host age, and having multiple surgical procedures during the graft placement.[50] Embedding suture knots within the host stroma instead of in the graft, eyes with larger graft beds in the host, and active blepharitis are significantly associated with KNV.[51] Other risks identified include atopic dermatitis, tear insufficiency, and short duration of graft storage.[52] The risk factors do not significantly change if the transplant is a first graft or a regraft.[53]

Optimizing surgical technique can minimize the incidence of KNV in transplant cases. Risk factors associated with KNV include shorter distance from the limbus of both the graft tissue and the sutures.[54] Use of nonmechanical trephination using an excimer laser may decrease the incidence of KNV within the 1st year.[55]

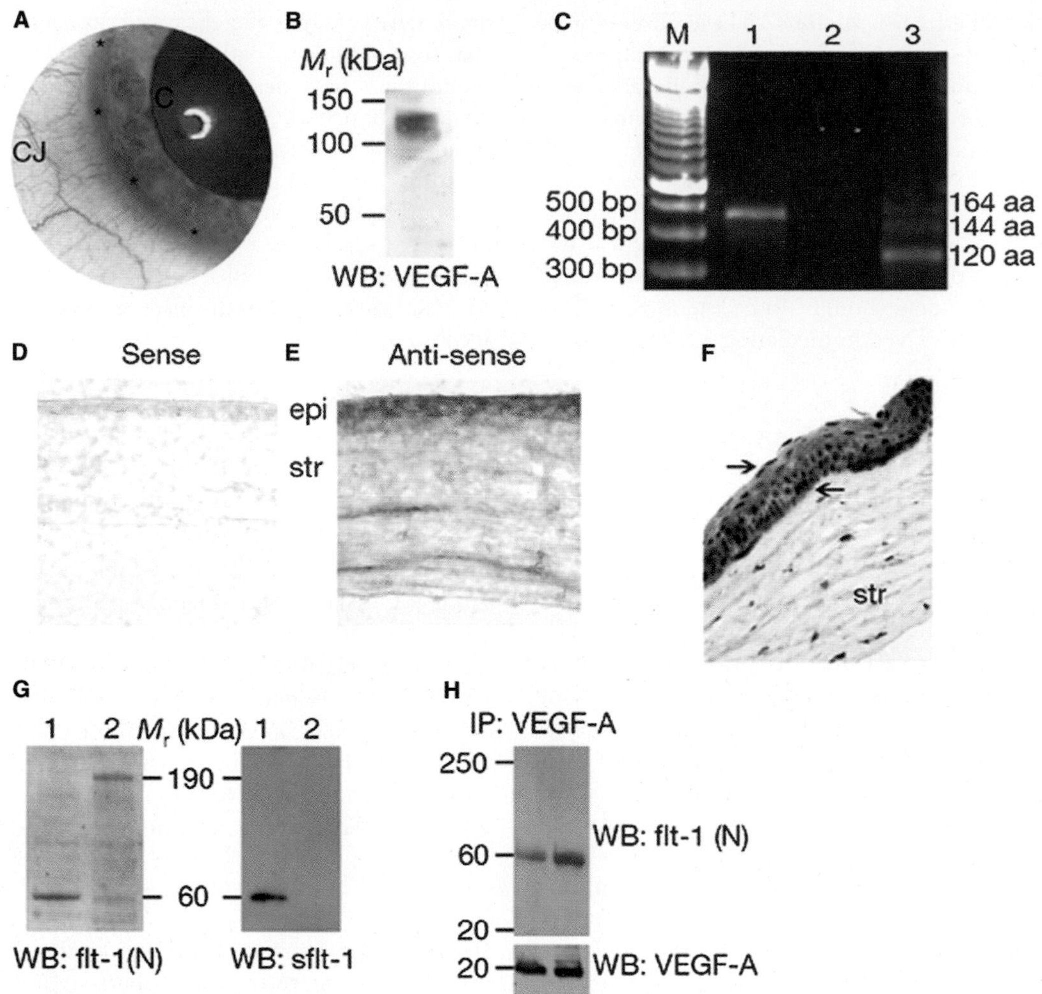

FIGURE 24.1. Avascular cornea contains sflt-1 bound to VEGF-A. **A**: Photo of human eye demonstrates abrupt termination of blood vessels in the conjunctiva (CJ) at its border with the cornea (C), the limbus (*asterisks*). **B**: Representative nonreducing Western blot of mouse cornea reveals immunoreactive bands of VEGF-A at 100 to 130 kDa corresponding to bound forms, and negligible immunoreactivity at 45 to 50 kDa corresponding to the free form. $n = 5$. **C**: sflt-1 (lane 1) and VEGF-A (lane 3) transcripts in mouse cornea identified by representative polymerase chain reaction with reverse transcription (RT-PCR). Lane 2 is water (template-negative) control. $n = 5$. bp, base pairs; aa, amino acids. **D, E**: sflt-1 mRNA detected by in situ hybridization in mouse corneal epithelium (epi) and stroma (str). Antisense RNA probes show purple-brown reactivity. Sense RNA probes show negligible reactivity. **F**: Immunolocalization (*brown*) of sflt-1 protein in mouse cornea. **G**: Representative reducing Western blots (WB) with an antibody against the amino (N) terminus of flt-1 that recognizes both mbflt-1 and sflt-1 and an antibody against the unique C terminus of sflt-1 show that mouse cornea (a) contains primarily sflt-1 (60 kDa), whereas the conjunctiva (b) contains mainly mbflt-1 (190 kDa). **H**: Representative Western blot of two independent mouse cornea samples immunoprecipitated (IP) with anti-VEGF-A antibody and immunoblotted (WB) with a biotinylated antibody against the N terminus of flt-1 that recognizes both mbflt-1 and sflt-1 shows that VEGF-A interacts with sflt-1 (60 kDa). Subsequent immunoblot with a biotinylated anti–VEGF-A antibody confirms the pull-down of VEGF-A by the immunoprecipitating antibody. $n = 6$. (Reproduced from Ambati., et al. *Nature.* 2006;443:993–997, with permission).

Donor tissue rejection occurs following the loss of immune privilege of the cornea. In animal studies, unless topical steroids were instituted sufficiently early, the course of neovascular response progressed to graft failure regardless of treatment.[56] The most profound outgrowth of KNV seems to occur in the 1st week following transplant and requires vigilant follow-up and aggressive treatment to avoid progression.[54] In mouse studies, short capillary growth began 1 day following cauterization and KNV peaked on days 4 and 5 and then regressed. Host immune cells access the corneal tissue and macrophages secrete VEGF,[57] which acts to swing the balance of growth factors in favor of angiogenesis. If treatment attempts fails, the rejection progresses to graft failure and necessitates subsequent transplants.

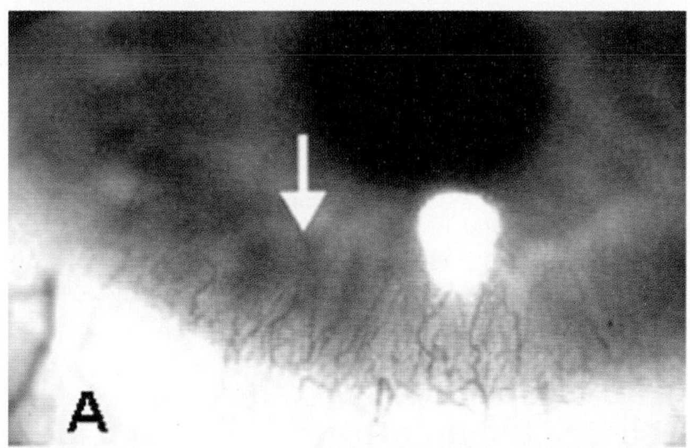

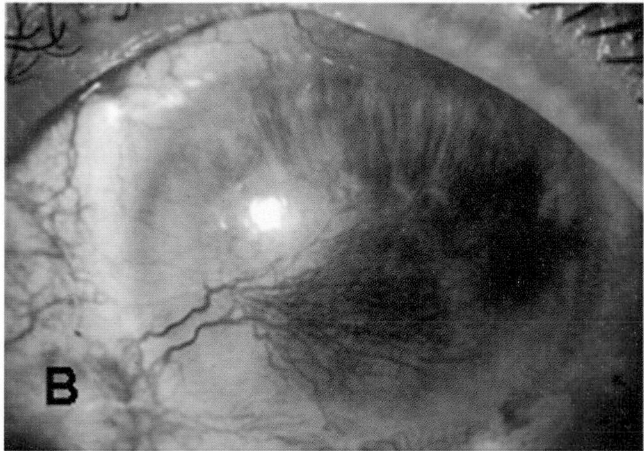

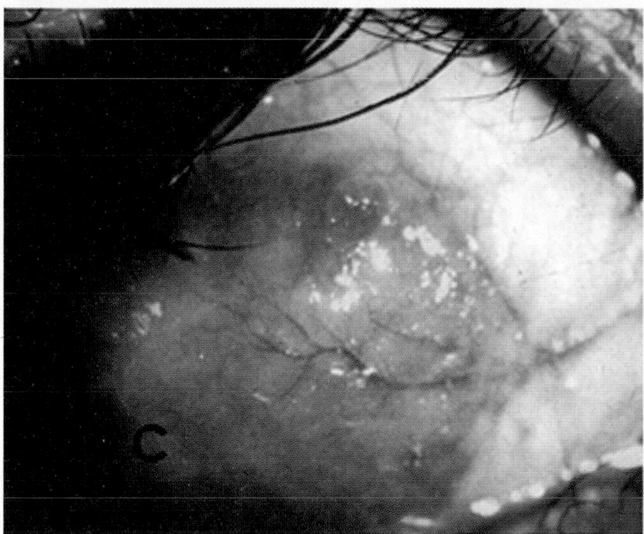

FIGURE 24.2. Common causes of corneal neovascularization. **A:** contact lens overwear, **B:** HSV keratitis and **C:** trachoma.

Ocular cicatricial pemphigoid is an autoimmune subepithelial blistering disorder.[58] The subepithelial bulla that forms can rupture and healing leads to scar formation. The immune reaction is a type II reaction with linear deposition of immunological factors in the epithelial basement membrane of the cornea. Most patients present later in the course of the disease. The prognosis is generally good when treatment is aimed at limiting inflammation and promoting healing. Systemic immunosuppressive therapy is the most important aspect of limiting disease progression. There are many extraocular manifestations of the disease that must be addressed as well.

Stevens-Johnson's (erythema multiforme major) is a severe immune reaction to an unknown pathogen involving mucous membranes. Many different causes have been implicated including infections with viruses, bacteria, and fungi or the use of certain medications. When severe, the skin lesions can last up to 6 weeks.[59] The eye is generally very dry and needs supportive lubrication. Systemic corticosteroids are used to treat and control acute disease.[60] Healing may lead to scar formation and lifelong sequelae.

Causes of acute conjunctivitis are either allergic or infectious. Allergic conjunctivitis is divided into both acute and chronic diseases. Acute allergic conjunctivitis includes both seasonal allergic conjunctivitis (SAC) and perennial allergic conjunctivitis (PAC). SAC is only seasonal while PAC generally presents all year with seasonal exacerbations of symptoms. Chronic atopic keratoconjunctivitis is a chronic inflammatory disease of the cornea and conjunctiva. A majority of patients have comorbid asthma or eczema.[61] Patients present with symptoms of intense itching, tearing, and blurred vision. Vernal keratoconjunctivitis is a recurrent inflammation that is associated with seasonal allergy, asthma, or eczema. Generally, the inflammation is worse in warmer months and remits in cooler months. For all of these conditions avoidance of the antigen stimulating the immune system is first-line therapy along with treatment of symptoms using artificial tears or cold compresses. Various medications can be used and selection depends on the patient's tolerance and severity of the symptoms.

Infectious

Many infectious organisms are directly associated with KNV.[62] Sixty percent of cases of keratoconjunctivitis have associated KNV.[63] These infectious diseases can be difficult to eradicate. Among the viral illnesses, the two main infections associated with KNV are in the herpes family of viruses: herpes zoster and herpes simplex. Bacterial causes include pseudomonas, *Chlamydia trachomatis,* and syphilis. Common fungal infections include Candida, Fusarium, and Aspergillus. Onchocerca volvulus infection is also known to induce KNV. All of these infections are associated with KNV in the literature. Now we will look at some common surface diseases that involve infect.

Infections including viral, bacterial, fungal, and parasitic can all lead to ocular surface injury. The fear of any of these infections is the progression to ulcerative keratitis. The most common pathogens of bacterial conjunctivitis include *Staphylococcus aureus*, *Streptococcus pneumoniae*, and *Haemophilus influenzae*. Treatment consists of topical antibiotic drops or ointments. Infection is generally self-limiting, but treatment can enhance recovery. Viral conjunctivitis is very common with adenovirus identified as the leading pathogen. In immunocompetent hosts the infection is self-limiting within 5 to 15 days.[64] Fungal and parasitic conjunctivitis are rare but require aggressive treatment to avoid corneal damage such as ulceration.

Neurotrophic keratopathy involves the loss of innervation to the cornea from the ophthalmic division of the trigeminal nerve. The absence of innervation to the cornea leads to decreased sensation and neurotrophic factors that normally support cell health.[65] The damage occurs commonly with varicella zoster and herpes simplex keratitis (HSV-1 more common than HSV-2). The nerve damage can lead to ulceration, melting, and perforation. The goal of treatment is to avoid the development of persistent epithelial defects, which can progress to ulceration, melting, and perforation necessitating keratoplasty. Treatment of epithelial defects includes lubrication and elimination of all topical toxicity. Ulcer treatment involves application of neuronal mediators including substance P and IGF-1.[66] Placing an amniotic membrane patch is used to decrease exposure and dryness, promoting wound healing.[67]

Traumatic Injury

In developed countries hypoxia-induced KNV is reported as a major cause of corneal loss leading to corneal transplant. As early as 1980, doctors recognized that wearing contact lenses for extended periods of time leads to corneal damage and KNV.[68] In 1983, a warning to patients fit with extended wear contact lenses was made.[69] These patients require frequent and diligent follow-up and should not be fitted with extended wear lenses if they are not able to manage their care properly. Many contact lenses causing a problem are too tight on patients. Any patient wearing contact lenses, regardless of the type needs follow-up eye exams to ensure proper use.[70] More commonly, KNV associated with contact lens use is more superficial. The hypoxia caused by wearing contact lenses for extended periods of time leads to chronic inflammation and the stimulation of growth factors that initiate new deep vessel growth.[71–73] Much of the vessel growth is superficial and generally responds well to medical treatment. Deeper vessel growth is more serious and can lead to hemorrhage, scarring, and loss of corneal transparency. Macrophages involved in the chronic inflammation play a role in the release of VEGF which stimulates the growth of new vessels. The presence of Macrophage Migration Inhibitory Factor (MIF), abundantly expressed in corneas with neovascularization, causes macrophages to infiltrate the cornea and secrete the angiogenic factors.[74]

KNV plays a role in wound repair in cases of trauma only when the angiogenic factors dominate the corneal environment.[13] Alkali burns occurring in patients involved in automobile accidents with deployment of airbags can lead to KNV.[75,76] This serious ocular injury is well treated if caught early following induction of the wound.

Alkali or acid injuries vary in the damage to the surface of the eye. The damage can vary from minor irritation of the eye to permanent visual loss. Alkali injuries are more common than acid injuries.[77] The common chemicals causing alkali injuries include ammonia, lye, potassium hydroxide, and magnesium hydroxide. Causes of acid injuries include sulfuric, sulfurous, hydrofluoric, acetic, and hydrochloric acid. Irrigating the surface of the eye following the insult as soon as possible will limit the damage. Damage is directly related to the exposure time of the chemical on the cornea. Removal of particles causing continued irritation and debridement of necrotic area promotes wound healing.

RESEARCH MODELS OF CORNEAL NEOVASCULARIZATION

Research of KNV necessitates creating various animal models that are reproducible and economic ways to investigate angiogensis and corneal neovasculariazation and to create theraputic targets:

Growth Factor–Induced KNV

Implantation of Hydron pellets induces development of angiogenesis in the cornea upon exposure to doses of bFGF or VEGF and sucralfate.[44]

With the number of people in the United States alone affected by KNV, the importance of recognizing and treating this condition in the early stages cannot be overemphasized. Studies are increasing throughout academia to find ways of preventing and treating KNV. While much is now known about the causes and associations of diseases with KNV, much more research is needed to increase our ability to slow its incidence.

Suture-induced Corneal Neovascularization

This model was produced by placing a silk suture centrally in pigmented mice corneas causing limbal vasculature to develop. This inflamatory response was found to correlate with the increased expression of matrix metalloproteinase-2 (MMP-2), a proteolytic enzyme that regulates angiogenesis. MMP-2–deficient mice exhibited significant delay of neovascularization in comparison with wild-type mice.[78]

Alkali Burns

In this model animal corneas were subjected to alkali-burning with NaOH and the effects of altering the eicosanoid precursor pool via dietary manipulation was monitored. The results of this study suggested that neovascular responses and chronic inflammation occurring in the clinical setting of severe structural damage may be modulated by nutritional alteration of the eicosanoid precursor pool. A similar in vivo model of alkali burn was used to monitor the process of corneal neovascularization from the early to the regressive stages.[79,80]

Spontaneous Vascularization

In this model, corneas of corn1 and Pax6$^{+/-}$ mice, which are found to be deficient in sflt-1, exhibited spontaneously vascularized corneas. Adminstration of recombinant sflt-1 restored corneal avascularity in these mice.[1] This model is similar to aniridia and spontaneous corneal neovascularization exhibited in humans with mutations in Pax6.

NEOVASCULARIZATION TREATMENT

Maintaining the avascular homeostatic state in the cornea has become a major focus of neovascularization research. Understanding the relationship between proangiogenic and antiangiogenic regulators has led to a number of antineovascularization pharmaceutical strategies. These therapeutic designs have targeted both the general inflammatory cascade and the inhibition of selective proangiogenic factors.

Steroids

In the clinic, steroids have remained the mainstay therapeutic strategy in the prevention of corneal neovascularization. Topical and subconjunctival administration of triamcinolone is known to inhibit corneal neovascularization.[81,82] However, steroids carry with them serious side effects including glaucoma, cataract formation, and an inherent risk of infection.[83] Likewise, corticosteroids sometimes are ineffective in inhibiting neovascularization, making alternative therapeutic strategies necessary.

VEGF Inhibitors

VEGF has been known to play a key role in angiogenesis in the human cornea. Comprised of five isoforms, VEGF promotes several steps within normal vascular growth including the induction of angiogenesis, endothelial cell proliferation, enhanced inflammatory response, proteolytic activities, and increased vascular permeability.[36,84,85]

Several cellular components within the human cornea have been found to produce VEGF when under inflammation or duress including corneal endothelial and epithelial cells, fibroblasts, macrophages, and limbal vessel vascular endothelial cells.[42,86,87] VEGF antagonists disrupt these pathways, thus decreasing or even preventing corneal neovascularization.

Bevacizumab and Ranibizumab

Bevacizumab is a full-length, recombinant monoclonal antibody that binds all VEGF isoforms (Fig. 24.3). First approved in 2004 as an antineovascularization strategy in the treatment of colon cancer, bevacizumab effectively inhibits the VEGF-receptor interaction, and thus inhibiting vascular permeability, and capillary formation.[88] A related compound, ranibizumab, is a high-affinity recombinant monoclonal antibody derived from the same parent murine antibody as bevacizumab. It is much smaller than the parent molecule and neutralizes all isoforms of VEGF-A.[89]

Bevacizumab and ranibizumab have seen extensive off-label use in the management of diabetic retinopathy and age-related maculopathy.[88,90] Initial reports in treating corneal neovascularization have shown bevacizumab to be safe and effective in both the animal model[85,91,92] and human clinical reports.[42]

Of specific clinical importance is the role that VEGF inhibitors may play in the prophylactic treatment of penetrating keratoplasty (PKP). The success of PKP is largely dependent on maintaining the immunoprivileged state of the cornea. Therapeutic strategies, therefore, have centered on maintaining corneal avascularity. Hindering neovascular access of the host immune system to the donor cornea will thereby inhibit antigen expression, migration of antigen-presenting cells, and modulation the host immune response.

Studies have investigated various drug delivery models of bevacizumab in neovascularization treatment. Two series consisting of patients with corneal neovascularization who effectively responded to bevacizumab eye drops have been described[93,94] (Fig. 24.4). However, difficulty that older patients may experience with the use of eye drops may make single injection a superior drug delivery method.[95] Subconjunctival administration of bevacizumab has been shown to inhibit corneal neovascularization in experimental rabbit models.[96] In human corneas, short-term results of subconjunctival injection of bevacizumab has been shown to be well tolerated and shows regression of corneal neovascularization[97,98] (Fig. 24.5).

It is now thought that bevacizumab not only mediates hemangiogenesis but also lymphangiogenesis.[85,22] The VEGF-A isotype plays a particularly important role in corneal lymphangiogenesis. This gives rise to the hope that bevacizumab may be of particular usefulness in preventing immune rejections after PKP as lymphangiogenesis is a component of graft rejection and in preventing tumor metastasis via lymphatic vessels.[43,52]

Both animal and human investigations of VEGF inhibition as a strategy to prevent corneal transplant rejection have been conducted. Recent studies have demonstrated posttransplant reduction of high-risk vascularity in the recipient corneal bed following bevacizumab monotherapy treatment.[11,72] Additionally, a recent case report showed successful regression of graft neovascularization with the use of subconjunctival bevacizumab combined with subconjunctival and topical steroid therapy.[79]

Not all results of preliminary corneal transplant rejection studies with bevacizumab have been favorable, however. One recent case series showed limitation of subconjunctival bevacizumab injections for vascularized rejecting corneal grafts, in which all three grafts eventually failed.[8]

Bevacizumab may also play a complementary role in preventing corneal neovascularization in herpetic stromal keratitis[95] as endothelium and stroma infected with herpes contain elevated levels of VEGF. In recurrent pterygium, bevacizumab may not be as effective. Short-term results of an initial study demonstrated that subconjunctival bevacizumab did not significantly induce regression of corneal vessels in recurrent pterygium.[99]

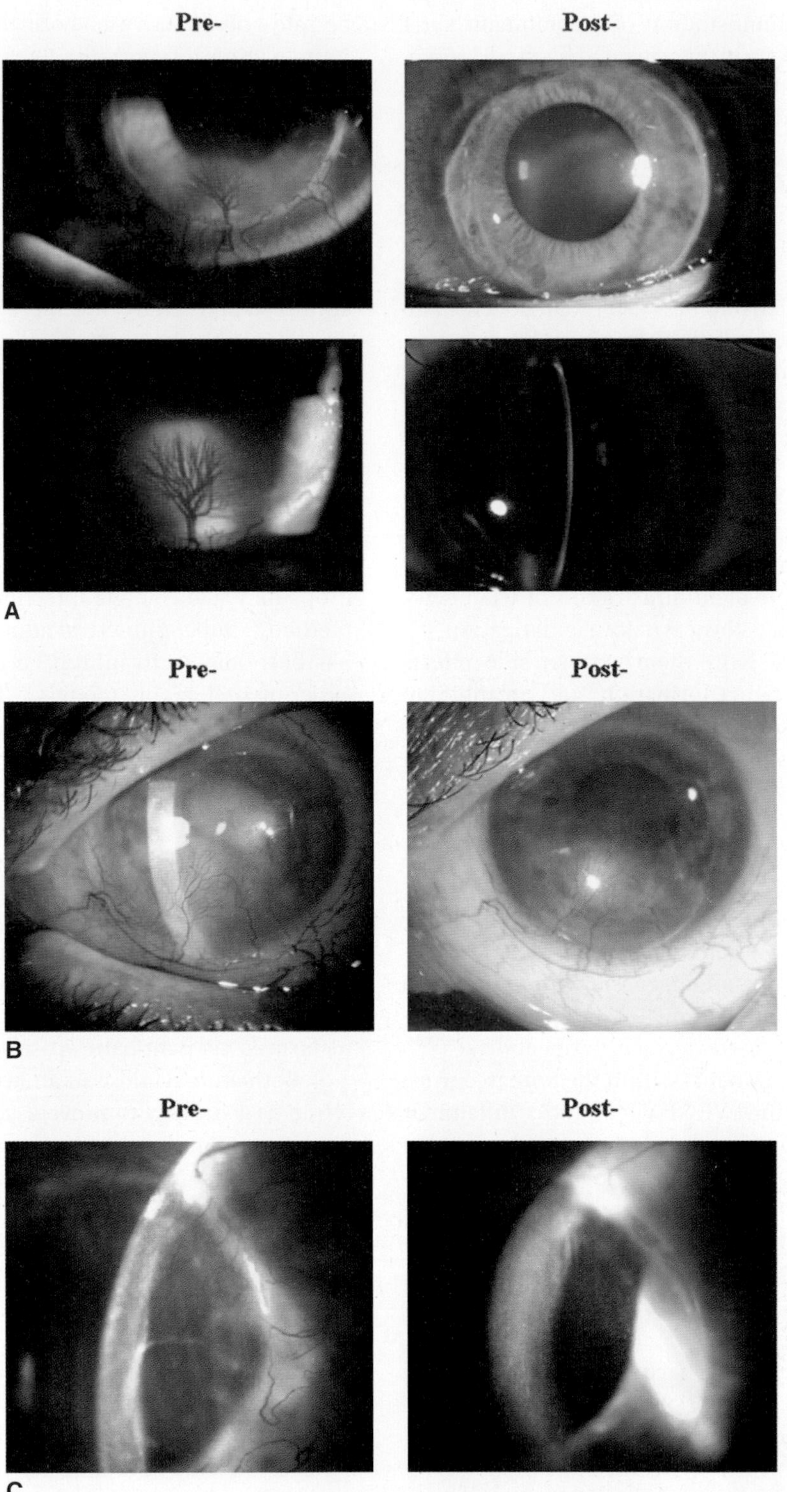

FIGURE 24.3. Bevacizumab therapy in corneal neovascularization showing pretreatment and posttreatment status (From author's own practice).

Inhibitors of MMP-2

Like other basement membranes in the body, Descemet membrane in the cornea consists of resilient sheets of rope-like collagen fibers, interlaced with proteoglycan and laminin. Likewise, corneal stoma is composed in part of dense interweaving collagen fibrils. Angiogenic invasion is dependent on the ability of invading vessels to breach the tissue architecture of the cornea. As growing capillaries crawl through connective tissue,

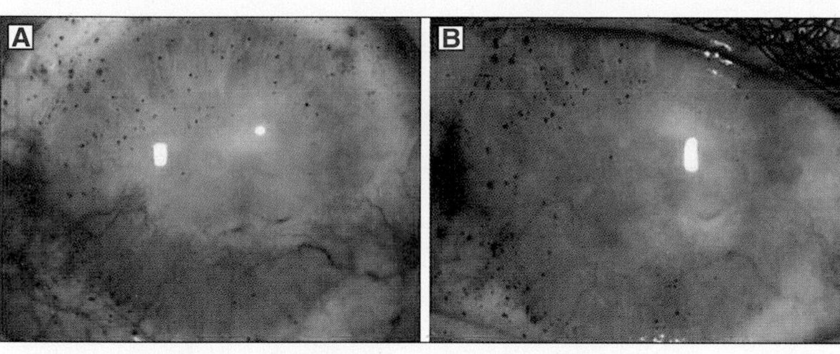

FIGURE 24.4. Topical bevacizumab therapy for corneal neovascularization. **A:** The patient's cornea is shown prior to topical bevacizumab treatment, displaying extensive neovascular vessels, most evident inferiorly. **B:** Dramatic reduction in vascularization resulted after 25 days of topical therapy. (Reproduced from DeStafeno K. *Arch Ophthalmol.* 2007;125:834–836, with permission).

specialized collagen proteinases called MMP-2 degrade collagen strands allowing capillary tubules to advance through basement membranes and dense connective protein matrixes.

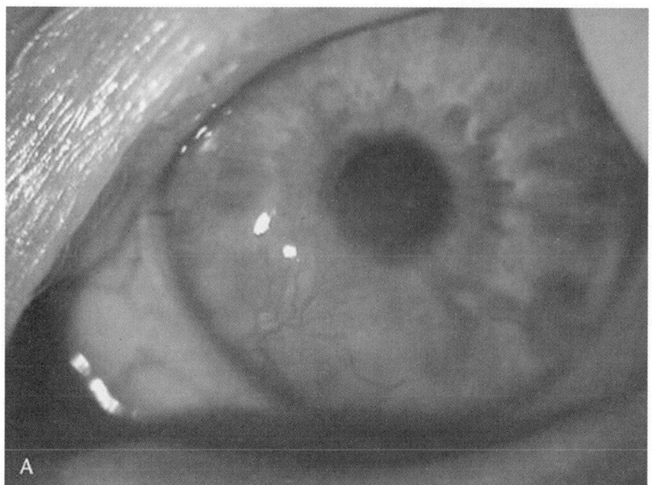

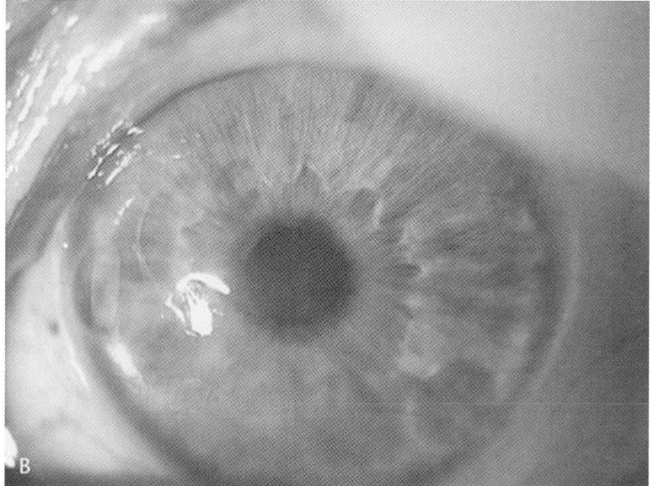

FIGURE 24.5. Subconjunctival bevacizumab injection for corneal neovascularization. Anterior-segment photograph of a patient (herpetic eye disease) (**A**) before bevacizumab injection (extent 5, centricity 3, density 2.5, proportion of vascularized cornea 12.61%) and (**B**) 1 week after the fourth injection (extent 2.5, centricity 1.75, density 1, proportion of vascularized cornea 5.5%). Note the significant, although not complete, regression of blood vessels.(Reproduced from Bahar I, et al. *Cornea.* 2008;27:142–147, with permission).

MMP-2 is therefore an attractive target in developing new neovascularization treatments.[78,100] Early investigations of corneal MMP-2 inhibition have been encouraging. Propolis extracts containing artepillin C and caffeic acid phenyl ester[101] have been shown to inhibit cell proliferation, migration, and capillary tube formation in the human cornea. Propolis reduced the number of newly formed vessels and inhibited expression of MMP-2 as well as VEGF production from various cells.[102] Doxycycline, an inhibitor of MMP-2, has also been found to effectively suppress corneal neovascularization while in combination with triamcinolone acetonide.[5]

Unregulated MMP-2 expression is also a culprit in cancer's ability to invade surrounding tissue. Specific chemotherapeutic strategies seeking to inactivate or inhibit MMP-2–facilitated tumor invasion have been successful in test models. One strategy is to utilize the natural inhibitors of MMP-2 proteinases, called tissue inhibitors of matrix metalloproteinases. Another strategy involves mimicking the propeptide activation domain of the protein, effectively maintaining MMP-2 in its inactive form. A similar strategy involves developing synthetic analogs that mimic the substrate of the enzyme, acting as active site inhibitors [*Oncologist*. 1999; 4(6):509–511]. Such chemotherapeutic strategies to impede the effects of MMP-2 may be of value in guiding corneal neovascularization pharmaceutical approaches.

Other Antineovascular Drugs

There are a number of other antineovascular drugs and compounds that have been proposed, exploiting a number of mechanisms. Heparin has demonstrated immunoreactivity with bFGF. Cyclosporin A[56] and nonsteroidal anti-inflammatory drugs[104] reduce interleukin (IL)-2–induced corneal neovascularization, methotrexate possibly inhibits both macrophage invasion during early angiogenesis and endothelial cell proliferation,[105] Tacrolimus (FK506) induces immunosuppression by inhibiting both T-lymphocyte signal transduction and IL-2 transcription,[106] and thalidomide inhibits bFGF- and VEGF-induced corneal neovascularization.[107,108] PEDF has recently been identified as an angiogenic inhibitor that typically aids in maintaining the quiescent vasculature in disease-free cornea and thus may be of therapeutic value in pathological neovascularization.[39]

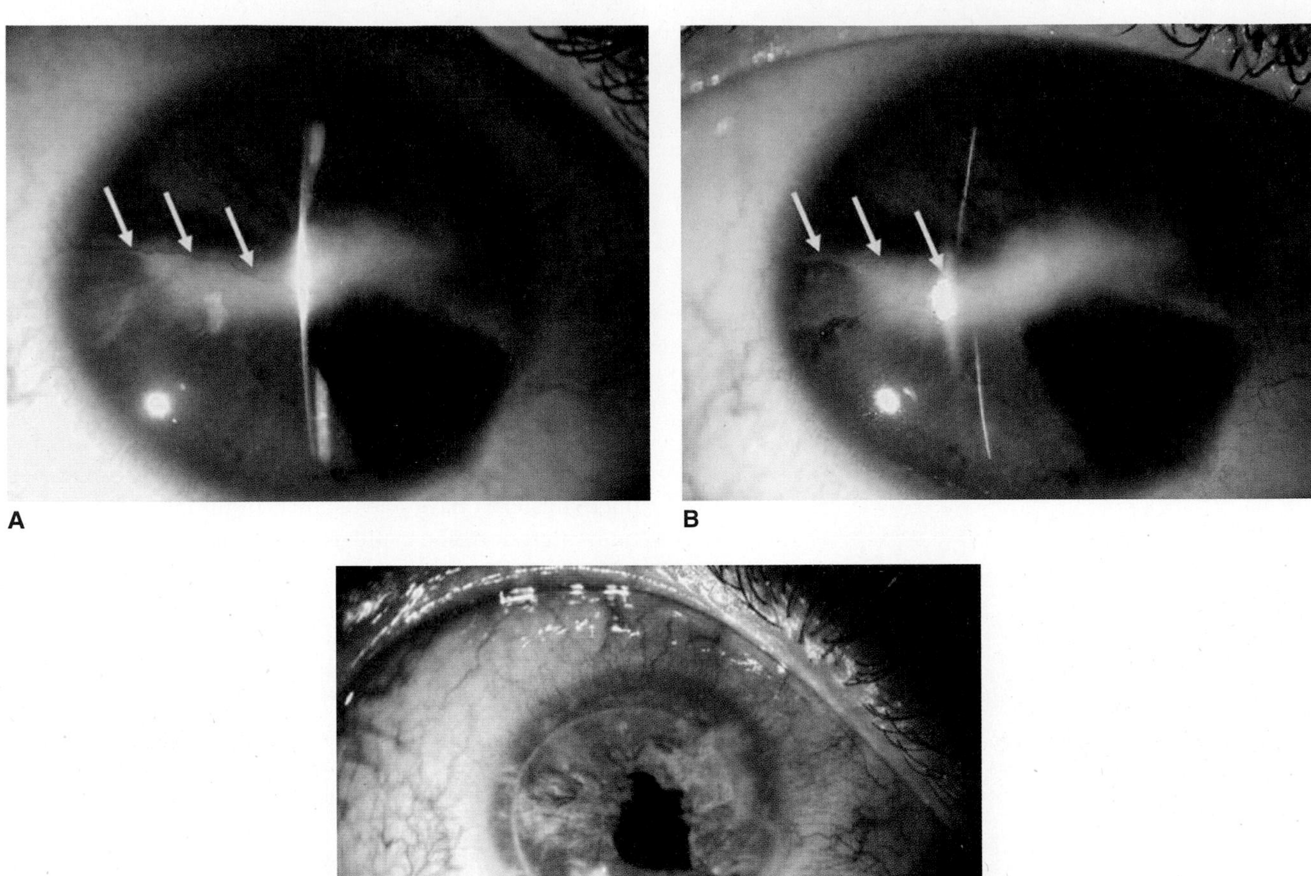

FIGURE 24.6. **A**: Slit lamp view of the right eye (patient A.K.) before bevacizumab and argon laser treatment: neovascularized central corneal scar with extensive anterior synechiae, aphakia, and traumatic/iatrogenic iris coloboma. The arrows indicate the main pathologic vessel. **B**: Slit lamp view of the right eye (patient A.K.) 4 weeks after bevacizumab and argon laser treatment: neovascularization is markedly reduced. The arrows indicate the former main pathologic vessel. **C**: Slit lamp view of the right eye (patient A.K.) 18 months after keratoplasty, irisplasty, vitrectomy, and intraocular bevacizumab injection: neovascularization did not return. The 8-mm corneal transplant is clear. (Reproduced from Gerten, et al. *Cornea*. 2008;27:1195–1199, with permission.)

Combination Treatments

Argon laser coagulation provides a potential treatment in closing pathologic blood vessels in the cornea.[109] Combination of bevacizumab injections and argon laser coagulation prior to PKP may be a promising tool to enhance transplant survival[110] (Fig. 24.6). A recent study demonstrated the inhibition of corneal neovascularization with topically administered combinations of triamcinolone acetonide with low molecular weight heparin.[83] Triamcinolone acetonide and doxycycline combinations also demonstrated efficient suppression of corneal neovascularization; yet these drugs were ineffective at similar concentrations used alone.[83]

CONCLUSION

The cornea is a highly complex transparent optical organ, which employs unique structural features and molecular mechanisms in order to maintain its function and transparency throughout life. The disruption of corneal integrity is thus affected by malfunctioning of any of the steps involved in the maintenance of structural architecture or the factors involved in prevention of angiogenesis and lymphangiogenesis. Corneal transparency which can be compromised by neovascularization is a prevalent health concern affecting millions. Recent research has promoted better understanding of factors, mechanisms, and causes of corneal neovascularization as well as treatment modalities.

However, much research is still needed to improve our understanding of this phenomenon.

KEY POINTS

- The cornea actively maintains an avascular state. The importance of corneal avascularity is underscored by its conservation across nearly all vertebrate species.
- The antiangiogenic state in cornea is maintained by factors that modify or are derived from components of the ECM, and a group of endothelial growth factors and other related signaling molecules known to regulate endothelial cell activation, vessel growth, and angiogenesis.
- Both VEGF-A and sFlt-1 are expressed at high levels in normal avascular corneal tissue.
- Causes of corneal neovascularization can be described in these categories: inflammatory (graft rejection, optimizing surgical technique, ocular cicatricial pemphigoid, Stevens-Johnson, and conjunctivitis), infectious (herpes zoster and herpes simplex, pseudomonas, chlamydia trachomatis and syphilis, and fungal infections), and trauma.
- Steroids have remained the mainstay therapeutic strategy in the prevention of corneal neovascularization.
- VEGF inhibitors like bevacizumab (both eye drops and subconjunctival injections) may have role as adjunct to improve prognosis in PKP.
- Bevacizumab is effective in acute KNV and has no toxicity. Chronic NV requires multiple therapy/injections. However, ghost vessels persist.
- Propolis extracts and doxycycline (inhibitors of MMP-2) have also been found to effectively suppress corneal neovascularization.
- A combination therapy of bevacizumab injections and argon laser coagulation prior to PKP may be a promising tool to enhance transplant survival.

REFERENCES

1. Ambati BK, Nozaki M, Singh N, et al. Corneal avascularity is due to soluble VEGF receptor-1. *Nature*. 2006;443 (7114):993–997.
2. Cursiefen C, Rummelt C, Jünemann A, et al. Absence of blood and lymphatic vessels in the developing human cornea. *Cornea*. 2006;25(6):722–726.
3. Cursiefen C, Chen L, Saint-Geniez M, et al. Nonvascular VEGF receptor 3 expression by corneal epithelium maintains avascularity and vision. *Proc Natl Acad Sci USA*. 2006;103(30):11405–11410.
4. Davanger M, Evensen A. Role of the pericorneal papillary structure in renewal of corneal epithelium. *Nature*. 1971; 229(5286):560–561.
5. Dua HS, Azuara-Blanco A. Limbal stem cells of the corneal epithelium. *Surv Ophthalmol*. 2000;44(5):415–425.
6. Dua HS, Joseph A, Shanmuganathan VA, et al. Stem cell differentiation and the effects of deficiency. *Eye*. 2003;17(8):877–885.
7. Dua HS, Kulkarni B, Singh R. Quest for limbal stem cells. *Clin Experiment Ophthalmol*. 2006;34(1):1–2.
8. Ebato B, Friend J, Thoft RA. Comparison of central and peripheral human corneal epithelium in tissue culture. *Invest Ophthalmol Vis Sci*. 1987;28(9):1450–1456.
9. Matsuda M, Ubels JL, Edelhauser HF. A larger corneal epithelial wound closes at a faster rate. *Invest Ophthalmol Vis Sci*. 1985;26(6):897–900.
10. Townsend WM. The limbal palisades of Vogt. *Trans Am Ophthalmol Soc*. 1991;89:721–756.
11. Tseng SC. Concept and application of limbal stem cells. *Eye*. 1989;3(Pt 2):141–157.
12. Ti SE, Grueterich M, Espana EM, et al. Correlation of long term phenotypic and clinical outcomes following limbal epithelial transplantation cultivated on amniotic membrane in rabbits. *Br J Ophthalmol*. 2004;88(3):422–427.
13. Azar DT. Corneal angiogenic privilege: angiogenic and antiangiogenic factors in corneal avascularity, vasculogenesis, and wound healing (an American Ophthalmological Society thesis). *Trans Am Ophthalmol Soc*. 2006;104:264–302.
14. Cornelius LA, Nehring LC, Harding E, et al. Matrix metalloproteinases generate angiostatin: effects on neovascularization. *J Immunol*. 1998;161(12):6845–6852.
15. Ferreras M, et al. Generation and degradation of human endostatin proteins by various proteinases. *FEBS Lett*. 2000;486(3):247–251.
16. Gabison E, Chang JH, Hernández-Quintela E, et al. Antiangiogenic role of angiostatin during corneal wound healing. *Exp Eye Res*. 2004;78(3):579–589.
17. Lin HC, Chang JH, Jain S, et al. Matrilysin cleavage of corneal collagen type XVIII NC1 domain and generation of a 28-kDa fragment. *Invest Ophthalmol Vis Sci*. 2001;42(11):2517–2524.
18. Warejcka DJ, Vaughan KA, Bernstein AM, et al. Differential conversion of plasminogen to angiostatin by human corneal cell populations. *Mol Vis*. 2005;11:859–868.
19. Kure T, Chang JH, Kato T, et al. Corneal neovascularization after excimer keratectomy wounds in matrilysin-deficient mice. *Invest Ophthalmol Vis Sci*. 2003;44(1):137–144.
20. Ambati BK, et al. Angiostatin inhibits and regresses corneal neovascularization. *Arch Ophthalmol*. 2002;120(8):1063–1068.
21. Lai LJ, Xiao X, Wu JH. Inhibition of corneal neovascularization with endostatin delivered by adeno-associated viral (AAV) vector in a mouse corneal injury model. *J Biomed Sci*. 2007;14(3):313–322.
22. Armstrong DJ, Hiscott P, Batterbury M, et al. Corneal stromal cells (keratocytes) express thrombospondins 2 and 3 in wound repair phenotype. *Int J Biochem Cell Biol*. 2002;34(6):588–593.
23. Cursiefen C, Massli S, Ng TF, et al. Roles of thrombospondin-1 and -2 in regulating corneal and iris angiogenesis. *Invest Ophthalmol Vis Sci*. 2004;45(4):1117–1124.
24. Sekiyama E, Nakamura T, Cooper LJ, et al. Unique distribution of thrombospondin-1 in human ocular surface epithelium. *Invest Ophthalmol Vis Sci*. 2006;47(4):1352–1358.

25. Jimenez B, Volpert OV, Crawford SE, et al. Signals leading to apoptosis-dependent inhibition of neovascularization by thrombospondin-1. *Nat Med*. 2000;6(1):41–48.
26. Simantov R, Febbraio M, Silverstein RL. The antiangiogenic effect of thrombospondin-2 is mediated by CD36 and modulated by histidine-rich glycoprotein. *Matrix Biol*. 2005; 24(1):27–34.
27. Lawler J. The functions of thrombospondin-1 and-2. *Curr Opin Cell Biol*. 2000;12(5):634–640.
28. Simantov R, Febbraio M, Crombie R, et al. Histidine-rich glycoprotein inhibits the antiangiogenic effect of thrombospondin-1. *J Clin Invest*. 2001;107(1):45–52.
29. Volpert OV, Tolsma SS, Pellerin S, et al. Inhibition of angiogenesis by thrombospondin-2. *Biochem Biophys Res Commun*. 1995;217(1):326–332.
30. Mwaikambo BR, Sennlaub F, Ong H, et al. Genetic ablation of CD36 induces age-related corneal neovascularization. *Cornea*. 2008;27(9):1037–1041.
31. Mwaikambo BR, Sennlaub F, Ong H, et al. Activation of CD36 inhibits and induces regression of inflammatory corneal neovascularization. *Invest Ophthalmol Vis Sci*. 2006;47(10):4356–4364.
32. Duenas Z, Torner L, Corbacho AM, et al. Inhibition of rat corneal angiogenesis by 16-kDa prolactin and by endogenous prolactin-like molecules. *Invest Ophthalmol Vis Sci*. 1999;40(11):2498–2505.
33. Clapp C, Torner L, Gutiérrez-Ospina G, et al. The prolactin gene is expressed in the hypothalamic-neurohypophyseal system and the protein is processed into a 14-kDa fragment with activity like 16-kDa prolactin. *Proc Natl Acad Sci USA*. 1994;91(22):10384–10388.
34. Mircheff AK, Warren DW, Wood RL, et al. Prolactin localization, binding, and effects on peroxidase release in rat exorbital lacrimal gland. *Invest Ophthalmol Vis Sci*. 1992;33(3):641–650.
35. Ochoa A, Montes de Oca P, Rivera JC, et al. Expression of prolactin gene and secretion of prolactin by rat retinal capillary endothelial cells. *Invest Ophthalmol Vis Sci*. 2001;42(7):1639–1645.
36. Chang JH, et al. Corneal neovascularization. *Curr Opin Ophthalmol*. 2001;12(4):242–249.
37. Becerra SP, Palmer I, Kumar A, et al. Overexpression of fetal human pigment epithelium-derived factor in *Escherichia coli*. A functionally active neurotrophic factor. *J Biol Chem*. 1993;268(31):23148–23156.
38. Ogata N, Wada M, Otsuji T, et al. Expression of pigment epithelium-derived factor in normal adult rat eye and experimental choroidal neovascularization. *Invest Ophthalmol Vis Sci*. 2002;43(4):1168–1175.
39. Dawson DW, Volpert OV, Gills P, et al. Pigment epithelium-derived factor: a potent inhibitor of angiogenesis. *Science*. 1999;285(5425):245–248.
40. Cai J, Jiang WG, Grant MB, et al. Pigment epithelium-derived factor inhibits angiogenesis via regulated intracellular proteolysis of vascular endothelial growth factor receptor 1. *J Biol Chem*. 2006;281(6):3604–3613.
41. Renard RA, et al. Eye phenotype of pigment epithelium-derived factor knockout mice. *Invest Ophthalmol Vis Sci*. 2003;44:2888.
42. Amano S, Rohan R, Kuroki M, et al. Requirement for vascular endothelial growth factor in wound- and inflammation-related corneal neovascularization. *Invest Ophthalmol Vis Sci*. 1998;39(1):18–22.
43. Cursiefen C, Chen L, Dana MR, et al. Corneal lymphangiogenesis: evidence, mechanisms, and implications for corneal transplant immunology. *Cornea*. 2003;22(3):273–281.
44. Kenyon BM, Voest EE, Chen CC, et al. A model of angiogenesis in the mouse cornea. *Invest Ophthalmol Vis Sci*. 1996;37(8):1625–1632.
45. Ponticelli S, Marasco D, Tarallo V, et al. Modulation of angiogenesis by a tetrameric tripeptide that antagonizes vascular endothelial growth factor receptor 1. *J Biol Chem*. 2008;283(49):34250–34259.
46. Ambati BK, Patterson E, Jani P, et al. Soluble vascular endothelial growth factor receptor-1 contributes to the corneal antiangiogenic barrier. *Br J Ophthalmol*. 2007;91(4):505–508.
47. Lee P, Wang CC, Adamis A. Ocular neovascularization: an epidemiologic review. *Surv Ophthalmol*. 1998;43(3): 245–269.
48. Kaminska GM, Niederkorn JY. Spontaneous corneal neovascularization in nude mice. Local imbalance between angiogenic and anti-angiogenic factors. *Invest Ophthalmol Vis Sci*. 1993;34(1):222–230.
49. Cursiefen C, Kuchle M, Naumann GO. Angiogenesis in corneal diseases: histopathologic evaluation of 254 human corneal buttons with neovascularization. *Cornea*. 1998;17(6):611–613.
50. Dua HS, Azuara-Blanco A. Corneal allograft rejection: risk factors, diagnosis, prevention, and treatment. *Indian J Ophthalmol*. 1999;47(1):3–9.
51. Dana MR, Schaumberg DA, Kowal VO, et al. Corneal neovascularization after penetrating keratoplasty. *Cornea*. 1995;14(6):604–609.
52. Kuchle M, Cursiefen C, Nguyen NX, et al. Risk factors for corneal allograft rejection: intermediate results of a prospective normal-risk keratoplasty study. *Graefes Arch Clin Exp Ophthalmol*. 2002;240(7):580–584.
53. Weisbrod DJ, Sit M, Naor J, et al. Outcomes of repeat penetrating keratoplasty and risk factors for graft failure. *Cornea*. 2003;22(5):429–434.
54. Lam VM, Nguyen NX, Martus P, et al. Surgery-related factors influencing corneal neovascularization after low-risk keratoplasty. *Am J Ophthalmol*. 2006;141(2):260–266.
55. Cursiefen C, Martus P, Nguyen NX, et al. Corneal neovascularization after nonmechanical versus mechanical corneal trephination for non-high-risk keratoplasty. *Cornea*. 2002;21(7):648–652.
56. Dana MR, Streilein JW. Loss and restoration of immune privilege in eyes with corneal neovascularization. *Invest Ophthalmol Vis Sci*. 1996;37(12):2485–2494.
57. Ogawa S, Yoshida S, Ono M, et al. Induction of macrophage inflammatory protein-1alpha and vascular endothelial growth factor during inflammatory neovascularization in the mouse cornea. *Angiogenesis*. 1999;3(4):327–334.
58. Chan LS, Ahmed AR, Anhalt GJ, et al. The first international consensus on mucous membrane pemphigoid: definition, diagnostic criteria, pathogenic factors, medical treatment, and prognostic indicators. *Arch Dermatol*. 2002;138(3):370–379.
59. Leonard JN, Hobday CM, Haffenden GP, et al. Immunofluorescent studies in ocular cicatricial pemphigoid. *Br J Dermatol*. 1988;118(2):209–217.
60. Tonnesen MG, Soter NA. Erythema multiforme. *J Am Acad Dermatol*. 1979;1(4):357–364.

61. Ono SJ, Abelson MB. Allergic conjunctivitis: update on pathophysiology and prospects for future treatment. *J Allergy Clin Immunol*. 2005;115(1):118–122.
62. Centifanto-Fitzgerald YM, Yamaguchi T, Kaufman HE, et al. Ocular disease pattern induced by herpes simplex virus is genetically determined by a specific region of viral DNA. *J Exp Med*. 1982;155(2):475–489.
63. Power WJ, Tugal-Tutkun I, Foster CS. Long-term follow-up of patients with atopic keratoconjunctivitis. *Ophthalmology*. 1998;105(4):637–642.
64. Thygeson P, Dawson CR. Trachoma and follicular conjunctivitis in children. *Arch Ophthalmol*. 1966;75(1):3–12.
65. Cavanagh HD, Colley AM. The molecular basis of neurotrophic keratitis. *Acta Ophthalmol Suppl*. 1989;192:115–134.
66. Tan MH, Bryars J, Moore J. Use of nerve growth factor to treat congenital neurotrophic corneal ulceration. *Cornea*. 2006;25(3):352–355.
67. Khokhar S, Natung T, Sony P, et al. Amniotic membrane transplantation in refractory neurotrophic corneal ulcers: a randomized, controlled clinical trial. *Cornea*. 2005;24(6):654–660.
68. Koniszewski G. Corneal neovascularization following short-term wear of soft contact lenses. *Klin Monatsbl Augenheilkd*. 1982;181(6):467–470.
69. Rakes JA. Corneal neovascularization from extended wear lenses. *J Am Optom Assoc*. 1983;54(3):259–261.
70. Wong AL, Weissman BA, Mondino BJ. Bilateral corneal neovascularization and opacification associated with unmonitored contact lens wear. *Am J Ophthalmol*. 2003;136(5):957–958.
71. Singh N, Higgins E, Amin S, et al. Unique homologous siRNA blocks hypoxia-induced VEGF upregulation in human corneal cells and inhibits and regresses murine corneal neovascularization. *Cornea*. 2007;26(1):65–72.
72. Nishida T, Yasumoto K, Morikawa Y, et al. Hard contact lens-induced corneal neovascularization treated by oxygenation. *Cornea*. 1991;10(4):358–360.
73. Singh N, Amin S, Richter E, et al. Flt-1 intraceptors inhibit hypoxia-induced VEGF expression in vitro and corneal neovascularization in vivo. *Invest Ophthalmol Vis Sci*. 2005;46(5):1647–1652.
74. Usui T, Yamagami S, Kishimoto S, et al. Role of macrophage migration inhibitory factor in corneal neovascularization. *Invest Ophthalmol Vis Sci*. 2007;48(8):3545–3550.
75. Allemann N, Chamon W, Silverman RH, et al. High-frequency ultrasound quantitative analyses of corneal scarring following excimer laser keratectomy. *Arch Ophthalmol*. 1993;111(7):968–973.
76. White JE, McClafferty K, Orton RB, et al. Ocular alkali burn associated with automobile air-bag activation. *CMAJ*. 1995;153(7):933–934.
77. Pfister RR. Chemical injuries of the eye. *Ophthalmology*. 1983;90(10):1246–1253.
78. Samolov B, Steen B, Seregard S, et al. Delayed inflammation-associated corneal neovascularization in MMP-2-deficient mice. *Exp Eye Res*. 2005;80(2):159–166.
79. Ormerod LD, Garsd A, Abelson MB, et al. Effects of altering the eicosanoid precursor pool on neovascularization and inflammation in the alkali-burned rabbit cornea. *Am J Pathol*. 1990;137(5):1243–1252.
80. Hayashi K, Ishibashi T. In vivo observations on experimental corneal neovascularization with a newly developed macroscope. *Graefes Arch Clin Exp Ophthalmol*. 1991;229(5):473–479.
81. Riazi-Esfahani M, Peyman GA, Aydin E, et al. Prevention of corneal neovascularization: evaluation of various commercially available compounds in an experimental rat model. *Cornea*. 2006;25(7):801–805.
82. Murata M, Shimizu S, Horiuchi S, et al. Inhibitory effect of triamcinolone acetonide on corneal neovascularization. *Graefes Arch Clin Exp Ophthalmol*. 2006;244(2):205–209.
83. Aydin E, Kivilcim M, Peyman GA, et al. Inhibition of experimental angiogenesis of cornea by various doses of doxycycline and combination of triamcinolone acetonide with low-molecular-weight heparin and doxycycline. *Cornea*. 2008;27(4):446–453.
84. Bock F, König Y, Dietrich T, et al. Inhibition of angiogenesis in the anterior chamber of the eye. *Ophthalmologe*. 2007;104(4):336–344.
85. Bock F, Onderka J, Dietrich T, et al. Bevacizumab as a potent inhibitor of inflammatory corneal angiogenesis and lymphangiogenesis. *Invest Ophthalmol Vis Sci*. 2007;48(6):2545–2552.
86. Gan L, Fagerholm P, Palmblad J. Vascular endothelial growth factor (VEGF) and its receptor VEGFR-2 in the regulation of corneal neovascularization and wound healing. *Acta Ophthalmol Scand*. 2004;82(5):557–563.
87. Philipp W, Speicher L, Humpel C. Expression of vascular endothelial growth factor and its receptors in inflamed and vascularized human corneas. *Invest Ophthalmol Vis Sci*. 2000;41(9):2514–2522.
88. Schmidt-Erfurth UM, Richard G, Augustin A, et al. Guidance for the treatment of neovascular age-related macular degeneration. *Acta Ophthalmol Scand*. 2007;85(5):486–494.
89. Ferrara N, Damico L, Shams N, et al. Development of ranibizumab, an anti-vascular endothelial growth factor antigen binding fragment, as therapy for neovascular age-related macular degeneration. *Retina*. 2006;26(8):859–870.
90. Avery RL, Pieramici DJ, Rabena MD, et al. Intravitreal bevacizumab (Avastin) for neovascular age-related macular degeneration. *Ophthalmology*. 2006;113(3):363–372.
91. Yoeruek E, Spitzer MS, Tatar O, et al. Safety profile of bevacizumab on cultured human corneal cells. *Cornea*. 2007;26(8):977–982.
92. Yoeruek E, Ziemssen F, Henke-Fahle S, et al. Safety, penetration and efficacy of topically applied bevacizumab: evaluation of eyedrops in corneal neovascularization after chemical burn. *Acta Ophthalmol*. 2008;86(3):322–328.
93. DeStafeno JJ, Kim T. Topical bevacizumab therapy for corneal neovascularization. *Arch Ophthalmol*. 2007;125(6):834–836.
94. Bock F, et al. Bevacizumab (Avastin) eye drops inhibit corneal neovascularization. *Graefes Arch Clin Exp Ophthalmol*. 2008;246(2):281–284.
95. Carrasco MA. Subconjunctival bevacizumab for corneal neovascularization in herpetic stromal keratitis. *Cornea*. 2008;27(6):743–745.
96. Papathanassiou M, Theodossiadis PG, Liarakos VS, et al. Inhibition of corneal neovascularization by subconjunctival bevacizumab in an animal model. *Am J Ophthalmol*. 2008;145(3):424–431.

97. You IC, Kang IS, Lee SH, et al. Therapeutic effect of subconjunctival injection of bevacizumab in the treatment of corneal neovascularization. *Acta Ophthalmol.* 2008.
98. Bahar I, Kaiserman I, McAllum P, et al. Subconjunctival bevacizumab injection for corneal neovascularization. *Cornea.* 2008;27(2):142–147.
99. Bahar I, Kaiserman I, McAllum P, et al. Subconjunctival bevacizumab injection for corneal neovascularization in recurrent pterygium. *Curr Eye Res.* 2008;33(1):23–28.
100. Kvanta A, Sarman S, Fagerholm P, et al. Expression of matrix metalloproteinase-2 (MMP-2) and vascular endothelial growth factor (VEGF) in inflammation-associated corneal neovascularization. *Exp Eye Res.* 2000;70(4): 419–428.
101. Totan Y, Aydin E, Cekic O, et al. Effect of caffeic acid phenethyl ester on corneal neovascularization in rats. *Curr Eye Res.* 2001;23(4):291–297.
102. Keshavarz M, Mostafaie A, Mansouri K, et al. Inhibition of corneal neovascularization with propolis extract. *Arch Med Res.* 2009;40(1):59–61.
103. Goodsell DS. The molecular perspective: Matrix Metalloproteinase 2. *Oncologist.* 1999;4:509-511.
104. Deutsch TA, Hughes WF. Suppressive effects of indomethacin on thermally induced neovascularization of rabbit corneas. *Am J Ophthalmol.* 1979;87(4):536–540.
105. Joussen AM, Kruse FE, Völcker HE, et al. Topical application of methotrexate for inhibition of corneal angiogenesis. *Graefes Arch Clin Exp Ophthalmol.* 1999;237(11):920–927.
106. Benelli U, Lepri A, Del Tacca M, et al. FK-506 delays corneal graft rejection in a model of corneal xenotransplantation. *J Ocul Pharmacol Ther.* 1996;12(4):425–431.
107. Abbas A, Khan B, Feroze AH, et al. Thalidomide prevents donor corneal graft neovascularization in an alkali burn model of corneal angiogenesis. *J Pak Med Assoc.* 2002;52(10):476–482.
108. Kenyon BM, Browne F, D'Amato RJ. Effects of thalidomide and related metabolites in a mouse corneal model of neovascularization. *Exp Eye Res.* 1997;64(6):971–978.
109. Gordon YJ, Mann RK, Mah TS, et al. Fluorescein-potentiated argon laser therapy improves symptoms and appearance of corneal neovascularization. *Cornea.* 2002;21(8):770–773.
110. Gerten G. Bevacizumab (avastin) and argon laser to treat neovascularization in corneal transplant surgery. *Cornea.* 2008;27(10):1195–1199.

CHAPTER 25

Neovascular Glaucoma

Hylton R. Mayer • James C. Tsai

INTRODUCTION

Neovascular glaucoma (NVG) is characterized by anterior chamber fibrovascular proliferation that causes elevated intraocular pressure (IOP). Significant and/or prolonged ocular hypertension (OHT) caused by NVG can result in glaucomatous optic neuropathy, varying degrees of visual field and vision loss, and ultimately blindness. Vascular endothelial growth factor (VEGF) and other angiogenic mediators play a key role in the development of anterior chamber neovascularization. The management of NVG requires a multifaceted approach to control IOP while decreasing or eliminating fibrovascular proliferation (Fig. 25.1). Recombinant anti-VEGF intraocular injections (off-label use for NVG) have become more commonly used in the management of NVG to dramatically and effectively eliminate clinically appreciable anterior segment neovascularization. Based on multiple anecdotal reports and a few small retrospective and prospective studies, the use of anti-VEGF agents for the management of NVG has improved clinicians' ability to treat patients with a historically difficult and devastating type of glaucoma.

CAUSES OF ANTERIOR CHAMBER NEOVASCULARIZATION

While many pathologic ocular processes can initiate fibrovascular proliferation, ischemic retinal disease is the most common cause of anterior chamber neovascularization (Table 25.1).[1] Proliferative diabetic retinopathy and central retinal vein occlusion are each responsible for about one third of cases of neovascularization of the iris (NVI).[2] Retinal ischemia from various disorders such as rhegmatogenous retinal detachment or vascular pathology account for the remaining one third of cases. Only about 3% of NVG cases are due to nonischemic causes, such as tumors or ocular inflammation.[2] The crystalline lens, lens capsule, and vitreous appear to act as natural barriers to the diffusion of angiogenic mediators into the anterior chamber; consequently, anterior segment neovascularization is often seen after vitrectomy or disruption of the posterior capsule in eyes with predisposing ocular pathology.[3,4,5,6] The ocular pathology causing NVG is typically obvious, identifiable by careful slit-lamp biomicroscopy, gonioscopy, and fundus examination. Occasionally, the etiology of NVG is unclear, and ancillary testing is necessary to detect occult pathology. Recognition of the underlying proangiogenic pathology is critical for successful treatment of NVG in order to effectively reduce the angiogenic mediators that promote anterior chamber neovascularization.

Microscopic analysis has revealed that the new, abnormal blood vessels arise from iris stromal vessels and spread onto the anterior iris surface.[7] Anterior segment neovascularization is characterized microscopically by thin, fenestrated blood vessels that grow in irregular patterns.[8,9,10] Clinical and microscopic analysis has identified fibrovascular tissue developing over anterior segment structures, including the trabecular meshwork and in intertrabecular spaces.[7,8,9,10,11]

CLINICOPATHOLOGIC STAGES

A spectrum of clinicopathologic stages may be identified in the development of NVG and can be useful for diagnostic classification, for developing treatment plans, and for prognostic direction (Fig. 25.2).[3] Anterior chamber neovascularization in the setting of normal IOP characterizes the preglaucoma stage. In the open-angle stage, IOP elevates when a fine fibrovascular membrane obstructs a gonioscopically open angle. The closed-angle stage occurs when the fibrovascular membrane contracts, causing varying degrees of peripheral anterior synechiae (PAS). Ultimately, obstruction of aqueous outflow causes elevated IOP, acutely or chronically, and is the primary mechanism by which glaucomatous optic neuropathy and ultimate visual field and vision loss may occur.

A high index of suspicion in the setting of common predisposing conditions, and a careful and comprehensive ocular exam, including gonioscopy, are necessary to detect NVI and/or neovascularization of the angle (NVA).

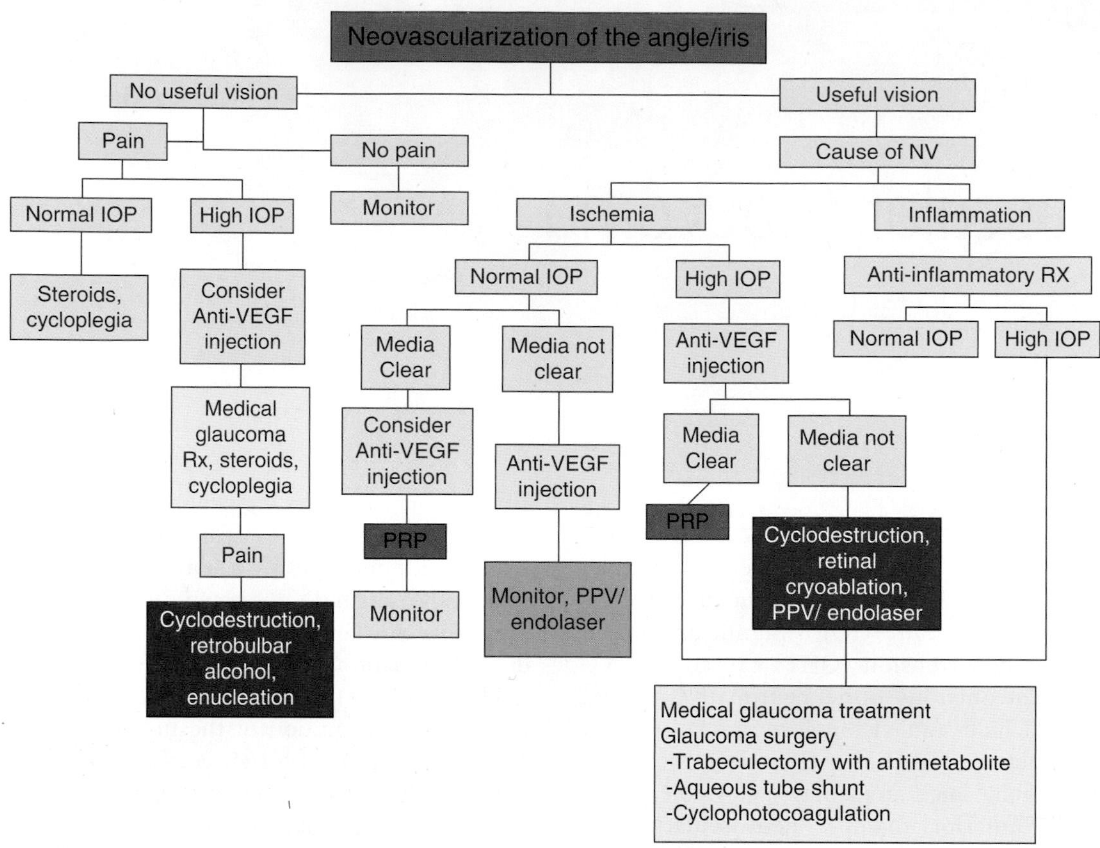

FIGURE 25.1. Algorithm regarding the management of neovascular glaucoma.

Iris or gonioscopic fluorescein angiography may be useful to detect NVI or NVA when rubeosis is not visualized by slit-lamp biomicroscopy.[12] Although NVI is typically appreciated prior to NVA, NVA may precede NVI in about 10% of eyes with retinal ischemia, highlighting the importance of gonioscopy in high-risk eyes.[13–15]

TREATMENT MODALITIES

Panretinal Photocoagulation

Panretinal photocoagulation (PRP) is the standard anti-angiogenic treatment for NVG caused by ischemic retinal disease.[16–19] Extensive PRP, usually 1,500 to 2,000 or more spots over two sessions, is necessary to decrease vasoproliferative factors.[20] PRP is believed to work by reducing the production of angiogenic mediators by the ablated and scarred retina.[21] In addition, PRP may work by creating a shunt through the scarred retinal tissue that improves oxygen delivery to the retina from the choroid.[22,23] While PRP is necessary for the long-term control of angiogenesis, it may take multiple sessions and 2 to 4 weeks after the laser therapy for regression of anterior chamber neovascularization, during which time aqueous outflow obstruction and synechial angle closure may persist or progress.[24] Intraocular anti-VEGF injections can offer rapid and effective adjunctive therapy to reduce anterior chamber neovascularization.

Anti-VEGF Drugs

Early anti-VEGF pharmacotherapy, either bevacizumab (Avastin [Genentech, South San Francisco, CA]) or ranibizumab (Lucentis [Genentech]), has been shown to promptly eliminate clinical evidence of anterior chamber neovascularization (Figs. 25.3–25.5).[25–29] Pathophysiologic analysis of trabecular meshwork sections, obtained at the time of trabeculectomy surgery from patients with NVG who received bevacizumab, demonstrated that despite clinical regression of NVA, neovascular tissue in angle structures persisted, but the remaining vascular tissue lacked normal fenestrations.[11] Early regression of angle neovascularization in the preglaucoma and open-angle stages of NVG can prevent the formation of PAS and preserve normal aqueous outflow routes. Maintenance of normal angle anatomy may eliminate the need for long-term IOP lowering therapy or may decrease the need for medical therapy or incisional surgery to treat NVG.[30,31]

IOP Control

In addition to reducing angiogenic mediators and anterior segment neovascularization, IOP control is important for short- and long-term ocular health. Topical IOP lowering therapy is typically rapidly increased to maximum tolerated medications, due to the refractory course of IOP control in patients with NVG. Barring contraindications

Table 25.1.

Diseases associated with neovascular glaucoma

Retinal ischemic diseases
Diabetes
Central retinal vein occlusion
Ocular ischemic syndrome/carotid occlusive disease
Central retinal artery occlusion
Retinal detachment
Leber congenital amaurosis
Coats disease
Eales disease
Sickle cell retinopathy
Retinal hemangioma
Persistent hyperplastic primary vitreous
Norrie disease
Wyburn-Mason
Carotid-cavernous fistula
Dural shunt
Stickler syndrome
X-linked retinoschisis
Takayasu aortitis
Juxtafoveal telangiectasia
Surgically induced
Carotid endarterectomy
Cataract extraction
Pars plana vitrectomy/lensectomy
Silicone oil
Scleral buckle
Neodymium: yttrium-aluminum-garnet capsulotomy
Laser coreoplasty
Tumors
Iris: melanoma, hemangioma, metastatic lesion
Ciliary body: ring melanoma
Retina: retinoblastoma, large cell lymphoma
Choroid: melanoma
Conjunctiva: squamous cell carcinoma
Radiation
External beam
Charged particle: proton, helium
Plaques
Photoradiation
Inflammatory diseases
Uveitis: chronic iridocyclitis, Behcet disease
Vogt-Koyanagi-Harada syndrome
Syphilitic retinitis
Sympathetic ophthalmia
Endophthalmitis
Miscellaneous
Vitreous wick syndrome
Interferon-α

Data from Sivak-Callcott JA, O'Day DM, Gass JDM, et al. Evidence-based recommendations for the diagnosis and treatment of neovascular glaucoma. *Ophthalmology*. 2001;108: 1767–1778.

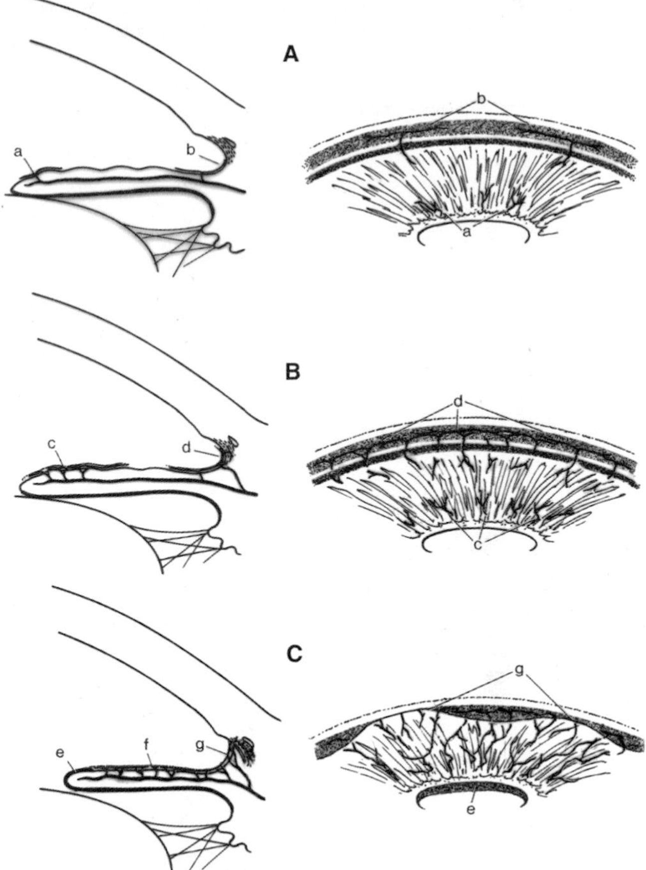

FIGURE 25.2. Clinicopathologic stages of neovascular glaucoma include (**A**) the preglaucoma stage with normal IOPs in the setting of iris (a) and angle neovascularization (b). **B:** The open-angle stage characterized by IOP elevation in the setting of iris neovascularization (c) and a fine fibrovascular membrane obstructing a gonioscopically open angle (d). **C:** The closed-angle stage occurs when the iris (f) and angle fibrovascular membrane contract, causing varying degrees of PAS (g) and ectropion uvea (e). (Reproduced from Allingham RR, Damji KF, Freedman S, et al. *Shields' Textbook of Glaucoma*. 5th ed. Philadelphia, PA: Lippincott Williams & Wilkins, 2004;330–335, with permission.)

related to allergies or systemic comorbidities, IOP control usually requires a combination of a beta-blocker, carbonic anhydrase inhibitor (CAI), and alpha-agonist. If these first-line medications do not adequately control IOP, a prostaglandin analog may occasionally be effective, despite decreased uveoscleral outflow due to peripheral anterior synechia or coexisting ocular inflammation. In a controlled study with adult patients, adding a systemic CAI to a topical CAI did not decrease aqueous production, although IOP lowering was appreciated in a similar study with pediatric patients.[32,33] In the authors' experience, the addition of a systemic CAI in a patient using a topical CAI occasionally lowers IOP, possibly from improved medication compliance/delivery. Often, a topical steroid and a cycloplegic agent are used to control associated ocular inflammation and pain. Despite aggressive antiangiogenic

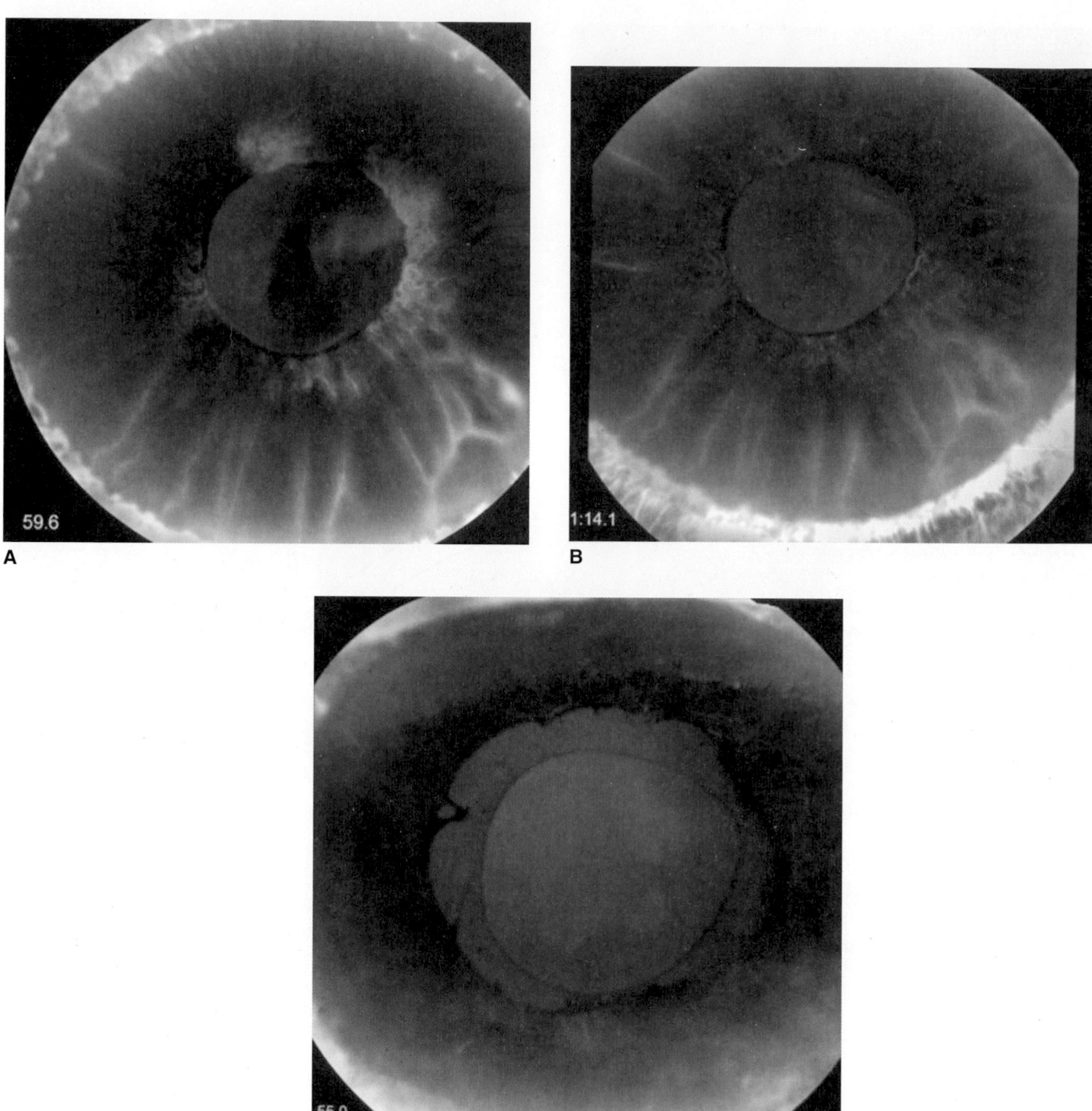

FIGURE 25.3. A: Iris fluorescein angiogram revealing florid rubeosis iridis before bevacizumab injection. **B:** Iris fluorescein angiogram showing marked improvement of rubeosis iridis 5 days after bevacizumab injection. **C:** Iris fluorescein angiogram demonstrating nearly resolved rubeosis 8 weeks after bevacizumab injection. (Reproduced from Davidorf, et al. *Retina.* 2006; 26:354–356, with permission.)

therapy and maximum IOP lowering medications, many patients present with or develop such extensive synechial angle closure that medical therapy alone is unable to adequately control IOP (Box 25.1).

Surgical Treatment

A trabeculectomy with antimetabolites is a reasonable consideration for surgically controlling IOP in the setting of NVG, although numerous studies have demonstrated poor long-term success, especially in young patients with diabetes.[34–38] Adjunctive use of anti-VEGF medications and tight control of proangiogenic factors have recently demonstrated decreased intraoperative complications such as hyphema and improved short-term outcomes after trabeculectomy with mitomycin C for patients with NVG.[39–43] In addition, anti-VEGF therapy

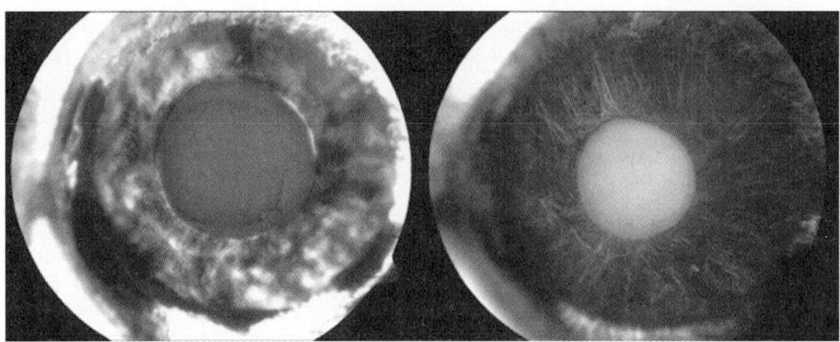

FIGURE 25.4. Iris rubeosis due to occlusive ischemic retinopathy. Iris fluorescein angiography of the right eye taken 5 days before (**Left**) and 2 days after (**Right**) intracameral injection of bevacizumab. Pictures were taken in the early phase (10 seconds) of angiography. (Reproduced from Grisanti, et al. *Am J Ophthalmol.* 2006;142:158–160, with permission.)

may result in decreased scarring and encapsulation of trabeculectomy blebs or glaucoma drainage implant blebs.[44,45] If IOP levels and optic nerve health permit, it may be reasonable and beneficial to delay any incisional surgery for 2 to 3 days after anti-VEGF injection, to wait for a reduction of anterior chamber neovascularization. In addition, anti-VEGF injections may be necessary postoperatively to control neovascularization and/or modulate wound healing.

Various glaucoma implants have been demonstrated to have similar long-term outcomes in the setting of NVG.[46–53] Baerveldt glaucoma implants are one type of glaucoma drainage device that have been used extensively for refractory glaucomas. Advantages of the Baerveldt implants are that they have a low profile and posterior bleb formation, a larger plate surface area that may result in lower rates of adjunctive medication necessary for IOP control, and no valve mechanism to that can malfunction. Because the Baerveldt implant lacks a valve mechanism, it is necessary to limit flow through the tube, prior to the encapsulation of the plate, to reduce *hypotony* and anterior chamber shallowing. A dissolvable ligature or a ligature and ripcord suture in the lumen of the tube can effectively reduce flow through the tube, resulting in a period of time, usually about 6 weeks, when the IOP may remain at preoperative levels. Many surgeons create slits in the tube lumen to lower IOP by allowing some venting of aqueous through the tube prior to release of the tube ligature. The authors currently prefer to place a glaucoma drainage implant, typically an Ahmed FP-7, when medical therapy fails to achieve safe IOPs. The Ahmed implant's valve mechanism enables predictable and effective early IOP lowering, especially in patients who may present with significantly elevated IOPs preoperatively and

BOX 25.1 Clinical Trials in Neovascular Glaucoma

1. Lucentis Vs. Mitomycin C During Glaucoma Surgery, Wills Eye: Recruiting
2. Ranibizumab in Preventing Failure of Ahmed Valve Glaucoma Surgery, UCSF.
3. Use of Ranibizumab with Mitomycin C During Trabeculectomy, Univ. Colorado.
4. Treatment of Failing Blebs with Ranibizumab, NYEEI.
5. Lucentis for New Onset Neovascular Glaucoma (NVG), University of Illinois.
6. Trabeculectomy With Mitomycin C Associated With Sub-Conjunctival Injection of Ranibizumab, Maisonneuve-Rosemont Hospital, Canada.
7. Rubeosis Anti-VEGF (RAVE) Trial for Ischemic Central Retinal Vein Occlusion, Greater Houston Retina Research.
8. Subconjunctival Bevacizumab to Prevent Bleb Failure after Glaucoma Filtration Surgery, Grewal Eye Institute, India.
9. Intravitreal Bevacizumab for Neovascular Glaucoma, Shaheed Beheshti, Iran.
10. Intraocular Bevacizumab (Avastin) for Rubeosis Iridis, Instituto de Olhos de Goiania, Brazil.
11. Bevacizumab for Central Retinal Vein Occlusion Study, St. Erik Eye Hospital, Sweden.
12. Subconjunctival Bevacizumab Effect on Bleb Vascularity, Rabin Medical Center, Israel.
13. Bleb Vascularity Change After Subconjunctival Injection Bevacizumab, Capital Medical University, China.
14. Does Adding Bevacizumab Therapy in Glaucoma Surgery Improve the Success of Needle Bleb Revisions? (Avastin), Wills Eye.

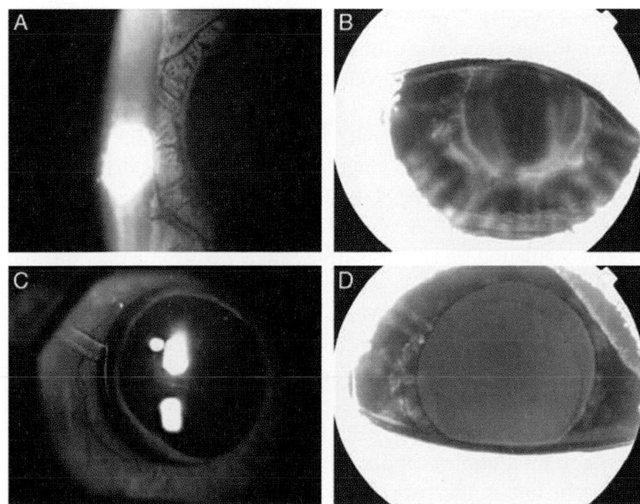

FIGURE 25.5. Iris rubeosis due to ocular ischemic syndrome (**A**). Regressed iris rubeosis 2 days after the intracameral bevacizumab injection and Ahmed glaucoma valve (AGV) implantation (**C**). Iris fluorescein angiography before (**B**) and 2 days after (**D**) intracameral bevacizumab injection and AGV implantation. (Reproduced from Shin, et al. *J Glaucoma.* 2009;18:589–594, with permission.)

who are likely to develop postoperative hypotony due to aqueous hyposecretion. Disadvantages of the Ahmed valve include the possibility of intrinsic valve dysfunction, blockage of the valve mechanism by blood or fibrin, and early exposure of the bleb to angiogenic and inflammatory mediators that may result in bleb encapsulation and failure.

If medical therapy inadequately controls IOP, the visual potential is poor, and/or the patient has significant social or medical contraindications to incisional surgery, cyclodestructive therapy is a reasonable option to control NVG.[54] The most widely employed cyclodestructive modality is via a transscleral diode laser. The laser energy can lower IOP by ablating the ciliary body, thereby decreasing aqueous production. The authors typically reserve cyclophotocoagulation as a last resort, due to a high rate of vision loss and the low but serious potential for phthisis, hypotony, and sympathetic ophthalmia.[55–59]

KEY POINTS

- Reduction or elimination of vision loss from NVG requires early diagnosis of anterior segment neovascularization, prompt identification of the etiology, effective reduction of angiogenic factors, and appropriate management of IOP.
- Further research into angiogenic mediators and the role of anti-VEGF agents in the management of NVG may help to improve clinicians' understanding and management of a historically refractory type of glaucoma (Box 25.2).

BOX 25.2 Clinical Significance

- Successful management of NVG requires a multifaceted approach to control IOP while decreasing or eliminating fibrovascular proliferation.
- The etiology of NVG is often obvious, but subspecialty evaluation (e.g., fluorescein angiography or B-scan ultrasound) may be necessary to identify the underlying cause.
- Early reduction of anterior segment neovascularization, utilizing anti-VEGF agents, may reduce ocular morbidity.
- Anti-VEGF agents may improve surgical outcomes.

REFERENCES

1. Sivak-Callcott JA, O'Day DM, Gass JDM, et al. Evidence-based recommendations for the diagnosis and treatment of neovascular glaucoma. *Ophthalmology*. 2001;108:1767–1778.
2. Brown GC, Magargal LE, Schachat A, et al. Neovascular glaucoma. Etiologic considerations. *Ophthalmology*. 1984;91:315–320.
3. Allingham RR, Damji KF, Freedman S, et al. *Shields' Textbook of Glaucoma*. 5th ed. Philadelphia: Lippincott Williams & Wilkins; 2004;330–335.
4. Aiello LM, Wang M, Liang G. Neovascular glaucoma and vitreous hemorrhage after cataract surgery in patients with diabetes mellitus. *Ophthalmology*. 1983;90:814–820.
5. Rice TA, Michels RG, Maguire MG, et al. The effect of lensectomy on the incidence of iris neovascularization and neovascular glaucoma after vitrectomy for diabetic retinopathy. *Am J Ophthalmol*. 1983;95:1–11.
6. Poliner LS, Christianson DJ, Escoffery RF, et al. Neovascular glaucoma after intracapsular and extracapsular cataract extraction in diabetic patients. *Am J Ophthalmol*. 1985;100:637–643.
7. Henkind P. Ocular neovascularization. *Am J Ophthalmol*. 1978;85:287–301.
8. Schulze RR. Rubeosis iridis. *Am J Ophthalmol*. 1967;63:487–495.
9. Anderson DM, Morin JD, Hunter WS. Rubeosis iridis. *Can J Ophthalmol*. 1971;6:183–188.
10. Peyman GA, Raichand M, Juarez CP, et al. Hypotony and experimental rubeosis iridis in primate eyes. A clinicopathologic study. *Graefes Arch Clin Exp Ophthalmol*. 1986;224:435–442.
11. Kubota T, Aoki R, Harada Y, et al. Trabecular meshwork in neovascular glaucoma eyes after the intravitreal injection of bevacizumab. *Br J Ophthalmol*. 2009;93:557–558.
12. Sanborn GE, Symes DJ, Magargal LE. Fundus-iris fluorescein angiography: evaluation of its use in the diagnosis of rubeosis iridis. *Ann Ophthalmol*. 1986;18:52–58 [Erratum in: Ann Ophthalmol 1986;18:155].
13. Blinder KJ, Friedman SM, Mames RN. Diabetic iris neovascularization. *Am J Ophthalmol*. 1995;120:393–395.
14. Baseline and early natural history report. The Central Vein Occlusion Study. *Arch Ophthalmol*. 1993;11:1087–1095.
15. Browning DJ, Scott AQ, Peterson CB, et al. The risk of missing angle neovascularization by omitting screening gonioscopy in acute central retinal vein occlusion. *Ophthalmology*. 1998;105:776–784.
16. Little HL, Rosenthal AR, Dellaporta A, et al. The effect of pan-retinal photocoagulation on rubeosis iridis. *Am J Ophthalmol*. 1976;81:804–809.
17. Wand M, Dueker DK, Aiello LM, et al. Effects of panretinal photocoagulation on rubeosis iridis, angle neovascularization, and neovascular glaucoma. *Am J Ophthalmol*. 1978;86:332–339.
18. Pavan PR, Folk JC, Weingeist TA, et al. Diabetic rubeosis and panretinal photocoagulation. A prospective, controlled, masked trial using iris fluorescein angiography. *Arch Ophthalmol*. 1983;101;882–884.
19. Hayreh SS, Klugman MR, Podhajsky P, et al. Argon laser panretinal photocoagulation in ischemic central retinal vein occlusion. A 10-year prospective study. *Graefes Arch Clin Exp Ophthalmol*. 1990;228:281–296.
20. Striga M, Ivanisevic M. Comparison between efficacy of full- and mild-scatter (panretinal) photocoagulation on the course of diabetic rubeosis iridis. *Ophthalmologica*. 1993;207:144–147.
21. Stitt AW, Gardiner TA, Archer DB. Retinal and choroidal responses to panretinal photocoagulation: an ultrastructural

perspective. *Graefe's Arch Clin Exp Ophthalmol.* 1995; 233:699–705.
22. Stefansson E. Oxygen and diabetic eye disease. *Graefes Arch Clin Exp Ophthalmol.* 1990;228:120–123.
23. Pournaras CJ. Retinal oxygen distribution. Its role in the physiopathology of vasoproliferative microangiopathies. *Retina.* 1995;15:332–347.
24. Duker JS, Brown GC. The efficacy of panretinal photocoagulation for neovascularization of the iris after central retinal artery obstruction. *Ophthalmology.* 1989;96:92–95.
25. Davidorf FH, Mouser JG, Derick RJ. Rapid improvement of rubeosis iridis from a single bevacizumab (Avastin) injection. *Retina.* 2006;26:354–356.
26. Kahook MY, Schuman JS, Noecker RJ. Intravitreal bevacizumab in a patient with neovascular glaucoma. *Ophthalmic Surg Lasers Imaging.* 2006;37:144–146.
27. Grisanti S, Biester S, Peters S, et al. Intracameral bevacizumab for iris rubeosis. *Am J Ophthalmol.* 2006;142:158–160.
28. Ichhpujani P, Ramasubramanian A, Kaushik S, et al. Bevacizumab in glaucoma: a review. *Can J Ophthalmol.* 2007;42: 812–815.
29. Ehlers JP, Spirn MJ, Lam A, et al. Combination intravitreal bevacizumab/panretinal photocoagulation versus panretinal photocoagulation alone in the treatment of neovascular glaucoma. *Retina.* 2008;28:696–702.
30. Wakabayashi T, Oshima Y, Sakaguchi H, et al. Intravitreal bevacizumab to treat iris neovascularization and neovascular glaucoma secondary to ischemic retinal diseases in 41 consecutive cases. *Ophthalmology.* 2008;115:1571–1580.
31. Beutel J, Peters S; the Bevacizumab Study Group, et al. Bevacizumab as adjuvant for neovascular glaucoma. *Acta Ophthalmol.* 2010;88:103–109.
32. Rosenberg LF, Krupin T, Tang LQ, et al. Combination of systemic acetazolamide and topical dorzolamide in reducing intraocular pressure and aqueous humor formation. *Ophthalmology.* 1998;105:88–92.
33. Sabri K, Levin AV. The additive effect of topical dorzolamide and systemic acetazolamide in pediatric glaucoma. *J AAPOS.* 2006;10:464–468.
34. Tsai JC, Feuer WJ, Parrish RK II, et al. 5-Fluorouracil filtering surgery and neovascular glaucoma. Long-term follow-up of the original pilot study. *Ophthalmology.* 1995;102:887–892.
35. Katz GJ, Higginbotham EJ, Lichter PR, et al. Mitomycin C versus 5-fluorouracil in high-risk glaucoma filtering surgery. Extended follow-up. *Ophthalmology.* 1995;102:1263–1269.
36. Kiuchi Y, Sugimoto R, Nakae K, et al. Trabeculectomy with mitomycin C for treatment of neovascular glaucoma in diabetic patients. *Ophthalmologica.* 2006;220:383–388.
37. Sisto D, Vetrugno M, Trabucco T, et al. The role of antimetabolites in filtration surgery for neovascular glaucoma: intermediate-term follow-up. *Acta Ophthalmol Scand.* 2007;85:267–271.
38. Takihara Y, Inatani M, Fukushima M, et al. Trabeculectomy with mitomycin C for neovascular glaucoma: prognostic factors for surgical failure. *Am J Ophthalmol.* 2009;147:912–918.
39. Kitnarong N, Chindasub P, Metheetrairut A. Surgical outcome of intravitreal bevacizumab and filtration surgery in neovascular glaucoma. *Adv Ther.* 2008;25:438–443.
40. Cornish KS, Ramamurthi S, Saidkasimova S, et al. Intravitreal bevacizumab and augmented trabeculectomy for neovascular glaucoma in young diabetic patients. *Eye.* 2009;23: 979–981.
41. Jue A. Angiogenesis: trabeculectomy and bevacizumab. *Semin Ophthalmol.* 2009;24:122–125.
42. Gupta V, Jha R, Rao A, Kong G, et al. The effect of different doses of intracameral bevacizumab on surgical outcomes of trabeculectomy for neovascular glaucoma. *Eur J Ophthalmol.* 2009;19:435–441.
43. Grewal DS, Jain R, Kumar H, et al. Evaluation of subconjunctival bevacizumab as an adjunct to trabeculectomy a pilot study. *Ophthalmology.* 2008;115:2141–2145.
44. Li Z, Van Bergen T, Van de Veire S, et al. Inhibition of Vascular Endothelial Growth Factor Reduces Scar Formation after Glaucoma Filtration Surgery. *Invest Ophthalmol Vis Sci.* 2009 [Epub ahead of print].
45. Guerriero E, Yu JY, Kahook MY, et al. Morphologic Evaluation Of Bevacizumab (Avastin) Treated Corneal Stromal Fibroblasts. *Invest Ophthalmol Vis Sci.* 2006;47:1642.
46. Tsai JC, Johnson CC, Dietrich MS. The Ahmed shunt versus the Baerveldt shunt for refractory glaucoma: A single-surgeon comparison of outcome. *Ophthalmology.* 2003;110:1814–1821.
47. Mermoud A, Salmon JF, Alexander P, et al. Molteno tube implantation for neovascular glaucoma. Long-term results and factors influencing the outcome. *Ophthalmology.* 1993;100: 897–902.
48. Every SG, Molteno AC, Bevin TH, et al. Long-term results of Molteno implant insertion in cases of neovascular glaucoma. *Arch Ophthalmol.* 2006;124:355–360.
49. Syed HM, Law SK, Nam SH, et al. Baerveldt-350 implant versus Ahmed valve for refractory glaucoma: A case-controlled comparison. *J Glaucoma.* 2004;13:38–45.
50. Ayyala RS, Zurakowski D, Monshizadeh R, et al. Comparison of double-plate Molteno and Ahmed glaucoma valve in patients with advanced uncontrolled glaucoma. *Ophthalmic Surg Lasers.* 2002;33:94–101.
51. Hong CH, Arosemena A, Zurakowski D, et al. Glaucoma drainage devices: a systematic literature review and current controversies. *Surv Ophthalmol.* 2005;50:48–60.
52. Schwartz KS, Lee RK, Gedde SJ. Glaucoma drainage implants: a critical comparison of types. *Curr Opin Ophthalmol.* 2006; 17:181–189.
53. Minckler DS, Vedula SS, Li TJ, et al. Aqueous shunts for glaucoma. *Cochrane Database Syst Rev.* 2006;:CD004918.
54. Yildirim N, Yalvac IS, Sahin A, et al. A comparative study between diode laser cyclophotocoagulation and the Ahmed glaucoma valve implant in neovascular glaucoma: a long-term follow-up. *J Glaucoma.* 2009;18:192–196.
55. Dickens C, Nguyen N, Mora J, et al. Long-term results of noncontact transscleral neodymium:YAG cyclophotocoagulation. *Ophthalmology.* 1995;102:1777–1781.
56. Shields MB, Shields SE. Noncontact transscleral Nd:YAG cyclophotocoagulation: a long-term follow-up of 500 patients. *Trans Am Ophthalmol Soc.* 1994;92:271–283.
57. Schlote T, Grüb M, Kynigopoulos M. Long-term results after transscleral diode laser cyclophotocoagulation in refractory posttraumatic glaucoma and glaucoma in aphakia. *Graefes Arch Clin Exp Ophthalmol.* 2007;246:405–410.
58. Lam S, Tessler HH, Lam BL, et al. High incidence of sympathetic ophthalmia after contact and noncontact neodymium:YAG cyclotherapy. *Ophthalmology.* 1992;99:1818–1822.
59. Edward DP, Brown SV, Higginbotham E, Jennings T, Tessler HH, Tso MO. Sympathetic ophthalmia following neodymium:YAG cyclotherapy. *Ophthalmic Surg.* 1989;20:544–546.

SECTION II

Practice

PART B

Future Therapies and Challenges

CHAPTER

26

Gene-Based Therapy in Ocular Angiogenesis

Sarah Parker Read • Siobhan M. Cashman • Rajendra Kumar-Singh

INTRODUCTION

Pathogenic growth of blood vessels occurs in virtually every compartment of the eye, including the choroid, retina, iris, and cornea (Table 26.1). In nearly every age group, the more common manifestations of vasoproliferative disorders account for major causes of blindness (for a complete review of ocular neovascular disorders see Ref. 1). Diabetic retinopathy is the leading cause of blindness in individuals 20 to 64 years of age, due primarily to abnormal blood vessel growth in the retina and macular edema.[2] Similarly, the leading cause of blindness among the elderly, wet age-related macular degeneration (AMD) involves neovascularization of the choroid, causing retinal detachment and eventual retinal degeneration.[3] Among children, retinopathy of prematurity (ROP), leading to vascularization of the retina and hemorrhage into the vitreous, is one of the most common causes of blindness.[4]

Though the underlying pathogenesis of these vasoproliferative disorders of the retina can differ, their final outcomes can be loosely divided into retinal neovascularization (RNV) and choroidal neovascularization (for review see Ref. 5). RNV is caused by the growth of blood vessels along the inner surface of the retina and can be a complicating factor in retinal ischemic events, such as occurs in diabetic retinopathy and ROP. In diabetic retinopathy, hyperglycemia leads to closure of retinal capillaries and decreased retinal perfusion. In ROP, stunting of the retinal vascular network results in insufficient blood flow to the peripheral retina. Ultimately, these ischemic events result in the activation of hypoxia inducible factor 1 (HIF-1),[6] which induces expression of vascular endothelial growth factor (VEGF) and other hypoxia-stimulated genes.[7] CNV involves the growth of blood vessels below the retinal pigment epithelium (RPE) and most commonly consists of proliferation from the choroidal plexus. However, blood vessels can occasionally sprout from the deep capillaries of the retina, a condition termed retinal angiomatous proliferation. In AMD, the etiology of angiogenic stimulation is less well understood (for reviews see Refs. 8 and 9) but appears to depend on the breakdown of Bruch membrane at the macula and, in the severe form, invasion of blood vessels through the RPE into the subretinal space.

CURRENT TREATMENT MODALITIES

Current treatments for AMD and diabetic retinopathy include laser photocoagulation and photodynamic therapy, both of which cauterize new blood vessels by scar tissue formation or destruction of tissue. However, this short-term treatment fails to address the underlying pathogenesis of blood vessel growth, often leading to a high incidence of disease recurrence. Almost half of AMD patients have been reported to exhibit persistent and recurrent neovascularization within 3 years of laser treatment.[10] In fact, laser treatment has been found to be detrimental compared to

Table 26.1.

Pathologic neovascularization occurs in various ocular tissues, including the cornea, iris, retina, and choroid

Tissue	Disease/Trauma
Cornea	Contact lens injury
	Trauma/alkali injury
	Infectious keratitis (trachoma)
Iris	Enucleation (i.e., retinoblastoma)
	Central retinal vein occlusion
	Diabetes mellitus or other forms of RNV
Retina	Proliferative diabetic retinopathy/other diabetic complications
	Retinopathy of prematurity
	Sickle cell retinopathy
	Central retinal vein occlusion
	Branch retinal vein occlusion
	Rare disorders (i.e., Eales disease)
Choroid	Age-related macular degeneration
	Myopia

no treatment in AMD patients with occult CNV, a condition in which leakage from blood vessels occurs in punctate areas in multiple distinct regions.[11] Such restrictions on current treatment highlight the need for the development of novel therapeutics to inhibit neovascularization.

While small molecule drugs are attractive due to increased stability and cost-effective large-scale production, preclinical data indicate that recombinant antiangiogenic proteins have fewer side effects and may be better suited for therapy.[12] Clinical trials over the past few years have begun to assess the efficacy of drugs injected into the vitreous of the eye and, as of 2008, more than 60 trials for the treatment of AMD were recruiting patients.[13] Currently, only two of these regimens have been approved for the treatment of wet AMD. In December 2004, the Food and Drug Administration (FDA) approved pegaptanib sodium (Macugen), an mRNA aptamer against a single VEGF isoform, for the treatment of wet AMD. However, only a subset of patients demonstrated improvements in visual acuity, leading to a subsequent decrease in popular use.[13] In 2006, the FDA approved ranibizumab (Lucentis), a modified humanized monoclonal antibody fragment against all VEGF-A isoforms. Lucentis has shown efficacy in halting the progression of disease and, in some cases, reversing vision loss.[13] Many of the therapies used to treat wet AMD are being evaluated for efficacy in other neovascular disorders.

LIMITATIONS OF CURRENT TREATMENTS

Aberrant blood vessel growth is critical to the pathogenesis of proliferative diabetic retinopathy and AMD. The chronic nature of both these disorders requires that inhibition of neovascularization be sustained over a long period of time, while the short half-life of many antiangiogenic molecules, such as pegaptanib and ranibizumab, necessitates repeat injection.[14] Though oral administration of antiangiogenic molecules has proven effective in inhibiting ocular neovascularization,[15] there are concerns over the consequences of long-term systemic exposure to antiangiogenic molecules[16]; for example, VEGF neutralizing molecules could disrupt the normal effects of VEGF on processes such as wound healing and endometriosis. Local administration of these molecules relies on repeat ocular injection, typically intravitreal, which brings with it several complications, such as endophthalmitis and retinal detachment, both of which have the potential for blinding.[16] While the risk with each injection is low, the cumulative risk over many years may be substantial.

Gene therapy has the potential to improve current therapies.[17] Long-term expression of the therapeutic protein would theoretically reduce administration of the treatment to a single event. By targeting specific tissues, and regulating gene expression, gene therapy allows for more precise control over exposure and dosing of the drug. The ability to deliver multiple transgenes could allow for the targeting of multiple steps or multiple pathways in the angiogenic process. In addition, recombinant proteins can be expensive to produce, so expression from gene therapy vectors has the potential to reduce cost. While there are many advantages associated with a gene therapy approach, a number of possible complications still limit application in the clinic, including immune reactions, integration into the host genome, cytotoxicity, and efficacy of transfection.

OCULAR TISSUE AS A TARGET FOR GENE THERAPY

The eye is uniquely suited to overcome barriers previously reported in gene therapy clinical trials. The eye is an immune privileged tissue and so injection does not evoke the normal humoral immune response that can preclude treatment with some vectors, especially viruses.[18] For example, injection of a normally immunogenic adenovirus into the subretinal space resulted in little systemic immune response, which could in turn allow for long-term transgene expression.[19] Intraocular injections primarily transfect local tissue with little diffusion of gene products into the systemic circulation. Ocular disorders typically occur bilaterally and the contralateral eye may act as an internal control. In addition, the translucency of the anterior portion of the eye allows for noninvasive monitoring of efficacy and toxicity of treatment.

Gene therapy approaches have demonstrated a high efficacy in the rescue of animal models of disease, ranging from single loss-of-function mutations in retinal degeneration models to complex acquired disorders (for review see Ref. 20). Gene replacement has proven effective in animal models of single gene disorders such as Leber congenital amaurosis (LCA)[21,22] and retinitis pigmentosa.[23–25] The expression of growth factors and signaling inhibitors has shown efficacy in preventing the pathogenic sequela in animal models of complex disorders such as retinal[26–28] and choroidal[27–31] neovascularization, experimental autoimmune uveoretinitis,[32] and experimental glaucoma.[33]

Recently, gene therapy clinical trials have shown positive outcomes in ocular disease[34] (Table 26.2). Neurotech Pharmaceuticals demonstrated that an intravitreal implant containing encapsulated cells transfected to secrete ciliary neurotrophic factor was safe for use in retinitis pigmentosa patients, with a subset of those treated showing improvement in visual acuity.[35] Virus-based clinical trials include retrovirus delivery of a dominant negative cyclin G1 construct for the treatment of superficial corneal opacity/corneal scarring,[36] adenovirus-based delivery of pigment epithelium–derived factor (PEDF) for the treatment of wet AMD[37] (see Box 26.1), adenovirus delivery of herpes simplex virus thymidine kinase for the treatment of refractory retinoblastoma,[38] and adeno-associated virus (AAV) delivery of the RPE65 gene for rescue of LCA.[39–41] No dose-limiting toxicities were observed after

Table 26.2.

Ocular gene therapy clinical trials

Therapy	Mechanism	Phase	Disease
AdV-Tk	HSV thymidine kinase expression with intravenously delivered ganciclovir	Phase 1	Refractive retinoblastoma
ADGVPEDF.11D	Adenovirus expressing PEDF	Phase 1	Wet AMD
Mx-dnG1	Retrovirus expressing dominant negative cyclin G1	Phase 1/2	Adjunctive therapy for superficial corneal opacity/corneal scarring
NT-501	Implant of encapsulated human NTC-201 cells releasing CNTF	Phase 2	Retinitis pigmentosa
		Phase 2	Visual impairment from AMD
rAAV2-CB-hRPE65	AAV expressing RPE65	Phase 1/2	Leber congenital amaurosis Type 2
AAV2-sFLT01	AAV expressing soluble FLT-1	Phase 1	Wet AMD

adenoviral injection in the retinoblastoma patients, with seven of the patients treated at the highest dose exhibiting resolution of the tumor.[38] Results from three different Phase 1 trials have shown short-term safety of the AAV viral vector in LCA patients,[39–41] with one study reporting modest improvement in visual acuity in all subjects.[39] In the latter study, further recovery of visual acuity was noted at the 1-year time point. Together, these trials have

BOX 26.1 Gene Therapy Phase 1 Clinical Trial: Adenovirus Mediated Expression of PEDF for the Treatment of Neovascular AMD

AMD is the leading cause of blindness in older adults in the United States,[3] with increasing incidence as the population ages. In 2006, Campochiaro et al.[37] published the results of a Phase 1 clinical trial for the treatment of AMD, the first gene therapy clinical trial for ocular angiogenesis. This study tests the use of a serotype 5 adenovirus (Ad5) expressing human pigment epithelium–derived factor (PEDF) (AdPEDF.11). Previously, studies in animal models have shown that injection of an earlier generation virus, AdPEDF.10, into the vitreous expresses high levels of PEDF protein 5 days postinjection. AdPEDF.11 has been shown to inhibit VEGF-induced CNV, laser-induced CNV, and hypoxia-induced RNV.[28] The inhibitory effect of AdPEDF.11 on laser-induced CNV was found to be over twofold higher when injected into the subretinal space.[28] Importantly, for the treatment of AMD patients, intravitreal injection of AdPEDF.11 was shown to cause regression of established laser-induced CNV.[152] In a pig model of laser-induced CNV, 10^9 particle units (PU) of AdPEDF.11 injected intravitreally caused a 38% reduction in neovascularization after 10 days.[134]

The initial Phase 1 trial was a dose escalation study, ranging from 10^6 to $10^{9.5}$ PU injected into the vitreous to evaluate potential toxicity of the vector. Previously, doses of 10^{10} PU or higher were shown to cause an increasingly severe inflammatory response in nonhuman primates.[162] Patients were monitored in 13 visits over a 12-month follow-up period. While there was mild transient inflammation in 25% of patients, no severe inflammation was noted, even at the highest dose tested. This agrees with previous Phase 1 results using adenovirus in which no toxicities were observed other than mild, controlled inflammation even up to 10^{10} PU, a higher dose than used with AdPEDF.11.[38] The increase in intraocular pressure observed in 6 of the 28 subjects was restored to normal using topical treatment. Serum adenoviral cultures were inconsistent, but remained low over time, and urine and sputum cultures were negative.

Fluorescein angiography was used to evaluate the size and leakage of the neovascular lesion. After 6 months, in the low-dose group (10^6–$10^{7.5}$ PU) 50% of patients showed stabilization or improvement in CNV lesion size and in the high-dose group (10^8–$10^{9.5}$ PU) 71% of patients showed stabilization or improvement in lesion size. While the median lesion size increased by 0.5 disk areas at 6 months and 1.0 disk areas at 12 months in the low-dose group, there was no increase in lesion size at either 6 or 12 months in the high-dose group. This appeared to correlate with functional tests in which patients in the high-dose group showed stable visual acuity over the 12-month period, whereas the low-dose group appeared to show deterioration of visual acuity at 6 and 12 months. Thus far, Phase 1 results using AdPEDF.11 indicate that at doses higher than 10^6 PU, long-term treatment of disease progression out to at least 12 months may be achieved. At this point, however, it is unclear if this is due to continued PEDF production, or the sustained effects of initial high PEDF expression that later turns off (AdPEDF.11 uses the CMV promoter, whose expression has been shown to decrease to undetectable levels after 90 days in the eye[144]). Taken with results from other gene therapy trials, there is strong support for the continuation of gene therapy strategies for the long-term treatment of ocular neovascular disorders such as AMD.

established gene therapy as a clinically viable approach in the treatment of ocular disease.

THERAPY TARGETS FOR OCULAR NEOVASCULARIZATION

Gene therapy strategies for the treatment of single gene disorders such as LCA, in which the genetic defect leading to pathology has been determined, are fairly straightforward. Development of potential therapeutic molecules in CNV and RNV, in which the molecular basis of the disease is more complex and less understood, has proven challenging.

Vascular Endothelial Growth Factor

Multiple lines of evidence suggest that VEGF plays a central role in the pathogenesis of ocular neovascularization. Patients with ischemic retinal disease and progression to RNV have been shown to exhibit a concurrent increase in VEGF in the ocular fluid.[13,42] In fact, VEGF has been shown to be both necessary and sufficient for induction of experimental neovascularization.[43–47] Drugs approved for the treatment of ocular angiogenesis, such as Lucentis, modulate VEGF, and anti-VEGF molecules delivered to animal models have shown significant reductions in both CNV and RNV.[48] These same molecules have shown comparable therapeutic efficiencies when delivered via a gene therapy approach. For example, a soluble VEGF receptor protein shown to prevent neovascularization[44] also does so when a transgene expressing the same protein is delivered.[49]

While current candidate molecules used in gene therapy experiments in the eye have focused primarily on VEGF inhibition, other inhibitors of angiogenesis have been identified. These include secreted angiostatic proteins, soluble receptors for proangiogenic factors, and complement inhibitors (for a review see Refs. 50 and 51). The relative efficacy and potency of these proteins are still under investigation.[52]

Secreted Angiostatic Factors

Secreted angiostatic factors are derived from naturally occurring proteins and therefore have the potential for a decreased immune response. One such protein, PEDF, was identified as a potent angiogenic inhibitor in the eye, with the ability to inhibit multiple proangiogenic factors.[53] PEDF is naturally produced by a number of different ocular cell types in humans, including the RPE and photoreceptors,[54] and loss of expression could at least partially contribute to disease. Downregulation of PEDF is known to occur in response to hypoxia[53] and expression of PEDF has been shown to be inversely correlated with age,[55] implicating it as a possible mediator of angiogenesis in AMD. PEDF has been reported to have neuroprotective properties[56] and has been shown to delay photoreceptor loss in a mouse model of retinal degeneration,[57] further enhancing its consideration as a therapeutic candidate.

Other endogenously secreted antiangiogenic molecules that have specific action against proliferating endothelial cells have been identified.[17] Angiostatin, a cleavage product of plasminogen,[58] has the ability to block capillary cell proliferation.[59] Endostatin is a proteolytic fragment of collagen XIII shown to inhibit VEGF-induced endothelial cell migration.[60] Additionally, endostatin has been shown to be inversely correlated with the severity of neovascularization in diabetic retinopathy.[61] In order for blood vessels to invade the retina in AMD, the barrier of the Bruch membrane must first be degraded. This is largely mediated by metalloproteinases (MMPs). Thus, inhibitors of MMPs, such as TIMP-3, have antiangiogenic properties.[62]

There is some evidence that indicates that angiostatic soluble factors work to inhibit angiogenesis with roughly the same efficiencies. In one study, AAV vectors were used to examine the efficacies of three secreted factors: PEDF, endostatin, and TIMP-3.[26] In an animal model of ocular neovascularization, all three molecules were able to significantly decrease the number of proliferating endothelial cells with efficacies ranging from 75% to 85%, though TIMP-3 appeared to be the least effective in this study.[26] In a separate study, AAV expression of PEDF and angiostatin inhibited the formation of neovascular nuclei by 74% and 78%, respectively.[63] While their potencies appear roughly comparable, it is worth noting that these proteins each inhibit angiogenesis via different mechanisms, so targeting multiple pathways by delivering multiple transgenes may allow for even greater antiangiogenic efficiency.

Soluble Receptors

Soluble receptors have also shown potency in inhibiting angiogenic signaling. The soluble form of the VEGF receptor has been shown to bind VEGF and block signaling.[64] Novel chimeric molecules of this receptor have been generated and shown to be effective in inhibiting neovascularization.[65] The Ang2 protein has been shown to be upregulated in surgically removed CNV membranes,[66] and the soluble form of its receptor Tie2 (ExTek) is shown to inhibit angiogenesis.[27,67]

A direct method of VEGF signaling inhibition is the knockdown of VEGF protein production itself, making it an ideal target for antisense RNA-mediated knockdown.[68] Two approaches have been used to deliver silencing RNA in the eye: delivery of small interfering siRNA against VEGF[69–71] and VEGF receptor 1.[72] Additionally, siRNA against HIF-1α, a hypoxia inducible factor that upregulates VEGF expression, has also been shown to be effective against in vivo angiogenesis.[73] In a recent report, siRNA activation of Toll-like receptor 3 (TLR3) led to inhibition of angiogenesis in two models of ocular neovascularization, independent of RNA sequence.[74] This implied that general mechanism of siRNA neovascular inhibition raises concerns over the exact mechanism of antiangiogenesis using intravitreal injection of naked anti-VEGF siRNA.[70,72] Such concerns could be addressed by expression of the antisense RNA within the cell using a gene therapy approach, thereby avoiding interaction of the siRNA with extracellular receptors. A short hairpin RNA (shRNA) targeting VEGF and expressed from an adenoviral vector has been shown to inhibit CNV,[75] thereby validating this approach.

The activation of endogenous antiangiogenic genes was recently shown to be an efficient inhibitor of ocular neovascularization.[76] In one study, AAV delivery of a zinc-finger transcription factor, engineered to upregulate PEDF gene expression, was able to reduce CNV after laser induction for up to 3 months.[76] The authors point to the use of this technology as a potential prophylactic treatment for at-risk AMD patients who have not yet developed neovascularization. Conversely, suppression of endogenous angiogenic factors would also inhibit neovascularization. The expression of GA-binding protein (GABP), a transcription factor that regulates the expression of VEGF and roundabout4 (Robo4), has been shown to decrease VEGF and Robo2 levels in vivo and inhibit angiogenesis.[77]

Complement Inhibitors

Recent work has shown that induction of the membrane attack complex (MAC), the final step in the complement cascade, is a critical mediator of laser-induced CNV.[78] Importantly, CD59, an inhibitor of MAC deposition, was found to be downregulated in laser-induced CNV, and CD59 null transgenics were more susceptible to CNV induction.[79] The potential for CD59 to inhibit CNV was confirmed by inhibition of MAC deposition and attenuation of laser-induced CNV after administration of a soluble CD59.[79] Adenovirus-mediated expression of membrane-bound human CD59 has been shown to prevent MAC deposition on the cornea and RPE of a murine ex vivo humanized model of AMD[80]; such an approach could further restrict the expression of a potent complement inhibitor to the relevant tissue. Polymorphisms in the complement factor H gene, an inhibitor of the alternative complement pathway, have been found to be associated with AMD.[81] Laser-induced CNV has been shown to be reduced by both recombinant factor H[82] and the protein thioredoxin-1,[83] which acts through an interaction with factor H, providing novel therapeutic avenues for treatment.

Other Molecules

Other proteins have been isolated and found to inhibit angiogenesis in vivo. For example, von Hippel-Lindau (VHL) protein, a mutant form of which causes the hereditary cancer syndrome von Hippel-Lindau, has been shown to decrease basal levels of VEGF transcripts in vitro when overexpressed in various cell types, including the RPE.[84] Adenovirus delivery of VHL transgene decreased VEGF expression and suppressed neovascularization in a nonhuman primate model of laser-induced branch retinal vein occlusion in vivo.[84] The anti-VEGF intraceptor gene (Flt23K) is a recombinant hybrid protein consisting of VEGFR-1/Flt-1 domains 2 and 3 (which bind VEGF) fused to the KDEL endoplasmic reticulum (ER) retention signal. KDEL binds ER proteins and prevents their secretion. Thus, upon expression, the anti-VEGF intraceptor binds VEGF intracellularly and sequesters it within the ER and has been shown to decrease ocular angiogenesis.[85]

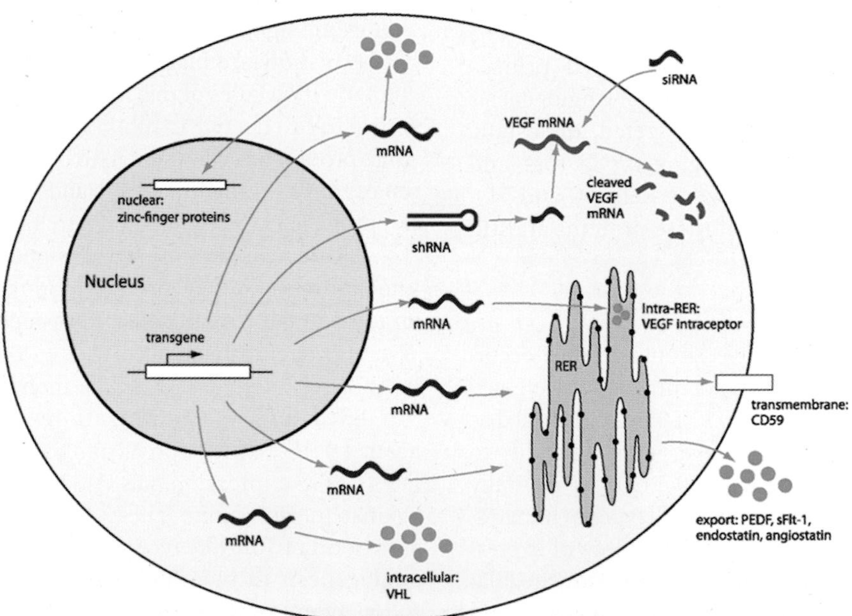

FIGURE 26.1. Gene therapy–mediated transgene expression targets molecules intracellularly and extracellularly. Targeted degradation of mRNA corresponding to angiogenic proteins, such as VEGF, has been demonstrated using shRNA and siRNA. Transgenic recombinant proteins can inhibit neovascularization by a variety of mechanisms, including sequestering VEGF protein in the RER (VEGF intraceptor), inhibition of MAC deposition on the cell surface (CD59), modulation of intracellular pathways (VHL), activation or inhibition of gene transcription (zinc-finger proteins), or secretion of antiangiogenic proteins (PEDF, sFlt-1). Gene therapy allows for inhibition of angiogenesis at many different locations by the expression of multiple transgenes. RER, rough endoplasmic reticulum; VEGF, vascular endothelial growth factor; PEDF, pigment epithelium–derived factor; VHL, von Hippel-Lindau protein.

A variety of molecules have been shown to inhibit angiogenesis in ocular tissue, ranging from soluble factors that bind VEGF directly to transmembrane molecules that inhibit neovascular initiation (Fig. 26.1). Many of these molecules have been tested via a gene therapy approach and proven successful in a wide array of animal models. A number of different gene therapy vectors have been tested in their ability to deliver these antiangiogenic factors and prevent neovascularization in vivo.

GENE DELIVERY VECTORS

There are many approaches to gene delivery in the eye that have shown efficacy in the rescue of animal models of disease. A number of different criteria must be considered when choosing an ideal vector for use in the clinic. Such factors include either nonspecific or site-specific integration in the host genome, lack of inflammation and immune response, specific transduction of target cells, large carrying

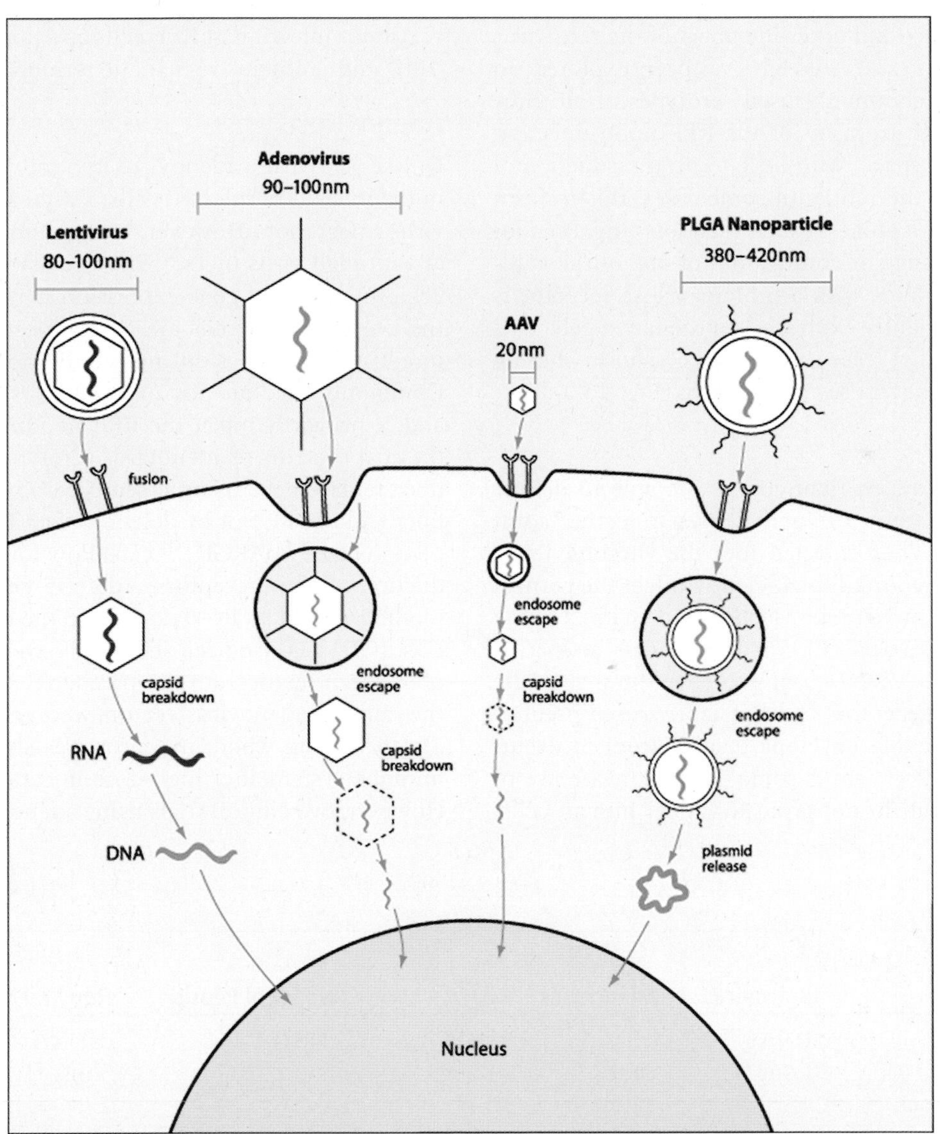

FIGURE 26.2. Vectors have different mechanisms of nuclear transgene delivery. While many vectors have been shown to transfect ocular tissue, only a few have demonstrated targeted transfection and inhibition of angiogenesis. Lentivirus, a member of the retrovirus family, fuses with the cell surface, eventually releasing its RNA genome, which is subsequently reverse-transcribed into DNA, transported to the nucleus, and integrated into the host genome. Adenovirus triggers endocytosis via interaction between the fiber protein and cell receptors. Within the endosome, capsid degradation is initiated, leading to endosomal escape and eventually release of viral DNA, which can then be transported to the nucleus. AAV entry proceeds by a similar mechanism binding the cell surface, triggering endocytosis and escape, and eventual trafficking to the nucleus. Within the nucleus, AAV must then mature the genome from single- to double-stranded DNA. PLGA nanoparticles are thought to bind receptors on the cell surface, trigger endocytosis and subsequent escape, release plasmid DNA into the cytoplasm, and finally transport of the DNA into the nucleus.

capacity, long-term expression, and high transfection efficiency (reviewed in Ref. 86). Transgene delivery can occur through a variety of mechanisms but involves targeting of the vector to a specific cell type, binding and uptake at the cell surface, escape from the endosome, release of DNA, and movement of DNA into the nucleus for transcription (Fig. 26.2). Despite differences in mechanism, a number of vectors have shown efficacy as gene delivery vehicles for the rescue of ocular neovascularization in animal models. For an overview of vectors, see Table 26.3.

Viruses are a common vector for ocular gene delivery, primarily because of their high transfection efficiency. In the eye, lentiviruses (and other members of the retrovirus family), adenovirus, and AAV have all been explored. In general, the most commonly used serotypes of all three viruses show a high tropism for the RPE upon injection into the subretinal space, with little to no transduction of other cell types in the retina. In some cases, this tropism can be overcome by a process called pseudotyping. Pseudotyping is the exchange or conjugation of one of the wild-type viral coat proteins with a protein whose receptor is known to be abundantly expressed on the target cell. This strategy has proved at least partially successful in altering the tropism of all the viruses listed above (Fig. 26.3).

Lentiviruses

In the postmitotic retina, lentiviruses are able to deliver genes to the RPE[87] but are inefficient at infecting adult photoreceptors.[88] When injected into the vitreous, lentiviruses have been reported to efficiently infect the corneal endothelium.[89] Lentiviruses pseudotyped with Equine Infections Anemia Virus (EIAV) or vesicular stomatitis virus glycoprotein (VSVG) coat proteins show sporadic infection of photoreceptors,[90–92] but lentiviruses pseudotyped with the Mokola envelope display tropism exclusively for the RPE.[92] There is some interest in the use of viral constructs that do not typically infect human cells, such as bovine immunodeficiency virus (BIV), which has been shown to stably infect the RPE after virus delivery into the subretinal space.[93] However, BIV still showed a lower transduction efficiency compared to similar experiments with Hd-Ad.[94] Lentiviruses have a cloning capacity of only approximately 7 kb and integrate into the host genome as part of their life cycle, which can lead to insertional mutagenesis and oncogenicity. Such an event led to the development of leukemia following ex vivo administration of the Moloney murine leukemia retrovirus in a clinical trial for SCID-X1.[95] Oxford Biomedica is currently developing an angiostatin and endostatin expressing lentivirus vector for infection of RPE cells as a potential treatment of AMD and proliferative diabetic retinopathy.

Adenovirus

Unlike lentivirus, adenovirus typically remains episomal in the nucleus of infected cells,[96] decreasing concerns over virus integration. However, integration has been reported at very high virus titers.[97] The necessity for integration to achieve long-term gene expression may not be relevant in the eye, in which cells are mostly postmitotic and therefore loss of episomes during cell division is not a concern. Commonly used adenovirus vectors, such as serotypes 2 and 5, primarily infect the RPE in adult retina.[98] Altering the coat proteins of adenovirus serotype 5 (Ad5) either by fiber replacement using a serotype 35 (Ad5/F35)[99] or 37 fiber (Ad5/F37)[100] or by deletion of an RGD domain in the penton base (AdΔRGD)[101] can allow for the efficient transduction of photoreceptors. Ad5/F35 virus with additional modification of an RGD domain to the knob portion (Ad5/F35 RGD) has also been shown to have increased duration of transgene expression compared to Ad5.[102] Concerns over the safety of adenovirus vectors were raised after the death of a patient in whom the virus was shown to trigger the immune system after high-dose injection into the liver.[103] However, two clinical trials using adenovirus vectors in the

Table 26.3.

Features of gene therapy vectors

	Retrovirus	Adenovirus	AAV	Nonviral Peptide	Nonviral Lipid	Physical
Transgene	RNA	dsDNA	ssDNA	dsDNA	dsDNA	dsDNA
Duration of expression	Long	Short	Long	Short	Short	Short
Delay in transgene expression	1 wk	2 d	1–4 wk	2 d	2 d	2 d
Average transgene cloning capacity	8 kB	8–36 kB	5 kB	High	High	High
Transfection efficiency	High	High	High	Low	Low	Medium
Primary cell target	RPE	Many	Many	RPE	RPE	RPE
Ease of production	High	High	Low	High	High	High
Immune reaction	Low	Low–high	Low	Low	Low	Low
Integration	High	Low	Possible	Low	Low	Low
Cytotoxicity	Low	Low	Low	Low	High	High

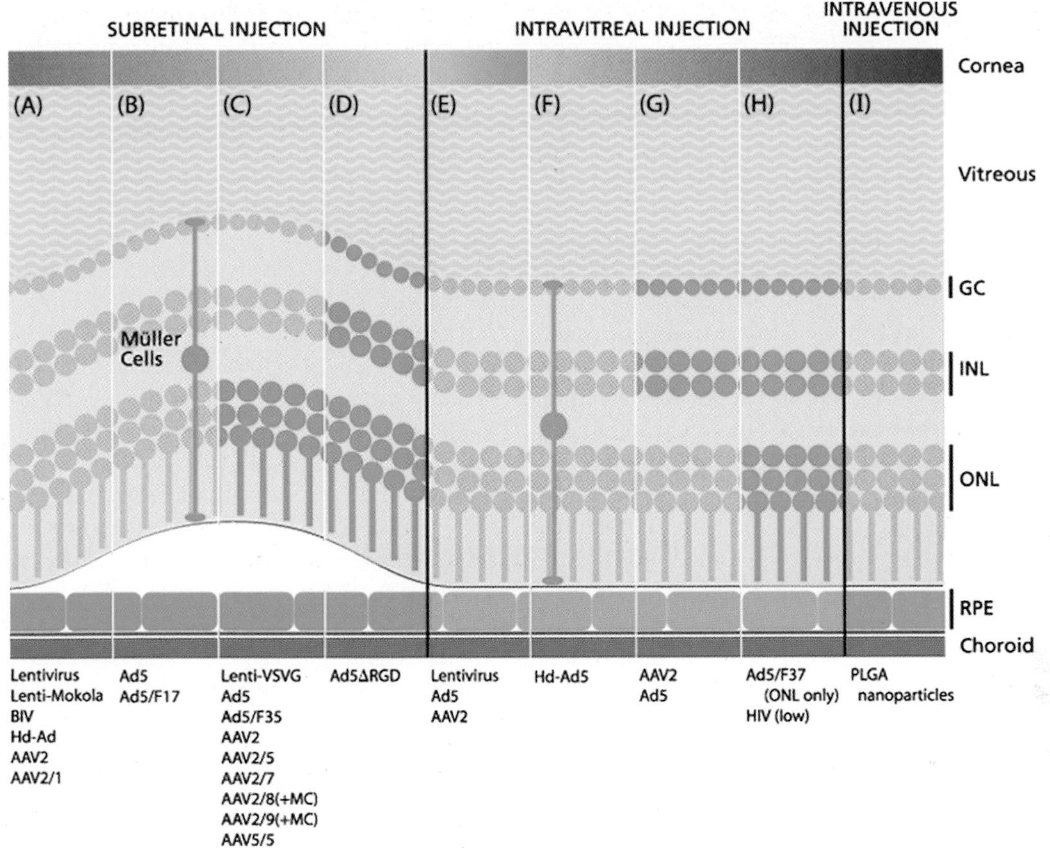

FIGURE 26.3. Pseudotyping and functionalization of gene therapy vectors can alter tissue tropism. While some vectors are consistently reported to show the same transfection patterns, others exhibit variable tropism potentially influenced by outside factors, such as transgene detection sensitivity, viral titer, and duration of incubation. (A) Transduction of primarily RPE after subretinal (SR) delivery of lentivirus,[88] lenti-Mokola,[92] BIV,[93] Hd-Ad,[94] AAV2, and AAV2/1.[92] (B) Transduction of RPE and Müller cells after SR delivery of Ad5[99,101] and Ad5/F17.[101] (C) Transduction of RPE and photoreceptors after SR delivery of lenti-VSVG,[92] Ad5,[84] Ad5/F35 (and Müller cells),[99] AAV2,[31,92,129,151] AAV2/5,[92,111] AAV2/7,[111] AAV2/8 (and Müller cells),[111] AAV2/9 (and Müller cells),[111] and AAV5/5.[92] (D) Transduction of RPE, photoreceptors, bipolar cells, and ganglion cells after SR delivery of Ad5ΔRGD.[101] (E) Transduction of the corneal epithelium after intravitreal (IV) delivery of lentivirus,[88] Ad5,[49,69,160] and AAV2.[129] (F) Transduction of Müller cells after IV delivery of Hd-Ad5.[109] (G) Transduction of ganglion cells after IV delivery of AAV2[31,49,92] and Ad5.[159] (H) Low transfection levels of ganglion cells, bipolar cells, and photoreceptors after IV delivery of HIV.[153] Transduction of photoreceptors after IV delivery of Ad5/F37.[100] (I) PLGA nanoparticles transfect the RPE after intravenous delivery.[85] AAV2/5, AAV2/1, and AAV5/5 show little transfection after IV delivery.[92] GC, ganglion cells; INL, inner nuclear layer; ONL, outer nuclear layer; RPE, retinal pigment epithelium.

eye have reported no adverse events or limiting toxicities other than mild inflammation that was easily managed.[37,38]

Adenoviruses have been developed to overcome a particular hurdle of viral gene therapy: that of limited cloning capacity. First-generation adenovirus only had a cloning capacity of approximately 7 kb, but the development of a helper-dependent (Hd) adenovirus has expanded that capacity to approximately 36 kb.[104–106] This allows for the incorporation of large upstream regulatory elements as well as the inclusion of multiple transgenes. Hd adenoviruses (Hd-Ad) contain only the inverted terminal repeats and packaging signal needed for replication and viral packaging. In first-generation adenovirus studies, the immune response to small amounts of viral gene expression was found to limit the duration of transgene expression.[107] However, Hd-Ad vectors have shown increased longevity of expression, up to 1 year, the longest time period tested.[108,109] Compared to first-generation adenovirus, a Hd-Ad expressing PEDF showed a substantially reduced cytokine/chemokine gene expression and inflammatory cell infiltrate, as well as a much longer duration of expression.[110]

Adeno-associated Virus

AAV is much smaller than adenovirus and has a cloning capacity of only approximately 4.8 kb. Like adenovirus serotype 5, the commonly used AAV serotype 2 primarily infects RPE. Pseudotyping of AAV2, by replacement of capsid proteins with those of other AAV serotypes, has proven effective in increasing infection of other tissues. For example, AAV2/8 and AAV2/9 transfect Müller cells and photoreceptors,[111] whereas AAV2/5, AAV2/7, and AAV5/5 have significantly increased photoreceptor transduction.[92,111] AAV is largely considered to be the least immunogenic viral vector and so is well suited for long-term therapy (reviewed in Refs. 112 and 113). It has been shown to exhibit long-term expression and rescue in animal models of LCA.[114] While inflammatory responses, neutralizing antibodies, and RPE atrophy have been reported after AAV delivery to the subretinal space of nonhuman primates,[115] after 1 year no adverse effects or toxicities have been documented in the clinical trial performed using AAV for the treatment of LCA. Wild-type AAV naturally recombines at a specific site in the human genome called AAVS1 on chromosome 19.[116] The *rep* protein that mediates recombination is deleted in recombinant AAV (rAAV) to increase the cloning capacity and, though rAAV remains primarily episomal, it has been shown to integrate randomly in human cells.[117] There is some evidence of AAV insertional mutagenesis in a mouse model of mucopolysaccharidosis type VII in which many of the animals developed hepatocellular carcinoma[118]; however, no such events have been documented in other animal models or in the AAV clinical trials for LCA.

Nonviral Gene Therapy

Nonviral gene therapy has the potential for decreased immune responses in the eye, in which even a very small amount of inflammation can exacerbate disease. Many strategies have been employed in the development of nonviral ocular gene therapy (for review see Ref. 119). However, in general, nonviral vectors have had low transduction efficiencies in the eye and there have been few examples of successful rescue of disease models. Nonviral strategies can be loosely grouped into chemical, including cationic lipids and peptides, and physical methods of delivery. Cationic lipids have been shown to cross the blood-retinal barrier and selectively transfect all cells in the eye via a rhodopsin promoter.[120–122] Subretinal delivery of Lipofectamine 2000 and NeuroPorter has shown efficient RPE delivery, although Lipofectamine demonstrated substantial toxicity.[123] Lipofectamine has been shown to successfully deliver antiangiogenic siRNA vectors in vivo when injected into the vitreous[73] while another lipoplex-based transfection reagent, FuGENE 6, has been used to deliver an angiostatic transcription factor to the cornea after subscleral injection.[77]

The PEGylated polylysine cationic peptide PEG-CK30 compacted DNA into elongated nanoparticles and has been shown to transfect many cell types in the retina at high levels.[124] PEG-CK30 is currently in clinical trials for gene delivery to the lungs of cystic fibrosis patients.[125] Recently, PEG-CK30 has been shown to partially rescue the peripherin/rds (slow degeneration) mouse model of retinitis pigmentosa.[126] Various mechanical approaches, such as electroporation[127] and electron avalanche transfection,[128] have shown efficacy in gene delivery, but are currently too toxic for clinical application.

One study recently showed evidence for nonviral gene therapy in the treatment of the laser-induced CNV model.[85] In this study, poly(lactic-co-glycolic acid) (PLGA) nanospheres, loaded with an anti-VEGF intraceptor gene (Flt23K), were functionalized with RGD and transferrin and shown to transfect the RPE when injected intravenously into the tail vein. The nanoparticles were shown to selectively transduce the laser-treated eye and had low efficiency of delivery to tissue outside the CNV lesion, perhaps overcoming concerns of systemic expression in intravenous delivery.

A number of different vectors, both viral and nonviral, have been designed for gene delivery to ocular tissue. While these vectors have been shown to demonstrate a wide range of tropism, tissue transduction also depends on the location of delivery and the cell types primarily exposed.

MODE OF DELIVERY AND THE TARGET CELL

The eye is unique in that (a) it is easily accessible for local administration of therapeutic genes and (b) isolation of the ocular tissues via the blood-retinal barrier allows for more targeted delivery of gene therapy vectors. Varying the location of administration can further restrict exposure to gene therapy vectors to a specific cell population. Additionally, current vectors not only transduce different cell types (as seen above) but also differ in their ability to penetrate ocular tissue. There are four different sites of injection that have shown efficacy in rescuing animal models of ocular neovascularization: the subretinal space, the vitreous, the periocular tissue, and the vasculature (including intramuscular and intravenous injection). The ideal mode of delivery depends on (a) the therapeutic factor being expressed, (b) the target tissue, and (c) the vector used for delivery.

Subretinal and intravitreal administration of the same vector can result in transfection of different cell types. In one study, upon injection into the vitreous, AAV2 was found to transfect many cells in the retina, primarily ganglion cells (GC) and the inner nuclear layer (INL), whereas in the same study, adenovirus 5 (Ad5) was shown to infect cells of the corneal endothelium, iris pigment epithelium, and ciliary epithelium.[49] Interestingly, though they transfected very different cell types, the two vectors had highly comparable levels of RNV reduction in an ROP model.[49] Although adenovirus infected cells were relatively farther away from the site of neovascularization, the soluble factor appeared able to diffuse across the vitreous at levels sufficient to inhibit blood vessel growth. Similarly, AAV expressing sFlt-1 delivered into the subretinal space at the equator of the eye was able to inhibit laser-induced neovascularization at the optic nerve, indicating that soluble factors are able to diffuse to the site of neovascularization even if not expressed proximal to the injury site.[129] While diffusion can lessen the importance of the injection location, the mode of delivery can also enhance the potency of the vector. For example, in a laser-induced CNV model, rescue using a PEDF expressing adenovirus increased from 33% to 70% after intravitreal versus subretinal injection.[28] The benefits of subretinal injection are not always clear; for example, AAV expressing PEDF demonstrated a reduction of laser-induced CNV of 33% when injected into the subretinal space, compared with 40% when injected into the vitreous.[31] Because subretinal injections are more invasive, any increase in potency may be outweighed by the risks associated with the injection, such as retinal detachment.

Though intravitreal injections are part of routine care for many patients with ocular neovascularization, they do carry risks for potentially blinding complications.[16] In contrast to subretinal and intravitreal injections, periocular injections are less invasive; however, they require the movement of material through the sclera and choroid in order to reach the inner structures of the eye. Periocular delivery involves the injection of material between the conjunctiva and the external surface of the sclera and avoids many complications of intraocular injections as the sclera itself is not injured.[130] Experiments using Green Fluorescent Protein (GFP) protein diffusion showed levels in the retina and RPE at levels comparable to intravitreal experiments, although the authors note that physiologically relevant proteins, like PEDF or sFlt-1, are larger than GFP and may have slower kinetics.[130] Naked siRNA against VEGFR-1 delivered via periocular injection diffused throughout the retina and inhibited neovascularization.[72] Subsequent studies examining gene delivery using adenovirus showed localization of LacZ along the sclera and outside surface of the orbit,[131] with diffusion of PEDF as far as the choroid and RPE.[131] In fact, periocular delivery of adenovirus expressing PEDF showed a significant increase in PEDF levels in the RPE and choroid compared to the same virus injected into the vitreous, although no PEDF was detected in the retina.[132] Periocular injection has proved effective in the rescue of CNV with an adenovirus expressing either PEDF[131,132] or sFlt-1,[132] as well as in the rescue of corneal angiogenesis using AAV expressing angiostatin.[133] Studies using a pig model of laser-induced CNV, in which scleral thickness and orbit size are more similar to humans, demonstrated that even under these conditions periocular injection of a PEDF expressing adenovirus results in a 77% reduction in CNV.[134] However, since PEDF was shown only to penetrate the RPE and choroid but not the retina, predictably periocular injection was unable to rescue an ROP model of RNV.[131,132] Thus, periocular gene delivery may not be a viable option for the treatment of retinal angiogenesis.

Intravenous administration is also an attractive delivery method for gene therapy since it avoids complications of intraocular delivery. However, systemic delivery of antiangiogenic molecules has the potential for side effects that may make them poorly tolerated. While injection of secreted gene therapy agents has shown efficacy in inhibiting ocular neovascularization, it has also shown a concomitant increase in serum levels of the protein.[27,30] Recent efforts have sought to target gene delivery specifically to the neovascular site, thus decreasing systemic exposure to the angiostatic protein. Evidence using functionalized nanoparticles[85] and pseudotyped AAV that target the vasculature indicate that intravenous injection may be a safe form of delivery. While restricting the site of exposure can increase transduction of specific cell types, transgenes can be further controlled by the use of promoters and enhancers that restrict the site of expression.

REGULATION OF GENE EXPRESSION

While gene therapy offers the potential for long-term drug delivery, sustained and unregulated expression of angiostatic factors could result in deleterious side effects to nearby tissue. VEGF mediates important housekeeping functions in the mature retina and acts as a survival factor for the vascular endothelium. Regulation of gene expression can be accomplished through a number of molecular mechanisms, including vector targeting of specific tissues, use of inducible promoters, and/or tissue response elements.

Targeting dividing cells may be a way to restrict tissue transfection to sites of neovascularization. In the laser-induced CNV model, adenovirus has been shown to preferentially infect the dividing RPE cells at the site of injury.[135] Integrins, such as $\alpha v\beta 3$, have been shown to be upregulated in neovascular blood vessels in proliferative diabetic retinopathy and AMD patients[136] and transferrin has been shown to be highly expressed in the retinas of AMD patients.[137] Capitalization of these properties by functionalization of nanospheres, with either a peptide that binds the $\alpha v\beta 3$ integrin or transferrin, has been shown to selectively increase transduction in neovascular ocular tissue.[85] Clinically, infants suffering from ROP have an initial state of hypoproliferation and there is concern that blanket antiangiogenic treatment could also block the healthy development of blood vessels. Developmental markers that distinguish between pathologic angiogenesis and normal blood vessel vasculogenesis may provide potential targets for gene therapy vectors.[138]

Tissue-specific promoters are another mechanism by which to target gene expression. Commonly used promoters such as the cytomegalovirus (CMV) enhancer-promoter and CMV enhancer-chicken beta-actin (CBA) promoter both drive expression in multiple cell types. Additionally, it should be noted that, while both the CMV and CBA promoters are considered ubiquitous, studies using Ad5 have shown that changing the transgene promoter from CMV to CBA dramatically increased photoreceptor expression.[101] Changing the promoter can ensure that gene expression is limited to a select cell population; however, large regulatory elements can exceed the cloning capacity of many viruses, especially AAV. Recently, smaller photoreceptor-specific promoters have been described that may circumvent the need for large regulatory elements, including a 470 bp[139] and a 235 bp promoter,[140] that limit expression to photoreceptors.

Inducible promoters allow for the selective activation of gene expression, often via an antibiotic response element. A few of these promoters have been described and have shown efficacy in the eye, such as the tetracycline inducible promoter expressed from either an adenovirus[109,141] or AAV[142] vector and the rapamycin inducible promoter expressed from an AAV vector.[143] The CMV promoter, while expressing a high level of transgene in most tissues, has been shown to have transient expression, with either little or no expression within a few weeks.[144] In a recent study, PEDF expression by the CMV promoter returned to baseline 90 days after adenoviral vector injection into the vitreous.[144] However, a systemic injection of all-trans retinoic acid was able to restimulate transgene expression and the level of reactivation was high enough to inhibit laser-induced CNV.[144] While the use of inducible promoters allows for tighter regulation of transgene expression, there are a number of drawbacks including the need for regular and more sensitive clinical observation for early detection of neovascularization, potentially inefficient drug penetration across the blood-retinal barrier, and the side effects of long-term antibiotic dosing.

An alternative to small molecule induced promoter regulation is the use of tissue response element promoters, which allow for transgene activation in response to the local tissue environment. Hypoxia is a driving stimulus for many antiangiogenic molecules and is a known pathogenic factor in ROP and diabetic retinopathy. Hypoxia response elements (HREs) tightly regulate gene expression to respond only to local tissue hypoxia. HREs regulate a number of different genes by binding hypoxia inducible factor 1α (HIF-1α), including VEGF.[145] The use of HRE sequences to regulate transgene expression has proven effective in other models of disease such as myocardial ischemia.[146] In experimental models of both RNV and CNV, HRE-mediated GFP expression from an AAV vector occurred only in sites of neovascularization during the early stages of angiogenesis.[147] Regulation using HRE and other tissue response regulatory sequences offers a promising tool to overcome potential complications of constitutive expression of antiangiogenic factors.

Table 26.4.

Gene therapy vectors used to rescue animal models of neovascularization

Vector	Site	Cells	Molecule	Model	Result	References
BIV	SR	RPE	Endostatin	VEGF-TG	Decreased RNV and permeability	(94)
HIV	IV	Low GC, INL, ONL	Angiostatin	ROP	90% decrease in RNV	(153)
Ad5	IV	CE, IPE	sFlt-1	ROP	56% decrease in RNV	(49)
Ad5 (second generation)	IV	GC, INL	sFlt-1	ROP	97.5% decrease in RNV	(159)
Ad5	IM		sFlt-1(fused to Ig Fc portion)	Laser	Decreased CNV and inflammation	(150)
Ad5 (second generation)	IV	CE, trabecular meshwork	sFlt-1	Corneal NV	80% decrease in corneal NV	(160)
Hd-Ad5	IV	MC	sFlt-1 (DOX)	ROP	60% decrease in RNV (dox dependent)	(109)
Ad5 (second generation)	PO	Extra-ocular tissue	PEDF	Laser	80% decreased CNV area	(131)
	PO			ROP	No reduction in RNV	
Ad/F35 RGD	IV	ND	PEDF	Laser	80% decrease in CNV	(102)
Ad5 (second generation)	PO	Extraocular tissue	sFlt-1	Laser	82% decrease in CNV, reduced permeability	(132)
	PO			ROP	No reduction in RNV	
	IV	ND		Laser	52% decrease in CNV	
Ad5 (second generation)	IV	ND	PEDF	Laser	33% decrease in CNV	(28)

Table 26.4.

Gene therapy vectors used to rescue animal models of neovascularization (*Continued*)

Vector	Site	Cells	Molecule	Model	Result	References
	IV			ROP	50% decrease in RNV	
	IV			VEGF-TG	80% decrease in RNV	
	SR	ND		Laser	70% decrease in CNV	
Ad5 (second generation)	IV	ND	PEDF	Laser	33% CNV regression	(152)
	SR	ND		Laser	50% CNV regression	
	SR			VEGF-TG	80% RNV regression	
Ad5 (second generation)	IV	CE	Anti-VEGF RNA	Corneal NV	Decreased VEGF levels, 86% decrease in NV	(69)
Ad5 (second generation)	SR	RPE	Anti-VEGF shRNA	Ad5-VEGF	84% CNV reduction	(75)
Hd-Ad5	SR	RPE	Endostatin (TAM)	VEGF-TG	Decreased RNV and permeability	(94)
Ad5 (second generation)	TV	liver	Endostatin	Laser	No detectable CMV	(30)
Ad5	IM					
	IM		ExTek	Laser	45% decrease in CNV	(27)
				ROP	47% decrease in RNV	
Ad5	SR	RPE, ONL	VHL	BRVO	Decreased RNV	(84)
AAV2	SR	RPE, ONL	sFlt-1	Laser	19% reduction in CNV	(129)
	IV	CE, IPE		Corneal NV	36% reduction in corneal NV	
AAV2 (P2 injection)	IV	GC, INL	sFlt-1	ROP	52% reduction in RNV	(49)
AAV2	SR	RPE, ONL	sFlt-1	VEGF-TG	85% decrease RNV, ERG rescue, decreased permeability	(151)
	SR			Laser (monkey)	No detectable CNV	
AAV2	SR	RPE, ONL	PEDF	Laser	33% decrease CNV area	(31)
	IV	GC			40% decrease CNV area	
AAV2/1	SR	RPE	PEDF	ROP	85% decrease in RNV	(26)
	SR		Endostatin		82% decrease in RNV	
	SR		TIMP-3		75% decrease in RNV	
AAV2	PO	Cornea	Endostatin	Corneal NV	No corneal NV	(161)
AAV2	SR	ND	PEDF	ROP	74% decrease NV cells	(63)
			Angiostatin		78% decrease NV cells	
AAV2	SR	ND	Angiostatin	Laser	40% reduction CNV area, rescue at 150 days postinjection	(29)
AAV2	PO	Extra-ocular tissue	Angiostatin	Corneal NV	Decreased corneal NV	(133)
AAV2	IV	GC, INL	ZFP-TF	Laser	Decreased CNV but not permeability, effect seen out to 3 months	(76)
	SR	RPE	Activating PEDF			
PGLA nanoparticles	TV	RPE	Anti-VEGF intra-ceptor	Laser	50%–75% reduction in CNV	(85)

(*Continued*)

Table 26.4.

Gene therapy vectors used to rescue animal models of neovascularization (*Continued*)

Vector	Site	Cells	Molecule	Model	Result	References
FuGENE 6	PO	Cornea	GABP	Corneal NV	Reduced VEGF and Robo4 expression, decreased corneal NV	(77)
Lipofectamine 2000	IV	Retina	siRNA against HIF-1 and VEGF	ROP	Decreased RNV	(73)
Direct injection	PO	GC, some INL, ONL	siRNA against VEGFR-1	Laser	45% reduction in NV	(72)
	IV	GC, some INL, ONL			66% reduction in NV	

Ad5, adenovirus; Ad5-VEGF, adenovirus expressing VEGF; BIV, bovine immunodeficiency virus; BRVO, multiple branch retinal vein occlusion; CE, corneal endothelium; CNV, choroidal neovascularization; DOX, doxycycline inducible; ExTek, soluble Ang2 receptor; GC, ganglion cells; Hd-Ad, helper-dependent adenovirus; Ig, immunoglobulin; IM, intramuscular; INL, inner nuclear layer (bipolar cell nuclei); IPE, iris pigment epithelium; IV, intravitreal; ND, not determined; NV, neovascular; ONL, outer nuclear layer (photoreceptor nuclei); PO, periocular; RNV, retinal neovascularization; ROP, retinopathy of prematurity hypoxic model; RPE, retinal pigment epithelium; SR, subretinal; TAM, tamoxifin inducible; TV, tail vein; VEGF-TG, VEGF transgenic; ZFP-TF, zinc-finger protein transcription factor.

ANIMAL MODELS AND RESCUE

A number of different animal models have been used to study ocular angiogenesis (for a complete review see Ref. 148). To date, a wide variety of vectors and transgenes have been shown to prevent angiogenesis using animal models of ocular neovascularization (Table 26.4). Gene therapy has shown efficacy in treating models of neovascularization in various tissues of the eye, including laser-induced disruption of Bruch membrane, hypoxia-induced RNV model of ROP, experimentally induced corneal angiogenesis, as well as VEGF overexpression (Table 26.5).

The laser-induced rupture of Bruch membrane via photocoagulation has proved to be the most reliable and reproducible model of CNV and is one of the primary models of ocular neovascularization. The use of the laser model has clarified many facets of CNV progression, including the importance of the RPE in maintaining the blood-retinal barrier, scarring, and angiogenesis. Unfortunately, there are a number of artifacts that complicate the laser model including RNV development, local inflammation, and glial pathology[149] Gene therapy expression of sFlt-1,[129,132,150,151] PEDF,[28,31,102,131,152] angiostatin,[29,153] endostatin,[30] the Ang2 receptor ExTek,[27] zinc-finger activation of PEDF expression,[76] siRNA targeting VEGF receptor (VEGFR-1),[72] and expression of a VEGF intraceptor[85] have all been shown to inhibit laser-induced CNV. AAV expression of sFlt-1 has been shown to rescue a transgenic model of CNV for up to 8 months.[151] This same construct has also demonstrated persistent expression out to 17 months in a nonhuman primate, the levels after 16 months being sufficient to inhibit all CNV postlaser induction.[151] Mice treated intravenously with the nonviral functionalized nanospheres were shown to have a 50% to75% decrease in CNV.[85] Additionally, the expression of PEDF from adenovirus has been shown to cause the regression of previously induced CNV (either by laser or VEGF overexpression) by induction of apoptosis in angiogenic vascular cells,[152] making it an attractive choice for patients with preestablished neovascular lesions.

While transgenic mice expressing VEGF in the RPE produce intra-CNV, the newly formed blood vessels do not penetrate Bruch membrane and there is no ERG reduction as seen in patients with severe late-stage AMD.[149] Overexpression of VEGF via virus-mediated delivery to the subretinal space led to marked neovascularization that penetrated Bruch membrane, proliferation of RPE cells, photoreceptor degeneration, and reduced ERG amplitude.[154] The delivery of basic fibroblast growth factor has also been shown to induce neovascularization.[155] VEGF overexpression models of CNV have been rescued using anti-VEGF therapy, such as shRNA targeting VEGF.[75] VEGF expression from a rhodopsin promoter induces neovascularization in the retina as well as increased permeability of the nascent blood vessels, which is an important part of the pathology of diabetic retinopathy that leads to retinal edema and detachment.[156,157] Gene therapy delivery of endostatin was shown to not only inhibit neovascularization but also increase the stability of blood vessels, resulting in reduced edema and detachment.[94] VEGF overexpression models of RNV have been rescued using sFlt-1,[151] PEDF,[28,152] and endostatin.[94]

Table 26.5.

Animal models of ocular neovasculariztion rescued via a gene therapy approach

Model	Therapeutic Transgenes
Hypoxia-induced RNV (ROP model)	sFlt-1
	PEDF
	Angiostatin
	Endostatin
	TIMP-3
	ExTek
	Anti-VEGF RNA
	Anti-HIF-1 RNA
Laser-induced CNV	sFlt-1
	PEDF
	Angiostatin
	Endostatin
	ExTek
	ZF-TF activating PEDF
	Anti-VEGFR-1 RNA
	Anti-VEGF intraceptor
VEGF transgenic (RNV)	sFlt-1
	PEDF
	Endostatin
VEGF virus infection (CNV)	Anti-VEGF shRNA
Corneal angiogenesis	sFlt-1
	Angiostatin
	Endostatin
	GABP
	anti-VEGF RNA

Models of diabetes, either spontaneous or streptozotocin-induced, fail to exhibit RNV common in diabetic retinopathy. The hypoxic model of RNV, however, offers a quantifiable model in which to study this process. Transient treatment with high oxygen levels results in a highly reproducible model of ischemia-induced RNV that is highly dependent on VEGF expression. Exposure of mouse pups to 75% oxygen for 5 days causes extensive retinal vessel stunting and capillary closure. When returned to room air, the attenuated vasculature causes relative hypoxia, resulting in retinal ischemia and VEGF-dependent RNV.[158] The neovascular response can be visualized by angiography and quantified histologically by counting the number of neovascular endothelial cell tufts projecting into the vitreous from the retinal vessels. Injection of siRNA targeting either VEGF or HIF-1α has proven effective in inhibiting RNV in the ROP model, with the largest effect occurring when both siRNA vectors are applied simultaneously.[73] Gene therapy expression of sFlt-1,[49,109,159] PEDF,[26,28,63] angiostatin,[63,153] endostatin,[26] TIMP-3,[26] the Ang2 inhibitor ExTek,[27] and siRNA targeting VEGF and HIF-1,[73] have been used to inhibit RNV in the hypoxia-induced model. For soluble factors, RNV appears to respond to diffusion of antiangiogenic molecules into the retina[132] and rescue does not appear to depend on the site of tissue transduction. For example, when either the ganglion cell layer and INL (using an AAV vector) or the corneal epithelium and iris pigment epithelium (using an adenovirus vector) were transduced with the sFlt-1 transgene in an ROP mouse model, a 52% and 56% reduction in RNV, respectively, was observed.[49]

Corneal angiogenesis is a model in which either a wound is applied to the surface of the cornea or a pellet of secreted VEGF is inserted into a pocket made in the corneal stroma. In both models blood vessels sprout from the limbus vessel network.[148] The area of these blood vessels can be easily quantified noninvasively over time. Vector-induced expression of sFlt-1,[129,160] angiostatin,[133] endostatin,[161] siRNA targeting VEGF,[69] and GABP[77] have all been shown to inhibit corneal neovascularization. GABP, a transcription factor that downregulates VEGF and Robo4, has been shown to decrease the expression of both factors as well as decrease the area of wound-induced corneal neovascularization.[77] Because extraocular secreted factors still contact the cornea, infection of the extraocular tissue via periocular injection has proven effective in delivering soluble factors such as angiostatin[133] and endostatin[161] to angiogenic corneal blood vessels.

KEY POINTS

- Current treatments for disorders of ocular angiogenesis do not address the underlying pathology or provide the required long-term treatment.
- Gene therapy is proving to be increasingly safe in clinical trials, including those addressing treatment of ocular disease, and neovascularization in particular.
- Targets for gene therapy include those employed by nonviral approaches, but a gene-based approach broadens the spectrum of potential targets.
- Selection of the most appropriate gene therapy vector will depend on a number of factors, including target tissue, therapeutic transgene being expressed, as well as the required duration and regulation of treatment.
- Use of transgene expression allows for opportunities in targeting and regulation of expression that can improve long-term safety.
- Gene therapy has shown a high degree of efficacy across a number of neovascular models and is a viable therapy in the treatment of vasoproliferative disorders.

SUMMARY

Gene therapy is an ideal treatment for chronic disorders such as AMD and diabetic retinopathy. As the population continues to age, the burden of chronic diseases will increase and so will the accumulated risk of drugs that require repeat administration. Gene therapy trials in the eye have demonstrated safety and efficacy in humans. Continued progress in vector and transgene development will hopefully translate experimental treatment into the standard of care for many chronic disorders.

REFERENCES

1. Lee P, Wang CC, Adamis AP. Ocular neovascularization: an epidemiologic review. *Surv Ophthalmol*. 1998;43:245–269.
2. Crawford TN, Alfaro DV III, Kerrison JB, etal. Diabetic retinopathy and angiogenesis. *Curr Diabetes Rev*. 2009;5:8–13.
3. Bressler NM, Bressler SB. Preventative ophthalmology. Age-related macular degeneration. *Ophthalmology*. 1995;102: 1206–1211.
4. Steinkuller PG, Du L, Gilbert C, et al. Childhood blindness. *J Aapos*. 1999;3:26–32.
5. Campochiaro PA. Retinal and choroidal neovascularization. *J Cell Physiol*. 2000;184:301–310.
6. Ozaki H, Yu AY, Della N, et al. Hypoxia inducible factor-1alpha is increased in ischemic retina: temporal and spatial correlation with VEGF expression. *Invest Ophthalmol Vis Sci*. 1999;40:182–189.
7. Kelly BD, Hackett SF, Hirota K, et al. Cell type-specific regulation of angiogenic growth factor gene expression and induction of angiogenesis in nonischemic tissue by a constitutively active form of hypoxia-inducible factor 1. *Circ Res*. 2003;93:1074–1081.
8. Ambati J, Ambati BK, Yoo SH, et al. Age-related macular degeneration: etiology, pathogenesis, and therapeutic strategies. *Surv Ophthalmol*. 2003;48:257–293.
9. de Jong PT. Age-related macular degeneration. *N Engl J Med*. 2006;355:1474–1485.
10. Macular Photocoagulation Study Group. Persistent and recurrent neovascularization after laser photocoagulation for subfoveal choroidal neovascularization of age-related macular degeneration. *Arch Ophthalmol*. 1994;112:489–499.
11. Soubrane G, Coscas G, Francais C, et al. Occult subretinal new vessels in age-related macular degeneration. Natural History and early laser treatment. *Ophthalmology*. 1990;97: 649–657.
12. Folkman J. Antiangiogenic gene therapy. *Proc Natl Acad Sci USA*. 1998;95:9064–9066.
13. Jager RD, Mieler WF, Miller JW. Age-related macular degeneration. *N Engl J Med*. 2008;358:2606–2617.
14. Mordenti J, Cuthbertson RA, Ferrara N, et al. Comparisons of the intraocular tissue distribution, pharmacokinetics, and safety of 125I-labeled full-length and Fab antibodies in rhesus monkeys following intravitreal administration. *Toxicol Pathol*. 1999;27:536–544.
15. Seo MS, Kwak N, Ozaki H, et al. Dramatic inhibition of retinal and choroidal neovascularization by oral administration of a kinase inhibitor. *Am J Pathol*. 1999;154:1743–1753.
16. van Wijngaarden P, Coster DJ, Williams KA. Inhibitors of ocular neovascularization: promises and potential problems. *Jama*. 2005;293:1509–1513.
17. Cao Y. Endogenous angiogenesis inhibitors and their therapeutic implications. *Int J Biochem Cell Biol*. 2001;33: 357–369.
18. Streilein JW. Unraveling immune privilege. *Science*. 1995; 270:1158–1159.
19. Bennett J, Pakola S, Zeng Y, et al. Humoral response after administration of E1-deleted adenoviruses: immune privilege of the subretinal space. *Hum Gene Ther*. 1996;7: 1763–1769.
20. Bainbridge JW, Tan MH, Ali RR. Gene therapy progress and prospects: the eye. *Gene Ther*. 2006;13:1191–1197.
21. Acland GM, Aguirre GD, Ray J et al. Gene therapy restores vision in a canine model of childhood blindness. *Nat Genet*. 2001;28:92–95.
22. Pawlyk BS, Smith AJ, Buch PK, et al. Gene replacement therapy rescues photoreceptor degeneration in a murine model of Leber congenital amaurosis lacking RPGRIP. *Invest Ophthalmol Vis Sci*. 2005;46:3039–3045.
23. Bennett J, Tanabe T, Sun D, et al. Photoreceptor cell rescue in retinal degeneration (rd) mice by in vivo gene therapy. *Nat Med*. 1996;2:649–654.
24. Schlichtenbrede FC, da Cruz L, Stephens C, et al. Long-term evaluation of retinal function in Prph2Rd2/Rd2 mice following AAV-mediated gene replacement therapy. *J Gene Med*. 2003;5:757–764.
25. Kumar-Singh R, Farber DB. Encapsidated adenovirus minichromosome-mediated delivery of genes to the retina: application to the rescue of photoreceptor degeneration. *Hum Mol Genet*. 1998;7:1893–1900.
26. Auricchio A, Behling KC, Maguire AM, et al. Inhibition of retinal neovascularization by intraocular viral-mediated delivery of anti-angiogenic agents. *Mol Ther*. 2002;6:490–494.
27. Hangai M, Moon YS, Kitaya N, et al. Systemically expressed soluble Tie2 inhibits intraocular neovascularization. *Hum Gene Ther*. 2001;12:1311–1321.
28. Mori K, Duh E, Gehlbach P, et al. Pigment epithelium-derived factor inhibits retinal and choroidal neovascularization. *J Cell Physiol*. 2001;188:253–263.
29. Lai CC, Wu WC, Chen SL, et al. Suppression of choroidal neovascularization by adeno-associated virus vector expressing angiostatin. *Invest Ophthalmol Vis Sci*. 2001;42:2401–2407.
30. Mori K, Ando A, Gehlbach P, et al. Inhibition of choroidal neovascularization by intravenous injection of adenoviral vectors expressing secretable endostatin. *Am J Pathol*. 2001; 159:313–320.
31. Mori K, Gehlbach P, Yamamoto S, et al. AAV-mediated gene transfer of pigment epithelium-derived factor inhibits choroidal neovascularization. *Invest Ophthalmol Vis Sci*. 2002;43:1994–2000.
32. Verwaerde C, Naud MC, Delanoye A, et al. Ocular transfer of retinal glial cells transduced ex vivo with adenovirus expressing viral IL-10 or CTLA4-Ig inhibits experimental autoimmune uveoretinitis. *Gene Ther*. 2003;10: 1970–1981.
33. Martin KR, Quigley HA, Zack DJ, et al. Gene therapy with brain-derived neurotrophic factor as a protection: retinal ganglion cells in a rat glaucoma model. *Invest Ophthalmol Vis Sci*. 2003;44:4357–4365.

34. Edelstein, M. (ed.). *J Gene Med.* 2007.
35. Sieving PA, Caruso RC, Tao W, et al. Ciliary neurotrophic factor (CNTF) for human retinal degeneration: phase 1 trial of CNTF delivered by encapsulated cell intraocular implants. *Proc Natl Acad Sci USA.* 2006;103:3896–3901.
36. Song JC, McDonnell PJ, Gordon EM, et al. Phase 1/2 evaluation of safety and efficacy of a matrix-targeted retroviral vector bearing a dominant negative cyclin G1 construct (Md-dnG1) as adjunctive intervention for superficial corneal opacity/corneal scarring. *Hum Gene Ther.* 2003;14:306–309.
37. Campochiaro PA, Nguyen QD, Shah SM, et al. Adenoviral vector-delivered pigment epithelium-derived factor for neovascular age-related macular degeneration: results of a phase 1 clinical trial. *Hum Gene Ther.* 2006;17: 167–176.
38. Chevez-Barrios P, Chintagumpala M, Mieler W, et al. Response of retinoblastoma with vitreous tumor seeding to adenovirus-mediated delivery of thymidine kinase followed by ganciclovir. *J Clin Oncol.* 2005;23:7927–7935.
39. Maguire AM, Simonelli F, Pierce EA, et al. Safety and efficacy of gene transfer for Leber's congenital amaurosis. *N Engl J Med.* 2008;358: 2240–2248.
40. Hauswirth WW, Aleman TS, Kaushal S, et al. Treatment of leber congenital amaurosis due to RPE65 mutations by ocular subretinal injection of adeno-associated virus gene vector: short-term results of a phase 1 trial. *Hum Gene Ther.* 2008;19:979–990.
41. Bainbridge JW, Smith AJ, Barker SS, et al. Effect of gene therapy on visual function in Leber's congenital amaurosis. *N Engl J Med.* 2008;358:2231–2239.
42. Aiello LP, Avery RL, Arrigg PG, et al. Vascular endothelial growth factor in ocular fluid of patients with diabetic retinopathy and other retinal disorders. *N Engl J Med.* 1994;331:1480–1487.
43. Spilsbury K, Garrett KL, Shen WY, et al. Overexpression of vascular endothelial growth factor (VEGF) in the retinal pigment epithelium leads to the development of choroidal neovascularization. *Am J Pathol.* 2000;157:135–144.
44. Aiello LP, Pierce EA, Foley ED, et al. Suppression of retinal neovascularization in vivo by inhibition of vascular endothelial growth factor (VEGF) using soluble VEGF-receptor chimeric proteins. *Proc Natl Acad Sci USA.* 1995;92: 10457–10461.
45. Pierce EA, Avery RL, Foley ED, et al. Vascular endothelial growth factor/vascular permeability factor expression in a mouse model of retinal neovascularization. *Proc Natl Acad Sci USA.* 1995;92:905–909.
46. Krzystolik MG, Afshari MA, Adamis AP, et al. Prevention of experimental choroidal neovascularization with intravitreal anti-vascular endothelial growth factor antibody fragment. *Arch Ophthalmol.* 2002;120:338–346.
47. Miller JW, Adamis AP, Shima DT, et al. Vascular endothelial growth factor/vascular permeability factor is temporally and spatially correlated with ocular angiogenesis in a primate model. *Am J Pathol.* 1994;145:574–584.
48. Husain D, Kim I, Gauthier D, et al. Safety and efficacy of intravitreal injection of ranibizumab in combination with verteporfin PDT on experimental choroidal neovascularization in the monkey. *Arch Ophthalmol.* 2005;123:509–516.
49. Bainbridge JW, Mistry A, De Alwis M, et al. Inhibition of retinal neovascularisation by gene transfer of soluble VEGF receptor sFlt-1. *Gene Ther.* 2002;9:320–326.
50. Campochiaro PA. Gene therapy for ocular neovascularization. *Curr Gene Ther.* 2007;7:25–33.
51. Campochiaro PA. Molecular targets for retinal vascular diseases. *J Cell Physiol.* 2007;210:575–581.
52. Kuo CJ, Farnebo F, Yu EY, et al. Comparative evaluation of the antitumor activity of antiangiogenic proteins delivered by gene transfer. *Proc Natl Acad Sci USA.* 2001;98: 4605–4610.
53. Dawson DW, Volpert OV, Gillis P, et al. Pigment epithelium-derived factor: a potent inhibitor of angiogenesis. *Science.* 1999;285:245–248.
54. Karakousis PC, John SK, Behling KC, et al. Localization of pigment epithelium derived factor (PEDF) in developing and adult human ocular tissues. *Mol Vis.* 2001;7:154–163.
55. Ogata N, Matsuoka M, Imaizumi M, et al. Decrease of pigment epithelium-derived factor in aqueous humor with increasing age. *Am J Ophthalmol.* 2004;137:935–936.
56. Taniwaki T, Becerra SP, Chader GJ, et al. Pigment epithelium-derived factor is a survival factor for cerebellar granule cells in culture. *J Neurochem.* 1995;64:2509–2517.
57. Cayouette M, Smith SB, Becerra SP, et al. Pigment epithelium-derived factor delays the death of photoreceptors in mouse models of inherited retinal degenerations. *Neurobiol Dis.* 1999;6:523–532.
58. O'Reilly MS, Holmgren L, Shing Y, et al. Angiostatin: a novel angiogenesis inhibitor that mediates the suppression of metastases by a Lewis lung carcinoma. *Cell.* 1994;79: 315–328.
59. Cao Y, Ji RW, Davidson D, et al. Kringle domains of human angiostatin. Characterization of the anti-proliferative activity on endothelial cells. *J Biol Chem.* 1996;271: 29461–29467.
60. Yamaguchi N, Anand-Apte B, Lee M, et al. Endostatin inhibits VEGF-induced endothelial cell migration and tumor growth independently of zinc binding. *Embo J.* 1999;18:4414–4423.
61. Noma H, Funatsu H, Yamashita H, et al. Regulation of angiogenesis in diabetic retinopathy: possible balance between vascular endothelial growth factor and endostatin. *Arch Ophthalmol.* 2002;120:1075–1080.
62. Moses MA, Sudhalter J, Langer R. Identification of an inhibitor of neovascularization from cartilage. *Science.* 1990;248: 1408–1410.
63. Raisler BJ, Berns KI, Grant MB, et al. Adeno-associated virus type-2 expression of pigmented epithelium-derived factor or Kringles 1–3 of angiostatin reduce retinal neovascularization. *Proc Natl Acad Sci USA.* 2002;99: 8909–8914.
64. Kong HL, Hecht D, Song W, et al. Regional suppression of tumor growth by in vivo transfer of a cDNA encoding a secreted form of the extracellular domain of the flt-1 vascular endothelial growth factor receptor. *Hum Gene Ther.* 1998; 9:823–833.
65. Pechan P, Rubin H, Lukason M, et al. Novel anti-VEGF chimeric molecules delivered by AAV vectors for inhibition of retinal neovascularization. *Gene Ther.* 2009;16:10–16.

66. Otani A, Takagi H, Oh H, et al. Expressions of angiopoietins and Tie2 in human choroidal neovascular membranes. *Invest Ophthalmol Vis Sci*. 1999;40:1912–1920.
67. Peters KG, Kontos CD, Lin PC, et al. Functional significance of Tie2 signaling in the adult vasculature. *Recent Prog Horm Res*. 2004;59:51–71.
68. Celec P, Yonemitsu Y. Vascular endothelial growth factor targeted RNA interference as a modulator of angiogenesis. *Biomed Pharmacother*. 2008;62:349–351.
69. Lai CM, Spilsbury K, Brankov M, et al. Inhibition of corneal neovascularization by recombinant adenovirus mediated antisense VEGF RNA. *Exp Eye Res*. 2002;75:625–634.
70. Reich SJ, Fosnot J, Kuroki A, et al. Small interfering RNA (siRNA) targeting VEGF effectively inhibits ocular neovascularization in a mouse model. *Mol Vis*. 2003;9:210–216.
71. Tolentino MJ, Brucker AJ, Fosnot J, et al. Intravitreal injection of vascular endothelial growth factor small interfering RNA inhibits growth and leakage in a nonhuman primate, laser-induced model of choroidal neovascularization. *Retina*. 2004;24:132–138.
72. Shen J, Samul R, Silva RL, et al. Suppression of ocular neovascularization with siRNA targeting VEGF receptor 1. *Gene Ther*. 2006;13:225–234.
73. Jiang J, Xia XB, Xu HZ, et al. Inhibition of retinal neovascularization by gene transfer of small interfering RNA targeting HIF-1alpha and VEGF. *J Cell Physiol*. 2009;218:66–74.
74. Kleinman ME, Yamada K, Takeda A, et al. Sequence- and target-independent angiogenesis suppression by siRNA via TLR3. *Nature*. 2008;452:591–597.
75. Cashman SM, Bowman L, Christofferson J, et al. Inhibition of choroidal neovascularization by adenovirus-mediated delivery of short hairpin RNAs targeting VEGF as a potential therapy for AMD. *Invest Ophthalmol Vis Sci*. 2006;47: 3496–3504.
76. Yokoi K, Zhang HS, Kachi S, et al. Gene transfer of an engineered zinc finger protein enhances the anti-angiogenic defense system. *Mol Ther*. 2007;15:1917–1923.
77. Yoon KC, Bae JA, Park HJ, et al. Subconjunctival gene delivery of the transcription factor GA-binding protein delays corneal neovascularization in a mouse model. *Gene Ther*. 2009;16:973–981.
78. Bora PS, Sohn JH, Cruz JM, et al. Role of complement and complement membrane attack complex in laser-induced choroidal neovascularization. *J Immunol*. 2005;174:491–497.
79. Bora NS, Kaliappan S, Jha P, et al. CD59, a complement regulatory protein, controls choroidal neovascularization in a mouse model of wet-type age-related macular degeneration. *J Immunol*. 2007;178:1783–1790.
80. Ramo K, Cashman SM, Kumar-Singh R. Evaluation of adenovirus-delivered human CD59 as a potential therapy for AMD in a model of human membrane attack complex formation on murine RPE. *Invest Ophthalmol Vis Sci*. 2008;49: 4126–4136.
81. Klein RJ, Zeiss C, Chew EY, et al. Complement factor H polymorphism in age-related macular degeneration. *Science*. 2005;308:385–389.
82. Rohrer B, Long Q, Coughlin B, et al. A targeted inhibitor of the alternative complement pathway reduces angiogenesis in a mouse model of age-related macular degeneration. *Invest Ophthalmol Vis Sci*. 2009;50:3056–3064.
83. Inomata Y, Tanihara H, Tanito M, et al. Suppression of choroidal neovascularization by thioredoxin-1 via interaction with complement factor H. *Invest Ophthalmol Vis Sci*. 2008;49:5118–5125.
84. Akiyama H, Tanaka T, Itakura H, et al. Inhibition of ocular angiogenesis by an adenovirus carrying the human von Hippel-Lindau tumor-suppressor gene in vivo. *Invest Ophthalmol Vis Sci*. 2004;45:1289–1296.
85. Singh SR, Grossniklaus HE, Kang SJ, et al. Intravenous transferrin, RGD peptide and dual-targeted nanoparticles enhance anti-VEGF intraceptor gene delivery to laser-induced CNV. *Gene Ther*. 2009;16:645–659.
86. Kumar-Singh R. Barriers for retinal gene therapy: separating fact from fiction. *Vision Res*. 2008;48:1671–1680.
87. Miyoshi H, Takahashi M, Gage FH, et al. Stable and efficient gene transfer into the retina using an HIV-based lentiviral vector. *Proc Natl Acad Sci USA*. 1997;94:10319–10323.
88. Bainbridge JW, Stephens C, Parsley K, et al. In vivo gene transfer to the mouse eye using an HIV-based lentiviral vector; efficient long-term transduction of corneal endothelium and retinal pigment epithelium. *Gene Ther*. 2001;8:1665–1668.
89. Challa P, Luna C, Liton PB, et al. Lentiviral mediated gene delivery to the anterior chamber of rodent eyes. *Mol Vis*. 2005;11:425–430.
90. Balaggan KS, Binley K, Esapa M, et al. Stable and efficient intraocular gene transfer using pseudotyped EIAV lentiviral vectors. *J Gene Med*. 2006;8:275–285.
91. Bemelmans AP, Bonnel S, Houhou L, et al. Retinal cell type expression specificity of HIV-1-derived gene transfer vectors upon subretinal injection in the adult rat:influence of pseudotyping and promoter. *J Gene Med*. 2005;7:1367–1374.
92. Auricchio A, Kobinger G, Anand V, et al. Exchange of surface proteins impacts on viral vector cellular specificity and transduction characteristics: the retina as a model. *Hum Mol Genet*. 2001;10:3075–3081.
93. Takahashi K, Luo T, Saishin Y, et al. Sustained transduction of ocular cells with a bovine immunodeficiency viral vector. *Hum Gene Ther*. 2002;13:1305–1316.
94. Takahashi K, Saishin Y, Saishin Y, et al. Intraocular expression of endostatin reduces VEGF-induced retinal vascular permeability, neovascularization, and retinal detachment. *Faseb J*. 2003;17:896–898.
95. Buckley RH. Gene therapy for SCID–a complication after remarkable progress. *Lancet*. 2002;360:1185–1186.
96. Russell WC. Update on adenovirus and its vectors. *J Gen Virol*. 2000;81:2573–2604.
97. Neumann R, Doerfler W. Integration of adenovirus type 2 DNA at a limited number of cellular sites in productively infected cells. *J Virol*. 1981;37:887–892.
98. Pang J, Cheng M, Stevenson D, et al. Adenoviral-mediated gene transfer to retinal explants during development and degeneration. *Exp Eye Res*. 2004;79:189–201.
99. Mallam JN, Hurwitz MY, Mahoney T, et al. Efficient gene transfer into retinal cells using adenoviral vectors: dependence on receptor expression. *Invest Ophthalmol Vis Sci*. 2004;45:1680–1687.
100. Von Seggern DJ, Aguilar E, Kinder K, et al. In vivo transduction of photoreceptors or ciliary body by intravitreal injection of pseudotyped adenoviral vectors. *Mol Ther*. 2003;7:27–34.

101. Cashman SM, McCullough L, Kumar-Singh R. Improved retinal transduction in vivo and photoreceptor-specific transgene expression using adenovirus vectors with modified penton base. *Mol Ther*. 2007;15:1640–1646.
102. Hamilton MM, Byrnes GA, Gall JG, et al. Alternate serotype adenovector provides long-term therapeutic gene expression in the eye. *Mol Vis*. 2008;14:2535–2546.
103. Marshall E. Gene therapy death prompts review of adenovirus vector. *Science*. 1999;286:2244–2245.
104. Kumar-Singh R, Chamberlain JS. Encapsidated adenovirus minichromosomes allow delivery and expression of a 14 kb dystrophin cDNA to muscle cells. *Hum Mol Genet*. 1996;5: 913–921.
105. Parks RJ, Chen L, Anton M, et al. A helper-dependent adenovirus vector system: removal of helper virus by Cre-mediated excision of the viral packaging signal. *Proc Natl Acad Sci USA*. 1996;93:13565–13570.
106. Haecker SE, Stedman HH, Balice-Gordon RJ, et al. In vivo expression of full-length human dystrophin from adenoviral vectors deleted of all viral genes. *Hum Gene Ther*. 1996; 7:1907–1914.
107. Reichel MB, Ali RR, Thrasher AJ, et al. Immune responses limit adenovirally mediated gene expression in the adult mouse eye. *Gene Ther*. 1998;5:1038–1046.
108. Kreppel F, Luther TT, Semkova I, et al. Long-term transgene expression in the RPE after gene transfer with a high-capacity adenoviral vector. *Invest Ophthalmol Vis Sci*. 2002;43:1965–1970.
109. Lamartina S, Cimino M, Roscilli G, et al. Helper-dependent adenovirus for the gene therapy of proliferative retinopathies: stable gene transfer, regulated gene expression and therapeutic efficacy. *J Gene Med*. 2007;9:862–874.
110. Chen P, Hamilton M, Thomas CA, et al. Persistent expression of PEDF in the eye using high-capacity adenovectors. *Mol Ther*. 2008;16:1986–1994.
111. Allocca M, Mussolino C, Garcia-Hoyos M, et al. Novel adeno-associated virus serotypes efficiently transduce murine photoreceptors. *J Virol*. 2007;81:11372–11380.
112. Surace EM, Auricchio A. Versatility of AAV vectors for retinal gene transfer. *Vision Res*. 2008;48:353–359.
113. Dinculescu A, Glushakova L, Min SH, et al. Adeno-associated virus-vectored gene therapy for retinal disease. *Hum Gene Ther*. 2005;16:649–663.
114. Narfstrom K, Katz ML, Ford M, et al. In vivo gene therapy in young and adult RPE65-/- dogs produces long-term visual improvement. *J Hered*. 2003;94:31–37.
115. Bennett J, Maguire AM, Cideciyan AV, et al. Stable transgene expression in rod photoreceptors after recombinant adeno-associated virus-mediated gene transfer to monkey retina. *Proc Natl Acad Sci USA*. 1999;96:9920–9925.
116. Kotin RM, Siniscalco M, Samulski RJ, et al. Site-specific integration by adeno-associated virus. *Proc Natl Acad Sci USA*. 1990;87:2211–2215.
117. Ponnazhagan S, Erikson D, Kearns WG, et al. Lack of site-specific integration of the recombinant adeno-associated virus 2 genomes in human cells. *Hum Gene Ther*. 1997;8:275–284.
118. Donsante A, Miller DG, Li Y, et al. AAV vector integration sites in mouse hepatocellular carcinoma. *Science*. 2007;317:477.
119. Andrieu-Soler C, Bejjani RA, de Bizemont T, et al. Ocular gene therapy: a review of nonviral strategies. *Mol Vis*. 2006; 12:1334–1347.
120. Zhang Y, Schlachetzki F, Li JY, et al. Organ-specific gene expression in the rhesus monkey eye following intravenous non-viral gene transfer. *Mol Vis*. 2003;9:465–472.
121. Zhu C, Zhang Y, Pardridge WM. Widespread expression of an exogenous gene in the eye after intravenous administration. *Invest Ophthalmol Vis Sci*. 2002;43:3075–3080.
122. Zhu C, Zhang Y, Zhang YF, et al. Organ-specific expression of the lacZ gene controlled by the opsin promoter after intravenous gene administration in adult mice. *J Gene Med*. 2004;6:906–912.
123. Kachi S, Oshima Y, Esumi N, et al. Nonviral ocular gene transfer. *Gene Ther*. 2005;12:843–851.
124. Farjo R, Skaggs J, Quiambao AB, et al. Efficient non-viral ocular gene transfer with compacted DNA nanoparticles. *PLoS One*. 2006;1:e38.
125. Konstan MW, Davis PB, Wagener JS, et al. Compacted DNA nanoparticles administered to the nasal mucosa of cystic fibrosis subjects are safe and demonstrate partial to complete cystic fibrosis transmembrane regulator reconstitution. *Hum Gene Ther*. 2004;15:1255–1269.
126. Cai X, Nash Z, Conley SM, et al. A partial structural and functional rescue of a retinitis pigmentosa model with compacted DNA nanoparticles. *PLoS One*. 2009;4:e5290.
127. Chalberg TW, Genise HL, Vollrath D, et al. phiC31 integrase confers genomic integration and long-term transgene expression in rat retina. *Invest Ophthalmol Vis Sci*. 2005; 46:2140–2146.
128. Chalberg TW, Vankov A, Molnar FE, et al. Gene transfer to rabbit retina with electron avalanche transfection. *Invest Ophthalmol Vis Sci*. 2006;47:4083–4090.
129. Lai YK, Shen WY, Brankov M, et al. Potential long-term inhibition of ocular neovascularisation by recombinant adeno-associated virus-mediated secretion gene therapy. *Gene Ther*. 2002;9:804–813.
130. Mac Gabhann F, Demetriades AM, Deering T, et al. Protein transport to choroid and retina following periocular injection: theoretical and experimental study. *Ann Biomed Eng*. 2007;35:615–630.
131. Gehlbach P, Demetriades AM, Yamamoto S, et al. Periocular injection of an adenoviral vector encoding pigment epithelium-derived factor inhibits choroidal neovascularization. *Gene Ther*. 2003;10:637–646.
132. Gehlbach P, Demetriades AM, Yamamoto S, et al. Periocular gene transfer of sFlt-1 suppresses ocular neovascularization and vascular endothelial growth factor-induced breakdown of the blood-retinal barrier. *Hum Gene Ther*. 2003;14:129–141.
133. Cheng HC, Yeh SI, Tsao YP, et al. Subconjunctival injection of recombinant AAV-angiostatin ameliorates alkali burn induced corneal angiogenesis. *Mol Vis*. 2007;13:2344–2352.
134. Saishin Y, Silva RL, Saishin Y, et al. Periocular gene transfer of pigment epithelium-derived factor inhibits choroidal neovascularization in a human-sized eye. *Hum Gene Ther*. 2005;16:473–478.
135. Lai CM, Shen WY, Constable IJ, et al. Preferential adenovirus-mediated transduction of cells at the sites of laser photocoagulation in the rat eye. *Curr Eye Res*. 1999;19:411–417.
136. Friedlander M, Theesfeld CL, Sugita M, et al. Involvement of integrins alpha v beta 3 and alpha v beta 5 in ocular neovascular diseases. *Proc Natl Acad Sci USA*. 1996;93: 9764–9769.

137. Chowers I, Wong R, Dentchev T, et al. The iron carrier transferrin is upregulated in retinas from patients with age-related macular degeneration. *Invest Ophthalmol Vis Sci*. 2006;47:2135–2140.
138. Beck L Jr, D'Amore PA. Vascular development: cellular and molecular regulation. *Faseb J*. 1997;11:365–373.
139. Glushakova LG, Timmers AM, Issa TM, et al. Does recombinant adeno-associated virus-vectored proximal region of mouse rhodopsin promoter support only rod-type specific expression in vivo? *Mol Vis*. 2006;12:298–309.
140. Khani SC, Pawlyk BS, Bulgakov OV, et al. AAV-mediated expression targeting of rod and cone photoreceptors with a human rhodopsin kinase promoter. *Invest Ophthalmol Vis Sci*. 2007;48:3954–3961.
141. Dejneka NS, Auricchio A, Maguire AM, et al. Pharmacologically regulated gene expression in the retina following transduction with viral vectors. *Gene Ther*. 2001;8:442–446.
142. McGee Sanftner LH, Rendahl KG, Quiroz D, et al. Recombinant AAV-mediated delivery of a tet-inducible reporter gene to the rat retina. *Mol Ther*. 2001;3:688–696.
143. Auricchio A, Rivera VM, Clackson T, et al. Pharmacological regulation of protein expression from adeno-associated viral vectors in the eye. *Mol Ther*. 2002;6:238–242.
144. McVey D, Hamilton MM, Hsu C, et al. Repeat administration of proteins to the eye with a single intraocular injection of an adenovirus vector. *Mol Ther*. 2008;16:1444–1449.
145. Semenza GL. Series introduction:tissue ischemia: pathophysiology and therapeutics. *J Clin Invest*. 2000;106:613–614.
146. Phillips MI, Tang Y, Schmidt-Ott K, et al. Vigilant vector: heart-specific promoter in an adeno-associated virus vector for cardioprotection. *Hypertension*. 2002;39:651–655.
147. Bainbridge JW, Mistry A, Binley K, et al. Hypoxia-regulated transgene expression in experimental retinal and choroidal neovascularization. *Gene Ther*. 2003;10:1049–1054.
148. Montezuma SR, Vavvas D, Miller JW. Review of the ocular angiogenesis animal models. *Semin Ophthalmol*. 2009;24:52–61.
149. Schwesinger C, Yee C, Rohan RM, et al. Intrachoroidal neovascularization in transgenic mice overexpressing vascular endothelial growth factor in the retinal pigment epithelium. *Am J Pathol*. 2001;158:1161–1172.
150. Honda M, Sakamoto T, Ishibashi T, et al. Experimental subretinal neovascularization is inhibited by adenovirus-mediated soluble VEGF/flt-1 receptor gene transfection: a role of VEGF and possible treatment for SRN in age-related macular degeneration. *Gene Ther*. 2000;7:978–985.
151. Lai CM, Shen WY, Brankov M, et al. Long-term evaluation of AAV-mediated sFlt-1 gene therapy for ocular neovascularization in mice and monkeys. *Mol Ther*. 2005;12:659–668.
152. Mori K, Gehlbach P, Ando A, et al. Regression of ocular neovascularization in response to increased expression of pigment epithelium-derived factor. *Invest Ophthalmol Vis Sci*. 2002;43:2428–2434.
153. Igarashi T, Miyake K, Kato K, et al. Lentivirus-mediated expression of angiostatin efficiently inhibits neovascularization in a murine proliferative retinopathy model. *Gene Ther*. 2003;10:219–226.
154. Wang F, Rendahl KG, Manning WC, et al. AAV-mediated expression of vascular endothelial growth factor induces choroidal neovascularization in rat. *Invest Ophthalmol Vis Sci*. 2003;44:781–790.
155. Kimura H, Sakamoto T, Hinton DR, et al. A new model of subretinal neovascularization in the rabbit. *Invest Ophthalmol Vis Sci*. 1995;36:2110–2119.
156. Okamoto N, Tobe T, Hackett SF, et al. Transgenic mice with increased expression of vascular endothelial growth factor in the retina: a new model of intraretinal and subretinal neovascularization. *Am J Pathol*. 1997;151:281–291.
157. Ohno-Matsui K, Hirose A, Yamamoto S, et al. Inducible expression of vascular endothelial growth factor in adult mice causes severe proliferative retinopathy and retinal detachment. *Am J Pathol*. 2002;160:711–719.
158. Smith LE, Wesolowski E, McLellan A, et al. Oxygen-induced retinopathy in the mouse. *Invest Ophthalmol Vis Sci*. 1994;35:101–111.
159. Rota R, Riccioni T, Zaccarini M, et al. Marked inhibition of retinal neovascularization in rats following soluble-flt-1 gene transfer. *J Gene Med*. 2004;6:992–1002.
160. Lai CM, Brankov M, Zaknich T, et al. Inhibition of angiogenesis by adenovirus-mediated sFlt-1 expression in a rat model of corneal neovascularization. *Hum Gene Ther*. 2001;12:1299–1310.
161. Lai LJ, Xiao X, Wu JH. Inhibition of corneal neovascularization with endostatin delivered by adeno-associated viral (AAV) vector in a mouse corneal injury model. *J Biomed Sci*. 2007;14:313–322.
162. Rasmussen H, Chu KW, Campochiaro P, et al. Clinical protocol. An open-label, phase 1, single administration, dose-escalation study of ADGVPEDF.11D (ADPEDF) in neovascular age-related macular degeneration (AMD). *Hum Gene Ther*. 2001;12:2029–2032.

CHAPTER 27

Endothelial Progenitor Therapy: Innately Beneficial, Innately Complicated

Matthew Neu • Ashay Bhatwadekar • Reinhold Medina • Alan Stitt • Maria Grant

INTRODUCTION

The notion of using endothelial progenitors to repair vasodegenerative vasculature in diabetic retinopathy is an interesting alternative to current treatment for retinopathy, the leading cause of visual impairment in the Western world.[1] This complication poses serious therapeutic problems and, even with current management regimens, continues to significantly reduce the quality of life for millions of people. Diabetic retinopathy is thought to be a result of hyperglycemia-induced retinal microvascular dysfunction, although there is growing evidence that a significant retinal neuroglial dysfunction also occurs during diabetes, perhaps in unison with vascular pathophysiology.[2] The vasodegenerative phase of diabetic retinopathy consists of significant autoregulatory dysfunction, blood flow abnormalities, premature death of capillary components, and eventually widespread nonperfusion of the inner retina.[3] Proliferative diabetic retinopathy ensues when the ischemic insult is sufficient to trigger retinal neovascularization, which is superimposed upon "background" retinopathy.

Currently available treatments for diabetic retinopathy such as panretinal laser photocoagulation, vitreoretinal surgery, and recently introduced vascular endothelial growth factor (VEGF) inhibitors are mainly focused on end stages of the disease. Importantly, these therapies do not address the primary pathology of retinal neurovascular degeneration during diabetes that precedes the sight-threatening neovascularization and diabetic macular edema. Fresh perspectives on the cellular and molecular mechanisms of diabetic retinopathy could lead to novel and much more effective prevention/reversal strategies. One exciting possible strategy is targeting the early and intermediate stages of vasodegeneration to enhance vessel repair, reverse ischemia, and prevent progression to the late, sight-threatening stages of diabetic retinopathy. For diabetic patients with an occluded retinal microvasculature, measures to preserve surviving vasculature and revascularize defunct capillary beds could extend the lifetime of the neuropile, reduce pathogenic output of vasoactive and neuropathic agents, and ensure retention of serviceable vision.

In the last decade, it has become established that endothelial progenitor cells (EPCs), as a minor subpopulation of the mononuclear cell fraction in peripheral blood, can be recruited to sites requiring vascular repair and contribute to the viability of the vasculature.[4] These cells are derived from the bone marrow or the vasculature itself and they form the basis for potential therapy based on inducing microvascular repair and/or "therapeutic angiogenesis"(Fig. 27.1). Current clinical trials have shown that intramyocardial injection/intracoronary infusion of autologous progenitor cells in patients with intractable angina/acute myocardial infarction is feasible, safe, and beneficial. The same scenario is also a possibility for treatment of retinal ischemia in diabetic retinopathy, and this review focuses on the latest research on the role of these progenitor populations in this complication. How can this knowledge, largely gained in other vascular beds, be exploited for the benefit of diabetic patients with this vision-threatening complication? The answer may lie in a synthesis of both clinical and basic perspectives now believed to dominate the field and new knowledge gained from advances in stem cell biology.

OVERVIEW OF ENDOTHELIAL PROGENITOR POPULATIONS

During the development of the embryo, local mesodermal precursors differentiate into vascular and endothelial cells (ECs) to form a primary vascular plexus, a process referred to as vasculogenesis.[5] This process of vasculogenesis was believed to occur only during embryonic development, but not in postnatal life. In the early 1960s, "GORE-TEX" grafts were developed. These artificial grafts were not re-endothelialized by ECs from the neighboring vessel but rather from circulation.[6] This gave rise to the idea that circulating cells could form capillaries de novo or serve to re-endothelialize damaged blood vessels. These initial observations were then explained by two groups reporting that human $CD34^+$ cells isolated from circulating peripheral blood, umbilical cord blood, and bone marrow

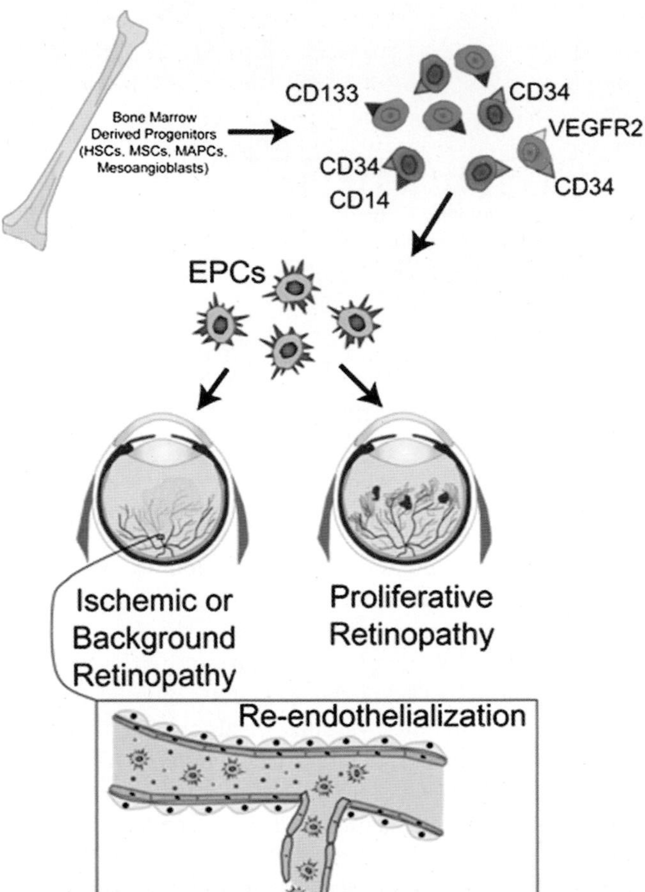

FIGURE 27.1. Role of EPCs in diabetic retinopathy. Bone marrow–derived EPCs in the peripheral circulation express combinations of many surface markers such as CD34, VEGFR2, and CD133. EPCs are home to sites of retinal ischemia and show capacity for repair of injured endothelium in the vasodegenerative stages of diabetic retinopathy. At the later vasoproliferative stages of diabetic retinopathy, EPCs in unison with resident ECs can participate in neovessel formation. Diabetes induces EPC dysfunction, under such circumstances CD14 cells expressing low CD34 can compensate for endothelial repair; however, progressive diabetes converts CD14 cells into an inflammatory, pro-oxidant, eNOS inhibitory, senescent phenotype generating cells that not only repair vasculature poorly but also actually hinder repair and function. HSCs, hematopoietic stem cells; MSCs, mesenchymal stem cells; MAPCs, multipotent adult progenitor cells.

could differentiate into ECs in vitro and in vivo in mouse models.[7,8] These studies launched the field that now has advanced to the therapeutic use of EPCs to enhance tissue and vascular repair in patients with ischemic conditions. Furthermore, different studies suggest that incorporation of bone marrow–derived cells occurs in blood vessels. These cells support the maintenance of such vessels[9] by healing wounds (Fig. 27.2),[10] areas of endothelial denudation,[11] induced hindlimb ischemia[12] and following experimental myocardial infarction.[13] Evidence from patients who have undergone bone marrow or peripheral blood stem cell transplantation shows that some ECs that line blood vessels in the recipient are of donor origin, pointing to the existence of circulating cells in the blood and bone marrow that contribute to endothelial turnover in blood vessels of humans.[14]

The use of "EPCs" has extended to a biomarker for vascular health. Clinical studies suggest an inverse correlation between the number of peripheral blood EPCs and the presence of atherosclerosis, an adverse cardiovascular risk score, level of cardiovascular dysfunction, or cardiovascular morbidity and mortality risk.[15] Also, the functions of EPCs such as cell adherence, migration, invasion, and vessel formation appear to be reduced in patients with increased cardiovascular risk factors and established cardiovascular disease.[16] Therefore, following the numbers of circulating EPCs may help in monitoring the effects of primary and secondary cardiovascular prevention strategies.

In spite of the growing number of reports on EPCs as a potential tool in regenerative medicine or a therapeutic target in oncology, contradicting results have been reported at the preclinical and clinical levels. Most of this confusion is due to varying definitions, identifications, and characterizations of the role of these cells in vascular homeostasis and disease. This chapter discusses these issues in depth and focuses on published studies as well as the authors' opinions on the potential role of these cells to correct retinal ischemia.

PROGENITOR CELLS IN DIABETES

Both Type 1 and Type 2 diabetic individuals with vascular complications would potentially benefit from cellular therapy with autologous cells. However, bone marrow–derived progenitors from diabetic patients are dysfunctional, producing fewer ECs with reduced proliferative and migratory potential.[17] Enhanced oxidative stress in diabetes contributes to progenitor dysfunction.[18] Accumulation of reactive oxygen species (ROS) increases cellular and replicative senescence in these progenitors as does increased angiotensin II, oxidized low-density lipoprotein (ox-LDL), and homocysteine. EPCs of diabetic origin show a reduced ability to integrate into EC tubes in vitro compared to EPCs of nondiabetic origin.[19–22] Vascularization is depressed when EPCs from diabetic mice are injected into normal mice.[23] Recently, it has been shown that activation of the HDL receptor is protective to EPCs by increasing eNOS,[24] whereas activation of the ox-LDL receptor downregulates eNOS, supporting a key role for NO in the function of progenitors.[25,26]

There is a significant depletion of ECs in retinal capillaries during diabetes. The endothelium can correct such loss through increased cell replication (whereby dead cells can be replaced by near neighbors); nevertheless, the concept of the "Hayflick limit" indicates that replicative senescence will occur more rapidly in diabetic retinal capillaries leading to acellular capillary formation. We

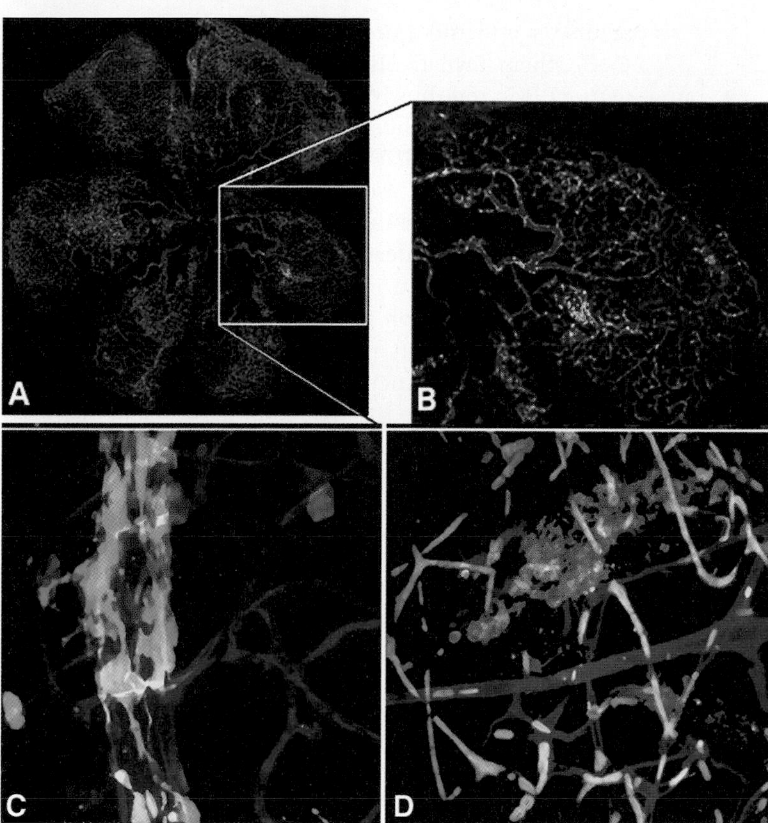

FIGURE 27.2. Fluorescence micrographs showing C57BL/6. *gfp* chimeric mice that underwent retinal ischemia. **A:** Typical whole retina from a treated eye. **B:** Areas with newly formed blood vessels are shown as small regions of green-yellow. **C:** An area depicting a parent vessel perfused with rhodamine-labeled dextran (*red*) with extravasations and initial tube formation by gfp^+ cells. **D:** Treated retina showing different stages of new capillary formation by gfp^+ cells. (Grant, et al. *Nat Med.* 2002;8:607–612.)

believe that development of acellular capillaries may be due to a diabetes-mediated dysfunction of EPCs, which manifests as failed attempts at repair of injured capillaries. This leads to the initiation and persistence of ischemia. Research conducted during the past 10 years has focused on understanding the basic mechanism responsible for the diabetes-associated defect in EPC function. Why is this important? Correcting these defects may allow the use of a diabetic patient's own EPCs for repair of their injured retinal and systemic vasculature as an autologous cell therapy strategy. Specifically in the retina, correction of this dysfunction could treat early and intermediate stages of vasodegeneration to enhance vessel repair, reverse ischemia, and prevent progression to the sight-threatening stages of diabetic retinopathy. However, if circulating cells such as EPCs are given at the "wrong" time, they could exacerbate diabetic retinopathy by contributing to proliferative retinopathy. Moreover, it has been suggested that transplanting some EPC populations into diabetic mice can provoke their differentiation to a proinflammatory and antiangiogenic phenotype and exacerbate ischemia.[27] Therefore, transplanting the wrong cell type (perhaps one carrying monocytic markers) into the diabetic retina could enhance differentiation toward an inflammatory cell fate and therefore promote retinopathic progression.

Thus, before EPCs can be used therapeutically in diabetic retinopathy to re-endothelialize acellular capillaries and eliminate retinal ischemia, several key questions must be answered. What triggers this phenotypic change in diabetic cells changing them from reparative cells to cells that are ineffectual at repair? What is the best reparative EPC population? Are some subpopulations more resistant to the injurious effects of diabetes? Should the bone marrow be a target for diabetic retinopathy therapy? What are the "component" cells that contribute to vasculogenesis in the adult? What strategies exist to assess the in vivo function of these diverse cell types?

Specifically in patients with vascular disorders such as diabetes, in vivo function is key. Moreover, confusion in defining functional characteristics and subpopulations of EPCs is due to variable approaches undertaken in research laboratories with regard to the source of the cell, (species and location: bone marrow or peripheral blood) the purification of the cell, the animal model or assay used to test the function of the cell, the method of detection of the cell in vivo and in vitro, and finally the actual interpretation of these studies.

PROGENITOR POPULATIONS DEFINED

There exist two main approaches to define and/or isolate cells with endothelial characteristics and regenerative capacity, as shown in Figure 27.3: culture selection from mononuclear cells (either from bone marrow or peripheral blood) or the use of a set of antibodies to various "identifying" markers of these cells.

Many groups have characterized endothelial precursors using a panel of immunological and nonimmunological

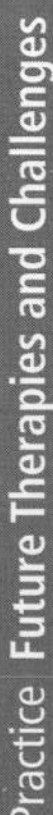

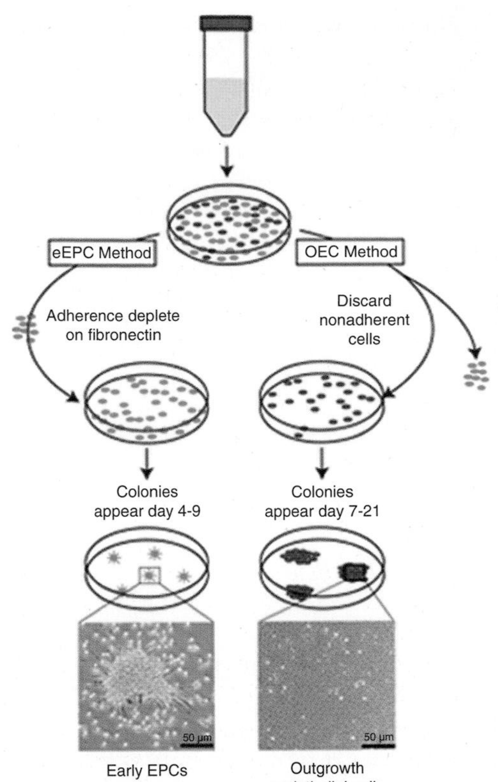

FIGURE 27.3. Isolation and culture of early and late EPCs: Mononuclear cells in presence of selective culture media and matrix (e.g., fibronectin) give rise to eEPCs at 7 to 10 days, whereas OECs are derived later in culture on collagen at 14 to 28 days in endothelial growth conditions. OECs subsequently reach confluence and form tubes on three-dimensional extracellular matrix.

markers in freshly isolated cells, followed by the use of these sorted cells in vitro or in vivo studies. This is the approach commonly used for the isolation of cells (from a patient's own bone marrow or peripheral blood) for cell therapy. The combination of CD34 and VEGFR-2 as surface markers remains the most common approach for the clinical isolation of these cells, but several other markers have been used to refine the identification of this therapeutic cell type. Some have described CD133 (prominin) as an additional marker,[28] particularly to identify the more "immature" EPCs. Considering the uncertainty as to the most reliable method to identify circulating EPCs, most studies employ either the CD34/VEGFR-2 combination or the CD34/CD133 set of markers to quantify circulating EPCs and to correlate their concentration to clinical conditions.[29–31]

However, turmoil developed in the field when Case et al. reported that isolated human umbilical cord blood or mobilized adult peripheral blood CD34$^+$VEGFR-2$^+$CD133$^+$ cells actually represent an enriched population of CD45$^+$ hematopoietic precursors rather than endothelial progenitors. They cleverly used in vitro hematopoiesis assays to show that CD34$^+$VEGFR-2$^+$CD133$^+$ were hematopoietic precursors and did not contribute to the formation of ECs.[32] Others have identified CD34$^+$CD45$^+$CD146$^+$ cells as the true EPCs and thus by using the hematopoietic marker CD45 with the endothelial progenitor markers CD34 and CD146 they believe that the optimal therapeutic cells can be identified. While Case and coworkers argue that these EPCs do not directly differentiate into ECs, they agree that these hematopoietic-derived cells contribute to vascular repair and do so in an indirect manner.[33–37] EPCs can be recruited to injured or angiogenic sites and secrete regulatory cytokines that promote vessel homeostasis and vascular repair. Whether these cells incorporate and differentiate directly into ECs has been highly dependent on the vascular bed. In this case, the retinal vasculature may be particularly unique and the contribution of the circulating cells may be more readily apparent in that the resident retinal vasculature is typically quiescent, making the circulating cell contribution highly apparent.[38] Thus, we strongly believe that the degree of EPC incorporation and contribution to neovessels may be influenced by competition between EPCs and the resident ECs during the vascular repair process.

When using animal models, the genetic background of the mouse, the type of vascular injury to be incurred, and the organ system to be challenged can all impact the outcome of EPC studies. For example, EPC contributions to tumor endothelium are highly dependent on tumor type, stage, and therapy.[39] The type of tissue injury may also be critical, because the cellular and molecular mechanisms of the neovascularization response may differ greatly. For example, laser occlusion of a vessel to induce ischemia may be very different than the thrombotic occlusion of a cardiac vessel in a patient having a myocardial infarction. Moreover, since the tissue "cues" are different, distinct specific cell subsets may be preferentially recruited. Thus, it is not surprising that conflicting results may ensue depending on the animal, the tissue, and the type of injury.

Bone marrow–derived CD14$^+$ monocytes also demonstrate potential to differentiate into endothelial-like cells.[40] Interestingly, although several independent groups have shown a clear development of an endothelial phenotype after selective culture, they have shown that the expression of monocytic antigens persisted following adopting this endothelial phenotype.[40,41] Several additional studies confirmed the overlap between ECs and monocyte phenotypes, suggesting that using traditional EC markers such as acLDL uptake, Ulex binding, CD31, CD105 (endoglin), CD144 (vascular endothelial cadherin), VEGFR-2, CD34, and Tie-2 may not be enough to distinguish between ECs and monocytes, and thus may not specifically identify EPCs.[42–44] Similarly, another group showed that cultured CD34$^-$CD14$^+$ peripheral blood mononuclear cells express Tie-2, VEGFR-2, CD144, von Willebrand factor (vWF), CD146, CD105, and eNOS.[41] Interestingly, another report suggested that CD14$^+$ monocytes, which express low levels of CD34 (undetectable with conventional techniques), may in fact contain the true progenitor cell population, with the greatest regenerative capacity.[45]

The failure to reliably characterize endothelial progenitors has generated some skepticism and confusion within the field of regenerative medicine. However, a recent study[46] and an excellent review by Schatteman et al.[47] have suggested that despite phenotypic overlap between various bone marrow–derived or circulating cell types, the endothelial phenotype can best be characterized by three features: eNOS expression, integration into tube-like structures formed by human umbilical vein endothelial cells (HUVECs), and stimulation of tube formation by HUVECs. It is suggested that these criteria might be the best in vitro method of judging the endothelial phenotype, regardless of the presence or absence of particular cell surface antigens. This simplified interpretation is significant, as it acknowledges the limitation of surface markers and affirms the importance of the identification of EPCs according to their potential to acquire functional properties of ECs.

In addition to the use of surface markers to isolate cells, the use of culture conditions can be used to identify EPC populations. Most investigators, out of sheer frustration in obtaining adequate numbers to sufficiently study EPCs in a disease model, use in vitro growth of mononuclear cells. Numerous assays have been developed to plate mononuclear cells in specific culture conditions to make putative EPCs differentiate into ECs,[7,8,48,49] expand ex vivo,[50,51] and to assay EPCs for colony forming capacity (Fig. 27.3).[52] Two major cell types have been shown to emerge out of these mononuclear cell cultures: cells that display a mixed endothelial-monocytic/hematopoietic phenotype,[4,53] which are referred to as "endothelial-like" monocytic cells or early EPCs (eEPCs), and cells with high proliferative potential that display typical endothelial characteristics, which are called outgrowth endothelial cells (OECs) or late EPCs.[51,54]

Both endothelial-like cells and OECs express similar surface markers such as CD31, lectin binding, vWF, and uptake of LDL.[4] However, recent studies have shown that "endothelial-like" cells co-express a set of endothelial surface markers[4,55,56] and have some characteristics of ECs, but do not form ECs in vivo. Further complicating matters, these cells may change their surface marker expression profile upon ex vivo culture and upon injection in vivo.[57] Thus, true EPCs need to form blood vessels in vitro and in vivo.

When considering what is really important in an EPC population, one has to consider the origins of the EPC and how the cells first characterized by Asahara et al. compare to the more recently identified OECs. Asahara et al. used a subset of $CD34^+$ hematopoietic progenitor cells.[7,58] They reported that peripheral blood mononuclear cells enriched for $CD34^+$ cells could differentiate into endothelial-like cells following culture on fibronectin in the presence of growth factors. After 7 days in culture, the fraction of cells co-expressing CD34 and VEGFR-2 increased. These cells also expressed other endothelial markers such as CD31 (platelet EC adhesion molecule-1, PECAM-1), tyrosine kinase with immunoglobulin-like and EGF-like domains 2 (Tie-2) and eNOS, incorporated acetylated low-density lipoprotein (acLDL), bound Ulex (UEA-1) lectin, and formed tube-like structures in vitro, supporting the contention that they possess the ability to differentiate into ECs. These findings were corroborated by Shi et al.[8]

Currently, culture selection involves the growth of peripheral blood mononuclear cells in selective medium and on either fibronectin coated dishes or collagen coated dishes.[59,60] The medium typically contains a cocktail of endothelial growth factors, such as VEGF, FGF-2, IGF-1, EGF as well as ascorbic acid and hydrocortisone. The medium is changed regularly (usually every 24–28 hours). It is not surprising that exposing cells to endothelial growth factors and placing them on matrixes that are known to "change" their appearance toward an endothelial phenotype will make them appear more "endothelial-like." These eEPCs have been most studied to date. eEPCs are those mainly derived from monocytes and do not proliferate long term but begin to gradually die after a few weeks in culture.[40,61] These characteristics are not indicative of what this population would do in vivo.

In contrast, late OECs usually begin growing after 2 weeks postisolation, eventually proliferate very rapidly, resemble microvascular ECs (with a cobblestone morphology), and have great proliferative potential[62,63] The distinction between these two cell types is reinforced by their expression of different markers. OECs do not express CD1a or CD14 and have a low expression of CD45, the panleukocyte marker.[64] The precise origin of the OEC is still in question, yet Yoder's group believes that the endothelium is the likely source of this progenitor and not the bone marrow.[4] The OEC represents one in a million mononuclear cells found in the circulation and thus can only be "identified" once it has grown out in culture.[22] However, little has been done with these cells in vivo and they have not been studied in humans as of yet.

Since most early studies of cell therapy in the heart and limbs employed eEPCs, there is abundant evidence that these transplanted cells can enhance revascularization,[65] although there is much debate about the precise mechanism of these effects. In contrast, OECs have been minimally studied in vivo.[56] Still their higher proliferative potential may be important when a large supply of regenerative cells is required. Therefore, OECs may have great utility as a cellular therapy.[47]

WHAT CAUSES EPC DYSFUNCTION IN DIABETIC PROGENITOR CELLS?

Much of our focus has been on explaining the migratory dysfunction that diabetic EPCs exhibit, as detailed in Figure 27.4. We have determined that this is due in part to reduced

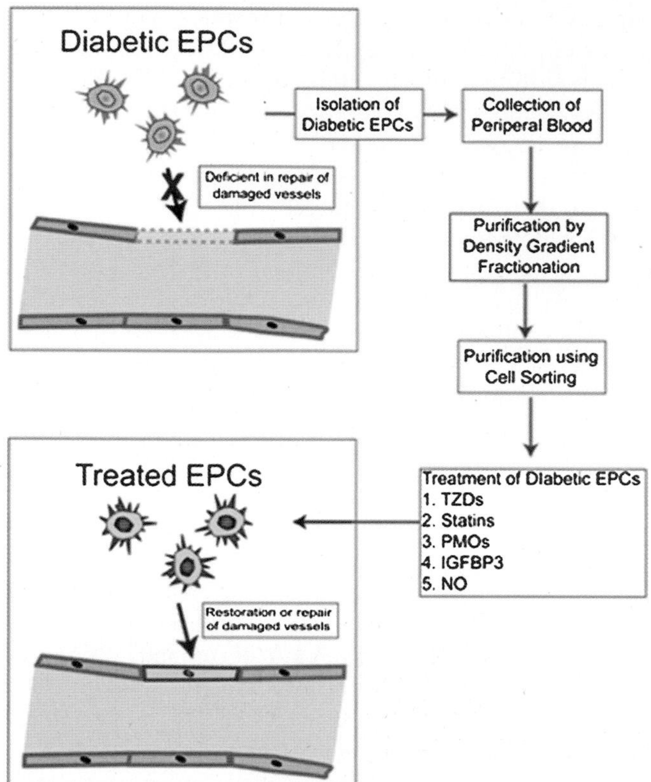

FIGURE 27.4. EPC dysfunction in diabetes. Healthy EPCs have proven ability to repair damaged endothelium by homing to sites of vascular damage and tissue ischemia. EPCs from diabetic donors lack this reparative ability due to inherent cytoskeletal defects and/or impaired signaling within defined transduction pathways. Ex vivo pharmacological manipulation of diabetic EPCs can restore this diabetic defects, improving their reparative ability prior to autologous therapeutic transfer.

nitric oxide availability. NO generation arises from the guanidine group of L-arginine and is a Nicotinamide adenine dinucleotide phosphate (NADPH)-dependent reaction catalyzed by a family of NOS. Three distinct isoforms of NOS, consisting of endothelial NOS (eNOS), neuronal NOS (nNOS), and inducible NOS (iNOS) are similar in structure and function, utilizing L-arginine, oxygen, and NADPH as substrates and requiring Flavin adenine dinucleotide (FAD), Flavin mononucleotide (FMN), calmodulin, and tetrahydrobiopterin as cofactors. The catalytic mechanism of NOS involves flavin-mediated electron transport from NADPH to the terminal heme, where oxygen is bound and incorporated into NO and citrulline.[66] Maintaining an adequate cellular supply of L-arginine is critical for normal vascular function. Deficiencies in L-arginine supply have been strongly implicated in vascular diseases, including diabetes.[67] If the supply of L-arginine or any cofactor does not meet the needs of active NOS, NOS becomes "uncoupled" and uses molecular oxygen as a substrate to form O_2^- instead of NO. An imbalance between L-arginine availability and NOS activity can occur when cellular transport of L-arginine is inhibited,[68] or when there is reduced recycling of L-citrulline back to L-arginine, or when an elevated catabolism of L-arginine by arginase exists.[69,70]

It has been demonstrated in a spontaneous rat model of Type 2 diabetes that eNOS was decreased while NADH oxidase, a major source of superoxide in the vascular endothelium, iNOS, and $ONOO^-$ were all increased in the retinal vasculature.[71] The shift in redox state in diabetes with increased ROS causes increased interaction of NO with O_2-, resulting in loss of bioavailable NO and formation of $ONOO^-$. The reduced NO and elevated $ONOO^-$ can lead to microvascular dysfunction in diabetes.[72–74] $ONOO^-$ is a potent oxidant that can attack many types of biological molecules; a high level of $ONOO^-$ initiates lipid peroxidation, hydroperoxides, nitration of amino acids such as tyrosine, oxidation of antioxidants such as ascorbic acid and α-tocopherol, and direct DNA damage. The increased oxidative stress associated with diabetes can limit tetrahydrobiopterin availability. Moreover, $ONOO^-$ formation affects tetrahydrobiopterin interaction with NOS,[75] leading to this "switch" or uncoupling of NOS from producing NO to producing O_2^-. Advanced glycation end products seen in diabetic individuals can also directly react with NO, diminishing NO bioavailability both in vitro and in vivo.[76]

In Type 1 diabetes, uncoupled eNOS has been found to be the major source of ROS generation,[77] and, when blocked, mouse models showed reduced retinal leukostasis, blood retinal breakdown, and reduced retinopathy.[78] Whereas nNOS is highly expressed in the retina, its role in diabetic retinopathy is still being determined. Interestingly, nNOS knockout mice still develop retinal leukostasis and blood-retinal barrier breakdown, suggesting that iNOS or eNOS may have a more central role in these particular aspects of diabetic retinopathy.[78] In a model of diabetic ketoacidosis, in which acetone is administered to a mouse, tissue damage is mediated by free radical generation via iNOS overexpression.[77] Diabetes-induced vascular dysfunction in rats has been prevented by administration of a specific inhibitor of iNOS, 1400W.[79,80]

Is Reduced Bioavailable NO Responsible for the Endothelial Progenitor Dysfunction Observed in Diabetic Retinopathy?

NO-mediated signaling pathways are essential for EPC mobilization from the bone marrow.[81–83] NO activates MMP-9, releasing soluble Kit ligand, which shifts EPCs and hematopoietic stem cells (HSCs) from a quiescent to a proliferative niche and stimulates rapid cell mobilization to the peripheral blood.[83,84] NO regulates migration of EPCs into ischemic sites[81,85–87] and their survival.[88] It has been shown that diabetic EPCs have decreased eNOS activity, and more importantly, that exogenous NO can correct the migratory defect in these cells.[89,90]

The impaired in vivo re-endothelialization capacity of human diabetic EPCs was restored by small interfering RNA silencing of NAD(P)H oxidase subunit p47(phox).[86] Preliminary data shows that pretreatment of diabetic $CD34^+VEGFR\text{-}2^+$ EPCs with apocynin or gp91ds-tat decreased superoxide production and increased NO availability. Pretreatment with apocynin or gp91ds-tat reversed the impaired migration of diabetic EPCs in response to SDF-1 and VEGF in vitro and enhanced their integration into ischemic retinal vasculature in vivo. Propofol, a peroxynitrite scavenger, inhibits NF-kB activation, increases NO production, and protects EPCs from apoptosis.[21,91,92] High glucose enhances EPC senescence and impairs migration and tube formation, and these effects can be ameliorated by co-incubation with the NO donor sodium nitroprusside and worsened by eNOS inhibition.[93] Diabetic EPC dysfunction was improved by the eNOS activator AVE9488[86,94] and with PPAR-γ agonists.[95,96] Specifically, these agonists promote differentiation, increase EPC number and migratory activity, and reduce EPC apoptotic rate.[97] Decreased NO can be due to increased oxidative degradation as well as reduced synthesis. ADMA, an analog of the amino acid L-arginine, inhibits the formation of NO and augments vascular oxidative stress, partly via eNOS uncoupling, resulting in higher superoxide radical generation. ADMA levels are increased in diabetes[98] and ADMA represses EPC proliferation, differentiation, and function in a concentration-dependent manner.[99] Dimethylarginine dimethylaminohydrolase (DDAH) enzymes inactivate ADMA and regulate NO production.[100] Overexpression of DDAH in vitro and in vivo increased NO production.[101]

BONE MARROW MICROENVIRONMENT IS DYSFUNCTIONAL IN DIABETES

The bone marrow (BM) stem cell niche is a specialized microenvironment that nurtures and regulates the stem cell pool. The release of EPCs from bone marrow follows a circadian pattern under the influence of norepinephrine (Fig. 27.5). Osteoblastic suppression and the release of norepinephrine from adrenergic neurons together contribute to EPC egress via downregulation of SDF-1 levels in bone marrow.[102,103] Interestingly, catecholamine neurotransmitters increase EPC mobilization, proliferation, colony formation, and engraftment.[104]

It has been shown that that diabetic bone marrow has large amounts of fat compared to bone marrow from healthy controls.[105] Adipocyte-rich marrow harbors a decreased number of progenitors and relatively quiescent stem cells. Mice that are genetically deficient in adipogenesis show accelerated hematopoietic recovery after bone marrow ablation, a phenomenon that can be reproduced pharmacologically in wild-type mice through PPAR-γ inhibition.[105] These results suggest a novel therapeutic approach to enhance hematopoietic engraftment after marrow or cord blood transplantation or to ameliorate aplasia in genetic bone marrow failure syndromes. Furthermore, this is a mechanism for the myelosuppression observed in patients treated with the PPAR-γ agonist rosiglitazone,[106–108] a diabetes drug known to increase marrow adiposity.[109]

Bone marrow adipocytes have a primarily suppressive effect on hematopoiesis within the bone marrow

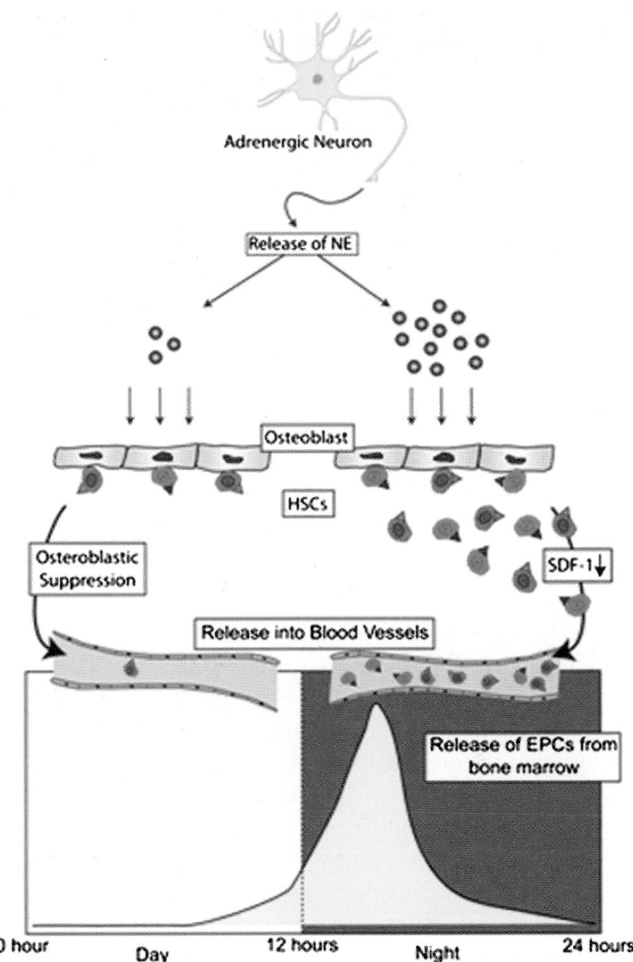

FIGURE 27.5. EPC release from bone marrow according to circadian cues: Norepinephrine from adrenergic neurons mediates osteoblastic suppression and reduction in SDF-1, which induces release of EPCs into peripheral blood from the bone marrow. EPCs are released in a diurnal manner with peak release in the early phases of the nightly cycle. Fewer EPCs are released in the "activity phase" during daytime.

microenvironment. Bone marrow adipocytes are less supportive of hematopoiesis in vitro than their undifferentiated stromal or preadipocytic counterparts, in part due to reduced production of growth factors such as granulocyte-macrophage colony-stimulating factor and granulocyte colony-stimulating factor.[110,111] Moreover, adipose tissue secretes neuropillin-1,[112] lipocalin 2,[113,114] adiponectin,[115] and Tumor Necrosis Factor (TNF)-α,[116,117] each of which can impair hematopoietic proliferation. Of note, TNF-α and adiponectin inhibit progenitor activity.[116,118] This suggests that adipocytes prevent hematopoietic progenitor expansion. Adipocytes and osteoblasts originate from mesenchymal stem cells within the bone marrow, where both compartments hold a reciprocal relationship.[118] Balancing the supportive role of the osteoblast in the HSC niche, it has been demonstrated that adipocytes act as negative regulators of hematopoiesis and that the diabetic fatty marrow has a deleterious effect on EPC function.[105]

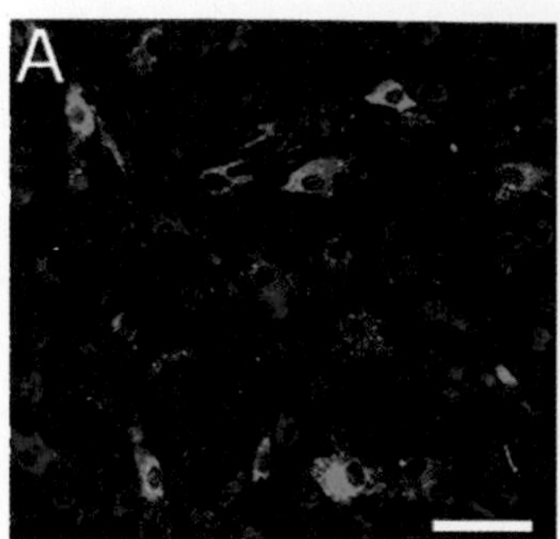

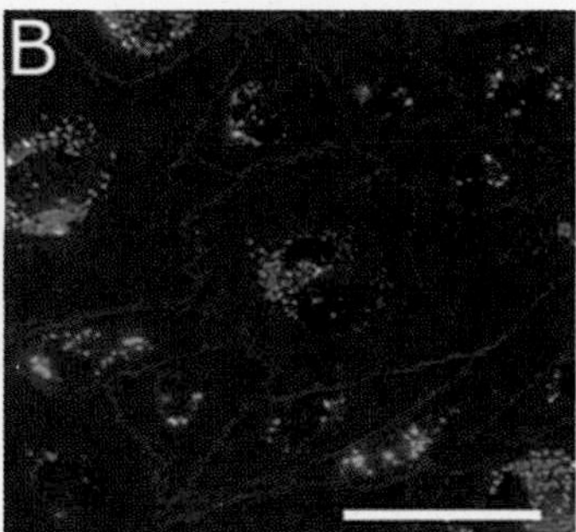

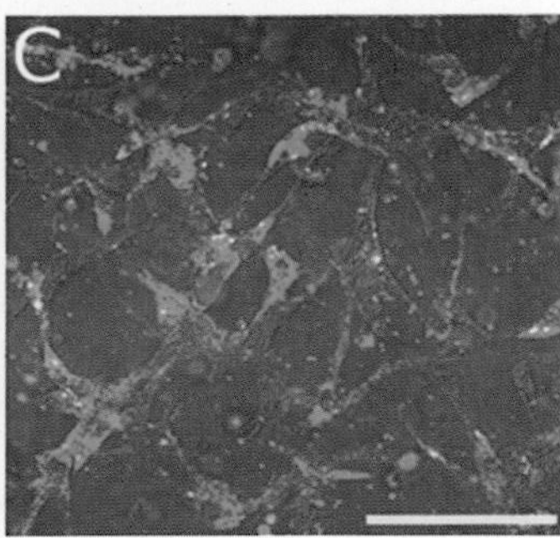

FIGURE 27.6. OECs fully incorporate into mature EC monolayers and tubes. **A:** OECs prelabeled in green incorporated into a retinal microvascular EC monolayer labeled in red. Scale bar: 100 μm. **B:** OECs marked with pink Qdots interact with human dermal microvascular ECs marked with green Qdots through adherens junctions (b catenin) stained in red. Scale bar: 50 μm. **C:** Cord blood-derived OECs were labeled in red and cocultured with retinal microvascular ECs labeled in green. OEC tubes incorporated into the mature EC network. Scale bar: 250 μm.

Thus, based on these observations, we conclude that eEPCs and OECs represent the cell populations with the greatest therapeutic utility and may provide the basis for an effective cell therapy for vasodegenerative disease in the retina.

A critical set of variables to consider when performing endothelial differentiation studies is that putative eEPCs might only give rise to endothelial-like cells depending on the exact combination of growth factors to which the cells have been exposed in vitro, and/or depending on the animal model used to assess postnatal vasculogenic activity, and/or the nature, extent, or method of delivery of the angiogenic stimulus applied in vivo. These important caveats, in what should be the most important criterion to validate EPC characteristics, make the study of these cells intriguing, but at the same time complicated. Therefore, further efforts should be focused on the development of a straightforward standard assay or set of assays that are accessible to all investigators to specifically define and validate the function of (candidate) EPCs. This would allow investigators to have a benchmark for comparison and a rationale for the examination and clinical translation of selected cell subsets in targeted clinical disorders.

Irrespective of whether they occur at appreciable levels in the in vivo situation, it could be considered that the OEC subpopulation could prove to have considerable value regarding cell therapy for diabetic retinopathy. This value is linked to several considerations: OECs do not express hematopoietic markers (CD14, CD45) but represent progenitors committed to the endothelial lineage. OECs possess significant potential for clonogenic expansion confronting issues around low abundance of cells. Finally, OECs can actively integrate into resident vascular endothelium (seen in Fig. 27.6) acting as "building blocks" that fully incorporate into the ischemic vasculature and directly contribute to vascular repair in the retina. In addition, because OECs have finite replicative capacity, these cells could be transplanted and supplement microvascular repair by the resident endothelium in a time-limited fashion. This offsets the obvious risk of introducing cells with infinite capacity to form blood vessels in human subjects.

CONCLUSION AND COMMENTS

An important drawback in the study of cultured cells is that eEPCs and OECs may have acquired or lost properties during culture that influence experimental outcomes. These cells always need to be compared back to their noncultured counterparts, the circulating cells from which they originate. Function (ability to generate vessels in vivo) and phenotype (surface markers) remain the "gold standards" of discrimination, and in vitro propagated cells may be culture artifacts compared to their in vivo counterpart.

BOX 27.1 Clinical Significance

- We conclude that eEPCs and OECs may represent the cell populations with the greatest therapeutic utility and may provide the basis for the most effective cell therapy for vasodegenerative disease in the retina.
- The eEPCs, we believe, are responsible for "provisional repair," that is transient repair preparing the environment for more durable repair, which is the function of the OECs. In healthy retina both populations participate in an ordered, temporal sequence with eEPCs homing in first, attracting the OECs later.
- In diabetes, dysregulation of NO is central to phenotypic transitions of these cells, which may be further influenced by the changing bone marrow microenvironment associated with diabetes.
- Ex vivo correction of the diabetes-induced defects in these cells, or systemic modulation of the bone marrow to correct the dysfunction of these cells will reduce the development of DR.

This issue should make all in vivo comparisons (studies) start with freshly isolated cells and then continue with the in vitro propagated populations for each individual. The researchers in this field should collectively accept all of these cells as EPC populations and refrain from attempting to choose one cell as the "winner" and discarding the rest. Instead of specifically profiling a patient's vascular reparative potential, all of these populations may be key and it is likely that combinations of these cells will be needed to optimally treat diabetic patients with vascular complications including degenerative retinopathy (Box 27.1).

KEY POINTS

- It has been a decade since EPCs were discovered but considerable debate remains about the phenotypic nature and cellular derivation of these cells. Defining correctly the population of EPCs is of considerable importance for their therapeutic use.
- Pharmacological manipulation of EPCs is necessary to correct diabetes-associated defects.
- Before clinical use of EPCs, it is necessary to titrate their dosing regimen to avoid unwanted responses such as accelerated proliferative retinopathy or, perhaps, increased incidence of malignancy.

REFERENCES

1. Fong DS, Sharza M, Chen W, et al. Vision loss among diabetics in a group model Health Maintenance Organization (HMO). *Am J Ophthalmol*. 2002;133:236–241.
2. Curtis TM, Gardiner TA, Stitt AW. Microvascular lesions of diabetic retinopathy: clues towards understanding pathogenesis? *Eye*. 2009;23:1496–1508.
3. Frank RN. Diabetic retinopathy. *N Engl J Med*. 2004;350: 48–58.
4. Yoder MC, Mead LE, Prater D, et al. Redefining endothelial progenitor cells via clonal analysis and hematopoietic stem/progenitor cell principals. *Blood*. 2007;109:1801–1809.
5. Carmeliet P. Mechanisms of angiogenesis and arteriogenesis. *Nat Med*. 2000;6:389–395.
6. Herring M, Gardner A, Glover J. A single-staged technique for seeding vascular grafts with autogenous endothelium. *Surgery*. 1978;84:498–504.
7. Asahara T, Murohara T, Sullivan A, et al. Isolation of putative progenitor endothelial cells for angiogenesis. *Science*. 1997;275:964–967.
8. Shi Q, Rafii S, Wu MH, et al. Evidence for circulating bone marrow-derived endothelial cells. *Blood*. 1998;92:362–367.
9. Lyden D, Hattori K, Dias S, et al. Impaired recruitment of bone-marrow-derived endothelial and hematopoietic precursor cells blocks tumor angiogenesis and growth. *Nat Med*. 2001;7:1194–1201.
10. Tepper OM, Capla JM, Galiano RD, et al. Adult vasculogenesis occurs through in situ recruitment, proliferation, and tubulization of circulating bone marrow-derived cells. *Blood*. 2005; 105:1068–1077.
11. Ii M, Takenaka H, Asai J, et al. Endothelial progenitor thrombospondin-1 mediates diabetes-induced delay in reendothelialization following arterial injury. *Circ Res*. 2006; 98:697–704.
12. Takahashi T, Kalka C, Masuda H, et al. Ischemia- and cytokine-induced mobilization of bone marrow-derived endothelial progenitor cells for neovascularization. *Nat Med*. 1999;5:434–438.
13. Jackson KA, Mi T, Goodell MA. Hematopoietic potential of stem cells isolated from murine skeletal muscle. *Proc Natl Acad Sci USA*. 1999;96:14482–14486.
14. Jiang S, Walker L, Afentoulis M, et al. Transplanted human bone marrow contributes to vascular endothelium. *Proc Natl Acad Sci USA*. 2004;101:16891–16896.
15. Fadini GP, de Kreutzenberg SV, Coracina A, et al. Circulating CD34+ cells, metabolic syndrome, and cardiovascular risk. *Eur Heart J*. 2006;27:2247–2255.
16. Tepper OM, Galiano RD, Capla JM, et al. Human endothelial progenitor cells from type II diabetics exhibit impaired proliferation, adhesion, and incorporation into vascular structures. *Circulation*. 2002;106:2781–2786.
17. Loomans CJ, van Haperen R, Duijs JM, et al. Differentiation of bone marrow-derived endothelial progenitor cells is shifted into a proinflammatory phenotype by hyperglycemia. *Mol Med*. 2009;15:152–159.
18. Donato AJ, Eskurza I, Silver AE, et al. Direct evidence of endothelial oxidative stress with aging in humans: relation to impaired endothelium-dependent dilation and upregulation of nuclear factor-kappaB. *Circ Res*. 2007;100:1659–1666.
19. Loomans CJ, de Koning EJ, Staal FJ, et al. Endothelial progenitor cell dysfunction: a novel concept in the pathogenesis of vascular complications of type 1 diabetes. *Diabetes*. 2004;53:195–199.
20. Funada J, Sekiya M, Hamada M, et al. Postprandial elevation of remnant lipoprotein leads to endothelial dysfunction. *Circ J*. 2002;66:127–132.
21. Imanishi T, Hano T, Sawamura T, et al. Oxidized low-density lipoprotein induces endothelial progenitor cell senescence, leading to cellular dysfunction. *Clin Exp Pharmacol Physiol*. 2004;31:407–413.
22. Zhu J, Xu ZK, Miao Y, et al. Changes of inducible protein-10 and regulated upon activation, normal T cell expressed and secreted protein in acute rejection of pancreas transplantation in rats. *World J Gastroenterol*. 2006;12:4156–4160.
23. Tamarat R, Silvestre JS, Le Ricousse-Roussanne S, et al. Impairment in ischemia-induced neovascularization in diabetes: bone marrow mononuclear cell dysfunction and therapeutic potential of placenta growth factor treatment. *Am J Pathol*. 2004;164:457–466.
24. Chang KH, Chan-Ling T, McFarland EL, et al. IGF binding protein-3 regulates hematopoietic stem cell and endothelial precursor cell function during vascular development. *Proc Natl Acad Sci USA*. 2007;104:10595–10600.
25. Ma FX, Zhou B, Chen Z, et al. Oxidized low density lipoprotein impairs endothelial progenitor cells by regulation of endothelial nitric oxide synthase. *J Lipid Res*. 2006;47: 1227–1237.

26. Shin T, Weinstock D, Castro MD, et al. Immunohistochemical localization of endothelial and inducible nitric oxide synthase within neurons of cattle with rabies. *J Vet Med Sci.* 2004;66:539–541.
27. Awad O, Dedkov EI, Jiao C, et al. Differential healing activities of CD34+ and CD14+ endothelial cell progenitors. *Arterioscler Thromb Vasc Biol.* 2006;26:758–764.
28. Kalka C, Masuda H, Takahashi T, et al. Vascular endothelial growth factor(165) gene transfer augments circulating endothelial progenitor cells in human subjects. *Circ Res.* 2000;86:1198–1202.
29. Cho HJ, Kim HS, Lee MM, et al. Mobilized endothelial progenitor cells by granulocyte-macrophage colony-stimulating factor accelerate reendothelialization and reduce vascular inflammation after intravascular radiation. *Circulation.* 2003;108:2918–2925.
30. George J, Herz I, Goldstein E, et al. Number and adhesive properties of circulating endothelial progenitor cells in patients with in-stent restenosis. *Arterioscler Thromb Vasc Biol.* 2003;23:e57–e60.
31. Ghani U, Shuaib A, Salam A, et al. Endothelial progenitor cells during cerebrovascular disease. *Stroke.* 2005;36: 151–153.
32. Case J, Mead LE, Bessler WK, et al. Human CD34+AC133+ VEGFR-2+ cells are not endothelial progenitor cells but distinct, primitive hematopoietic progenitors. *Exp Hematol.* 2007;35:1109–1118.
33. Grant MB, May WS, Caballero S, et al. Adult hematopoietic stem cells provide functional hemangioblast activity during retinal neovascularization. *Nat Med.* 2002;8:607–612.
34. Ziegelhoeffer T, Fernandez B, Kostin S, et al. Bone marrow-derived cells do not incorporate into the adult growing vasculature. *Circ Res.* 2004;94:230–238.
35. Fazel S, Cimini M, Chen L, et al. Cardioprotective c-kit+ cells are from the bone marrow and regulate the myocardial balance of angiogenic cytokines. *J Clin Invest.* 2006;116: 1865–1877.
36. Takakura N, Watanabe T, Suenobu S, et al. A role for hematopoietic stem cells in promoting angiogenesis. *Cell.* 2000;102:199–209.
37. Bailey AS, Jiang S, Afentoulis M, et al. Transplanted adult hematopoietic stems cells differentiate into functional endothelial cells. *Blood.* 2004;103:13–19.
38. Nakao A, Mimura H, Fujisawa K, et al. Generalized peritonitis due to spontaneously perforated pyometra presenting as pneumoperitoneum: report of a case. *Surg Today.* 2000;30:454–457.
39. Nolan DJ, Ciarrocchi A, Mellick AS, et al. Bone marrow-derived endothelial progenitor cells are a major determinant of nascent tumor neovascularization. *Genes Dev.* 2007;21:1546–1558.
40. Fernandez Pujol B, Lucibello FC, Gehling UM, et al. Endothelial-like cells derived from human CD14 positive monocytes. *Differentiation.* 2000;65:287–300.
41. Harraz M, Jiao C, Hanlon HD, et al. CD34- blood-derived human endothelial cell progenitors. *Stem Cells.* 2001;19: 304–312.
42. Schmeisser A, Garlichs CD, Zhang H, et al. Monocytes coexpress endothelial and macrophagocytic lineage markers and form cord-like structures in Matrigel under angiogenic conditions. *Cardiovasc Res.* 2001;49:671–680.
43. Schmeisser A, Strasser RH. Phenotypic overlap between hematopoietic cells with suggested angioblastic potential and vascular endothelial cells. *J Hematother Stem Cell Res.* 2002;11:69–79.
44. Rohde E, Malischnik C, Thaler D, et al. Blood monocytes mimic endothelial progenitor cells. *Stem Cells.* 2006;24:357–367.
45. Romagnani P, Annunziato F, Liotta F, et al. CD14+CD34low cells with stem cell phenotypic and functional features are the major source of circulating endothelial progenitors. *Circ Res.* 2005;97:314–322.
46. Loomans CJ, Wan H, de Crom R, et al. Angiogenic murine endothelial progenitor cells are derived from a myeloid bone marrow fraction and can be identified by endothelial NO synthase expression. *Arterioscler Thromb Vasc Biol.* 2006;26:1760–1767.
47. Schatteman GC, Dunnwald M, Jiao C. Biology of bone marrow-derived endothelial cell precursors. *Am J Physiol Heart Circ Physiol.* 2007;292:H1–H18.
48. Bompais H, Chagraoui J, Canron X, et al. Human endothelial cells derived from circulating progenitors display specific functional properties compared with mature vessel wall endothelial cells. *Blood.* 2004;103:2577–2584.
49. Friedrich EB, Walenta K, Scharlau J, et al. CD34-/CD133+/ VEGFR-2+ endothelial progenitor cell subpopulation with potent vasoregenerative capacities. *Circ Res.* 2006;98:e20–e25.
50. Sharpe EE III, Teleron AA, Li B, et al. The origin and in vivo significance of murine and human culture-expanded endothelial progenitor cells. *Am J Pathol.* 2006;168: 1710–1721.
51. Ingram DA, Mead LE, Tanaka H, et al. Identification of a novel hierarchy of endothelial progeitor cells using human peripheral and umbilical cord blood. *Blood.* 2004;104: 2752–2760.
52. Hill JM, Zalos G, Halcox JP, et al. Circulating endothelial progenitor cells, vascular function, and cardiovascular risk. *N Engl J Med.* 2003;348:593–600.
53. Rehman J, Li J, Orschell CM, et al. Peripheral blood "endothelial progenitor cells" are derived from monocyte/ macrophages and secrete angiogenic growth factors. *Circulation.* 2003;107:1164–1169.
54. Griese DP, Ehsan A, Melo LG, et al. Isolation and transplantation of autologous circulating endothelial cells into denuded vessels and prosthetic grafts: implications for cell-based vascular therapy. *Circulation.* 2003;108:2710–2715.
55. Timmermans F, Van Hauwermeiren F, De Smedt M, et al. Endothelial outgrowth cells are not derived from CD133+ cells or CD45+ hematopoietic precursors. *Arterioscler Thromb Vasc Biol.* 2007;27:1572–1579.
56. Yoon CH, Hur J, Park KW, et al. Synergistic neovascularization by mixed transplantation of early endothelial progenitor cells and late outgrowth endothelial cells: the role of angiogenic cytokines and matrix metalloproteinases. *Circulation.* 2005;112:1618–1627.
57. Amatschek S, Kriehuber E, Bauer W, et al. Blood and lymphatic endothelial cell-specific differentiation programs are stringently controlled by the tissue environment. *Blood.* 2007;109:4777–4785.
58. Asahara T, Takahashi T, Masuda H, et al. VEGF contributes to postnatal neovascularization by mobilizing bone marrow-derived endothelial progenitor cells. *Embo J.* 1999; 18:3964–3972.

59. Gulati R, Jevremovic D, Peterson TE, et al. Diverse origin and function of cells with endothelial phenotype obtained from adult human blood. *Circ Res*. 2003;93:1023–1025.
60. Gulati R, Jevremovic D, Peterson TE, et al. Autologous culture-modified mononuclear cells confer vascular protection after arterial injury. *Circulation*. 2003;108:1520–1526.
61. Eggermann J, Kliche S, Jarmy G, et al. Endothelial progenitor cell culture and differentiation in vitro: a methodological comparison using human umbilical cord blood. *Cardiovasc Res*. 2003;58:478–486.
62. Hur J, Yoon CH, Kim HS, et al. Characterization of two types of endothelial progenitor cells and their different contributions to neovasculogenesis. *Arterioscler Thromb Vasc Biol*. 2004; 24:288–293.
63. Delorme B, Basire A, Gentile C, et al. Presence of endothelial progenitor cells, distinct from mature endothelial cells, within human CD146+ blood cells. *Thromb Haemost*. 2005; 94:1270–1279.
64. Gehling UM, Ergun S, Schumacher U, et al. In vitro differentiation of endothelial cells from AC133-positive progenitor cells. *Blood*. 2000;95:3106–3112.
65. Crosby JR, Kaminski WE, Schatteman G, et al. Endothelial cells of hematopoietic origin make a significant contribution to adult blood vessel formation. *Circ Res*. 2000;87:728–730.
66. Sobrevia L, Mann GE. Dysfunction of the endothelial nitric oxide signalling pathway in diabetes and hyperglycaemia. *Exp Physiol*. 1997;82:423–452.
67. Weyrich AS, Ma XL, Lefer AM. The role of L-arginine in ameliorating reperfusion injury after myocardial ischemia in the cat. Circulation 1992;86:279–288.
68. Kaesemeyer WH, Ogonowski AA, Jin L, et al. Endothelial nitric oxide synthase is a site of superoxide synthesis in endothelial cells treated with glyceryl trinitrate. *Br J Pharmacol*. 2000;131:1019–1023.
69. Berkowitz DE, White R, Li D, et al. Arginase reciprocally regulates nitric oxide synthase activity and contributes to endothelial dysfunction in aging blood vessels. *Circulation*. 2003;108:2000–2006.
70. Jean C, Rome S, Mathe V, et al. Metabolic evidence for adaptation to a high protein diet in rats. *J Nutr*. 2001;131:91–98.
71. Ellis EA, Guberski DL, Hutson B, et al. Time course of NADH oxidase, inducible nitric oxide synthase and peroxynitrite in diabetic retinopathy in the BBZ/WOR rat. *Nitric Oxide*. 2002;6:295–304.
72. Szabo C, Mabley JG, Moeller SM, et al. Part I: pathogenetic role of peroxynitrite in the development of diabetes and diabetic vascular complications: studies with FP15, a novel potent peroxynitrite decomposition catalyst. *Mol Med*. 2002;8:571–580.
73. Kobayashi T, Taguchi K, Takenouchi Y, et al. Insulin-induced impairment via peroxynitrite production of endothelium-dependent relaxation and sarco/endoplasmic reticulum Ca(2+)-ATPase function in aortas from diabetic rats. *Free Radic Biol Med*. 2007;43:431–443.
74. Camici GG, Schiavoni M, Francia P, et al. Genetic deletion of p66(Shc) adaptor protein prevents hyperglycemia-induced endothelial dysfunction and oxidative stress. *Proc Natl Acad Sci USA*. 2007;104:5217–5222.
75. Munzel T, Sayegh H, Freeman BA, et al. Evidence for enhanced vascular superoxide anion production in nitrate tolerance. A novel mechanism underlying tolerance and cross-tolerance. *J Clin Invest*. 1995;95:187–194.
76. Bucala R, Tracey KJ, Cerami A. Advanced glycosylation products quench nitric oxide and mediate defective endothelium-dependent vasodilatation in experimental diabetes. *J Clin Invest*. 1991;87:432–438.
77. Stadler K, Bonini MG, Dallas S, et al. Direct evidence of iNOS-mediated in vivo free radical production and protein oxidation in acetone-induced ketosis. *Am J Physiol Endocrinol Metab*. 2008;295:E456–E462.
78. Leal EC, Manivannan A, Hosoya K, et al. Inducible nitric oxide synthase isoform is a key mediator of leukostasis and blood-retinal barrier breakdown in diabetic retinopathy. *Invest Ophthalmol Vis Sci*. 2007;48:5257–5265.
79. Nagareddy PR, Xia Z, McNeill JH, et al. Increased expression of iNOS is associated with endothelial dysfunction and impaired pressor responsiveness in streptozotocin-induced diabetes. *Am J Physiol Heart Circ Physiol*. 2005;289:H2144–H2152.
80. Cheng X, Cheng XS, Kuo KH, et al. Inhibition of iNOS augments cardiovascular action of noradrenaline in streptozotocin-induced diabetes. *Cardiovasc Res*. 2004;64:298–307.
81. Aicher A, Zeiher AM, Dimmeler S. Mobilizing endothelial progenitor cells. *Hypertension*. 2005;45:321–325.
82. Heissig B, Hattori K, Dias S, et al. Recruitment of stem and progenitor cells from the bone marrow niche requires MMP-9 mediated release of kit-ligand. *Cell*. 2002;109:625–637.
83. Heissig B, Werb Z, Rafii S, et al. Role of c-kit/Kit ligand signaling in regulating vasculogenesis. *Thromb Haemost*. 2003; 90:570–576.
84. Shintani S, Murohara T, Ikeda H, et al. Augmentation of postnatal neovascularization with autologous bone marrow transplantation. *Circulation*. 2001;103:897–903.
85. Dimmeler S, Fleming I, Fisslthaler B, et al. Activation of nitric oxide synthase in endothelial cells by Akt-dependent phosphorylation. *Nature*. 1999;399:601–605.
86. Sorrentino SA, Bahlmann FH, Besler C, et al. Oxidant stress impairs in vivo reendothelialization capacity of endothelial progenitor cells from patients with type 2 diabetes mellitus: restoration by the peroxisome proliferator-activated receptor-gamma agonist rosiglitazone. *Circulation*. 2007;116:163–173.
87. Thum T, Fraccarollo D, Schultheiss M, et al. Endothelial nitric oxide synthase uncoupling impairs endothelial progenitor cell mobilization and function in diabetes. *Diabetes*. 2007;56:666–674.
88. Vasa M, Breitschopf K, Zeiher AM, et al. Nitric oxide activates telomerase and delays endothelial cell senescence. *Circ Res*. 2000;87:540–542.
89. Li Calzi S, Purich DL, Hee Chang K, et al. Carbon Monoxide and Nitric Oxide Mediate Cytoskeletal Reorganization in Microvascular Cells via Vasodilator-Stimulated Phosphoprotein (VASP) Phosphorylation: Evidence for Blunted Responsiveness in Diabetes. *Diabetes*. 2008;57:2488–2494.
90. Segal MS, Shah R, Afzal A, et al. Nitric oxide cytoskeletal-induced alterations reverse the endothelial progenitor cell migratory defect associated with diabetes. *Diabetes*. 2006;55:102–109.
91. Gao J, Zhao WX, Zhou LJ, et al. Protective effects of propofol on lipopolysaccharide-activated endothelial cell barrier dysfunction. *Inflamm Res*. 2006;55:385–392.
92. Luo T, Xia Z, Ansley DM, et al. Propofol dose-dependently reduces tumor necrosis factor-alpha-Induced human umbilical vein endothelial cell apoptosis: effects on Bcl-2 and Bax expression and nitric oxide generation. *Anesth Analg*. 2005;100:1653–1659.

93. Chen YS, Chen KH, Liu CC, et al. Propofol-induced vascular permeability change is related to the nitric oxide signaling pathway and occludin phosphorylation. *J Biomed Sci*. 2007; 14:629–636.
94. Sasaki K, Heeschen C, Aicher A, et al. Ex vivo pretreatment of bone marrow mononuclear cells with endothelial NO synthase enhancer AVE9488 enhances their functional activity for cell therapy. *Proc Natl Acad Sci USA*. 2006;103:14537–14541.
95. Dimmeler S, Aicher A, Vasa M, et al. HMG-CoA reductase inhibitors (statins) increase endothelial progenitor cells via the PI 3-kinase/Akt pathway. *J Clin Invest*. 2001;108:391–397.
96. Landmesser U, Engberding N, Bahlmann FH, et al. Statin-induced improvement of endothelial progenitor cell mobilization, myocardial neovascularization, left ventricular function, and survival after experimental myocardial infarction requires endothelial nitric oxide synthase. *Circulation*. 2004;110:1933–1939.
97. Verma S, Szmitko PE, Anderson TJ. Endothelial function: ready for prime time? *Can J Cardiol*. 2004;20:1335–1339.
98. Forstermann U, Munzel T. Endothelial nitric oxide synthase in vascular disease: from marvel to menace. *Circulation*. 2006; 113:1708–1714.
99. Thum T, Bauersachs J. Spotlight on endothelial progenitor cell inhibitors: short review. *Vasc Med*. 2005;10 Suppl 1:S59–S64.
100. Achan V, Broadhead M, Malaki M, et al. Asymmetric dimethylarginine causes hypertension and cardiac dysfunction in humans and is actively metabolized by dimethylarginine dimethylaminohydrolase. *Arterioscler Thromb Vasc Biol*. 2003;23:1455–1459.
101. Dayoub H, Achan V, Adimoolam S, et al. Dimethylarginine dimethylaminohydrolase regulates nitric oxide synthesis: genetic and physiological evidence. *Circulation*. 2003;108:3042–3047.
102. Katayama Y, Battista M, Kao WM, et al. Signals from the sympathetic nervous system regulate hematopoietic stem cell egress from bone marrow. *Cell*. 2006;124:407–421.
103. Mendez-Ferrer S, Lucas D, Battista M, et al. Haematopoietic stem cell release is regulated by circadian oscillations. *Nature*. 2008;452:442–447.
104. Spiegel A, Shivtiel S, Kalinkovich A, et al. Catecholaminergic neurotransmitters regulate migration and repopulation of immature human CD34+ cells through Wnt signaling. *Nat Immunol*. 2007;8:1123–1131.
105. Naveiras O, Nardi V, Wenzel PL, et al. Bone-marrow adipocytes as negative regulators of the haematopoietic microenvironment. *Nature*. 2009;460:259–263.
106. Digman C, Borto D, Nasraway SA, Jr. Hyperglycemia in the critically ill. *Nutr Clin Care* 2005;8:93–101.
107. Maaravi Y, Stessman J. Mild, reversible pancytopenia induced by rosiglitazone. *Diabetes Care*. 2005;28:1536.
108. Berria R, Glass L, Mahankali A, et al. Reduction in hematocrit and hemoglobin following pioglitazone treatment is not hemodilutional in Type II diabetes mellitus. *Clin Pharmacol Ther*. 2007;82:275–281.
109. Lazarenko OP, Rzonca SO, Hogue WR, et al. Rosiglitazone induces decreases in bone mass and strength that are reminiscent of aged bone. *Endocrinology*. 2007;148: 2669–2680.
110. Nishikawa S, Kumar PK, Jeoung YH, et al. Chemical probing studies of the hepatitis delta virus (HDV) genomic ribozyme. *Nucleic Acids Symp Ser*. 1993:119–120.
111. Corre J, Barreau C, Cousin B, et al. Human subcutaneous adipose cells support complete differentiation but not self-renewal of hematopoietic progenitors. *J Cell Physiol*. 2006;208:282–288.
112. Belaid-Choucair Z, Lepelletier Y, Poncin G, et al. Human bone marrow adipocytes block granulopoiesis through neuropilin-1-induced granulocyte colony-stimulating factor inhibition. *Stem Cells*. 2008;26:1556–1564.
113. Miharada K, Hiroyama T, Sudo K, et al. Lipocalin 2-mediated growth suppression is evident in human erythroid and monocyte/macrophage lineage cells. *J Cell Physiol*. 2008;215:526–537.
114. Yan QW, Yang Q, Mody N, et al. The adipokine lipocalin 2 is regulated by obesity and promotes insulin resistance. *Diabetes*. 2007;56:2533–2540.
115. Yokota T, Oritani K, Takahashi I, et al. Adiponectin, a new member of the family of soluble defense collagens, negatively regulates the growth of myelomonocytic progenitors and the functions of macrophages. *Blood*. 2000;96: 1723–1732.
116. Zhang Y, Harada A, Bluethmann H, et al. Tumor necrosis factor (TNF) is a physiologic regulator of hematopoietic progenitor cells: increase of early hematopoietic progenitor cells in TNF receptor p55-deficient mice in vivo and potent inhibition of progenitor cell proliferation by TNF alpha in vitro. *Blood*. 1995;86:2930–2937.
117. Hotamisligil GS, Shargill NS, Spiegelman BM. Adipose expression of tumor necrosis factor-alpha: direct role in obesity-linked insulin resistance. *Science*. 1993;259: 87–91.
118. DiMascio L, Voermans C, Uqoezwa M, et al. Identification of adiponectin as a novel hemopoietic stem cell growth factor. *J Immunol*. 2007;178:3511–3520.

CHAPTER 28

Drug Delivery to the Posterior Segment: Challenges

Prithvi Mruthyunjaya

In proangiogenic diseases such as neovascular age-related macular degeneration (ARMD) and diabetic retinopathy (DR), there is growing interest in delivery of targeted therapeutic agents to the posterior segment. Even if a new therapeutic agent is found to be active in preclinical studies to specific retinal structures or disease states, the challenge remains to bring the agent to the target site in safe and effective concentrations.[1] Furthermore, finding delivery methods to minimize administration frequency while maintaining therapeutic drug concentrations at the target tissue may help modulate the disease while minimizing side effects from repeated delivery.

BARRIERS TO DRUG DELIVERY

Drugs must enter the eye through a specified route, maintain its active biochemical properties (bioactivity), achieve a therapeutic concentration at its target site, and sustain an effective concentration to counteract the disease process. Despite identification of the best agents to treat posterior segment diseases, there are numerous physical and physiologic barriers to achieving sustained and therapeutic drug concentrations at the retina and choroid. Barrier functions work to inhibit entry of the agent into the eye, specifically the retina and vitreous, while clearance mechanisms remove drugs that may have been successfully delivered. In addition, the disease state itself may alter both barrier and clearance mechanisms, thereby altering expected drug concentrations and duration of contact with target structures.

The ocular surface is the most anterior barrier to ocular drug penetration. Aqueous tears dilute and flush topically administered medications into the lacrimal drainage system. The tear film volume is approximately 5 to 7 μL, which is replaced almost continuously.[2] However, the volume of a typical eye drop (25–50 μL) is typically cleared by bulk flow through the nasolacrimal duct in 5 minutes, leaving insufficient time for effective ocular penetration. Systemic absorption may also occur at the conjunctival and lacrimal sac via local capillaries or through sinus mucosal absorption.[3]

The cornea provides a structural and biochemical barrier to drug delivery. Apical corneal tight junctions can limit paracellular drug passage. However, inefficient, transcorneal permeation remains a major route of topical drug entry into the anterior chamber. Biochemical mechanisms within the cornea, including efflux pumps, peptide transporters, and multidrug resistance proteins, further limit transport from the ocular surface into the eye. The result is that <3% of the drug volume of a topically administered agent will enter into the anterior segment, which may not allow for therapeutic concentrations to effectively enter the eye.[4–6]

The blood-ocular barrier is the predominant deterrent to achieving therapeutic posterior segment drug concentrations via systemic, topical, or periocular administration. The anterior blood-aqueous barrier (BAB) is formed by the endothelial cells within the anterior uveal tract (iris and ciliary body), limiting plasma albumin and hydrophilic drugs from entering the aqueous humor.[3,7] The BAB may significantly reduce intraocular concentrations of drugs that are designed to enter the eye through anterior pathways (conjunctival or topically).

The blood-retina barrier limits diffusion of drugs and targeted agents delivered through (BRB) a systemic or periocular route. There are two components of the Blood-Retinal Barrier (BRB): the retinal pigment epithelium (RPE) (outer barrier) and the tight junctions of the retinal vascular endothelial cells (inner barrier). The highly perfused choriocapillaris have abundant fenestrations, which provide minimal resistance to the transport of molecules into the choroid. However, the Retinal pigment epithelium (RPE) itself, with the exception of its homeostatic function of allowing selective passage of nutrients and removal of waste products between the choroid, restricts movement of particles.[6,8] The retinal vascular endothelium also has a low permeability tolerance and, typically, only highly lipophilic compounds can penetrate this inner blood-ocular barrier.[6] As only a fraction of the systemic blood volume flushes through the eye, very small quantities of systemically delivered drugs can be detected within the eye.[2,9]

When a drug reaches the posterior segment (retina or vitreous), it may be eliminated by two routes: anterior elimination involves drainage through the trabecular meshwork and by bulk flow aqueous turnover, while posterior elimination requires the drug to penetrate through the blood-retinal barrier and then actively or passively transported out of the eye. Elimination through these routes favors small, lipophilic molecules and may be altered by systemic medications.[2,3]

Ocular disease states may influence posterior segment drug entry and elimination. Posterior segment inflammation may have opposing effects on drug elimination based on the biochemical properties of the agent. For example, in the setting of inflammation, elimination of aminoglycoside can be increased, whereas beta-lactam antibiotics can be decreased due to permeability and active transport mechanisms.[2] In retinal vascular diseases such as DR, damage to retinal vascular endothelium may enhance drug permeability and limit clearance, thereby increasing retinal drug concentrations. Similarly, in choroidal neovascular diseases such as neovascular ARMD, disruption of RPE outer barrier function may enhance drug entry and limit elimination.

ROUTES OF DRUG DELIVERY

Numerous routes have been proposed and used to deliver drugs to the posterior segment in attempts to control retinal vascular and neovascular diseases. These routes include (a) systemic delivery, (b) topical administration, (c) periocular administration, (d) transscleral delivery, and (e) intravitreal administration. Each method has its own advantages and disadvantages, which will be discussed.

Systemic Delivery

Systemic drug delivery to the posterior segment involves oral or intravenous drug administration. Patient compliance, systemic absorption, and first-pass drug metabolism determine the bioavailability of the drug as it is transported to the eye through blood vessels. Drug access to the posterior segment requires penetration across the blood-ocular barrier, which may typically occur with lipophilic drugs. Alternatively, drugs may diffuse into the posterior chamber through a concentration gradient from the anterior chamber and aqueous humor. These penetration mechanisms are constantly being thwarted by normal elimination mechanisms, resulting in an inefficient method of attaining therapeutic intraocular drug concentrations. In order to combat these barrier and elimination forces, high drug doses or frequent systemic administration is necessary to produce therapeutic ocular concentrations. The drawback to this method is the increased exposure of the drug to the systemic circulation.

In patients with DR, oral agents have been used to target upregulated protein kinase C (PKC) as a method to reduce vascular permeability and mediate concurrent overexpression vascular endothelial growth factor (VEGF) expression.[10,11] PKC412 is an oral nonspecific multikinase inhibitor that blocks VEGF-1 and VEGF-2 receptors, Platelet-derived growth factor receptors (PDGF), and several PKC isoforms. In a double-masked, randomized, variable dose, controlled clinical trial of 141 patients with diabetic macular edema, oral doses of 100 mg/d significantly reduced macular thickening and improved visual acuity.[12,13] Liver toxicity was a possible concern, limiting its continued systemic use. Ruboxistaurin mesylate (LY333531) is a specific PKC-beta isoform inhibitor that was tested in a 36-month randomized, placebo-controlled trial of 685 patients with nonproliferative DR. A significant risk reduction (40%) in sustaining moderate vision loss and preventing progression of foveal macular edema was demonstrated.[14–17]

Choroidal neovascularization in ARMD has been established as a VEGF-driven pathologic response to angiogenic signaling.[18] Initial antiangiogenic strategies utilized selective VEGF-165 isoform inhibition by intravitreal injections of pegaptanib sodium (Macugen, OSI/Eyetech, New York, NY).[19,20] Data from examination of extracted choroidal neovascular membranes demonstrated multiple isoforms of VEGF, including 121 and 110, exist within these lesions but could not be blocked with pegaptanib sodium alone.[21] Bevacizumab (Avastin, Genentech, Inc., South San Francisco, California) is a full-length, humanized monoclonal antibody with two active binding sites that can bind and inhibit all active VEGF-A isoforms. Prior to the Food and Drug Administration (FDA) approval of ranibizumab (Lucentis, Genentech, Inc., South San Francisco, California) for neovascular ARMD, systemic administration of bevacizumab was studied in the Phase 1/2 Systemic Avastin for Neovascular AMD (SANA) Study. In an open-label, uncontrolled study, 18 patients with subfoveal choroidal neovascularization were given intravenous bevacizumab infusions (5 mg/kg) at study entry and an additional one to two injections in the subsequent 4 weeks. No adverse events were noted and there was mild, but controllable, elevation in systemic blood pressure. Visual acuity improved and central retinal thickness decreased through 24 weeks with few re-treatments after the initial series.[22,23] These examples demonstrate the feasibility of some systemic agents to reach effective ocular concentrations, but with nonocular side effects.

Topical Delivery

Eye drop formulations of medications designed to treat posterior segment diseases have the distinct advantages of easy, noninvasive delivery (Fig. 28.1). However, as discussed above, the tear film and cornea pose a formidable barrier to absorption through the ocular surface. Once through the corneal layers, the drug may diffuse into the aqueous humor and travel around the lens zonules into the vitreous humor where it may contact the retina. Alternatively, noncorneal entry by a topical drug may occur either directly through the pars plana into the vitreous cavity or directly across the sclera and into the vitreous cavity after traversing the choroid, RPE, and retina.[6] Just entering the

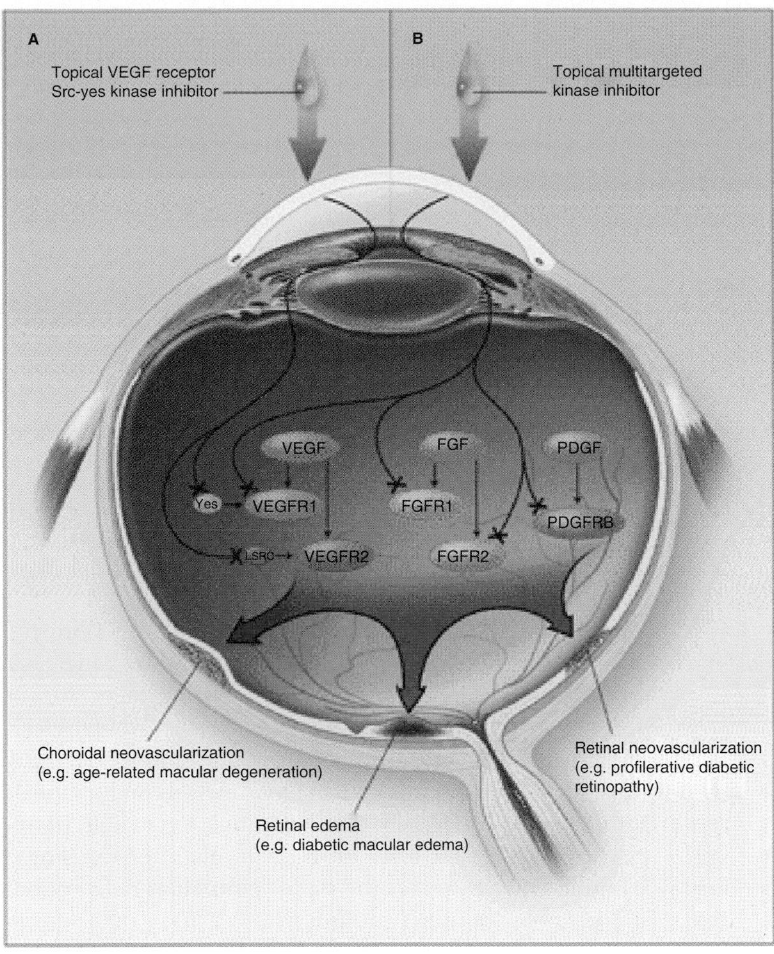

FIGURE 28.1. Topical use of kinase inhibitors. Retinal edema and neovascularization of the choroid and retina are the primary causes of vision loss in most developed countries. Multiple mechanisms mediate these changes, including pathways involving vascular endothelial growth factor (VEGF), platelet-derived growth factor (PDGF), and fibroblast growth factor (FGF) receptor kinases. These growth factors bind a variety of receptors, including VEGFR1, VEGFR2, FGFR1, FGFR2, and PDGFRβ. A recent study by Scheppke et al.[24] showed that topical application of a VEGF receptor Src–Yes kinase inhibitor can essentially eliminate retinal edema in animals (**Panel A**). A similar study by Doukas et al.[25] showed that a topical multitargeted kinase inhibitor of VEGF, PDGF, and FGF pathways can reduce choroidal neovascularization and retinal edema in animals (**Panel B**). Note the corneal penetration and proposed diffusion of the drug into the vitreous cavity. (Reproduced from Aiello. *N Engl J Med.* 2008;359:967, with permission.)

eye by a topically placed drug compound does not ensure adequate bioavailability to attain therapeutic efficacy at the retinal or choroidal target site. A concentration gradient is required to allow for diffusion into the posterior segment, but drug clearance mechanisms via aqueous outflow and biochemical drug inactivation may quickly reduce anterior chamber concentrations. Repeated installation of high concentration eye drops may help ensure this gradient, but may also increase the risk of local or systemic toxicity.[7]

Despite these challenges, studies are underway to determine the efficacy of topical drops for ocular neovascular diseases focusing on protein kinase inhibition. These drugs may bind a variety of receptors that mediate signaling pathways used for cell proliferation, blocking apoptosis, and vascular remodeling. A unique feature of this drug class is the inhibitory effect on multiple VEGF family members including VEGFR1, VEGFR2, FGFR1, FGFR2, and PDGFR-B.[18] In preclinical studies, Scheppke et al. reported the use of a topical VEGFR2–Src kinase inhibitor in knockout mice, which reduced both VEGF-induced vascular permeability and laser-induced vein occlusion-associated macular edema in rabbits.[24] Using a different topical multikinase inhibitor that targeted VEGF, PDGF, and FGF, Doukas et al. noted reduced vascular leakage and reduction of choroidal neovascularization in rodent models.[25] Another agent, pazopanib (GlaxoSmithKline), has demonstrated choroidal neovascularization (CNV) inhibitory effects in a murine model with activity against VEGFR1, VEGFR2, VEGFR3, PDGFR, c-Kit, and FGF.[26] Phase 1 studies with topical delivery of pazopanib are currently underway.[27]

Periocular Delivery

Periocular delivery utilizes passage of the drug through the outer scleral eye wall to reach choroidal, retinal, and vitreous targets. Drugs have been delivered into the sub-Tenon, retrobulbar, episcleral, intrascleral, or suprachoroidal locations. Many of these locations, especially retrobulbar and sub-Tenon space, can be easily accessed in the clinic setting and have been used for many years to delivery periocular steroids that have been shown to have a therapeutic effect. These delivery techniques all have the advantage of avoiding direct intraocular penetration or wound creation to place the drug or drug delivery device. The relatively large surface area of the sclera and the expandable orbital tissues allows for long-acting drug depots to be placed in these locations, creating opportunities for more sustained release through

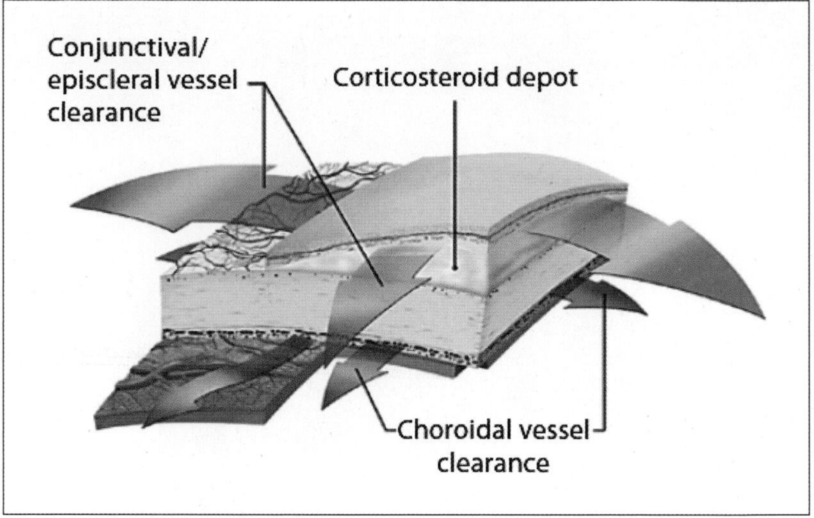

FIGURE 28.2. Subconjunctival drug depots are cleared by both periocular (conjunctival and episcleral vessels and lymphatics) and choroidal vascular channels. (Reproduced from Lee SS, Robinson MR. *Ophthal Res.* 2009;41:124, with permission.)

the sclera. Further, the local administration may limit systemic toxicity as the drug is delivered close to its target site (Fig. 28.2).

Transscleral Delivery

It is estimated that only 1% of drug placed on the episcleral surface will enter the retina and vitreous.[28] The ocular tissues (sclera, choroid, and RPE) constitute a physical barrier to drug penetration by pharmacokinetic modeling and from a protein transport data.[29,30] However, in vitro and in vivo studies have demonstrated that the sclera is permeable to low- and high-molecular weight compounds as well as other novel drug formulations such as single-strand oligonucleotides, large molecular immunoglobulins, and adenoviral vectors coding for antiangiogenic proteins as large as 50 to 75 kDa.[31–37] Scleral permeability appears to decrease with increasing molecular weight and molecular radius, with the latter being more predictive for transscleral passage.[29,31]

Clearance mechanisms must also be considered in determining the low retinal and vitreous concentrations obtained after periocular drug delivery. Such mechanisms have been implicated, for example, in the lack of clinical superiority in the use of periocular depot of anecortave acetate, an angiostatic steroid formulation, compared to verteporfin photodynamic therapy in neovascular ARMD patients.[28,38]

The choroid and choriocapillaris represent high-flow vascular beds that may contribute to bulk drug elimination. However, cryotherapy elimination of the choroid in rabbits or in vitro did not enhance vitreous concentration after a periocular steroid injection, suggesting the importance of conjunctival and lymphatic drainage.[39–41] Kim et al. utilized magnetic resonance imaging to follow the movement of gadolinium–diethylenetriamine pentaacetic acid (Gd–DTPA) from an episcleral implant placed in rabbit eyes and found Gd–DTPA accumulation in the buccal lymph nodes. In periocular delivery studies, following euthanasia, intravitreal drug concentrations increase, suggesting preferential transscleral permeability in the absence of lymphatic, conjunctival, and choroidal clearance mechanism.[29,42,43] Robinson et al. demonstrated the importance of the conjunctival blood vessels and lymphatics in the rabbit eye, by demonstrating detectable triamcinolone acetonide (TA) vitreous levels after excising a conjunctival window at the site of periocular delivery, but not in eyes with intact conjunctiva.[29,39]

Several approaches have been reported to enhance intraocular drug availability following periocular delivery, which focus on minimizing or eliminating clearance mechanisms (Fig. 28.3). Drug-releasing episcleral exoplants provide higher and more sustained scleral drug concentration gradients, which allow greater transscleral diffusion despite normal conjunctival and lymphatic clearance mechanisms. Device construction with polymeric coatings may help shield the drug core from washout from the periocular tissues and lymphatics. A flexible, refillable silicone device that was sutured to rabbit eyes demonstrated increased retina and vitreous sodium fluorescein compared to a periocular injection. The unique device sheltered the drug from the conjunctiva and only allowed direct contact with the sclera.[44] In a similar concept, a nonbioerodible polyvinyl alcohol (PVA)–betamethasone episcleral exoplant allowed preferential delivery into the rabbit retina-choroid rather than the vitreous.[45] Using a novel synthetic polymer, poly(methylidene malonate) (PMM2.12), 8 × 1 mm TA discs were coated and sutured to the scleral surface to allow therapeutic intravitreal levels in rabbit eyes for up to 5 to 8 weeks.[46]

Intrascleral implants typically place a drug reservoir under a scleral flap adjacent to the inner scleral lamella or into the suprachoroidal space and have generally been well tolerated in animal studies. In theory, such placement reduces periocular clearance and brings the drug in closer

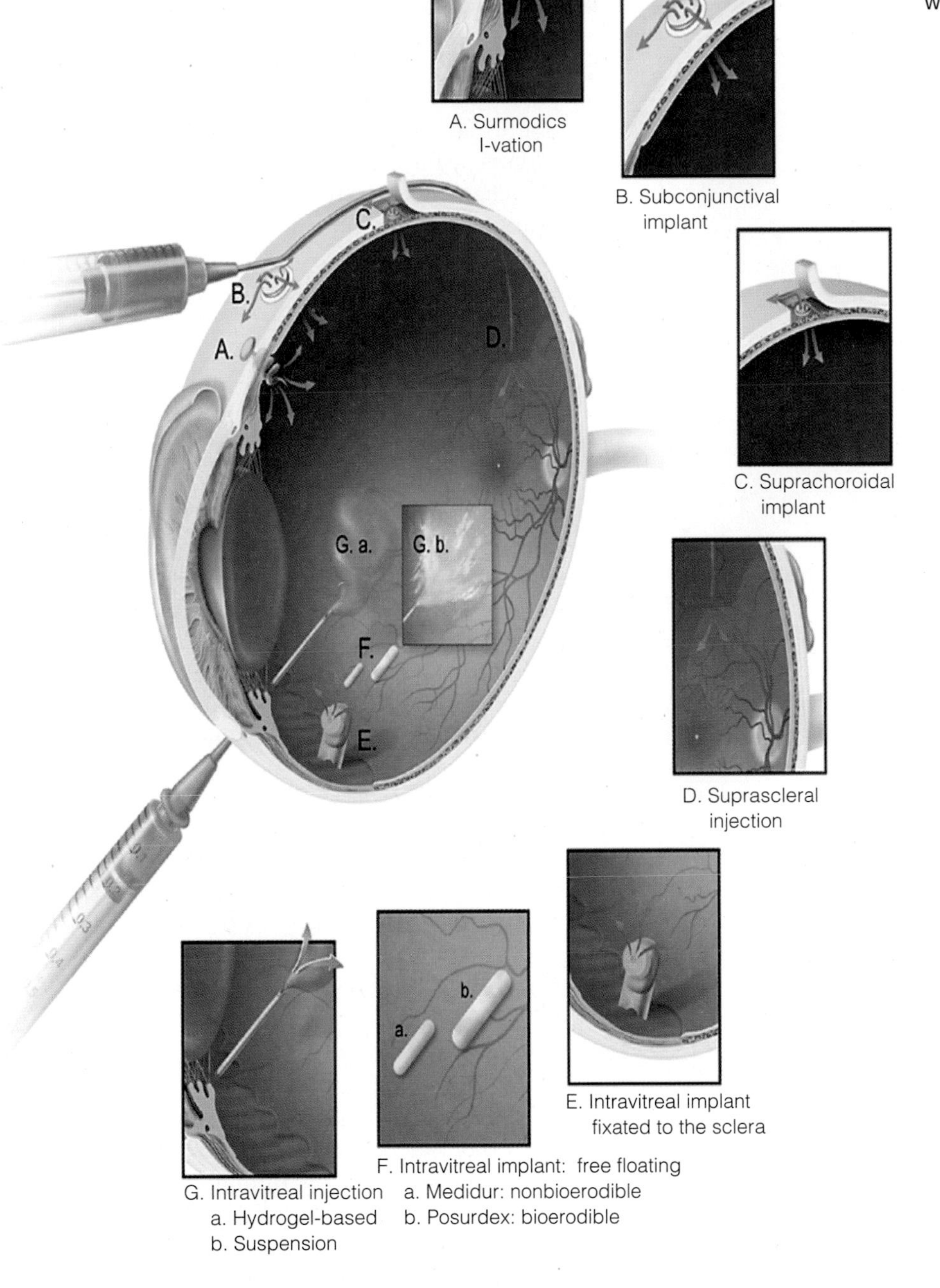

FIGURE 28.3. Various routes and systems of drug delivery for posterior segment disorders. (Reproduced from Lee SS, Robinson MR. *Ophthal Res.* 2009;41:124, with permission.)

contact with the choroid and retina, potentially favoring increased intraocular drug concentrations.

Corticosteroids and anti-inflammatory agents have been married with polymeric coatings with intrascleral delivery approaches in order to target posterior uveitis. A biodegradable poly(D,L-lactide) (PLA) coated betamethasone pellet was devised and found to have a biphasic in vitro release profile over 50 days. The implant was placed into a scleral pocket, shielding it from the conjunctiva and lymphatics, in rabbits and was able to deliver higher drug concentrations to the retina/choroid than in the vitreous. Over an 8-week period, drug levels at each of these locations were within the therapeutic range to treat intraocular inflammation. Placement with respect to anterior or posterior scleral location influenced drug concentrations detected in the anterior chamber, vitreous and posterior pole regions.[45,47–49] In a rabbit model of experimental uveitis, a 6.4-mg PLA-TA intrascleral implant was found to effectively suppress intraocular inflammation for 1 month.[50] A cyclosporine-A (CsA) drug core was

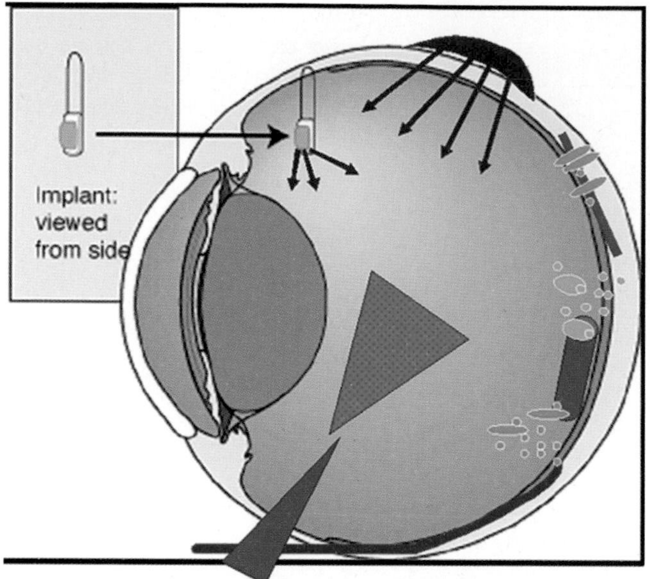

FIGURE 28.4. Various sites of ocular drug delivery implants. (Courtesy of Glenn J. Jaffe, MD.)

pelleted and coated with a PVA polymer placed through an intrascleral wound, compared to episcleral placement, and was found to have greater and more sustained intraocular concentrations in equine eyes. In a clinical application, these intrascleral CsA implants helped to control reflares and preserve visual function in horses with equine recurrent uveitis.[51,52] In a novel surgical delivery system, Olsen et al. developed an illuminated microcannula system for suprachoroidal drug delivery. The system allowed for consistent suprachoroidal TA placement in pigs under direct visualization with measured and sustained intraocular tissue drug concentrations (Fig. 28.4).[53]

Intravitreal Delivery

Directly placing drugs into the vitreous cavity has the distinct advantage of bringing high drug concentrations within close proximity to target tissues such as the retina and choroid. The property of the drug itself, including solubility, hydophilicity, and diffusion properties in the vitreous will determine final concentration in the vitreous and further help determine penetration into the retina and choroid.[2] In proangiogenic diseases such as DR and ARMD, intravitreal delivery of corticosteroid and anti-VEGF therapies have demonstrated remarkable clinical efficacy and enjoyed widespread adaptation. Direct intravitreal injection is the most common technique employed for intravitreal delivery, though new technologies are being applied to obtain higher and more sustained intraocular drug concentrations. The benefits of higher drug concentration aside, intravitreal delivery does have the risk of increased complications and side effects including cataract progression, secondary glaucoma, and toxic and infectious inflammatory reactions.[54–64]

Antiangiogenic agents have been used to target conditions such as ARMD, proliferative DR, and retinal vascular occlusions.[65] Currently, anti-VEGF agents used in clinical practice include pegaptanib sodium (Macugen, OSI Pharmaceuticals, Melville, New York), ranibizumab (Lucentis, Genentech, Inc, South San Francisco, CA), VEGF Trap-Eye (Regeneron Pharmaceuticals, Tarrytown, New York, NY), and bevacizumab (Avastin, Genentech, Inc, South San Francisco, CA).[66–69] The clinical use of these agents by intravitreal injection has been discussed in previous chapters throughout. A variety of corticosteroid agents are used to treat complications of DR, retinal vascular occlusions, and macular degeneration, among other conditions and include TA (Kenalog-40 [Bristol Meyers Squibb, Peapack, New York, NY], Trivaris [Allergan, Inc., USA], and Triesence [Alcon, Inc., USA]), dexamethasone, and fluocinolone acetonide (FA).[8]

SUSTAINED RELEASE DEVICES

A sustained release drug delivery platform for chronic ocular diseases like neovascular AMD or diabetic macular edema provides prolonged and controlled drug delivery. Most devices have a predetermined release rate over the lifespan of the device that can delivery drug over a period of weeks to years. Such platforms eliminate the need for frequent redosing, as currently required with intravitreal anti-VEGF and TA injection therapy, thereby avoiding repeated "peak and trough" pharmacokinetics. Instead, the constant drug levels at the target tissue may actually impact on the natural course of the disease by decreasing disease duration or severity by yet unknown mechanisms. Further, these systems eliminate the need for frequent (e.g., monthly or quarterly) re-dosing, which is more convenient and may eliminate potential procedure-related complications. Downsides to maintaining prolonged and sustained steroid concentrations include more pronounced, even accelerated, development of side effects.

These devices are categorized in several ways: choice of drug core used (bioerodible vs. nonerodible, see Table 28.1), device delivery technique (implantation and secured to eye vs. insertion through small gauge opening), and type of drug delivered (e.g., corticosteroids such as TA, dexamethasone, or FA). A new category includes cellular production based (e.g., Encapsulated Cell Technology [Neurotech, Lincoln, Rhode Island]) versus drug reservoir based.

Two general types of platforms are available for sustained release drug delivery to the posterior segment. The first has a polymer-coated, nonbiodegradable drug core that is implanted into the eye and replaced once the drug reservoir is empty. Such a device has the potential for extended duration of drug delivery and thereby potential for better disease control. However, the device may require removal and reimplantation for continuing therapy beyond the lifespan of drug release. A second type of device has a

Table 28.1.

Comparison of bioerodible and nonbioerodible sustained release devices

Typical Features	Nonbioerodible Drug Core Implants	Bioerodible Drug Core Inserts
Duration of delivery	Longer (months to years)	Shorter (weeks to months)
Steady-state drug concentrations	Can be equivalent based on technology	
Size	Can be equivalent based on technology	
Side effects	More severe	Less severe
Ability to control disease in short term	Equivalent	
Ability to control disease in long term	Superior	Inferior
Replacement	Removal/reinsertion	Introduction of new insert
Examples	Retisert and Iluvien (FA)	Ozurdex (dexamethasone), I-vation (TA)

bioerodible core that is covered or coated by a polymer material. The dissolution of the polymer allows drug elution into an aqueous phase typically in an initial burst and then at a design-specific rate until the polymer and drug have completely dissolved.[70] Such devices are inserted into the eye and provide more consistent drug levels than that detected with topical or intravitreal injections, but typically have a shorter lifespan of delivery compared to the nonbiodegradable implants (Fig. 28.5). This implies that the ability to control a long-term disease may not be as effective as the longer duration implants and may require reapplication (Table 28.2).

Fluocinolone-Based Devices

FA is a synthetic fluorinated corticosteroid with low aqueous solubility, making it useful as a dissolving drug reservoir. Iluvien (pSivida Inc., Watertown, Massachusetts, and licensed to Alimera Sciences, Inc., Alpharetta, Georgia) is the latest generation FA sustained release intravitreal implant designed for in-office implantation. The Iluvien platform is based on the Retisert (Bausch & Lomb, Rochester, New York, NY) FA intravitreal implant, which remains the only FDA-approved sustained release steroid device in ophthalmic clinical practice and is labeled to treat noninfectious uveitis.[71–73]

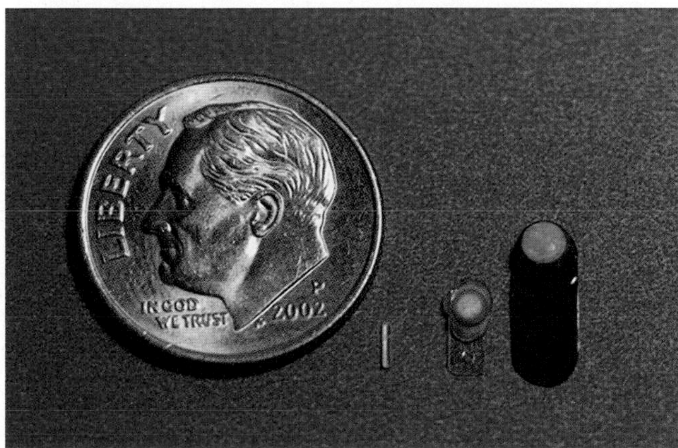

FIGURE 28.5. Comparison of relative sizes of (left to right) Iluvien, Retisert, and Vitrasert nonbiodegradable implants in relation to a quarter. (Courtesy of Sivida, Inc.)

With the Retisert, a 0.5 mg FA drug core is coated with a silicone PVA laminate and has a release opening covered by PVA.[74] It is attached to a PVA suture tab, which allows it to be secured to the sclera through a pars plana operative incision. It is designed to release 0.59 μg of FA per day for approximately 3 years.[72,73]

The Retisert DME Study 002 enrolled adult subjects with DME at least one disc area in size that involved the central fovea, despite at least 1 prior macular laser in the study eye more than 3 months prior to entry. Subjects were randomized to undergo either standard of care (SOC), consisting of macular grid laser or observation, or insertion of FA implants that released at 0.5 or 2.0 μg/d. The primary endpoint was resolution of edema at the macular center as determined by a masked reading center. Enrollment into the 2.0 μg/d group was discontinued early in the study. At 24 months, macular edema completely resolved in the FA-treated, compared to SOC, groups (54% vs. 29%, respectively, $p < 0.05$). Importantly, VA significantly improved by at least three lines in 37% of FA-treated eyes compared to 14% of SOC eyes.[75–77]

The second study (Retisert DME 005) enrolled 197 adult subjects with diffuse DME. Resolution of retinal thickening at the macular center was the primary endpoint. Subjects were randomized to receive a 0.59 FA Retisert implant or SOC in a 2:1 ratio. At 36 months, complete resolution of edema was significantly greater in

Table 28.2.

Available ocular implantable drug delivery devices

Brand	Manufacturer	Drug	Dose	Duration	Approved Indication
Nonbioerodible drug core					
Vitrasert	pSivida, licensed to Bausch & Lomb	Ganciclovir	0.45 mg	8 mo	CMV retinitis
Retisert	pSivida, licensed to Bausch & Lomb	Fluocinolone acetonide	0.59 mg	3 y	Noninfectious uveitis
Iluvien	pSivida, licensed to Alimera	Fluocinolone acetonide	0.5 or 0.2 μg/d	18–36 mo	*Pending*
I-vation	SurModics	Triamcinolone acetonide	1 or 3 μg/d	2 y	*Pending*
Bioerodible drug core					
Ozurdex	Allergan	Dexamethasone	350 or 700 μg	6 mo	Macular edema from retinal vein occlusion
Other devices					
NT-501	Neurotech Pharmaceuticals	Ciliary neurotrophic factor	800 ng per 1 × 10^6 cells/d	18 mo	*Pending*

the FA group compared to the SOC group (58% vs. 30%, respectively; $p < 0.001$). VA also improved by greater than three lines in a higher percentage of FA-treated eyes (28% vs. 15%, respectively). In addition, the Retisert DME trials also recorded that overall DR severity scales were less severe in treated eyes compared to SOC, suggesting that the sustained steroid therapy has a more global role in mediating angiogenic factors in diabetic eye disease than previously appreciated.[75–77]

Ocular serious adverse events in both studies were similar in the implanted eyes and were attributed to the ocular side effect profile of glucocorticoids. Significant intraocular pressure (IOP) elevation developed in 32% and 35% of patients at 2 and 3 years, respectively. Rates of retinal detachment, endophthalmitis, and device explantation remained very low.[75–77]

Ahmad et al. determined that pretreatment visual acuity and postimplantation resolution of edema correlated with maximal postimplantation acuity, while duration of diabetes and severity of DME both inversely correlated with posttreatment acuity. The pretreatment presence of large macular cysts was associated with greater reduction of central foveal thickness.[78,79]

The Iluvien implant consists of a 180-μg FA drug core surrounded by a 3.5-mm polyimide-coated cylinder. Once cured, PVA end caps are applied, which regulate the drug release rate. Two different release-rate implants are currently in clinical trials: 0.5 and 0.2 μg/d. The implant is then delivered into the vitreous base region through a 25-gauge needle attached to a modified tuberculin syringe as an office-based procedure.[79] The 0.5 and 0.2 μg/d implants are predicted to release FA for 1.5 and 3 years, respectively.[80,81]

The rationale for the use of Iluvien implants in phase 3 DME trials is based on two separate 4-year, randomized, multicenter phase 2b/3 clinical trials with the Retisert FA delivery platform in DME patients. The Flucocinolone Acetonide in Diabetic Macular Edema (FAME) study is a randomized, double-masked, parallel group, multicenter, dose-finding safety and efficacy study that compares the 0.5 and 0.2 μg/d injectable Iluvien implants with a sham injection. The study includes two doses of FA, as the Retisert DME study provided safety and efficacy data for the 0.5 μg/d dose, but it is unknown whether the 0.2 μg/d dose would be as effective but with a lower side effect profile.[79] The FAME study seeks to enroll 450 patients in two parallel trials (total 900 patients) worldwide. The primary endpoints are the proportion of patients with at least a three-line improvement in ETDRS acuity at 18 and 36 months compared to baseline and proportion of subjects with at least a two-step worsening in the ETDRS DR scale. Secondary objectives include determining which is an optimal FA dose to treat DME and minimizing side effects.[79]

Dexamethasone Based Devices

The dexamethasone drug delivery system (Ozurdex, Allergan, CA) is a nonreservoir-based, biodegradable delivery system. The small cylindrical device uses a lactic and glycolic acid polymer matrix that binds the water soluble drug. As the matrix dissolves in an aqueous environment, the drug is released in a linear release format. No visible device matrix or drug is seen after dissolution. Currently, two drug doses are being tested clinically: 350 and 700 µg. Drug has been detected into the vitreous up to 6 months after insertion. The office-based insertion procedure utilizes a unique trigger activated applicator with a needle tip to facilitate device insertion.

A 6-month phase 2 study of 315 patients with persistent macular edema and best acuity of 20/40 to 20/200 demonstrated an improvement in of at least 10 letters in a significantly greater proportion than patients who were observed. Both doses had a favorable response but with a trend toward better vision gain in the 700-µm device. Angiography and optical coherence tomography (OCT) testing paralleled the vision response. The intraocular pressure response (3%–6% of treated eyes) appeared to be lower than that reported with the fluocinolone devices. The Ozurdex device is currently FDA approved to treat macular edema from retinal vein occlusion.[8,82]

Triamcinolone-Based Device

Triamcinolone-based systems have the benefit of clinical familiarity with the expected response in many macular diseases. I-vation TA (SurModics, Irvine, CA) is a novel delivery system that coats triamcinolone over a helical coil-shaped implantation device. The helical shape increases potential surface area for drug coating. The device has a proprietary construction and coating that combines polybutyl methacrylate and PVA, which are used to control the rate and duration of drug release. The drug can be released for 6 to 12 months and is loaded to hold 925 µg of TA.

The drug device is implanted in the office. A conjunctival opening is followed by use of a 25-gauge needle to make a small sclerostomy. The device is then inserted through the sclerostomy. The device has the advantage of being able to be easily removed and replaced when drug release is completed.

In a prospective, phase 1 study of 31 patients with DME implanted with two release rates of the I-vation implant (Sustained Triamcinolone Release for the Inhibition of Diabetic Macular Edema [STRIDE] study), at 24 months 64% to 72% of patients had improved visual acuity with a decrease in central retinal thickening inversely related to the drug release rate. Cataract progression and minimal intraocular pressure increase were noted.[83] The phase 2b study was stopped prior to completion.

MICROPARTICLE ENCAPSULATION

An alternative intravitreal sustained delivery platform is encapsulation of the drug with biocompatible materials into either microparticles (1–1,000 µm) or nanoparticles (1–1,000 nm). Once delivered via intravitreal injection, the coatings slowly dissolve, thereby releasing the encapsulated drug into the vitreous cavity. The sustained release mechanism extends the drug half-life and reduces the need for repeated injection. It has the advantage of easy administration compared to other implantable sustained release devices. The particles themselves can produce vitreous clouding. Poly (lactic-co-glycolic) Acid (PLGA) microspheres containing an anti-VEGF RNA aptamer (EYE001) had sustained in vitro release of 2 µg/d over a 20-day period.[84] Bevacizumab was encapsulated into nanoparticle liposomes, two-layer vesicles used to encapsulate the drug, which dissolve to release the drug after intravitreal injection. Rabbit studies demonstrated ocular safety and immediate high intravitreal levels, which reduced by 100-fold over 40 days, but still resulted in therapeutic levels for nearly 6 weeks after a single administration.[85]

KEY POINTS

- Numerous routes of drug delivery may be used to deliver bioactive drug concentrations to the posterior segment.
- Various physiologic ocular barriers work to reduce intraocular drug concentrations.
- Innovations to overcome or eliminate these ocular barriers and clearance mechanisms may help enhance drug concentrations.
- Sustained release devices provide longer duration therapeutic drug delivery, which may reduce the "peak and trough" effect from repeated intravitreal injections.

REFERENCES

1. Gaudana R, Jwala J, Boddu SH, et al. Recent perspectives in ocular drug delivery. *Pharm Res*. 2009;26:1197–1216.
2. Ashton P. Retinal drug delivery. In: *Intraocular Drug Delivery*. Jaffe GJ, Ashton P, Pearson PA, eds. New York, NY: Taylor & Francis Group; 2006:1–26.
3. Urtti A. Challenges and obstacles of ocular pharmacokinetics and drug delivery. *Adv Drug Deliv Rev*. 2006;58:1131–1135.
4. Grass GM, Robinson JR. Relationship of chemical structure to corneal penetration and influence of low-viscosity solution on ocular bioavailability. *J Pharm Sci*. 1984;73:1021–1027.
5. Grass GM, Robinson JR. Mechanisms of corneal drug penetration. II: Ultrastructural analysis of potential pathways for drug movement. *J Pharm Sci*. 1988;77:15–23.
6. Hughes PM, Olejnik O, Chang-Lin JE, et al. Topical and systemic drug delivery to the posterior segments. *Adv Drug Deliv Rev*. 2005;57:2010–2032.
7. Del Amo EM, Urtti A. Current and future ophthalmic drug delivery systems. A shift to the posterior segment. *Drug Discov Today*. 2008;13:135–143.
8. Mansoor S, Kuppermann BD, Kenney MC. Intraocular sustained-release delivery systems for triamcinolone acetonide. *Pharm Res*. 2009;26:770–784.
9. Antonetti DA, Gardner TW, Barber AJ. Blood-retinal barrier. In: *Intraocular Drug Delivery*. Jaffe GJ, Ashton P, Pearson PA, eds. New York, NY: Taylor & Francis Group; 2006:27–40.

10. Rana ZA, Pearson PA. Pharmacologic treatment in diabetic macular edema. In: *Intraocular Drug Delivery*. Jaffe GJ, Ashton P, Pearson PA, eds. New York, NY: Taylor & Francis Group; 2006:291–300.
11. Frank RN. Potential new medical therapies for diabetic retinopathy: protein kinase C inhibitors. *Am J Ophthalmol*. 2002; 133:693–698.
12. Campochiaro PA. Reduction of diabetic macular edema by oral administration of the kinase inhibitor PKC412. *Invest Ophthalmol Vis Sci*. 2004;45:922–931.
13. Fabbro D, Ruetz S, Bodis S, et al. PKC412–a protein kinase inhibitor with a broad therapeutic potential. *Anticancer Drug Design*. 2000;15:17–28.
14. Aiello LP, Davis MD, Girach A, et al. Effect of ruboxistaurin on visual loss in patients with diabetic retinopathy. *Ophthalmology*. 2006;113:2221–2230.
15. Aiello LP. The potential role of PKC beta in diabetic retinopathy and macular edema. *Surv Ophthalmol*. 2002;47 Suppl 2:S263–S269.
16. Aiello LP, Clermont A, Arora V, et al. Inhibition of PKC beta by oral administration of ruboxistaurin is well tolerated and ameliorates diabetes-induced retinal hemodynamic abnormalities in patients. *Invest Ophthalmol Vis Sci*. 2006; 47:86–92.
17. Strom C, Sander B, Klemp K, et al. Effect of ruboxistaurin on blood-retinal barrier permeability in relation to severity of leakage in diabetic macular edema. *Invest Ophthalmol Vis Sci*. 2005;46:3855–3858.
18. Aiello LP. Targeting intraocular neovascularization and edema–one drop at a time. *N Engl J Med*. 2008;359:967–969.
19. Eyetech Study Group. Preclinical and phase 1A clinical evaluation of an anti-VEGF pegylated aptamer (EYE001) for the treatment of exudative age-related macular degeneration. *Retina*. 2002;22:143–152.
20. Eyetech Study Group. Anti-vascular endothelial growth factor therapy for subfoveal choroidal neovascularization secondary to age-related macular degeneration: phase 2 study results. *Ophthalmology*. 2003;110:979–986.
21. Lopez PF, Sippy BD, Lambert HM, et al. Transdifferentiated retinal pigment epithelial cells are immunoreactive for vascular endothelial growth factor in surgically excised age-related macular degeneration-related choroidal neovascular membranes. *Invest Ophthalmol Vis Sci*. 1996;37: 855–868.
22. Michels S, Rosenfeld PJ, Puliafito CA, et al. Systemic bevacizumab (Avastin) therapy for neovascular age-related macular degeneration twelve-week results of an uncontrolled open-label clinical study. *Ophthalmology*. 2005;112:1035–1047.
23. Moshfeghi AA, Rosenfeld PJ, Puliafito CA, et al. Systemic bevacizumab (Avastin) therapy for neovascular age-related macular degeneration: twenty-four-week results of an uncontrolled open-label clinical study. *Ophthalmology*. 2006; 113:e2001–e2012.
24. Scheppke L, Aguilar E, Gariano RF, et al. Retinal vascular permeability suppression by topical application of a novel VEGFR2/Src kinase inhibitor in mice and rabbits. *J Clin Investig*. 2008;118:2337–2346.
25. Doukas J, Mahesh S, Umeda N, et al. Topical administration of a multi-targeted kinase inhibitor suppresses choroidal neovascularization and retinal edema. *J Cell Physiol*. 2008; 216:29–37.
26. Takahashi K, Saishin Y, Saishin Y, et al. Suppression and regression of choroidal neovascularization by the multitargeted kinase inhibitor pazopanib. *Arch Ophthalmol*. 2009;127: 494–499.
27. Chang LK. Overview of emerging molecular therapies for neovascular AMD. *Ret Physician*. 2009.
28. Csaky KG. Hurdles and prospects for episclearl drug delivery. *Ret Physician*. 2009.
29. Ranta VP, Urtti A. Transscleral drug delivery to the posterior eye: prospects of pharmacokinetic modeling. *Adv Drug Deliv Rev*. 2006;58:1164–1181.
30. Mac Gabhann F, Demetriades AM, Deering T, et al. Protein transport to choroid and retina following periocular injection: theoretical and experimental study. *Ann Biomed Eng*. 2007;35:615–630.
31. Ambati J, Canakis CS, Miller JW, et al. Diffusion of high molecular weight compounds through sclera. *Invest Ophthalmol Vis Sci*. 2000;41:1181–1185.
32. Cruysberg LP, Nuijts RM, Geroski DH, et al. The influence of intraocular pressure on the transscleral diffusion of high-molecular-weight compounds. *Invest Ophthalmol Vis Sci*. 2005; 46:3790–3794.
33. Shuler RK Jr, Dioguardi PK, Henjy C, et al. Scleral permeability of a small, single-stranded oligonucleotide. *J Ocul Pharmacol Ther*. 2004;20:159–168.
34. Jonas JB, Kreissig I, Spandau UH, et al. Infectious and noninfectious endophthalmitis after intravitreal high-dosage triamcinolone acetonide. *Am J Ophthalmol*. 2006;141:579–580.
35. Demetriades AM, Deering T, Liu H, et al. Trans-scleral delivery of antiangiogenic proteins. *J Ocul Pharmacol Ther*. 2008;24:70–79.
36. Gehlbach P, Demetriades AM, Yamamoto S, et al. Periocular injection of an adenoviral vector encoding pigment epithelium-derived factor inhibits choroidal neovascularization. *Gene Ther*. 2003;10:637–646.
37. Gehlbach P, Demetriades AM, Yamamoto S, et al. Periocular gene transfer of sFlt-1 suppresses ocular neovascularization and vascular endothelial growth factor-induced breakdown of the blood-retinal barrier. *Hum Gene Ther*. 2003;14: 129–141.
38. Russell SR, Hudson HL, Jerdan JA. Anecortave acetate for the treatment of exudative age-related macular degeneration—a review of clinical outcomes. *Surv Ophthalmol*. 2007;52 Suppl 1:S79–S90.
39. Robinson MR, Lee SS, Kim H, et al. A rabbit model for assessing the ocular barriers to the transscleral delivery of triamcinolone acetonide. *Exp Eye Res*. 2006;82:479–487.
40. Lee SS, Robinson MR. Novel drug delivery systems for retinal diseases. A review. *Ophthal Res*. 2009;41:124–135.
41. Olsen TW, Edelhauser HF, Lim JI, et al. Human scleral permeability. Effects of age, cryotherapy, transscleral diode laser, and surgical thinning. *Invest Ophthalmol Vis Sci*. 1995;36:1893–1903.
42. Kim H, Robinson MR, Lizak MJ, et al. Controlled drug release from an ocular implant: an evaluation using dynamic three-dimensional magnetic resonance imaging. *Invest Ophthalmol Vis Sci*. 2004;45:2722–2731.
43. Ghate D, Brooks W, McCarey BE, et al. Pharmacokinetics of intraocular drug delivery by periocular injections using ocular fluorophotometry. *Invest Ophthalmol Vis Sci*. 2007;48:2230–2237.

44. Pontes de Carvalho RA, Krausse ML, Murphree AL, et al. Delivery from episcleral exoplants. *Invest Ophthalmol Vis Sci.* 2006;47:4532–4539.
45. Kato A, Kimura H, Okabe K, et al. Feasibility of drug delivery to the posterior pole of the rabbit eye with an episcleral implant. *Invest Ophthalmol Vis Sci.* 2004;45:238–244.
46. Felt-Baeyens O, Eperon S, Mora P, et al. Biodegradable scleral implants as new triamcinolone acetonide delivery systems. *Int J Pharm.* 2006;322:6–12.
47. Okabe K, Kimura H, Okabe J, et al. Ocular tissue distribution of betamethasone after anterior-episcleral, posterior-episcleral, and anterior-intrascleral placement of nonbiodegradable implants. *Retina.* 2007;27:770–777.
48. Okabe K, Kimura H, Okabe J, et al. Intraocular tissue distribution of betamethasone after intrascleral administration using a non-biodegradable sustained drug delivery device. *Invest Ophthalmol Vis Sci.* 2003;44:2702–2707.
49. Okabe J, Kimura H, Kunou N, et al. Biodegradable intrascleral implant for sustained intraocular delivery of betamethasone phosphate. *Invest Ophthalmol Vis Sci.* 2003;44:740–744.
50. Shin JP, Park YC, Oh JH, et al. Biodegradable intrascleral implant of triamcinolone acetonide in experimental uveitis. *J Ocul Pharmacol Ther.* 2009;25:201–208.
51. Gilger BC, Salmon JH, Wilkie DA, et al. A novel bioerodible deep scleral lamellar cyclosporine implant for uveitis. *Invest Ophthalmol Vis Sci.* 2006;47:2596–2605.
52. Gilger BC, Michau TM, Salmon JH. Immune-mediated keratitis in horses: 19 cases (1998–2004). *Vet Ophthalmol.* 2005; 8:233–239.
53. Olsen TW, Feng X, Wabner K, et al. Cannulation of the suprachoroidal space: a novel drug delivery methodology to the posterior segment. *Am J Ophthalmol.* 2006;142:777–787.
54. Bonini-Filho MA, Jorge R, Barbosa JC, et al. Intravitreal injection versus sub-Tenon's infusion of triamcinolone acetonide for refractory diabetic macular edema: a randomized clinical trial. *Invest Ophthalmol Vis Sci.* 2005;46:3845–3849.
55. Chieh JJ, Roth DB, Liu M, et al. Intravitreal triamcinolone acetonide for diabetic macular edema. *Retina.* 2005;25:828–834.
56. Jonas J, Heatley G, Spaide R, et al. Intravitreal triamcinolone acetonide and secondary ocular hypertension. *J Glaucoma.* 2005;14:168–171.
57. Jonas JB, Martus P, Degenring RF, et al. Predictive factors for visual acuity after intravitreal triamcinolone treatment for diabetic macular edema. *Arch Ophthalmol.* 2005;123: 1338–1343.
58. Martidis A, Duker JS, Greenberg PB, et al. Intravitreal triamcinolone for refractory diabetic macular edema. *Ophthalmology.* 2002;109:920–927.
59. Massin P, Audren F, Haouchine B, et al. Intravitreal triamcinolone acetonide for diabetic diffuse macular edema: preliminary results of a prospective controlled trial. *Ophthalmology.* 2004;111:218–224; discussion 224–215.
60. Sutter FK, Simpson JM, Gillies MC. Intravitreal triamcinolone for diabetic macular edema that persists after laser treatment: three-month efficacy and safety results of a prospective, randomized, double-masked, placebo-controlled clinical trial. *Ophthalmology.* 2004;111:2044–2049.
61. Fintak DR, Shah GK, Blinder KJ, et al. Incidence of endophthalmitis related to intravitreal injection of bevacizumab and ranibizumab. *Retina.* 2008;28:1395–1399.
62. Jonas JB, Kamppeter BA, Harder B, et al. Intravitreal triamcinolone acetonide for diabetic macular edema: a prospective, randomized study. *J Ocul Pharmacol Ther.* 2006; 22:200–207.
63. Moshfeghi DM, Kaiser PK, Bakri SJ, et al. Presumed sterile endophthalmitis following intravitreal triamcinolone acetonide injection. *Ophthal Surg Lasers Imaging.* 2005;36:24–29.
64. Moshfeghi DM, Kaiser PK, Scott IU, et al. Acute endophthalmitis following intravitreal triamcinolone acetonide injection. *Am J Ophthalmol.* 2003;136:791–796.
65. Peyman GA, Lad EM, Moshfeghi DM. Intravitreal injection of therapeutic agents. *Retina (Philadelphia, Pa).* 2009;29: 875–912.
66. Brown DM, Kaiser PK, Michels M, et al. Ranibizumab versus verteporfin for neovascular age-related macular degeneration. *N Engl J Med.* 2006;355:1432–1444.
67. Rosenfeld PJ. Intravitreal avastin: the low cost alternative to lucentis? *Am J Ophthalmol.* 2006;142:141–143.
68. Rosenfeld PJ, Brown DM, Heier JS, et al. Ranibizumab for neovascular age-related macular degeneration. *N Engl J Med.* 2006;355:1419–1431.
69. Gragoudas ES, Adamis AP, Cunningham ET Jr, et al. Pegaptanib for neovascular age-related macular degeneration. *N Engl J Med.* 2004;351:2805–2816.
70. Kuppermann BD. Drug delivery strategies for combination ophthalmic treatments. *Retina.* 2009;29:S24–S26.
71. Jaffe GJ, Ben-Nun J, Guo H, et al. Fluocinolone acetonide sustained drug delivery device to treat severe uveitis. *Ophthalmology.* 2000;107:2024–2033.
72. Jaffe GJ, Martin D, Callanan D, et al. Fluocinolone acetonide implant (Retisert) for noninfectious posterior uveitis: thirty-four-week results of a multicenter randomized clinical study. *Ophthalmology.* 2006;113:1020–1027.
73. Jaffe GJ, Yang CH, Guo H, et al. Safety and pharmacokinetics of an intraocular fluocinolone acetonide sustained delivery device. *Invest Ophthalmol Vis Sci.* 2000;41:3569–3575.
74. Mruthyunjaya P, Khalatbari D, Yang P, et al. Efficacy of low-release-rate fluocinolone acetonide intravitreal implants to treat experimental uveitis. *Arch Ophthalmol.* 2006;124:1012–1018.
75. Pearson P, Baker CW, Eliott D, et al. Fluocinolone acetonide intravitreal implant in patients with diabetic macular edema: 12 month results. *Invest Ophthalmol Vis Sci.* 2003;44: E-abstract 4288.
76. Pearson P, Levy B, Comstock T, et al. Fluocinolone acetonide intravitreal implant to treat diabetic macular edema: 3-year results of a multi-center clinical trial. *Invest Ophthalmol Vis Sci.* 2006; 47:E-abstract 5442.
77. Pearson P, Levy B, Fluconolone Acetonide Implant Study G. Fluocinolone acetonide intravitreal implant to treat diabetic macular edema: 2-year results of a multi-center clinical trial. *Invest Ophthalmol Vis Sci.* 2005;46:E-abstract 4673.
78. Ahmad S, Stinnett SS, Jaffe GJ. Pre-treatment prognosticators of response to a fluocinolone acetonide implant for diabetic macular edema. *Invest Ophthalmol Vis Sci.* 2006;47: E-abstract 979.
79. Mruthyunjaya P, Jaffe GJ. The medidur implant. *Ret Physician.* September 2007 edition.
80. See RF, Peairs JJ, Srivastava S, et al. Safety and drug release profile of injectable intravitreal sustained-release fluocinolone acetonide device. *Invest Ophthalmol Vis Sci.* 2006;47: E-abstract 5119.

81. Srivastava S, Mruthyunjaya P, Wiser J, et al. Intravitreal sustained-release fluocinolone acetonide device to treat severe experimental uveitis. *Invest Ophthalmol Vis Sci*. 2005;46: E-abstract 3536.
82. Kuppermann BD, Blumenkranz MS, Haller JA, et al. Randomized controlled study of an intravitreous dexamethasone drug delivery system in patients with persistent macular edema. *Arch Ophthalmol*. 2007;125:309–317.
83. Dugel PU, Eliott D, Cantrill HL, et al. I-Vation TA: 24-month clinical results of the phase 1 saftey and preliminary efficacy study. *Invest Ophthalmol Vis Sci*. 2009;50:E-abstract 4332.
84. Carrasquillo KG, Ricker JA, Rigas IK, et al. Controlled delivery of the anti-VEGF aptamer EYE001 with poly-(lactic-co-glycolic)acid microspheres. *Invest Ophthalmol Vis Sci*. 2003;44:290–299.
85. Abrishami M, Ganavati SZ, Soroush D, et al. Preparation, characterization, and in vivo evaluation of nanoliposomes-encapsulated bevacizumab (avastin) for intravitreal administration. *Retina*. 2009;29:699–703.

CHAPTER

29

Financial and Regulatory Implications of Anti-angiogenic Drugs

George A. Williams

INTRODUCTION

The advent of anti–vascular endothelial growth factor (VEGF) therapy for neovascular age-related macular degeneration has prevented blindness in tens of thousands of people. However, the costs of these drugs are beyond anything seen before in ophthalmic drug therapeutics. An analysis of the financial implications of retinal drugs must include not only an evaluation of the direct costs of the drugs and the costs associated with their administration but also the cost savings that accrue from their clinical benefit. This chapter discusses the financial and regulatory issues associated with retinal drugs.

The development of photodynamic therapy with verteporfin and pegaptanib sodium for neovascular age-related macular degeneration introduced ophthalmologists to the financial and regulatory implications of physician-administered drugs. The financial implications of physician-administered drugs can be considered from both a microeconomic and a macroeconomic perspective. The microeconomic perspective involves the cost to the patient and the ophthalmologist. The macroeconomic perspective considers the costs to society and the health care system. Together, these costs present significant and difficult issues.

COSTS TO PATIENTS

The economic burden of antiangiogenic therapy to the patient can be considerable.

Under Medicare, physician-administered drugs are paid for by Part B and therefore patients are responsible for 20% of the allowable reimbursement for both the drug and the physician services associated with administering the drug. For ranibizumab, this can total nearly $500. The need for repeated treatment in most patients multiplies the economic burden. Fortunately, a majority of Americans have supplemental insurance to cover co-payment costs. However, the recent economic problems are beginning to adversely affect some patients' access to supplemental insurance coverage. Many drug companies have programs through independent foundations to assist financially eligible patients with drug-related co-payments. Although the preliminary experience with these programs has been generally positive, their long-term viability is unknown. There are also significant indirect costs associated with antiangiogenic therapy related to the frequency of treatment and follow-up such as transportation, parking, time away from work for the patient or more commonly their family members, or even loss of a job. The net result is that antiangiogenic therapy can create a substantial economic burden for many patients.

An analysis of a "typical" patient on antiangiogenic treatment readily demonstrates the costs involved. If we assume that a patient with active neovascular age-related macular degeneration (AMD) is seen every 4 to 6 weeks and receives six injections per year, we can calculate the costs associated with such a treatment regimen. Each office visit costs approximately $150 with the evaluation and management service combined with a unilateral optical coherence tomography. At eight visits per year, this cost is $1,200. If a patient receives two unilateral fluorescein angiograms per year, this adds $235. Six injections of ranibizumab per year cost approximately $12,200. The total for such a "typical" patient is $13,635. Obviously, the cost increases if more visits or injections are required or if the patient has bilateral disease.

COSTS TO OPHTHALMOLOGISTS

For ophthalmologists, antiangiogenic therapy also creates significant economic problems. Practice management issues related to increased patient volume and drug costs are considerable. The increased patient volume may require additional office and clinical personnel as well as more office space or office hours. The costs of drugs such as ranibizumab distort practice accounting and demand detailed tracking of accounts payable and receivable. For some practices, drug costs can become the leading cost in the practice. Under current Medicare regulations, the allowable reimbursement for retinal drugs is paid at 106%

of the average sales price (ASP) of the respective drug. This 6% margin is expected to cover the costs of an efficient provider for the drug ordering, billing, and inventory. The ASP is determined quarterly by Medicare based on reports from the drug manufacturer, which provide the net revenue per unit dose of the drug. The net revenue is the actual sales price minus any rebates, discounts, or fees paid to distributors or physicians. Thus, the ASP is often less than the actual cost of the drug to the ophthalmologist. Although, the ASP can change every 3 months, the physician cost for the drug rarely reflects the changes in net revenue and therefore physicians rarely receive the full 6% margin. Also, state and local sales taxes or gross revenue taxes on drug revenues can further decrease the reimbursement to the ophthalmologist. In the first quarter of 2009, the allowable reimbursement for ranibizumab was $2,036. The cost of ranibizumab is $1,950. Therefore, the true margin is not 6% but only 4%. This of course assumes that the ophthalmologist receives payment from both Medicare (80%) and the co-payment (20%). If not, the ophthalmologist loses over $400 per treatment. Typically, there is no problem with the Medicare's 80% payment, but the 20% co-payment is sometimes a problem due to the vagaries of secondary insurance coverage or patients' inability to pay. Ophthalmologists are then placed in the uncomfortable position of losing money per treatment. This can create an adversarial situation that may compromise the patient-ophthalmologist relationship. It is therefore critical that ophthalmologists explain to their patients the financial implications of antiangiogenic treatment.

Typically, the ophthalmologist purchases the drug from suppliers or directly from the manufacturer. Although this can be done on a just-in-time basis, most physicians carry an inventory of the drug to provide same-day convenience for their patients. However, maintaining an inventory of expensive drugs entails considerable financial risk. This can create a conflict between accounts payable and accounts receivable.

The 20% co-pay requirement by Medicare can create significant problems for both patients and their physicians. The co-pay results in substantial out-of-pocket liabilities for patients without secondary coverage. For expensive drugs that are used on a monthly basis, this rapidly results in large balances. Regardless of whether or not the patient is able to pay off these balances, the physician is responsible for payment to the distributor or manufacturer. This creates a conflict between the physician and patient, which can damage the therapeutic relationship. Even when patients have secondary coverage for the co-pay, physicians may remain in financial jeopardy. Unfortunately, many secondary insurers have inconsistent and irregular payment policies concerning Part B drugs. This is particularly common with Medicare Advantage plans, which in 2008 covered 22% of Medicare beneficiaries.

At the macroeconomic level, antiangiogenic therapy is most commonly used for neovascular age-related macular degeneration, a disease with a large and increasing case number resulting in increased utilization of physician services, imaging, and drugs. It is clear that the direct costs of antiangiogenic treatment will total billions of dollars per year and contribute to the continuing escalation in health care costs.

The financial burden to the overall health care system from Part B antiangiogenic drugs was 4% of the total Part B drug costs in 2007. Even more impressive is that it represented 13% of the $5.4 billion spent for all of ophthalmology. This trend is seen throughout all of Medicare. In 1997, Part B drugs cost $2.8 billion compared to physician payments of $31.9 billion or 8.6%. In 2007, Part B drugs cost $16.3 billion compared to physician payments of $60 billion or 27%. Thus, from 1997 to 2007, physician payments increased 88% compared to a 582% increase for Part B drugs.

Physician services associated with administration of antiangiogenic drugs have exploded over the past several years. In 2000, the number of intravitreal injections given to Medicare beneficiaries was 3000. In 2008, this had increased to nearly 1 million. This alone increased Medicare costs over $180 million. As expected, imaging studies have also increased from 3.1 million in 2004 to 6.8 million in 2007. This increase is primarily due to antiangiogenic therapy and costs an additional $155 million. Other studies such as fluorescein angiography have also increased.

This growth in physician services, imaging, and drug costs adversely affects the sustainable growth rate (SGR), which is used to determine the yearly revaluation of physician reimbursement. Although the costs directly associated with antiangiogenic therapy are a small contributor to the overall effect, they are indicative of the problems inherent in the SGR system. In fact, the American Medical Association (AMA) has repeatedly cited the increased costs associated with antiangiogenic therapy for neovascular age-related macular degeneration as a factor in the overall growth in physician services. The AMA estimated that in 2007 these costs were $300 million, not counting the cost of the drugs. However, the AMA has also described the benefits of antiangiogenic therapy to Medicare beneficiaries as "priceless." Although there is widespread consensus that the SGR system is fatally flawed and that a new payment update mechanism is needed, at the time of this writing, the SGR system remains in effect.

COST CUTTING

One obvious way to decrease the cost of antiangiogenic therapy is to use less expensive drugs. The use of bevacizumab instead of ranibizumab has the potential to save billions of dollars. In order to determine the potential savings associated with bevacizumab, several assumptions are necessary. The simplest model assumes equal efficacy, safety, and injection frequency between bevacizumab and ranibizumab. In 2008, the US sales for ranibizumab were $875 million, which equates to 450,000 injections per year. Market and physician surveys suggest that in 2008, approximately 40% of patients treated with antiangiogenic therapy for neovascular AMD received ranibizumab. This is consistent with the approximately 1 million intravitreal injections in the Medicare population. Therefore, the use of bevacizumab at approximately $40 per injection compared to the $2,031 per injection cost of ranibizumab may have saved approximately $1 billion in direct drug costs.

Although the direct costs of antiangiogenic therapy are substantial, the indirect costs of untreated or undertreated neovascular AMD with attendant blindness, disability, and lost productivity are even greater. People with visual loss from neovascular AMD have a lower employment than unaffected people. The employment rate for people afflicted with visual loss from AMD is 44% for those with mild visual limitation and 31% for those with severe visual limitation due to neovascular AMD and/or geographic atrophy compared to 78% of those unaffected. Additionally, people with advanced AMD earn less money compared to people without disability. In 1997, the mean wage for a person with no disability was $31,182. The mean wage for a person with mild visual loss was 30% less and for a person with severe visual loss it was 38% less. A detailed analysis of the economic loss to the gross domestic product (GDP) of the United States estimated the total loss from advanced AMD to be $29.8 billion. A study on the effect of AMD upon the Canadian GDP found similar results when adjusted for the population difference.[1]

Furthermore, vision loss leads to higher nonocular-related medical costs due to depression, injury from falls, skilled nursing facility utilization, and long-term care utilization. A study examining the association between vision loss and medical care costs in Medicare beneficiaries concluded that persons with vision loss incur significantly higher costs than those with normal vision. Approximately 90% of these costs are nonocular-related medical costs. This study estimated that blindness and vision loss resulted in $2.14 billion in nonocular-related medical costs in 2003.[2] Treatments such as antiangiogenic therapy, which can prevent or reverse vision loss, can reduce these costs. Therefore, any analysis of the costs of antiangiogenic therapy must consider the huge indirect costs associated with vision loss.

REGULATORY ISSUES

The pharmacotherapy of blinding retinal disease is replete with examples of off-label drug use. The history of this off-label drug use is testimony to the innovation, persistence, and even courage of ophthalmologists in their continuing efforts to improve vision for those afflicted with retinal disease. Sometimes, off-label drug use is employed to treat relatively rare conditions such as endophthalmitis or uveitis for which a Food and Drug Administration (FDA) label is unlikely. Other times, off-label drugs are used to treat common disorders such as diabetic retinopathy or age-related macular degeneration. The advent of ocular photodynamic therapy with verteporfin in 2000 initiated a new era in the management of age-related macular degeneration. Although this novel therapy provided a safe and effective treatment for many patients with previously untreatable subfoveal choroidal neovascularization, the FDA label restricted its use to predominantly classic neovascular lesions. This limited label was used as the basis for the Centers for Medicare and Medicaid Services (CMS) coverage as outlined in a National Coverage Determination (NCD).[3] Although this NCD was the first exposure for many ophthalmologists to the confusing and arcane regulations that govern off-label drug use, most ophthalmologists had been using approved drugs off-label for years for the treatment of endophthalmitis, uveitis, proliferative vitreoretinopathy, and cystoid macular edema. Even the use of preoperative and postoperative antibiotics for endophthalmitis prophylaxis is off-label.

An understanding of the issues involving off-label drug use requires a review of the FDA label process.[4] The FDA is a public health agency whose mission is to oversee the use and marketing of regulated medical products. The FDA reviews the toxicology and clinical research from Phase 1, Phase 2, and Phase 3 studies, which is presented in an Investigational New Drug (IND) application and, when appropriate, approves a drug for use and marketing. When a drug is approved, the FDA issues a label that describes and defines the drug's specific medical indication(s), dose, dosage form, side effects, and chemical structure. For some drugs, the FDA may include a "black box" warning in the label to emphasize potential complications associated with severe morbidity or mortality. The format of the FDA label has received widespread criticism for its confusing and almost impenetrable structure and syntax. Recently, FDA announced a more "user-friendly" format designed to facilitate use by both patients and physicians.[5] Although this new format is an improvement, it remains suboptimal.

Any use of a drug not listed in the label is considered off-label. Off-label uses include giving an approved drug for a disease or indication other than that for which it is approved; at a different dose, frequency, or route of administration than specified in the label; or to treat a child when the product is approved to treat only adults. However, the use of an approved product by physicians is not restricted by the FDA to the limitations of the label. Physicians are allowed to use FDA-approved drugs in the treatment of an individual patient as medical practice. The FDA recognizes that off-label use of drugs by physicians is often appropriate and may represent the standard of care. The most obvious example of off-label drug use constituting the standard of care in ophthalmology is the use of intravitreal antibiotics for endophthalmitis, despite the fact that no antibiotics are approved for intravitreal injection or for the treatment of endophthalmitis. The FDA has issued specific guidance on off-label drug use.

> "Good medical practice and the best interests of the patient require that physicians use legally available drugs, biologics and devices according to their best knowledge and medical judgment. If physicians use a product for an indication not in the approved labeling, they have the responsibility to be well-informed about the product, to base its use on firm scientific rationale and on sound medical evidence and to maintain records on the product's use and effects. Use of a marketed product in this manner when the intent is in the practice of medicine does not require the submission of an Investigational New Drug Application........or review by an Institutional Review Board (IRB). However, the institution at which the product will be used may, under its own authority, require IRB review or other institutional oversight."[5]

In addition to the FDA, medical organizations such as the AMA and the American Academy of Ophthalmology are on record supporting off-label drug use when there is appropriate evidence-based medicine, expert consensus opinion, or unmet medical need.[6,7] The American Medical Association policy on off-label drug use is "The AMA confirms its strong support for the autonomous clinical decision-making authority of a physician and that a physician may lawfully use an FDA approved drug product or medical device for an unlabeled indication when such use is based on sound scientific evidence and sound medical opinion."[7]

If the FDA recognizes off-label drug use as appropriate and if the FDA does not regulate medical practice in the treatment of an individual patient, what role does the FDA play in off-label drug use? One important role is that the FDA precludes drug sponsors from marketing drugs to physicians or patients for off-label use. "Pharmaceutical manufacturers cannot proactively discuss off-label uses, nor may they distribute written materials (promotional pieces, reprints of articles, etc.) that mention off-label use."[8] Therefore, the FDA label has important marketing implications because pharmaceutical companies are not allowed to market drugs for off-label use. Currently, this limitation applies to any formal marketing such as media advertising or drug detail information. Recently, the FDA has proposed a controversial relaxation on the restrictions for the marketing of off-label indications.[9] Regardless of the status of off-label marketing, the FDA does not restrict other parties such as physicians or specialty societies from discussing off-label uses or distributing written materials concerning them.

The FDA also becomes involved in off-label drug use when the drug is in "investigational use." The term "investigational use" suggests the use of an approved drug in the context of a clinical study protocol. When the primary intent of the investigational use is to develop information about a drug's safety or efficacy, or if the off-label use involves a route of administration or dosage level or use in a subject population or other factor that significantly increases the risks associated with the use of the drug, submission of an IND is required.[4] Physicians can obtain the IND application (form 1571) from the Internet.[5] Most investigational review boards will require an IND for a clinical trial involving off-label drug use.

Another regulatory issue involving off-label drugs is the formulation of ophthalmic preparations by compounding pharmacies. Any drug product prepared by a compounding pharmacy is considered by the FDA to be either off-label or a new drug.[10] Compounding pharmacies are licensed by individual states to provide drugs to individual patients at the prescription request of a physician. In ophthalmology, compounding pharmacies provide multiple drugs for retinal pharmacotherapy such as antibiotics, corticosteroids, and bevacizumab. Compounding pharmacies prepare approved drugs at dosages that are relevant for ocular administration and prepare preservative-free drugs. Although the FDA states "Traditional compounding typically is used to prepare medications that are not available commercially....," the FDA has recently expressed concerns about the legality of some compounding pharmacy practices related to retinal pharmacotherapy.[11] These issues are related primarily to the marketing of compounded retinal drugs and the need for a patient-specific prescription for each dose. The role of the FDA in regulating the state-controlled compounding pharmacies is also a concern. At the time of this writing, these issues are under litigation. As a result, legislation has been introduced in Congress to clarify the role of the FDA in the regulation of compounding pharmacies. The implications of this legislation to retinal pharmacotherapy are unknown.

The legal implications of off-label drug use primarily involve risk management issues. The keys to addressing these risk management issues are patient selection and informed consent. As discussed above, FDA approval status does not necessarily define appropriate medical practice, nor does the FDA regulate medical practice. Medical practice is the therapeutic relationship between a physician and an individual patient. The physician must decide what the appropriate medical care is for each patient and this decision must fall within the standard of care. The question then becomes "When does off-label drug use become the standard of care?" The answer depends on who is defining the standard of care. Payers may use specific definitions of the standard of care to establish coverage determinations, which are discussed later. From a risk management perspective involving malpractice, a jury, judge, or arbitrator determines whether treatment is within the standard of care. This determination is based upon such factors as supporting authoritative literature, expert consensus, scientific rationale, and local or national medical practice patterns.

An important factor in establishing the standard of care is informed consent. This is particularly critical with off-label drug use. The Ophthalmic Mutual Insurance Company (OMIC) recommends that physicians inform patients about the off-label status of a proposed treatment.[12] The discussion should include the known and potential unknown risks as well as the rationale for the off-label drug use. The physician should also discuss why any available FDA-approved or CMS-covered therapies are not appropriate. This discussion should be well documented in the medical record. OMIC also recommends that a specific off-label informed consent be used. OMIC provides a specific consent for bevacizumab and triamcinolone acetonide with useful suggestions concerning patient selection, preparation of the medication, and informed consent and documentation.[12] Recently, the off-label use of bevacizumab for retinopathy of prematurity has raised concerns. This treatment must be considered investigational and should be performed only in the context of an approved clinical trial with an IND from the FDA.

Another difficult issue concerning off-label drug use concerns coverage for the drug and associated services. In ophthalmology, this usually means coverage by Medicare, which can be established either by the local Medicare carrier via a local carrier decision or by CMS as an NCD. The Medicare Benefit Policy Manual provides that individual carriers may establish on a case-by-case basic coverage for off-label drug use based upon their assessment of the medical indication as reasonable and necessary.

> "FDA approved drugs for indications other than what is indicated on the official label may be covered under Medicare if the carrier determines the use to be medically accepted, taking into consideration the major drug compendia, authoritative medical literature and for accepted standards of medical practice….." [13]

Some carriers have outlined criteria that they consider when determining coverage of off-label drug use on a case-by-case basis. These criteria consider the following factors:

1. Whether alternative treatments were tried before considering off-label use
2. Whether there are published recommendations from specialty societies or in other authoritative based guidelines
3. Whether authoritative medical literature supports the off-label use. Such literature must include peer-reviewed publications that demonstrate efficacy. Such studies may not include case reports, opinions, book chapters, or abstracts.
4. Whether there is other evidence of broad scientific support
5. Whether the use is an accepted standard of medical practice[14]

For some off-label drug use such as the use of intravitreal antibiotics for endophthalmitis, the above criteria are easily satisfied. For other off-label treatments, the evidence is less compelling. As a result, there are variable coverage policies between Medicare carriers concerning off-label retinal pharmacotherapy. Currently, there is considerable controversy involving the off-label use of anti-VEGF agents such as pegaptanib sodium, ranibizumab, and bevacizumab. All Medicare carriers cover pegaptanib sodium and ranibizumab for the labeled treatment of neovascular age-related macular degeneration. All but one of the Medicare carriers covers bevacizumab for the off-label treatment of neovascular age-related macular degeneration as well. However, the coverage for other off-label uses such as proliferative diabetic retinopathy, diabetic macular edema, retinal vascular occlusions, and neovascular glaucoma is variable. This irregular coverage is frustrating to both ophthalmologists and patients since many of these conditions have no approved or consistently effective therapy. Medicare carriers often look to professional organizations such as the American Academy of Ophthalmology for guidance on these coverage issues. The American Academy of Ophthalmology in turn looks to the scientific literature for appropriate evidence to support recommendations for coverage particularly in situations of unmet medical need. The strong support of the American Academy of Ophthalmology for the use of off-label bevacizumab was instrumental in obtaining Medicare coverage.[6]

CMS can establish a national coverage mandate to all Medicare carriers through an NCD. CMS uses an NCD to determine whether an item or service is "reasonable and necessary." While there is no statutory or regulatory definition of "reasonable and necessary," CMS has generally interpreted the term to mean that the item or service should improve health outcomes for Medicare beneficiaries.[13] CMS may consider an NCD when

1. There are questions about the safety, effectiveness, or appropriateness of a therapy including off-label use of drugs.
2. Local coverage policies are inconsistent.
3. There is wide variation in billing practices not related to variation in clinical need.
4. The health technology represents a substantial clinical advance and is likely to result in significant health benefits if it diffuses more rapidly to all patients for whom it is indicated.

To address the above issues, CMS relies on generally accepted principles of evidenced-based medicine.[13] For drug coverage, an NCD typically requires strong evidence from clinical trials on safety and efficacy for the indication. Interestingly, FDA approval of the indication is not required for CMS coverage. This is the case for the coverage of photodynamic therapy with verteporfin for the treatment of occult with no classic and minimally classic subfoveal choroidal neovascularization and evidence of recent disease progression.[3] This indication is not listed in the verteporfin FDA label. However, this NCD is based on multiple clinical trials, an independent review by CMS of the clinical trial data, and the recommendation of a Medicare Carrier Advisory Committee. Such a process typically takes a year or longer.

A relatively new mechanism by which CMS may cover off-label drug use is through a clinical trial. To be eligible for coverage, the clinical trial must meet a variety of requirements including the following:

1. The principal purpose of the trial should be to test whether the intervention improves the participant's health outcome.
2. The trial should either be well supported by available scientific and medical information or be intended to clarify or establish the health outcomes of interventions already in common clinical use.
3. The trial must not duplicate existing studies.
4. The trial must be appropriately designed and sponsored by a credible organization.

One obvious way to conduct such a trial is through the National Eye Institute and such trials on off-label drug use are in progress and include the Comparison of Age-related Macular Degeneration Treatment Trials (CATT) and the Diabetic Retinopathy Clinical Research Network.[15] Such trials will be useful as CMS develops further policies for comparative effectiveness studies. The concept of comparative effectiveness is likely to become an important factor in Medicare payment policy.

Thus, off-label drug use in ophthalmology is at the discretion of the local Medicare carriers and coverage will depend on whether the carrier considers the off-label drug use reasonable and necessary. The Medicare Carrier Manual states that if a medication is determined not to be reasonable and necessary, the carrier excludes the entire charge including any charges for services that were primarily for the purpose of administering a noncovered medication. This means that for intravitreal injection of a therapeutic agent if the drug is not covered, then neither is the injection.

Considering the above aspects of off-label drug coverage, how should ophthalmologists proceed when they believe off-label drug is in a patient's best interest? For Medicare beneficiaries, ophthalmologists should seek specific guidance from their local Medicare carrier. If the carrier declines coverage, the ophthalmologist may bill the patient for noncovered services associated with the off-label drug use by using an Advance Beneficiary Notice (ABN). The necessary ABN form is available on the CMS Web site, cms.medicare.gov. The use of an ABN requires that the patient be informed about why the proposed treatment is not covered by Medicare and that the ABN form is signed prior to the performance of the service. The ABN form is then submitted to the local Medicare carrier with the bill on form 1500 using either the GA or GY modifier. Physicians should contact their local carrier to determine which modifier is preferred and to confirm how the carrier handles the ABN process. With an appropriate ABN, physicians can bill the patient for the noncovered services. For payers other than Medicare, ophthalmologists must contact the individual payer to determine payment policy for off-label retinal pharmacotherapy. Many payers have established payment policy based on the above discussed criteria.

KEY POINTS

- With the continued development of new and more effective drugs for retinal disease, off-label drug use will escalate as ophthalmologists attempt to optimize treatment outcomes.
- This is particularly true for combination therapies in which drugs with different mechanisms of action are combined to improve visual outcomes and minimize complications.
- This increase in off-label drug use carries the responsibility to establish both safety and efficacy in order to allow off-label drugs to become evidence-based treatments.

REFERENCES

1. Brown MM, Brown GC, Stein JD, et al. Age-related macular degeneration: Economic burden and value-based medicine analysis. *Can J Ophthalmol.* 2005;40(3):277.
2. Javitt JC, Zhou Z, Wilke RJ. Association between vision loss and higher medical care costs in Medicare beneficiaries. Costs are greater for those with progressive vision loss. *Ophthalmology.* 2007;114:238.
3. CMS Manual System. Pub 100-03. Medicare National Coverage Determinations. April 1, 2004. Change request 3191.
4. Feinsod M, Chambers WA. A primer on successfully navigating the waters of the Food and Drug Administration. *Ophthalmology*. 2004;111:1801–1806.
5. www.fda.gov
6. American Academy of Ophthalmology, www.aao.org
7. Patient access to treatments prescribed by their physician. H-120.988 www.ama-assn.org
8. U.S. Food and Drug Administration. Off-label and investigational use of marketed drugs. Biologics and medical devices. www.fda.gov/oc/ohrt/irbs/offlabel.html
9. U.S. Food and Drug Administration. Good reprint practices for the distribution of medical journal articles and medical or scientific reference publications on un-approved new uses of approved drugs and approved or cleared medical devices: draft guidance, Feb 2008. Fed Regist. 2008:74(34):9342. http://www.fda.gov/oc/op/goodreprint.html.
10. Psaty BM, Ray W. FDA guidance on Off-label promotion and the state of literature from sponsors. *JAMA.* 2008;299: 1949–1951.
11. www.fda.gov/foi/warning_letters/g6147d.htm
12. www.omic.com
13. CMS Draft Guidance for NCDS's, www.cms.gov March 9, 2005.
14. Off-label use of non-oncology drugs and biologicals LCD No. L18709 AdminiStar Federal, Inc (February 10, 2005)
15. www.clinicaltrials.gov. Updated: 6/3/09 11:10 AM.

CHAPTER 30

The Future of Anti-Angiogenic Therapy

Anthony P. Adamis

Until recently, the treatment of ocular neovascular diseases such as age-related macular degeneration (AMD) and diabetic retinopathy (DR) has focused on ablative laser-based approaches to retard the loss of vision. In response to almost four decades of research into the cellular and molecular mechanisms underlying physiological and pathological angiogenesis, this situation is changing rapidly, with therapies offering the promise not only of maintaining vision but also of actually improving it. Currently, two agents, both targeting vascular endothelial growth factor (VEGF), have received clinical approval for treatment of AMD and more are in development as discussed in the accompanying chapters of this book. In addition, a number of new candidate agents offer promise, some of which are already in clinical trials.

Given the rather remarkable efficacy of the anti-VEGF drugs, especially in light of the therapies that preceded them, drugs addressing new pathways most likely will be used in combination with an anti-VEGF drug. One notable example in clinical development, and described below, is the anti–platelet-derived growth factor (anti-PDGF) aptamer. When used in combination with ranibizumab, preliminary indications are that anti-PDGF aptamer leads to the regression of choroidal neovascularization (CNV), an effect not ordinarily seen with anti-VEGF therapy alone. Early clinical data suggest that the regression of choroidal neovascular vessels translates to a visual outcome.

Another major advance toward which the field is progressing with some urgency is sustained-release technology for drug delivery. Monthly injections are a significant treatment burden for patients and physicians alike. Sustained-release formulations that allow the treatment frequency to be reduced to every 4 to 6 months will open new vistas in the treatment of chronic angiogenic diseases such as DR. Since many retinal diseases play out over years, sustained-release formulations will allow patients to be treated continuously and for longer periods of time, potentially improving visual outcomes. More patients also will find the treatments acceptable. In addition, sustained-release technology will facilitate an approach to prophylactic therapy. For example, a patient with CNV in one eye with high-risk phenotypic characteristics in the second eye could be treated with a sustained-release formulation of an antiangiogenic drug to prevent the initiation of CNV. As effective as the anti-VEGF drugs are, the phase 3 ranibizumab trials report visual acuities of 20/50 or worse in up to 60% of patients if treatment is initiated after the onset of CNV. A prophylactic approach therefore could lead to a substantial reduction in vision loss and blindness, thereby addressing an important unmet medical need. The future also will see the increased use of genetic testing to identify patients at risk. With the identification of new "at risk" genotypes, a simple blood test could distinguish those patients who are most likely to benefit from prophylactic therapy. Clinical trials enrolling patients possessing "at risk" genotypes will focus therapy on those who are most likely to benefit.

This chapter necessarily focuses on the molecular pathways and inflammatory processes that contribute to pathological angiogenesis. Molecules considered to be endogenous inhibitors of angiogenesis and those known for mediating physiological processes other than angiogenesis that only recently have been found to affect the development of ocular neovascularization are discussed. Some of these molecules will very likely form the basis of future antiangiogenic therapy in ophthalmology.

PLATELET-DERIVED GROWTH FACTOR

The four PDGF species, PDGF-A through PDGF-D, which usually occur as homodimers, are ligands for their cognate receptor tyrosine kinases, PDGFR-α and PDGFR-β.[1,2] Many studies on the role of PDGF in angiogenesis have focused on PDGF-B acting through PDGFR-β and have identified a central role for PDGF-B in the physiology of the pericytes and smooth muscle cells (collectively known as mural cells) that surround the developing blood vessels. This signaling is essential not only for pericyte proliferation and recruitment to the vasculature[3] but also for the maintenance of blood vessel coverage.[4] In the eye, gene knockout of PDGF-B[5] as well as the administration of an inhibitor of PDGFR[6] resulted in incomplete pericyte coverage of the retinal vasculature leading to proliferative retinopathy. PGDF-B signaling is not restricted to pericytes but also promotes endothelial cell proliferation[7–9] and the development of capillary tubes.[8]

Given the importance of PDGF for the pericyte component of blood vessels, it might be expected that a combinatorial approach involving joint inhibition of both PDGF and VEGF signaling would be an especially effective approach to inhibiting neovascularization. Preclinical experiments have supported this prediction. In three different mouse models of ocular neovascularization, VEGF signaling was most important for newly developing blood vessels in contrast to PDGF-B inhibition, which affected the more mature vessels; combined VEGF and PDGF-B inhibition proved synergistic (Fig. 30.1).[10] This approach is now being investigated clinically in a phase 1 clinical trial (NCT00569140; Ophthotech, New York, NY) involving the drug E10030, a DNA aptamer directed against PDGF-B, as an intravitreally administered agent given alone or in combination with ranibizumab as a treatment for neovascular AMD. Preliminary results indicate that it is well tolerated and that at a 3-month follow-up the majority of subjects showed regression of CNV and gained three or more lines of visual acuity.[11]

MEDIATORS OF INFLAMMATION

The development of ocular neovascularization bears many of the hallmarks of an inflammatory process whose full nature is still being elucidated; this link appears to be relevant not only for AMD but also for other neovascular syndromes, such as retinopathy of prematurity (ROP) and DR. Several different types of data support the importance of inflammatory cells and factors classically associated with inflammatory processes. These include (a) both genetic and experimental data supporting a role of the complement

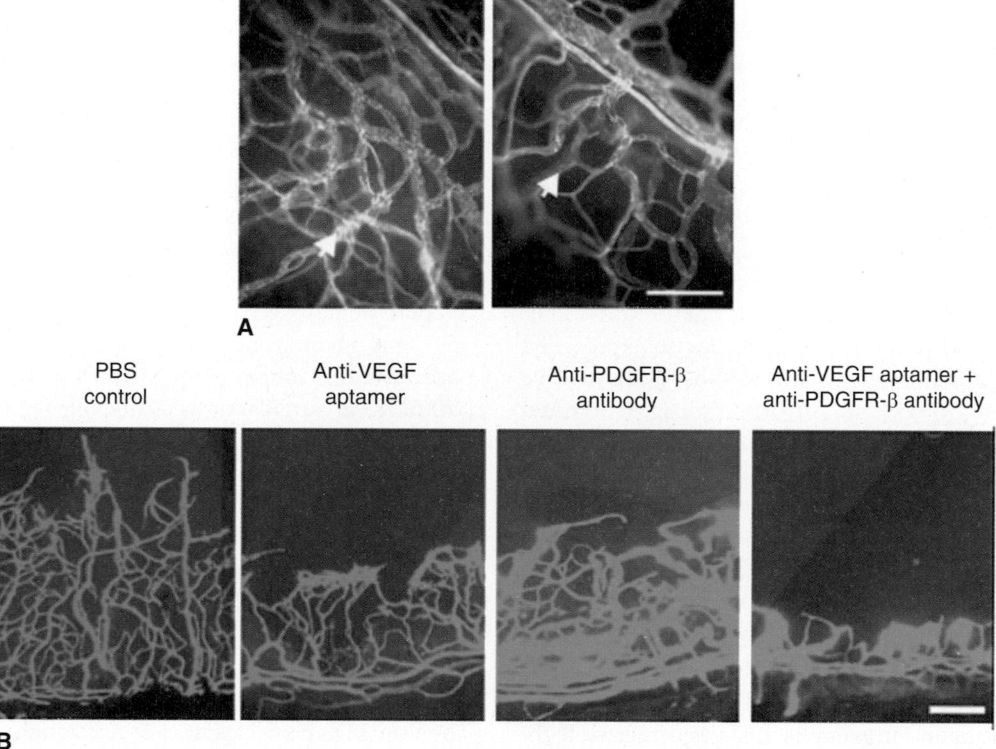

FIGURE 30.1. The role of platelet-derived growth factor (PDGF)-B on blood vessel growth and mural cell coverage in a corneal neovascularization model. **A:** Endothelial cells were labeled by staining with lectin (*green*) and mural cells were stained with an antibody against smooth muscle actin (*red*). Starting at 10 days following corneal injury, mice received daily intraperitoneal injections of an anti–PDGFR-β antibody or phosphate-buffered saline (PBS) and were sacrificed at 20 days postinjury. Treatment with the anti–PDGF-β antibody led to reduced mural cell coverage compared to controls (*arrows*). Scale bar: 20 μm. **B:** Following induction of corneal injury, mice received daily intraperitoneal injections of one of the following: PBS, a polyethylene-glycolated anti-VEGF aptamer, an anti–PDGFR-β antibody, or both the anti-VEGF aptamer and the anti–PDGFR-β antibody. Neovasculature (*green*) was stained by fluorescein isothiocyanate-concanavalin A. Neovascularization was significantly reduced by the anti-VEGF aptamer compared with either PBS or the anti–PDGFR-β antibody ($p < 0.01$); inhibition of both VEGF and PDGF-B signaling led to a further significant reduction ($p < 0.05$) compared to inhibition of VEGF signaling alone. Scale bar: 100 μm. (Adapted from Jo, et al., *Am J Pathol.* 2006;168:2036–2053, with permission.)

cascade[12,13]; (b) the presence of macrophages in surgically excised choroidal neovascular membranes,[14,15] together with the dependence of experimentally induced ocular neovascularization on the migration of macrophages (Fig. 30.2)[16–19]; (c) the clinical findings that an antibody against tumor necrosis factor-α (TNF-α), an inflammatory cytokine, can alleviate symptoms of AMD[20]; and (d) evidence that the influx of inflammatory cells is central to the attack on the retinal vasculature and the resulting ischemic neovascularization that are characteristic of DR.[21]

Given the importance of anti-VEGF therapies for current treatment protocols, it is of particular interest that VEGF itself is known to act as a potent inflammatory cytokine in models of both ischemic neovascularization[17] and DR-associated retinal pathology.[21–23] The data supporting the importance of other inflammatory mediators in promoting ocular neovascularization offer the hope that they too may prove to be attractive therapeutic targets. Several of these mediators of inflammation are discussed in this section.

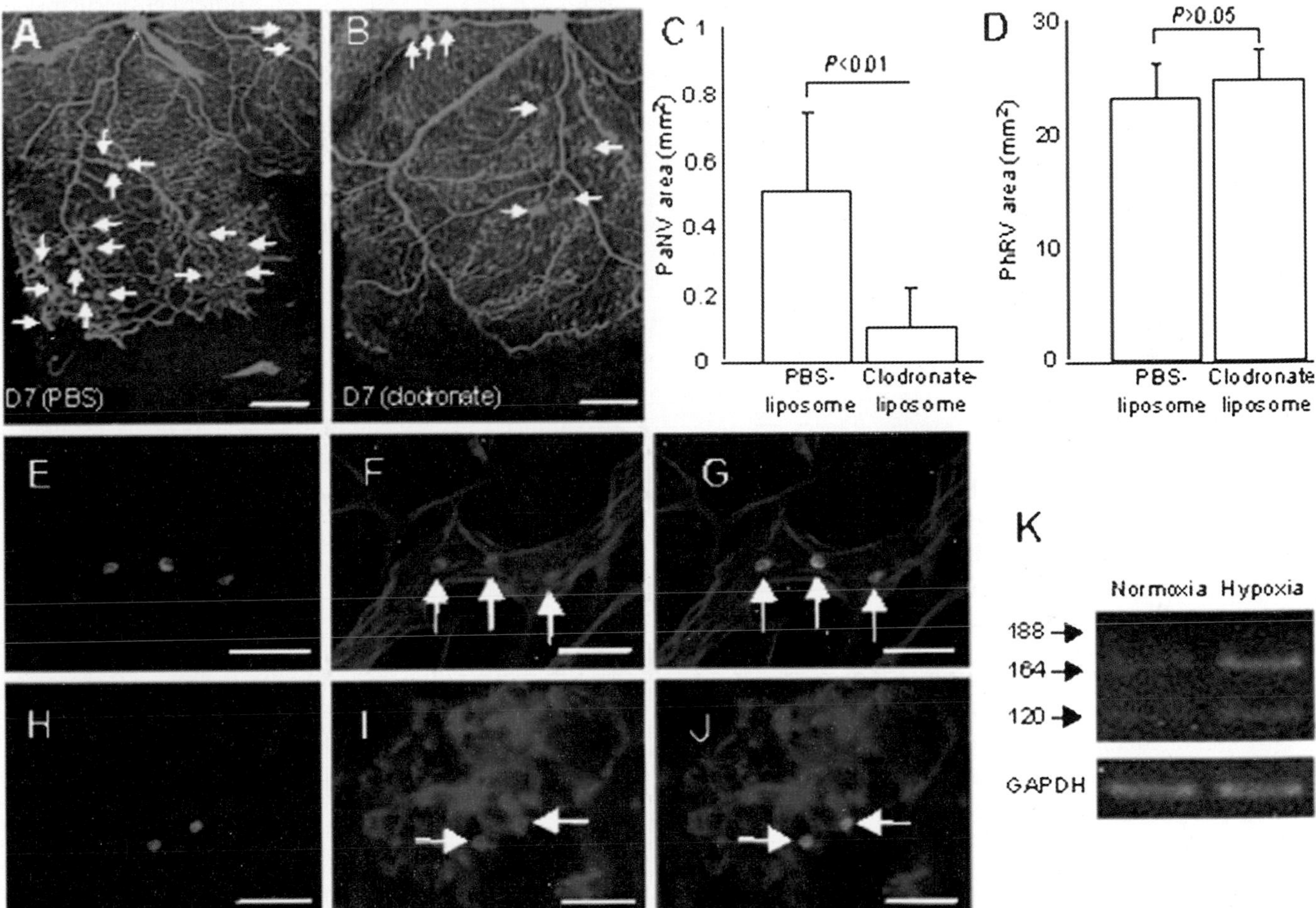

FIGURE 30.2. Monocytes contribute to pathological retinal neovascularization. In an ROP model, postnatal day zero (P0) rats were maintained for 10 days in 80% oxygen, interrupted daily by 30 minutes in room air, followed by a progressive return to 80% oxygen. This treatment led to an avascular retina. On P10, corresponding to study day 0 (D0), retinal revascularization was induced by maintaining the rats in room air for an additional 7 days (D7). **A–C:** At D7, pathological neovascularization (PaNV; *arrows* in **A** and **B**) was significantly inhibited by treatment with clodronate liposomes compared to control liposomes ($n = 8$ for both treatments; means ± standard deviation). **D:** Physiological neovascular area (PhRV) was not significantly affected by treatment with clodronate liposomes ($p > 0.05$). **E–J:** Influx of monocytes was observed just before and during pathological neovascularization **(H–J).** Monocytes were labeled with a fluorescein-conjugated antibody to CD13 **(E** and **H)**, while rhodamine-conjugated concanavalin A was used to label the retinal vasculature and adherent leukocytes **(F** and **I)**. As shown by superposition of these figures **(G** and **J)**, the concanavalin A and CD13 staining colocalized, indicating that the adherent leukocytes were monocytes. **K:** In cultured peripheral blood monocytes obtained from retinopathologic rats at D7, exposure to hypoxia (1% oxygen) led to a marked increase in the expression of VEGF mRNA compared to exposure to normoxia (21% oxygen). Scale bars: **(A** and **B)** 0.5 mm and **(E–J)** 50 μm. (Reproduced from Ishida, et al. *J Exp Med.* 2003;198:483–489, with permission.)

Complement Factors C3a, C5a, and CD59

Evidence supporting a role for the complement system in ocular neovascularization has come from both clinical and preclinical data. Genetic studies have identified specific haplotypes of complement factor H, a regulatory component of the complement cascade, as a significant risk factor for AMD.[12,13] In addition, complement factors C3a and C5a have attracted particular interest as promoters of pathological ocular neovascularization. These factors accumulate in drusen of AMD patients, and this accumulation also is observed experimentally in mice after induction of CNV by laser wounding.[24] Inhibition of experimental CNV is inhibited by the genetic ablation of the receptors for C3a and C5a[24] or of C3 itself,[25] as well as by complement depletion with cobra venom.[25] As intravitreal injection of these factors was found to upregulate VEGF expression,[24] the degree to which their induction of CNV is mediated through VEGF-independent pathways remains to be determined. A phase 1 trial (NCT00709527; Ophthotech) is underway to assess the utility of ARC1905, an aptamer against C5, given either alone or in combination with ranibizumab as a treatment for neovascular AMD. Another phase 1 trial is examining the effect of POT-4, an analog of the potent C3 inhibitor compstatin,[26] as an intravitreal treatment for AMD (NCT00473928; Potentia, Pharmaceuticals, Louisville, KY).

Other studies of the molecular mechanisms of the complement system have found that CD59, a regulatory component, could directly inhibit neovascularization. When expressed from adenovirus-expressing transgene in a mouse model system, CD59 inhibited the deposition of membrane attack complexes on the retinal pigment epithelium (RPE).[27] Direct administration of a CD59 fusion protein, either intravitreally or intraperitoneally, significantly inhibited the induction of CNV by laser wounding, while in the converse experiment, genetic ablation of CD59 enhanced the development of CNV.[28]

Tumor Necrosis Factor-α

TNF-α is a potent proinflammatory cytokine known to be involved in a variety of nonimmune regulatory functions as well.[29,30] These include a role in promoting angiogenesis that may be mediated, at least in part, through upregulation of molecules such as VEGF[31]and its receptor, VEGF receptor-2 (VEGFR2),[32] as well as PDGF-B.[33] Preclinical studies in rodent models have demonstrated the efficacy of agents targeting TNF-α in reducing laser-induced CNV.[34,35] In addition, two small case series reported that intravenous administration of infliximab, an anti–TNF-α monoclonal antibody, provided visual benefits for patients with neovascular AMD[20] and diabetic macular edema.[36] A small-scale study employing intravitreal injections of infliximab has also been encouraging,[37] with the intravitreal approach being evaluated in a phase 1 trial involving patients with AMD and diabetic macular edema (NCT00695682; Retina Research Foundation, Houston, Texas).

Integrins

The integrins comprise a large family of membrane-bound cellular receptors, each consisting of an α and a β subunit, that mediate signaling through cell-cell contact or by interacting with components of the extracellular matrix.[38] The $\alpha_5\beta_1$ integrin is of particular interest as a therapeutic target, with small molecule inhibitors of the $\alpha_5\beta_1$ integrin having demonstrated efficacy in preclinical studies of ocular neovascularization.[39–41] These include JSM6427, which suppressed retinal neovascularization caused by ischemia[39] as well as laser-induced CNV when administered systemically,[40] and JSM5562, which inhibited corneal neovascularization.[41] Intravitreal administration of JSM6427 also produced a dose-dependent reduction in clinically significant lesions in a laser-induced CNV model in monkeys without any related ocular adverse effects or evidence of systemic accumulation.[42] JSM6427 is in a phase 1 trial (NCT00536016; Jerini AG, New York, NY) for the treatment of neovascular AMD. Volociximab, a monoclonal antibody that targets the $\alpha_5\beta_1$ integrin, also was found to inhibit experimentally induced CNV in monkeys[43] and is being evaluated in a phase 1 trial for the treatment of neovascular AMD (NCT00782093; Ophthotech).

Mammalian Target of Rapamycin

Mammalian target of rapamycin (mTOR) is a component of a heterotrimeric protein kinase that signals through two protein complexes, mTORC1 and mTORC2, to regulate a variety of processes, including angiogenesis[44] and inflammation.[45] Rapamycin inhibits the formation of mTORC1[44] and has been shown to reduce VEGF expression in RPE cells[46] and to inhibit ocular angiogenesis in various preclinical models, including CNV as well as retinal and corneal neovascularization.[47–49] Rapamycin also has been found to inhibit VEGF-induced vascular permeability.[50] Similar findings with respect to ocular neovascularization and VEGF-induced vascular permeability have been reported for Palomid 529, another mTOR inhibitor that inhibits both mTORC1 and mTORC2 pathways.[51–52]

Clinical trials are investigating the utility of rapamycin for the treatment of neovascular AMD. In a phase 1 study of intravitreal or subconjunctival rapamycin, rapamycin was well tolerated and associated with improvements in both visual acuity and retinal thickness[53]; this study is being continued as a phase 2 trial (NCT00712491, MacuSight, Union City, CA). In addition, another phase 2 trial is examining the use of subconjunctival rapamycin in combination with intravitreal ranibizumab (NCT00766337; MacuSight), while oral rapamycin is being compared in a phase 2 trial (NCT00304954; National Eye Institute, Bethesda, Maryland) to two anti-inflammatory agents (infliximab and daclizumab) given intravenously; both of these trials are for the treatment of AMD.

Placental Growth Factor

Placental growth factor (PlGF) is a protein structurally related to VEGF that is also a ligand for VEGF receptor-1 (VEGFR1). PlGF is involved in a wide range of physiological processes[54,55] such as recruitment of endothelial progenitor cells[56] and modulation of immune system responses.[57] PlGF has been implicated in pathological angiogenesis related to inflammation and ischemia,[58] including laser-induced CNV.[59] The role of PlGF in ocular angiogenesis may involve recruitment of monocytes[60] that appear to be required for the maximal induction of ischemia-induced ocular neovascularization.[22] VEGF-TRAP, a fusion protein containing the VEGF binding domains of VEGFR1 and VEGFR2 and that correspondingly targets both VEGF and PlGF, is currently in phase 3 trials (NCT00509795, Regeneron, Tarrytown, New York, NY; NCT00637377, Bayer, Leverkusen, Germany) for the treatment of neovascular AMD.

Pigment Epithelium-derived Factor

Pigment epithelium-derived factor (PEDF) is a secreted glycoprotein that acts as a natural inhibitor of angiogenesis[61,62] and ocular inflammation.[63] In many respects, it acts in direct opposition to VEGF, downregulating ischemia-induced VEGF expression in the retina[64] and inhibiting VEGF-induced proliferation[65] and endothelial permeability.[66] In contrast to VEGF's actions as an endothelial survival factor,[67] PEDF induces endothelial cell apoptosis.[68–70] In preclinical models of ischemia-induced retinal neovascularization, PEDF proved inhibitory whether administered intravitreally,[65] systemically,[68] or by expression from an intraocularly injected adenovirus.[71] Some findings have proved contradictory, however, in that CNV induced by laser wounding was inhibited at low PEDF doses but actually increased at higher doses.[72] The full elucidation of these dose-response issues will be required to permit further exploitation of PEDF as an inhibitor of CNV. To date, PEDF has been examined in one phase 1 trial (NCT00109499; Genvec, Gaithersburg, MA) in which an intravitreally administered adenovirus vector was used to express PEDF in patients with AMD with encouraging results.[73]

Renin/Angiotensin System

Evidence implicates the renin/angiotensin system in the development of inflammatory ocular neovascularization. In the classic renin/angiotensin pathway, the sequential action of renin and angiotensin-converting enzyme (ACE) ultimately yields angiotensin II, which then activates its type 1 and type 2 receptors.[74] Blocking ACE activity was found to inhibit laser-induced CNV.[75] Intraperitoneal injection of telmisartan, a blocker of the angiotensin II type 1 receptor (AT1-R), also has been found to inhibit both corneal neovascularization[76] and laser-induced CNV,[77] as well as ischemia-induced pathological neovascularization[78]; physiological retinal vascularization was not affected.[78] As angiotensin II has been shown to upregulate VEGF expression[79] while telmisartan reduced both leukocyte influx and expression of VEGFR1,[78] it was suggested that blocking the AT1-R ultimately affected VEGF-mediated monocyte influx.[78]

In addition, an entirely different pathway involving the action of prorenin with its receptor may regulate ocular neovascularization in that administration of a decoy peptide to block this receptor led to inhibition of pathological neovascularization in the ischemic retinopathy model[80] and of laser-induced CNV.[81] Furthermore, the decoy peptide further inhibited CNV even if the AT1-R was ablated, showing that the actions of the decoy peptide were not simply a result of preventing the generation of angiotensin II.[81]

Angiopoietins

Angiopoietin-1 (Ang1) and angiopoietin-2 (Ang2) are both ligands for the Tie-2 receptor tyrosine kinase, through whose actions they regulate the development and remodeling of the vascular system.[82] Usually, although not always, they act in an antagonistic manner, with Ang2 acting as a proinflammatory agent, destabilizing vascular endothelial cells and facilitating their response to transient signaling.[83] In contrast, Ang1 provides a continuous stabilizing signal to the quiescent vasculature and in general exerts an anti-inflammatory action.[83]

These differences are exemplified in the interactions of Ang1 and Ang2 with VEGF. In transgenic model systems in which the expression of Ang1 and VEGF can be induced simultaneously, these two molecules act cooperatively in promoting angiogenesis. However, the vessels so induced are much less permeable than those induced by VEGF alone,[84] owing to the inhibition by Ang1 of the VEGF-induced internalization of vascular endothelial cadherin, a key component of tight junctions VEGF.[85] Similarly, overexpression of Ang1 inhibited the development of retinal neovascularization as well as CNV induced by laser wounding,[86] suggesting that Ang1 could provide a therapeutic option for AMD.

In contrast, the interactions of Ang2 with VEGF tend to be destabilizing, with overexpression of Ang 2 furthering the promotion of endothelial cell permeability[87] and of ocular neovascularization,[88,89] although in the context of low levels of VEGF, Ang2 actually induced the regression of the neovascularization.[89] This latter action has led to the suggestion that combinatorial therapy, in which an anti-VEGF agent is administered together with Ang2, might hold promise in treating CNV.[90]

Vascular Adhesion Protein-1

Vascular adhesion protein-1 (VAP-1) is a cell-surface glycoprotein expressed on endothelial cells that is involved in leukocyte recruitment during inflammation.[91] In a recent study of laser-induced CNV in rats, VAP-1 was found to be upregulated and expressed in choroidal vessels; the blockade of VAP-1 by the injection of a specific VAP-1 inhibitor (U-V002) resulted in reduced CNV together with a lower expression of inflammatory markers such as TNF-α, monocyte chemoattractant protein-1, and intercellular adhesion molecule-1.[92]

ENDOGENOUS INHIBITORS OF ANGIOGENESIS

Investigations into the mechanisms mediating both physiological and pathological angiogenesis have identified a number of endogenous inhibitors, many of which are proteolytic fragments of larger molecules. The present discussion focuses on those for which a role in regulating ocular neovascularization has already been established. In contrast to molecules such as VEGF, for which therapeutic agents are used to block their action, these proteins are being examined as potential therapeutic agents in their own right.

Endostatin

Endostatin, a proteolytic fragment of collagen XVIII, is a potent endogenous inhibitor of angiogenesis.[93,94] Endostatin is localized in Bruch membrane and in the choriocapillaris; patients with AMD show markedly reduced levels of immunoreactivity in these tissues.[95] In a murine model of laser-induced CNV, the genetic ablation of collagen XVIII/endostatin led to significantly larger lesions, while in the converse experiment, intraperitoneal administration of endostatin in wild-type mice almost totally eliminated the formation of lesions.[96] Similar reductions in laser-induced CNV were observed when endostatin was overexpressed from a transgene,[97,98] and in another murine model, ischemia-induced retinal neovascularization was significantly reduced by intravitreally injected endostatin.[99] Taken together, these findings suggest that endostatin, especially as an intravitreal agent, could provide a viable therapeutic option in treating AMD.

Angiostatin

Angiostatin, a name collectively given to various proteolytic fragments of plasminogen, is another endogenous inhibitor of angiogenesis,[63,100] acting as a proapoptotic factor on endothelial cells while also inhibiting their migration and tube formation.[101] Data very similar to those for endostatin suggest that angiostatin could prove a useful therapeutic agent. In a murine oxygen-induced retinopathy model, both systemic and intravitreal administration of angiostatin inhibited the pathological neovascularization without affecting physiological vascularization.[102] In addition, both preretinal neovascularization induced by retinal vein occlusion[103] and CNV induced by laser wounding[98–104] were significantly inhibited by the expression of angiostatin from transgenes carried on viral vectors.

Thrombospondin-1

Thrombospondin-1 (TSP-1) is one of five related members of a glycoprotein family that is involved in physiological processes that include angiogenesis, wound healing, and blood coagulation.[105] In angiogenesis, TSP-1 has been found to inhibit endothelial cell proliferation, adhesion, and migration[106] and to promote endothelial cell apoptosis.[107] It is synthesized by numerous ocular cell types,[108] including the RPE,[109] but, like endostatin, its presence has been detected in much lower amounts in the RPE and choriocapillaris of patients with AMD than in normal controls.[95] In rodent preclinical models, TSP-1 significantly reduced ischemia-induced neovascularization whether injected intravitreally[110] or when expressed from a transgene.[111]

$VEGF_{xxx}b$ Isoforms

$VEGF_{xxx}b$ denotes a family of VEGF isoforms that, compared to those that have been the focus of most investigations,[112] have an altered carboxyl terminus owing to alternative splicing. As a result, these isoforms can bind VEGFR2 but do not initiate downstream signaling and thus serve as endogenous competitive inhibitors of VEGF.[113] This inhibition has been demonstrated to have important physiological consequences. For example, the downregulation of $VEGF_{xxx}b$ has been correlated with the occurrence of malignancies.[113] $VEGF_{xxx}b$ isoforms have been measured in the ocular fluids of human subjects; in diabetic patients with proliferative DR, they comprised only 12% of the total VEGF in the vitreous compared with 64% in control subjects, suggesting that the altered ratio contributed to the development of DR.[114] Moreover, administration of recombinant $VEGF_{xxx}b$ was found to inhibit blood vessel growth in mouse models of corneal[115] and retinal[116] neovascularization. Taken together, these findings suggest that isoforms of the $VEGF_{xxx}b$ family may play an important role in regulating VEGF signaling and that the efficacy of anti-VEGF agents thus may depend on the local VEGF isoform expression pattern. As a naturally occurring inhibitor, the $VEGF_{xxx}b$ family ultimately could prove to be useful as therapeutic agents.

Tryptophanyl-tRNA Synthetase Fragment

Tryptophanyl-tRNA synthetase fragment (T2-TrpRS) is a natural cleavage product of tryptophanyl-tRNA synthetase,[117] which was shown to inhibit both physiological retinal angiogenesis and VEGF-induced angiogenesis in murine models[117]; in an ROP model, intravitreal T2-TrpRS dramatically inhibited preretinal pathological tuft formation and facilitated physiological vascularization of the obliterated retinal vasculature.[118] The mechanisms underlying these differing actions are unclear; one possible action as an antiangiogenic agent may be through binding to vascular-endothelial cadherin, a component of intercellular junctions between endothelial cells.[119] Recently, a combination of T2-TrpRS plus an anti-VEGF aptamer and an αvβ3 integrin antagonist proved to be especially potent in the inhibition of neonatal retinal angiogenesis and in obliterating tumor vasculature in murine models[120]; in addition, the combination of T2-TrpRS and an anti-VEGF aptamer proved highly effective as an inhibitor of pathological neovascularization in an ROP model.[120]

NOVEL TARGETS FOR INHIBITION

In addition to the molecular targets that have emerged from focused investigations into the mechanisms underlying pathological angiogenesis, interesting candidates originally identified as acting in other physiological processes have since been found to play roles in regulating angiogenesis as well.

Erythropoietin

Aside from its established role in promoting erythropoiesis, erythropoietin also is important for neuroprotection[121] and recently has been found to protect RPE cells against oxidative damage[122,123] and to promote angiogenesis through recruitment of endothelial precursor cells and upregulation of VEGF.[124] Studies also support the relevance of erythropoietin in mediating ocular neovascularization. In addition to clinical findings demonstrating elevated ocular levels of erythropoietin in conditions such as proliferative DR,[125] preclinical studies with murine models have demonstrated reductions in retinal neovascularization using intravitreal injections of either a soluble erythropoietin receptor[125] or a small interference RNA directed against erythropoietin.[126] These studies suggest that interference with erythropoietin signaling may be a viable strategy for treating AMD, though clearly the protective actions of erythropoietin for both neurons and the RPE mandate careful monitoring of potential adverse events.

Nicotinic Acetylcholine Receptors

Nicotinic acetylcholine receptors are known principally as the mediators of synaptic transmission, yet they also have been found to regulate ocular neovascularization. In cultured cells, nicotine was found to stimulate endothelial cell proliferation, migration, and tube formation[127] and to upregulate the expression of VEGF[128] and VEGFR2.[129] Orally administered nicotine increased the severity of laser-induced CNV,[130,131] an effect mediated partly by the increased recruitment of bone marrow precursor cells.[132] Additionally, subcutaneous administration of mecamylamine, an inhibitor of nicotinic acetylcholine receptors, blocked CNV induction (Fig. 30.3).[131] Topical administration of mecamylamine as a treatment for AMD is being examined in a phase 2 trial (NCT00607750; CoMentis, South San Francisco, California).

Notch

The Notch family of cell-surface proteins mediates a wide variety of developmental processes including the nervous system, the kidney, and the vascular system. Notch is activated by cognate ligands of the Jagged and Delta families, both of which are themselves membrane bound, so that signaling requires cell-cell contact.[133–135] Using rodent models of retinal vascular development, Notch signaling, initiated by its ligand Delta-like 4 (Dll4), has been identified as an important mechanism in regulating the angiogenic sprouting that is induced by VEGF.[135,136] In these experiments, inhibition of the Notch pathway leads to increased formation of tip cells,[137] proliferation of endothelial cells,[138] and enhanced vessel branching (Fig. 30.4).[139] In addition, Notch signaling has recently been found to interact with PDGF-B signaling by upregulating the synthesis of PDGFR-β,[140] an action that may be important in the Notch-mediated regulation of mural cell differentiation.[141] Given the complexity of these various actions, further work will be required to exploit the involvement of Notch in strategies for inhibiting pathological angiogenesis.

Slit/Roundabout 4

The Slit family of secreted ligands acts by activating a family of membrane receptors, including Roundabout 4 (Robo4). Originally implicated in neuronal patterning, Slit/Robo4 signaling acts to regulate angiogenesis[142–144] and has been shown to antagonize such processes as VEGF-induced endothelial cell migration and tube formation.[145] Intraocular injection of Slit2 inhibited pathological ocular neovascularization in both retinal and choroidal murine models, effects that were not observed if Robo4 was genetically ablated.[145] These findings suggest that Slit, or a modified version of it, could prove to be a useful therapeutic agent.

CONCLUSIONS

The continuing research effort into the mechanisms underlying the pathophysiology of AMD has provided potential therapeutic strategies involving the targeting of key molecular regulators of neovascularization. The challenge remaining is to move these strategies into the clinic; given the established utility of therapies targeting VEGF, it will be of particular interest to assess which of these new approaches can be employed in combination with anti-VEGF agents to provide maximal benefits in preserving and improving vision.

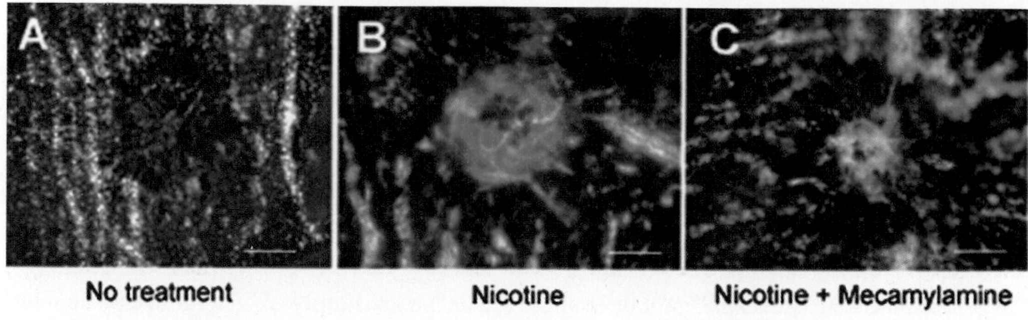

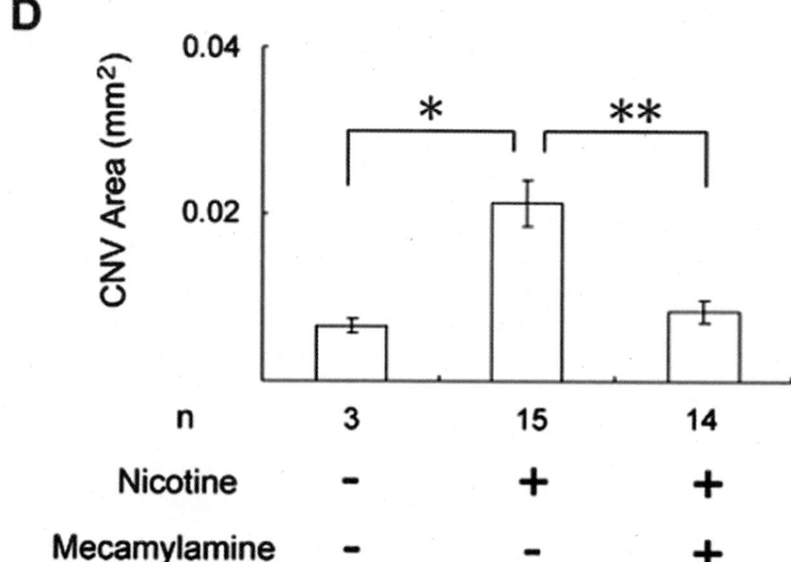

FIGURE 30.3. Mecamylamine blocks nicotine-induced stimulation of CNV. Six-week-old C57BL/6 mice were given 100 g/mL nicotine in their drinking water, and each underwent implantation of an osmotic pump that released mecamylamine or vehicle subcutaneously. After 2 days, these mice and a control group of three mice that did not receive any nicotine experienced a rupture of Bruch membrane at three locations in each eye. Fourteen days after laser, the mice were perfused with fluorescein-labeled dextran, and the area of CNV at Bruch membrane rupture sites was measured by image analysis. Compared with CNV lesions in untreated mice that did not receive nicotine **(A)**, the lesions appeared larger in mice that received nicotine and underwent implantation of pumps that released only vehicle **(B)** but not in mice that received nicotine and mecamylamine **(C)**. Measurement of the area of CNV by image analysis confirmed that nicotine caused a significant increase in lesion size that was completely blocked by mecamylamine **(D)**. $*p = 0.006470142$; $**p = 0.007367749$; analysis of variance with Dunnett adjustment for multiple comparisons. (Reproduced from Kiuchi, et al. *Invest Ophthalmol Vis Sci.* 2008;49:1705–1711, with permission).

FIGURE 30.4. Inhibition of Delta-like 4 signaling leads to increased vessel mass. Compared to wild-type (Wt) mice **(A)**, retinal vessels stained at postnatal day 5 in mice for which Delta-like 4 (dll4) was heterozygously ablated **(B)** show hyperbranching within the vascular plexus (a, artery; v, vein). Retinal vessels were stained with isolectin B_4. Scale bar: 250 μm. (Adapted from Suchting, et al. *Proc Natl Acad Sci USA.* 2007;104:3225–3230, with permission.)

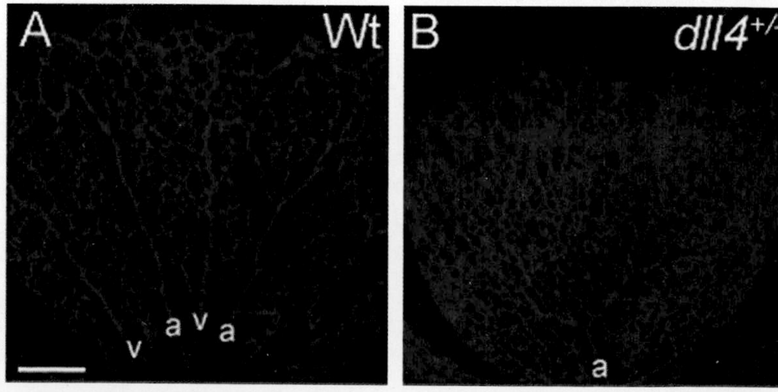

KEY POINTS

- Extensive investigation into the mechanisms controlling angiogenesis has led to the identification of a variety of proangiogenic and antiangiogenic factors active in ocular neovascularization that may serve as therapeutic targets.
- Certain of these, such as PDGF-B, have been shown to be especially effective when used in combination with anti-VEGF agents in preclinical models; clinical testing of this combination is under way.
- It is now well established that ocular neovascular diseases such as AMD have an inflammatory basis, suggesting a wide array of molecular targets that may have therapeutic potential. These include components of the complement system, TNF-α, integrins, and many others.
- Naturally occurring endogenous inhibitors of angiogenesis such as endostatin, angiostatin, and TSP-1 also may have potential as therapeutic agents, although they have not yet been explored clinically. Finally, novel targets include erythropoietin and nicotinic acetylcholine receptors, among others.
- The field of angiogenesis research, particularly as it relates to the understanding of ocular neovascular diseases, is at a very promising juncture with many new potential targets of treatment on the horizon.

REFERENCES

1. Heldin CH, Westermark B. Mechanism of action and in vivo role of platelet-derived growth factor. *Physiol Rev.* 1999; 79:1283–1316.
2. Andrae J, Gallini R, Betsholtz C. Role of platelet-derived growth factors in physiology and medicine. *Genes Dev.* 2008; 22:1276–1312.
3. Hellstrom M, Kalen M, Lindahl P, et al. Role of PDGF-B and PDGFR-beta in recruitment of vascular smooth muscle cells and pericytes during embryonic blood vessel formation in the mouse. *Development.* 1999;126:3047–3055.
4. Sennino B, Falcon BL, McCauley D, et al. Sequential loss of tumor vessel pericytes and endothelial cells after inhibition of platelet-derived growth factor B by selective aptamer AX102. *Cancer Res.* 2007;67:7358–7367.
5. Enge M, Bjarnegard M, Gerhardt H, et al. Endothelium-specific platelet-derived growth factor-B ablation mimics diabetic retinopathy. *EMBO J.* 2002;21:4307–4316.
6. Wilkinson-Berka JL, Babic S, De Gooyer T, et al. Inhibition of platelet-derived growth factor promotes pericyte loss and angiogenesis in ischemic retinopathy. *Am J Pathol.* 2004;164:1263–1273.
7. Beitz JG, Kim IS, Calabresi P, et al. Human microvascular endothelial cells express receptors for platelet-derived growth factor. *Proc Natl Acad Sci USA.* 1991;88:2021–2025.
8. Battegay EJ, Rupp J, Iruela-Arispe L, et al. PDGF-BB modulates endothelial proliferation and angiogenesis in vitro via PDGF beta-receptors. *J Cell Biol.* 1994;125:917–928.
9. Marx M, Perlmutter RA, Madri JA. Modulation of platelet-derived growth factor receptor expression in microvascular endothelial cells during in vitro angiogenesis. *J Clin Invest.* 1994;93:131–139.
10. Jo N, Mailhos C, Ju M, et al. Inhibition of platelet-derived growth factor B signaling enhances the efficacy of anti-vascular endothelial growth factor therapy in multiple models of ocular neovascularization. *Am J Pathol.* 2006;168: 2036–2053.
11. Boyer DS. Combined inhibition of platelet derived (PDGF) and vascular endothelial (VEGF) growth factors for the treatment of neovascular age-related macular degeneration (NV-AMD) – results of a phase 1 study. *Invest Ophthalmol Vis Sci.* 2009;50:E-Abstract 1260.
12. Jager RD, Mieler WF, Miller JW. Age-related macular degeneration. *N Engl J Med.* 2008;358:2606–2617.
13. Bora NS, Jha P, Bora PS. The role of complement in ocular pathology. *Semin Immunopathol.* 2008;30:85–95.
14. Grossniklaus HE, Cingle KA, Yoon YD, et al. Correlation of histologic 2-dimensional reconstruction and confocal scanning laser microscopic imaging of choroidal neovascularization in eyes with age-related maculopathy. *Arch Ophthalmol.* 2000;118:625–629.
15. Grossniklaus HE, Ling JX, Wallace TM, et al. Macrophage and retinal pigment epithelium expression of angiogenic cytokines in choroidal neovascularization. *Mol Vis.* 2002; 8: 119–126.
16. Sakurai, E, Anand A, Ambati BK, et al. Macrophage depletion inhibits experimental choroidal neovascularization. *Invest Ophthalmol Vis Sci.* 2003;44:3578–3585.
17. Ishida S, Usui T, Yamashiro K, et al. VEGF164-mediated inflammation is required for pathological, but not physiological, ischemia-induced retinal neovascularization. *J Exp Med.* 2003;198:483–489.
18. Espinosa-Heidmann DG, Suner IJ, et al. Macrophage depletion diminishes lesion size and severity in experimental choroidal neovascularization. *Invest Ophthalmol Vis Sci.* 2003; 44:3586–3592.
19. Tsutsumi C, Sonoda KH, Egashira K, et al. The critical role of ocular-infiltrating macrophages in the development of choroidal neovascularization. *J Leukoc Biol.* 2003;74: 25–32.
20. Markomichelakis NN, Theodossiadis PG, Sfikakis PP. Regression of neovascular age-related macular degeneration following infliximab therapy. *Am J Ophthalmol.* 2005; 139:537–540.
21. Adamis AP, Berman AJ. Immunological mechanisms in the pathogenesis of diabetic retinopathy. *Semin Immunopathol.* 2008;30:65–84.
22. Ishida S, Usui T, Yamashiro K, et al. VEGF164 is proinflammatory in the diabetic retina. *Invest Ophthalmol Vis Sci.* 2003; 44:2155–2162.
23. Adamis AP. Is diabetic retinopathy an inflammatory disease? *Br J Ophthalmol.* 2002;86:363–365.
24. Nozaki M, Raisler BJ, Sakurai E, et al. Drusen complement components C3a and C5a promote choroidal neovascularization. *Proc Natl Acad Sci USA.* 2006;103:2328–2333.
25. Bora PS, Sohn JH, Cruz JM, et al. Role of complement and complement membrane attack complex in laser-induced choroidal neovascularization. *J Immunol.* 2005;174: 491–497.

26. Ricklin D, Lambris JD. Compstatin: a complement inhibitor on its way to clinical application. *Adv Exp Med Biol.* 2008; 632:273–292.
27. Ramo K, Cashman SM, Kumar-Singh R. Evaluation of adenovirus-delivered human CD59 as a potential therapy for AMD in a model of human membrane attack complex formation on murine RPE. *Invest Ophthalmol Vis Sci.* 2008;49: 4126–4136.
28. Bora NS, Kaliappan S, Jha P, et al. CD59, a complement regulatory protein, controls choroidal neovascularization in a mouse model of wet-type age-related macular degeneration. *J Immunol.* 2007;178:1783–1790.
29. Hehlgans T, Pfeffer K. The intriguing biology of the tumour necrosis factor/tumour necrosis factor receptor superfamily: players, rules and the games. *Immunology.* 2005;115:1–20.
30. Sethi G, Sung B, Aggarwal BB. TNF: a master switch for inflammation to cancer. *Front Biosci.* 2008;13:5094–5107.
31. Hangai M, He S, Hoffmann S, et al. Sequential induction of angiogenic growth factors by TNF-alpha in choroidal endothelial cells. *J Neuroimmunol.* 2006;171:45–56.
32. Giraudo E, Primo L, Audero E, et al. Tumor necrosis factor-alpha regulates expression of vascular endothelial growth factor receptor-2 and of its co-receptor neuropilin-1 in human vascular endothelial cells. *J Biol Chem.* 1998;273: 22128–22135.
33. Sainson RC, Johnston DA, Chu HC, et al. TNF primes endothelial cells for angiogenic sprouting by inducing a tip cell phenotype. *Blood.* 2008;111:4997–5007.
34. Shi X, Semkova I, Muther PS, et al. Inhibition of TNF-alpha reduces laser-induced choroidal neovascularization. *Exp Eye Res.* 2006;83:1325–1334.
35. Olson JL, Courtney RJ, Mandava N. Intravitreal infliximab and choroidal neovascularization in an animal model. *Arch Ophthalmol.* 2007;125:1221–1224.
36. Sfikakis PP, Markomichelakis N, Theodossiadis GP, et al. Regression of sight-threatening macular edema in type 2 diabetes following treatment with the anti-tumor necrosis factor monoclonal antibody infliximab. *Diabetes Care.* 2005; 28:445–447.
37. Theodossiadis PG, Liarakos VS, Sfikakis PP, et al. Intravitreal administration of the anti-tumor necrosis factor agent infliximab for neovascular age-related macular degeneration. *Am J Ophthalmol.* 2009;147:825–830, 830e1.
38. Avraamides CJ, Garmy-Susini B, Varner JA. Integrins in angiogenesis and lymphangiogenesis. *Nat Rev Cancer.* 2008; 8:604–617.
39. Maier AK, Kociok N, Zahn G, et al. Modulation of hypoxia-induced neovascularization by JSM6427, an integrin alpha5beta1 inhibiting molecule. *Curr Eye Res.* 2007;32: 801–812.
40. Umeda N, Kachi S, Akiyama H, et al. Suppression and regression of choroidal neovascularization by systemic administration of an alpha5beta1 integrin antagonist. *Mol Pharmacol.* 2006;69:1820–1828.
41. Muether PS, Dell S, Kociok N, et al. The role of integrin alpha(5)beta(1) in the regulation of corneal neovascularization. *Exp Eye Res.* 2007;85:356–365.
42. Zahn G, Vossmeyer D, Stragies R, et al. Preclinical evaluation of the novel small molecule integrin a5β1 inhibitor JSM6427 in monkey and rabbit models of choroidal neovascularization. *Arch Ophthalmol.* 2009;127:1329–1335.
43. Ramakrishnan V, Bhaskar V, Law DA, et al. Preclinical evaluation of an anti-alpha5beta1 integrin antibody as a novel anti-angiogenic agent. *J Exp Ther Oncol.* 2006;5: 273–286.
44. Guertin DA, Sabatini DM. Defining the role of mTOR in cancer. *Cancer Cell.* 2007;12:9–22.
45. Weichhart T, Costantino G, Poglitsch M, et al. The TSC-mTOR signaling pathway regulates the innate inflammatory response. *Immunity.* 2008;29:565–577.
46. Stahl A, Paschek L, Martin G, et al. Rapamycin reduces VEGF expression in retinal pigment epithelium (RPE) and inhibits RPE-induced sprouting angiogenesis in vitro. *FEBS Lett.* 2008;582:3097–3102.
47. Dejneka NS, Kuroki AM, Fosnot J, et al. Systemic rapamycin inhibits retinal and choroidal neovascularization in mice. *Mol Vis.* 2004;10:964–972.
48. Kwon YS, Kim JC. Inhibition of corneal neovascularization by rapamycin. *Exp Mol Med.* 2006;38:173–179.
49. Shi W, Gao H, Xie L, et al. Sustained intraocular rapamycin delivery effectively prevents high-risk corneal allograft rejection and neovascularization in rabbits. *Invest Ophthalmol Vis Sci.* 2006;47:3339–3344.
50. Kleinman DM, Kim DD, Nivaggioli T, et al. Sirolimus inhibits VEGF-induced microvascular hyperpermeability. *Invest Ophthalmol Vis Sci.* 2007;48:E-Abstract 1422.
51. Sherris D, Bora NS, Bora PS, et al. Palomid 529, a non-steroidal small molecule anti-angiogenic agent inhibits retinal and subretinal neovascularization by inhibiting the Akt/mTOR pathway. *Invest Ophthalmol Vis Sci.* 2008;49: E-Abstract 3766.
52. Xue Q, Hopkins B, Perruzzi C, et al. Palomid 529, a novel small-molecule drug, is a TORC1/TORC2 inhibitor that reduces tumor growth, tumor angiogenesis, and vascular permeability. *Cancer Res.* 2008;68:9551–9557.
53. Dugel PU, Quiroz-Mercado H, Kleinman DM, et al. Interim analysis of a randomized dose-escalation trial of locally-administered sirolimus to treat choroidal neovascularization secondary to age-related macular degeneration. *Invest Ophthalmol Vis Sci.* 2008;49:E-Abstract 582.
54. Ribatti D. The discovery of the placental growth factor and its role in angiogenesis: a historical review. *Angiogenesis.* 2008;11:215–221.
55. Fischer C, Mazzone M, Jonckx B, et al. FLT1 and its ligands VEGFB and PlGF: drug targets for anti-angiogenic therapy? *Nat Rev Cancer.* 2008;8:942–956.
56. Li B, Sharpe EE, Maupin AB, et al. VEGF and PlGF promote adult vasculogenesis by enhancing EPC recruitment and vessel formation at the site of tumor neovascularization. *FASEB J.* 2006;20:1495–1497.
57. Lin YL, Liang YC, Chiang BL. Placental growth factor down-regulates type 1 T helper immune response by modulating the function of dendritic cells. *J Leukoc Biol.* 2007;82: 1473–1480.
58. Carmeliet P, Moons L, Luttun A, et al. Synergism between vascular endothelial growth factor and placental growth factor contributes to angiogenesis and plasma extravasation in pathological conditions. *Nat Med.* 2001;7:575–583.
59. Rakic JM, Lambert V, Devy L, et al. Placental growth factor, a member of the VEGF family, contributes to the development of choroidal neovascularization. *Invest Ophthalmol Vis Sci.* 2003;44:3186–3193.

60. Clauss M, Weich H, Breier G, et al. The vascular endothelial growth factor receptor Flt-1 mediates biological activities. Implications for a functional role of placental growth factor in monocyte activation and chemotaxis. *J Biol Chem.* 1996;271:17629–17634.
61. Dawson DW, Volpert OV, Gillis P, et al. Pigment epithelium-derived factor: a potent inhibitor of angiogenesis. *Science.* 1999;285:245–248.
62. Filleur S, Nelius T, de Riese W, et al. Characterization of PEDF: a multi-functional serpin family protein. *J Cell Biochem.* 2009;106:769–775.
63. Zhang SX, Ma JX. Ocular neovascularization: implication of endogenous angiogenic inhibitors and potential therapy. *Prog Retin Eye Res.* 2007;26:1–37.
64. Zhang SX, Wang JJ, Gao G, et al. Pigment epithelium-derived factor downregulates vascular endothelial growth factor (VEGF) expression and inhibits VEGF-VEGF receptor 2 binding in diabetic retinopathy. *J Mol Endocrinol.* 2006;37:1–12.
65. Duh EJ, Yang HS, Suzuma I, et al. Pigment epithelium-derived factor suppresses ischemia-induced retinal neovascularization and VEGF-induced migration and growth. *Invest Ophthalmol Vis Sci.* 2002;43:821–829.
66. Yamagishi S, Abe R, Jinnouchi Y, et al. Pigment epithelium-derived factor inhibits vascular endothelial growth factor-induced vascular hyperpermeability both in vitro and in vivo. *J Int Med Res.* 2007;35:896–899.
67. Alon T, Hemo I, Itin A, et al. Vascular endothelial growth factor acts as a survival factor for newly formed retinal vessels and has implications for retinopathy of prematurity. *Nat Med.* 1995;1:1024–1028.
68. Stellmach V, Crawford SE, Zhou W, et al. Prevention of ischemia-induced retinopathy by the natural ocular antiangiogenic agent pigment epithelium-derived factor. *Proc Natl Acad Sci USA.* 2001;98:2593–2597.
69. Chen L, Zhang SS, Barnstable CJ, et al. PEDF induces apoptosis in human endothelial cells by activating p38 MAP kinase dependent cleavage of multiple caspases. *Biochem Biophys Res Commun.* 2006;348:1288–1295.
70. Ho TC, Chen SL, Yang YC, et al. PEDF induces p53-mediated apoptosis through PPAR gamma signaling in human umbilical vein endothelial cells. *Cardiovasc Res.* 2007;76:213–223.
71. Mori K, Gehlbach P, Ando A, et al. Regression of ocular neovascularization in response to increased expression of pigment epithelium-derived factor. *Invest Ophthalmol Vis Sci.* 2002;43:2428–2434.
72. Apte RS, Barreiro RA, Duh E, et al. Stimulation of neovascularization by the anti-angiogenic factor PEDF. *Invest Ophthalmol Vis Sci.* 2004;45:4491–4497.
73. Campochiaro PA, Nguyen QD, Shah SM, et al. Adenoviral vector-delivered pigment epithelium-derived factor for neovascular age-related macular degeneration: results of a phase 1 clinical trial. *Hum Gene Ther.* 2006;17:167–176.
74. Wilkinson-Berka JL. Prorenin and the (pro)renin receptor in ocular pathology. *Am J Pathol.* 2008;173:1591–1594.
75. Nagai N, Oike Y, Izumi-Nagai K, et al. Suppression of choroidal neovascularization by inhibiting angiotensin-converting enzyme: minimal role of bradykinin. *Invest Ophthalmol Vis Sci.* 2007;48:2321–2326.
76. Usui T, Sugisaki K, Iriyama A, et al. Inhibition of corneal neovascularization by blocking the angiotensin II type 1 receptor. *Invest Ophthalmol Vis Sci.* 2008;49:4370–4376.
77. Nagai N, Oike Y, Izumi-Nagai, K et al. Angiotensin II type 1 receptor-mediated inflammation is required for choroidal neovascularization. *Arterioscler Thromb Vasc Biol.* 2006;26:2252–2259.
78. Nagai N, Noda K, Urano T, et al. Selective suppression of pathologic, but not physiologic, retinal neovascularization by blocking the angiotensin II type 1 receptor. *Invest Ophthalmol Vis Sci.* 2005;46:1078–1084.
79. Shi RZ, Wang JC, Huang SH, et al. Angiotensin II induces vascular endothelial growth factor synthesis in mesenchymal stem cells. *Exp Cell Res.* 2009;315:10–15.
80. Satofuka S, Ichihara A, Nagai N, et al. Role of nonproteolytically activated prorenin in pathologic, but not physiologic, retinal neovascularization. *Invest Ophthalmol Vis Sci.* 2007; 48:422–429.
81. Satofuka S, Ichihara A, Nagai N, et al. (Pro)renin receptor promotes choroidal neovascularization by activating its signal transduction and tissue renin-angiotensin system. *Am J Pathol.* 2008;173:1911–1918.
82. Eklund L, Olsen BR. Tie receptors and their angiopoietin ligands are context-dependent regulators of vascular remodeling. *Exp Cell Res.* 2006;312:630–641.
83. Fiedler U, Augustin HG. Angiopoietins: a link between angiogenesis and inflammation. *Trends Immunol.* 2006;27: 552–558.
84. Thurston G, Suri C, Smith K, et al. Leakage-resistant blood vessels in mice transgenically overexpressing angiopoietin-1. *Science.* 1999;286:2511–2514.
85. Gavard J, Patel V, Gutkind JS. Angiopoietin-1 prevents VEGF-induced endothelial permeability by sequestering Src through mDia. *Dev Cell.* 2008;14:25–36.
86. Nambu H, Nambu R, Oshima Y, et al. Angiopoietin 1 inhibits ocular neovascularization and breakdown of the blood-retinal barrier. *Gene Ther.* 2004;11:865–873.
87. Peters S, Cree IA, Alexander R, et al. Angiopoietin modulation of vascular endothelial growth factor: effects on retinal endothelial cell permeability. *Cytokine.* 2007;40:144–150.
88. Asahara T, Chen D, Takahashi T, et al. Tie2 receptor ligands, angiopoietin-1 and angiopoietin-2, modulate VEGF-induced postnatal neovascularization. *Circ Res.* 1998;83: 233–240.
89. Oshima Y, Oshima S, Nambu H, et al. Different effects of angiopoietin-2 in different vascular beds: new vessels are most sensitive. *FASEB J.* 2005;19:963–965.
90. Hanahan D. Signaling vascular morphogenesis and maintenance. *Science.* 1997;277:48–50.
91. Salmi M, Jalkanen S. A 90-kilodalton endothelial cell molecule mediating lymphocyte binding in humans. *Science.* 1992;257:1407–1409.
92. Noda K, She H, Nakazawa T, et al. Vascular adhesion protein-1 blockade suppresses choroidal neovascularization. *FASEB J.* 2008;22:2928–2935.
93. O'Reilly MS, Boehm T, Shing Y, et al. Endostatin: an endogenous inhibitor of angiogenesis and tumor growth. *Cell.* 1997; 88:277–285.
94. Marneros AG, Olsen BR. Physiological role of collagen XVIII and endostatin. *FASEB J.* 2005;19:716–728.
95. Bhutto IA, Uno K, Merges C, et al. Reduction of endogenous angiogenesis inhibitors in Bruch's membrane of the submacular region in eyes with age-related macular degeneration. *Arch Ophthalmol.* 2008;126:670–678.

96. Marneros AG, She H, Zambarakji H, et al. Endogenous endostatin inhibits choroidal neovascularization. *FASEB J.* 2007;21:3809–3818.
97. Takahashi K, Saishin Y, Saishin Y, et al. Intraocular expression of endostatin reduces VEGF-induced retinal vascular permeability, neovascularization, and retinal detachment. *FASEB J.* 2003;17:896–898.
98. Balaggan KS, Binley K, Esapa M, et al. EIAV vector-mediated delivery of endostatin or angiostatin inhibits angiogenesis and vascular hyperpermeability in experimental CNV. *Gene Ther.* 2006;13:1153–1165.
99. Zhang M, Yang Y, Yan M, et al. Downregulation of vascular endothelial growth factor and integrinbeta3 by endostatin in a mouse model of retinal neovascularization. *Exp Eye Res.* 2006;82:74–80.
100. Wahl ML, Kenan DJ, Gonzalez-Gronow M, et al. Angiostatin's molecular mechanism: aspects of specificity and regulation elucidated. *J Cell Biochem.* 2005;96:242–261.
101. Claesson-Welsh L, Welsh M, Ito N, et al. Angiostatin induces endothelial cell apoptosis and activation of focal adhesion kinase independently of the integrin-binding motif RGD. *Proc Natl Acad Sci USA.* 1998;95:5579–5583.
102. Drixler TA, Borel Rinkes IH, Ritchie ED, et al. Angiostatin inhibits pathological but not physiological retinal angiogenesis. *Invest Ophthalmol Vis Sci.* 2001;42:3325–3330.
103. Lai CC, Wu WC, Chen SL, et al. Recombinant adeno-associated virus vector expressing angiostatin inhibits preretinal neovascularization in adult rats. *Ophthalmic Res.* 2005;37:50–56.
104. Lai CC, Wu WC, Chen SL, et al. Suppression of choroidal neovascularization by adeno-associated virus vector expressing angiostatin. *Invest Ophthalmol Vis Sci.* 2001;42:2401–2407.
105. Adams JC, Lawler J. The thrombospondins. *Int J Biochem Cell Biol.* 2004;36:961–968.
106. Esemuede N, Lee T, Pierre-Paul D, et al. The role of thrombospondin-1 in human disease. *J Surg Res.* 2004;122:135–142.
107. Nör JE, Mitra RS, Sutorik MM, et al. Thrombospondin-1 induces endothelial cell apoptosis and inhibits angiogenesis by activating the caspase death pathway. *J Vasc Res.* 2000;37:209–218.
108. Hiscott P, Paraoan L, Choudhary A, et al. Thrombospondin 1, thrombospondin 2 and the eye. *Prog Retin Eye Res.* 2006;25:1–18.
109. Miyajima-Uchida H, Hayashi H, Beppu R, et al. Production and accumulation of thrombospondin-1 in human retinal pigment epithelial cells. *Invest Ophthalmol Vis Sci.* 2000;41:561–567.
110. Shafiee A, Penn JS, Krutzsch HC, et al. Inhibition of retinal angiogenesis by peptides derived from thrombospondin-1. *Invest Ophthalmol Vis Sci.* 2000;41:2378–2388.
111. Wu Z, Wang S, Sorenson CM, et al. Attenuation of retinal vascular development and neovascularization in transgenic mice over-expressing thrombospondin-1 in the lens. *Dev Dyn.* 2006;235:1908–1920.
112. Ferrara N. Vascular endothelial growth factor: basic science and clinical practice. *Endocr Rev.* 2004;25:581–611.
113. Harper SJ, Bates DO. VEGF-A splicing: The key to anti-angiogenic therapeutics? *Nat Rev Cancer.* 2008;8:880–887.
114. Perrin RM, Konopatskaya O, Qiu Y, et al. Diabetic retinopathy is associated with a switch in splicing from anti- to pro-angiogenic isoforms of vascular endothelial growth factor. *Diabetologia.* 2005;48:2422–2427.
115. Woolard J, Wang WY, Bevan HS, et al. VEGF165b, an inhibitory vascular endothelial growth factor splice variant: mechanism of action, in vivo effect on angiogenesis and endogenous protein expression. *Cancer Res.* 2004;64:7822–7835.
116. Konopatskaya O, Churchill AJ, Harper SJ, et al. VEGF165b, an endogenous C-terminal splice variant of VEGF, inhibits retinal neovascularization in mice. *Mol Vis.* 2006;12:626–632.
117. Otani A, Slike BM, Dorrell MI, et al. A fragment of human TrpRS as a potent antagonist of ocular angiogenesis. *Proc Natl Acad Sci USA.* 2002;99:178–183.
118. Banin E, Dorrell MI, Aguilar E, et al. T2-TrpRS inhibits preretinal neovascularization and enhances physiological vascular regrowth in OIR as assessed by a new method of quantification. *Invest Ophthalmol Vis Sci.* 2006;47:2125–2134.
119. Tzima E, Reader JS, Irani-Tehrani M, et al. VE-cadherin links tRNA synthetase cytokine to anti-angiogenic function. J Biol Chem 2005;280:2405–2408.
120. Dorrell MI, Aguilar E, Scheppke L, et al. Combination angiostatic therapy completely inhibits ocular and tumor angiogenesis. *Proc Natl Acad Sci USA.* 2007;104:967–972.
121. Bartesaghi S, Marinovich M, Corsini E, et al. Erythropoietin: a novel neuroprotective cytokine. *Neurotoxicology.* 2005;26:923–928.
122. Gawad AE, Schlichting L, Strauß O, et al. Antiapoptotic properties of erythropoietin: novel strategies for protection of retinal pigment epithelial cells. *Eye.* 2009;23:2245–2250.
123. Wang ZY, Shen LJ, Tu LL, et al. Erythropoietin protects retinal pigment epithelial cells from oxidative damage. *Free Radic Biol Med.* 2009;72:448–450.
124. Nakano M, Satoh K, Fukumoto Y, et al. Important role of erythropoietin receptor to promote VEGF expression and angiogenesis in peripheral ischemia in mice. *Circ Res.* 2007;100:662–669.
125. Watanabe D, Suzuma K, Matsui S, et al. Erythropoietin as a retinal angiogenic factor in proliferative diabetic retinopathy. *N Engl J Med.* 2005;353:782–792.
126. Chen J, Connor KM, Aderman CM, et al. Erythropoietin siRNA suppresses retinal neovascularization in a mouse model of proliferative retinopathy. *Invest Ophthalmol Vis Sci.* 2009;50:1329–1335.
127. Park YJ, Lee T, Ha J, et al. Effect of nicotine on human umbilical vein endothelial cells (HUVECs) migration and angiogenesis. *Vascul Pharmacol.* 2008;49:32–36.
128. Zhang Q, Tang X, Zhang ZF, et al. Nicotine induces hypoxia-inducible factor-1alpha expression in human lung cancer cells via nicotinic acetylcholine receptor-mediated signaling pathways. *Clin Cancer Res.* 2007;13:4686–4694.
129. Shin VY, Wu WK, Chu KM, et al. Nicotine induces cyclooxygenase-2 and vascular endothelial growth factor receptor-2 in association with tumor-associated invasion and angiogenesis in gastric cancer. *Mol Cancer Res.* 2005;3:607–615.
130. Suñer IJ, Espinosa-Heidmann DG, Marin-Castano ME, et al. Nicotine increases size and severity of experimental choroidal neovascularization. *Invest Ophthalmol Vis Sci.* 2004;45:311–317.

131. Kiuchi K, Matsuoka M, Wu JC, et al. Mecamylamine suppresses basal and nicotine-stimulated choroidal neovascularization. *Invest Ophthalmol Vis Sci*. 2008;49:1705–1711.
132. Hou HY, Wang YS, Xu JF, et al. Nicotine promotes contribution of bone marrow-derived cells to experimental choroidal neovascularization in mice. *Exp Eye Res*. 2008;86:983–990.
133. Gridley T. Notch signaling in vascular development and physiology. *Development*. 2007;134:2709–2718.
134. Roca C, Adams RH. Regulation of vascular morphogenesis by Notch signaling. *Genes Dev*. 2007;21:2511–2524.
135. Siekmann AF, Covassin L, Lawson ND. Modulation of VEGF signalling output by the Notch pathway. *Bioessays*. 2008;30:303–313.
136. Sainson RC, Harris AL. Regulation of angiogenesis by homotypic and heterotypic Notch signalling in endothelial cells and pericytes: from basic research to potential therapies. *Angiogenesis*. 2008;11:41–51.
137. Hellstrom M, Phng LK, Hofmann JJ, et al. Dll4 signalling through Notch1 regulates formation of tip cells during angiogenesis. *Nature*. 2007;445:776–780.
138. Lobov IB, Renard RA, Papadopoulos N, et al. Delta-like ligand 4 (Dll4) is induced by VEGF as a negative regulator of angiogenic sprouting. *Proc Natl Acad Sci USA*. 2007;104:3219–3224.
139. Suchting S, Freitas C, le Noble F, et al. The Notch ligand Delta-like 4 negatively regulates endothelial tip cell formation and vessel branching. *Proc Natl Acad Sci USA*. 2007;104:3225–3230.
140. Jin YH, Kim H, Oh M, et al. Regulation of Notch1/NICD and Hes1 expressions by GSK-3 alpha/beta. *Mol Cells*. 2009;27:15–19.
141. Wang T, Baron M, Trump D. An overview of Notch3 function in vascular smooth muscle cells. *Prog Biophys Mol Biol*. 2008;96:499–509.
142. Eichmann A, Makinen T, Alitalo K. Neural guidance molecules regulate vascular remodeling and vessel navigation. *Genes Dev*. 2005;19:1013–1021.
143. Acevedo LM, Weis SM, Cheresh DA. Robo4 counteracts VEGF signaling. *Nat Med*. 2008;14:372–373.
144. Legg JA, Herbert JM, Clissold P, et al. Slits and Roundabouts in cancer, tumour angiogenesis and endothelial cell migration. *Angiogenesis*. 2008;11:13–21.
145. Jones CA, London NR, Chen H, et al. Robo4 stabilizes the vascular network by inhibiting pathologic angiogenesis and endothelial hyperpermeability. *Nat Med*. 2008;14:448–453.

Index

Page numbers followed by "b" indicate boxes; those in *italics* indicate figures; those followed by "t" indicate tables.

S

T

U

V